METHODS IN MOLECULAR BIOLOGY

Series Editor
John M. Walker
School of Life and Medical Sciences
University of Hertfordshire
Hatfield, Hertfordshire, UK

For further volumes:
http://www.springer.com/series/7651

For over 35 years, biological scientists have come to rely on the research protocols and methodologies in the critically acclaimed *Methods in Molecular Biology* series. The series was the first to introduce the step-by-step protocols approach that has become the standard in all biomedical protocol publishing. Each protocol is provided in readily-reproducible step-by-step fashion, opening with an introductory overview, a list of the materials and reagents needed to complete the experiment, and followed by a detailed procedure that is supported with a helpful notes section offering tips and tricks of the trade as well as troubleshooting advice. These hallmark features were introduced by series editor Dr. John Walker and constitute the key ingredient in each and every volume of the *Methods in Molecular Biology* series. Tested and trusted, comprehensive and reliable, all protocols from the series are indexed in PubMed.

Trypanosomatids

Methods and Protocols

Edited by

Paul A. M. Michels

School of Biological Sciences, University of Edinburgh, Edinburgh, UK

Michael L. Ginger

School of Applied Sciences, University of Huddersfield, Huddersfield, UK

Dan Zilberstein

Faculty of Biology, Technion–Israel Institute of Technology, Haifa, Israel

Humana Press

Editors
Paul A. M. Michels
School of Biological Sciences
University of Edinburgh
Edinburgh, UK

Michael L. Ginger
School of Applied Sciences
University of Huddersfield
Huddersfield, UK

Dan Zilberstein
Faculty of Biology
Technion–Israel Institute of Technology
Haifa, Israel

ISSN 1064-3745 ISSN 1940-6029 (electronic)
Methods in Molecular Biology
ISBN 978-1-0716-0296-6 ISBN 978-1-0716-0294-2 (eBook)
https://doi.org/10.1007/978-1-0716-0294-2

Cover illustration: Scanning electron micrograph of Angomonas deanei in early cytokinesis, cleavage furrow indicates two daughter cells ready for division with two externalised flagella. Courtesy of Drs. Carolina Catta-Preta and Cristina Motta (Chapter 26).

This Humana imprint is published by the registered company Springer Science+Business Media, LLC, part of Springer Nature.
The registered company address is: 1 New York Plaza, New York, NY 10004, U.S.A.

Preface

Around the turn of the twentieth century, parasitic protists were identified as causal agents of three groups of serious human diseases in tropical and subtropical countries in different parts of the world: sleeping sickness—or human African trypanosomiasis (HAT)—in The Gambia [1], and subsequently in what was then North-East Rhodesia (now Zimbabwe) [2] and elsewhere; Chagas disease—or American trypanosomiasis—first in Brazil and then in large parts of Latin-America [3]; and visceral leishmaniasis, in India and then Tunisia [4]. These parasites were *Trypanosoma brucei gambiense*, *Trypanosoma brucei rhodesiense*, *Trypanosoma cruzi*, *Leishmania donovani*, and *Leishmania infantum*. Recognition of other *Leishmania* species responsible for the considerably different manifestations of leishmaniasis seen in many countries of different continents occurred steadily throughout the twentieth century, and novel pathogenic *Leishmania* species have continued to be discovered during the first two decades of the twenty-first century [4]. Coincident with the discoveries that apparently related trypanosomatid parasites were responsible for diverse (and serious) tropical diseases, a striking commonality in the mode of disease transmission was also recognized: these parasites were transmitted between people by specific blood-feeding insects.

Large populations were—and still are—at risk of sleeping sickness, Chagas disease, or leishmaniasis. However, biological understanding of the parasites that cause these diseases and advances in dealing with the resultant health problems occurred at a slow pace for much of the last century. Some treatments for the diseases were developed (e.g., the antimonials introduced in the 1920s to treat leishmaniasis; suramin and melarsoprol, introduced in 1922 and 1949, respectively, to treat sleeping sickness). However, these and other medicines used to treat trypanosomatid diseases were not adequate: the medicines were little efficacious and often highly toxic. Indeed, there remains no medicine that can be used to treat effectively chronic forms of Chagas disease. Moreover, of the twentieth century pharmaceutical companies that arose and invested in research to develop drugs and vaccines for various human and veterinary infectious diseases, the trypanosomatid-borne diseases remained largely unexplored because they typically affected people living in impoverished regions. Thus, there was little economic incentive for the pharma industry to invest in such research. However, from the 1960s onwards, trypanosomatids started to attract the interest of academic laboratories, both in affluent countries, such as the USA, Japan, or within Europe, and the Global South where trypanosomatid diseases are typically endemic. This new interest was in part due to curiosity for peculiar aspects of the parasites, such as their large mitochondrial DNA content or the antigenic variation of *T. brucei*, and in part it related to the wider health burden these parasites posed. Addressing the latter aspect was to a large extent made possible by the "Special Programme for Research and Training in Tropical Diseases" (TDR), created in 1974 by the World Health Organization (WHO), with cosponsoring by the United Nations Development Programme (UNDP), the World Bank, and UNICEF. TDR set out to conduct research on a defined group of neglected, tropical diseases, including those caused by the three trypanosomatid parasites (TriTryp) aimed at developing new tools to help control them and to train scientists and strengthen institutions from the endemic countries, so that they could play a major role in this endeavor [5, 6]. From the 1980s, research of the parasites and possibilities to combat the diseases was further boosted by support for collaboration between teams from countries in the north and those from countries in the south afflicted by the diseases, enabling multidisciplinary approaches, by organizations like the European Economic Community (later the European Union), the National Institutes of Health (NIH) in the USA, and later also various philanthropic organizations. Crucially, research supported by these and other initiatives has seen the introduction of a few new medicines into the clinic (e.g., eflornithine to treat sleeping sickness; amphotericin B and miltefosine to treat leishmaniasis), often through the repurposing of medicines developed to treat other diseases (for reviews, *see* [7, 8]), and there is optimism in some quarters that eradication of sleeping sickness as a public health concern may be possible within the next 10–15 years [9].

Initial research from university laboratories resulted in the acquisition of a wealth of data about the biology, cellular and molecular biology, and biochemistry of trypanosomatids. Many novelties were discovered, about macromolecules, subcellular structures, and biological mechanisms, either unique to trypanosomatids or previously not yet detected in other, well-studied eukaryotic organisms like mammals, plants, and yeasts. Examples of such novelties included mechanisms for expression of the large number of genes for variable surface glycoproteins (VSGs) responsible for antigenic variation in *T. brucei*; the unique form of nuclear DNA modification by base J; polycistronic transcripts and trans-splicing; glycophosphatidylinositol (GPI) anchors used for the attachment of proteins to the plasma membrane; the unique structure and peculiar replication processes of these parasites' mitochondrial genomes (or kinetoplast DNA); U-insertion/deletion editing of transcripts produced from mitochondrial gene expression; peroxisome-related organelles containing glycolytic enzymes called glycosomes; acidocalcisomes; a trypanothione-based system for combatting reactive oxygen species, and still others (for—in some cases personal—accounts of various of these discoveries, *see* [10–13]). Moreover, novel approaches and methods were applied in these early stages of trypanosomatid research that, at that time, were not yet standardly used elsewhere, such as structure-based drug design (reviewed in [14]) and metabolic control analysis of entire pathways using in silico models [15] and, at later stages, also in vivo systems [16].

Several methodological developments in the 1990s and early 2000s were crucial for further progress in the research of trypanosomatids: the development of new or optimization of existing in vitro culture systems to enable growth, differentiation, or genetic manipulation of parasites; the huge improvement of methods for sequencing of DNA and bioinformatics that also enabled the determination and analysis of the TriTryp genome sequences [17]; the subsequent introduction of other -omics methodologies such as transcriptomics, proteomics, and metabolomics; and the finding of RNAi in *T. brucei* [18] just after, and independently of its discovery in *Caenorhabditis elegans*, followed by its application in trypanosomes for gene function analysis and latterly the development of genome-wide RNAi library screens and an RNAi target sequencing (RIT-seq) approach for high-throughput phenotyping of trypanosomes [19–21].

The most recent development of CRISPR/Cas9 for in situ targeted mutagenesis has successfully been adopted for use in all TriTryps [22–24]. Unlike mammals, the microhomology-mediated end joining (MMEJ) mechanism is somewhat more flexible in trypanosomatid genomes as it allows accumulating mutations of up to several kilobases distal to the breakpoint junction targeted by gRNA. Therefore, targeting gRNA to a specific sequence does not necessarily indicate location of mutation [25].

The recent exploration of biodiversity, involving the sequencing of genomes of many diverse organisms, has also drastically changed the ideas about eukaryotic evolution and the place of trypanosomatids within the tree of life. While for a long time, these protists were considered organisms that branched early in evolution from a single eukaryotic trunk [26], more recent studies indicate that eukaryotes are comprised of several supergroups which each diverged early and evolved independently from a "Last Eukaryotic Common Ancestor" (LECA) [27, 28]. The trypanosomatids belong to a phylum Euglenozoa within the supergroup Excavata, and the Excavata supergroup is comprised only of protists. This offers an explanation for the many novelties found in trypanosomatids when compared to animals and yeasts, which are both present in another supergroup (Opisthokonta), or plants, which are part of the supergroup Archaeplastida.

It is the differences in biology and molecular mechanisms between trypanosomatids and the people they infect that opens many perspectives for the development of anti-trypanosomatid drugs. It also implies a necessity to develop many unique research approaches and methods. In this volume of Methods in Molecular Biology, a large number of methods currently being used in research of different trypanosomatid parasites are presented. The research on trypanosomatids covers many disciplines, from organismal biology to molecular mechanisms; it also involves different species that, although clearly evolutionarily related and belonging to a single family, show many differences in their biology and the pathologies they cause. For each parasite, research is often done on the different stages of their complex life cycles, and the parasite interaction(s) with either insect vector or mammalian host. Much of the ongoing research is eventually aimed at the development of vaccines and drugs to prevent or cure the diseases caused by these parasites. Accordingly, some chapters of this volume will present methods highly specific for one species, while other chapters will deal with methods that can be applied straightforwardly to different parasites or, when described for one species, may readily be adapted for use on others. Some methods described cover the interaction(s) of the parasites with either the insect vector or a mammalian host, or the isolation of the parasites from either host or vector. In addition, methods used to test the efficacy of candidate anti-trypanosomatid drugs within in vitro growth assays or in vivo within mice are presented; a standardized vaccination protocol for the analysis of protective immunity in trypanosome-infected mice is also provided.

Motility is important for the establishment of infection and the survival of trypanosomatids and thus, protocols for motility analysis of trypanosomes are provided. Also relevant for the survival of trypanosomes within the host are the trypanolytic factors (TLFs), a topic for which methodological procedures are given for TLF isolation. Resistance of trypanosomatid parasites against drugs is increasingly a major public health problem, warranting the inclusion of a chapter about methods for the identification of chemo-resistant isolates in *Leishmania* using specific cellular markers. Other chapters will present improved methods for culturing of parasites and the facilitation of the in vitro differentiation of *Leishmania* spp. and *T. brucei*, and transfection of pleomorphic *T. brucei*. Various microscopy approaches used in structural and cell biology analyses of trypanosomatid cells, including the interaction of a subset of (non-pathogenic) trypanosomatids with their intriguing, cell-cycle entrained bacterial endosymbionts, are also provided.

A number of chapters address different molecular biological methods currently being applied to trypanosomatids: methods for high-throughput sequencing, next-generation analysis of trypanosomatid genome stability and instability, DNA repair in cell extracts, forward genetics using RNAi, ribosome profiling, the isolation and analysis of RNA–protein complexes and the use of CRISPR/Cas9 technology for gene editing.

Signal transduction is covered in several chapters, which focus on different aspects and different methods, including protocols for CRISPR/Cas9, (phospho)proteomics, and kinase and phosphatase assays

Concerning biochemistry, several chapters describe methods for the analysis of proteomes and phosphoproteomes, as well as metabolomes. Protocols are presented for the purification of organelles including flagella, extracellular vesicles, mitochondria, glycosomes, and acidocalcisomes and for the isolation of protein complexes. In addition, a chapter is devoted to metabolic control analysis for drug target prioritization; this chapter is illustrated with the example of trypanothione metabolism of *T. cruzi.*

Of course, the chapters cover only a fraction of all methodologies being used in research of these parasites, and progress in science will lead to new methodologies to be developed in the future. Undoubtedly, updating of existing protocols and development of new ones will be needed in due time. Nonetheless, we hope that the methods described in this volume will be useful for the community of researchers working on trypanosomatids and that their application will lead to the acquisition of new knowledge and, eventually, better treatment of trypanosomatid-borne diseases. Despite all efforts in the last few decades, the introduction of some new medicines and combination therapies plus promising prospects in preclinical work with some parasites—the currently available drugs have still major drawbacks, drug resistance is increasingly an issue, and vaccines are not available.

Finally, we thank all of the authors for the time they have taken to prepare articles and their patience during the editing process.

Edinburgh, UK *Paul A. M. Michels*
Huddersfield, UK *Michael L. Ginger*
Haifa, Israel *Dan Zilberstein*

References

1. Steverding D (2008) The history of African trypanosomiasis. Parasit Vectors 1(1):3. https://doi.org/10.1186/1756-3305-1-3
2. Stephens JWW, Fantham HB (1910) On the peculiar morphology of a trypanosome from a case of sleeping sickness and the possibility of its being a new species (*T. rhodesiense*). Roy Soc Proc B 83:28–33. https://doi.org/10.1098/rspb.1910.0064
3. Steverding D (2014) The history of Chagas disease. Parasit Vectors 10;7:317. https://doi.org/10.1186/1756-3305-7-317
4. Steverding D (2017) The history of leishmaniasis. Parasit Vectors 10(1):82. https://doi.org/10.1186/s13071-017-2028-5
5. Reeder JC, Guth JA (2015) What have we learned from 40 years of supporting research and capacity building? PLoS Negl Trop Dis 9(1):e3355. https://doi.org/10.1371/journal.pntd.0003355
6. Ogundahunsi OA, Vahedi M, Kamau EM et al (2015) Strengthening research capacity—TDR's evolving experience in low- and middle-income countries. PLoS Negl Trop Dis 9(1):e3380. https://doi.org/10.1371/journal.pntd.0003380
7. Andrews KT, Fisher G, Skinner-Adams TS (2014) Drug repurposing and human parasitic protozoan diseases. Int J Parasitol Drugs Drug Resist 4(2):95–111
8. Kaiser M, Mäser P, Tadoori LP, Ioset JR, Brun R (2015) Antiprotozoal activity profiling of approved drugs: a starting point towards drug repositioning. PLoS One 10(8):e0135556. https://doi.org/10.1371/journal.pone.0135556

9. Franco JR, Cecchi G, Priotto G et al (2018) Monitoring the elimination of human African trypanosomiasis: update to 2016. PLoS Negl Trop Dis 12(12):e0006890. https://doi.org/10.1371/journal.pntd.0006890
10. Borst P (2016) Maxi-circles, glycosomes, gene transposition, expression sites, transsplicing, transferrin receptors and base J. Mol Biochem Parasitol 205(1–2):39–52
11. Simpson L (2011) A personal scientific odyssey. Protist 162(1):188–206
12. Englund PT (2014) A passion for parasites. J Biol Chem 289(49):33712–33729
13. Matthews KR (2015) 25 years of African trypanosome research: from description to molecular dissection and new drug discovery. Mol Biochem Parasitol 200(1–2):30–40
14. Hol WG (2015) Three-dimensional structures in the design of therapeutics targeting parasitic protozoa: reflections on the past, present and future. Acta Crystallogr F Struct Biol Commun 71 (5):485–499
15. Bakker BM, Michels PA, Opperdoes FR, Westerhoff HV (1997) Glycolysis in bloodstream form Trypanosoma brucei can be understood in terms of the kinetics of the glycolytic enzymes. J Biol Chem 272(6):3207–3215
16. Haanstra JR, Gerding A, Dolga AM et al (2017) Targeting pathogen metabolism without collateral damage to the host. Sci Rep 7:40406. https://doi.org/10.1038/srep40406
17. El-Sayed NM, Myler PJ, Blandin G, et al (2005) Comparative genomics of trypanosomatid parasitic protozoa. Science 309 (5733):404–409
18. Ngô H, Tschudi C, Gull K, Ullu E (1998) Double-stranded RNA induces mRNA degradation in Trypanosoma brucei. Proc Natl Acad Sci U S A 95(25):14687–14692
19. Wang Z, Morris JC, Drew ME, Englund PT (2000) Inhibition of Trypanosoma brucei gene expression by RNA interference using an integratable vector with opposing T7 promoters. J Biol Chem 275 (51):40174–40179
20. Morris JC, Wang Z, Drew ME, Englund PT (2002) Glycolysis modulates trypanosome glycoprotein expression as revealed by an RNAi library. EMBO J 21;4429–4438
21. Alsford S, Turner DJ, Obado SO et al (2011) High-throughput phenotyping using parallel sequencing of RNA interference targets in the African trypanosome. Genome Res 21(6):915–924
22. Beneke T, Madden R, Makin L et al (2017) A CRISPR Cas9 high-throughput genome editing toolkit for kinetoplastids. R Soc Open Sci 4(5):170095. https://doi.org/10.1038/srep4040610.1098/rsos.170095
23. Zhang WW, Lypaczewski P, Matlashewski G (2017) Optimized CRISPR-Cas9 genome editing for Leishmania and its use to target a multigene family, induce chromosomal translocation, and study DNA break repair mechanisms. mSphere 2(1):e00340-16. https://doi.org/10.1128/mSphere.00340-16
24. Lander N, Chiurillo MA (2019) State-of-the-art CRISPR/Cas9 technology for genome editing in trypanosomatids. J Eukaryot Microbiol in press. https://doi.org/10.1111/jeu.12747
25. Goldman-Pinkovich A, Kannan S, Nitzan-Koren R, et al (2019) The hunger games: sensing host arginine is essential for Leishmania parasite virulence. bioRxiv 751610. https://doi.org/10.1101/751610
26. Sogin ML, Elwood HJ, Gunderson JH (1986) Evolutionary diversity of eukaryotic small-subunit rRNA genes. Proc Natl Acad Sci U S A 83(5):1383–1387
27. Adl SM, Simpson AG, Lane CE et al (2012) The revised classification of eukaryotes. J Eukaryot Microbiol 59(5):429–493
28. Adl SM, Bass D, Lane CE et al (2019) Revisions to the classification, nomenclature, and diversity of eukaryotes. J Eukaryot Microbiol 66(1):4–119

Contents

Contributors

HÉCTOR ACOSTA • *Laboratorio de Enzimología de Parásitos, Facultad de Ciencias, Universidad de Los Andes, Mérida, Venezuela*

MAYKE BEZERRA ALENCAR • *Laboratory of Biochemistry of Tryps – LaBTryps, Department of Parasitology, Institute of Biomedical Sciences, University of São Paulo, São Paulo, SP, Brazil*

JUAN D. ALFONZO • *Department of Microbiology, The Ohio State University, Columbus, OH, USA; The Ohio State Biochemistry Program, The Ohio State University, Columbus, OH, USA; The Center for RNA Biology, The Ohio State University, Columbus, OH, USA*

SARAH L. ALLINSON • *Division of Biomedical and Life Sciences, Faculty of Health and Medicine, Lancaster University, Lancaster, UK*

GUILLERMO D. ALONSO • *Laboratorio de Señalización y Mecanismos Adaptativos en Tripanosomátidos, Instituto de Investigaciones en Ingeniería Genética y Biología Molecular "Dr. Héctor N. Torres" (INGEBI), Buenos Aires, Argentina*

LYSANGELA RONALTE ALVES • *Laboratório de Regulação da Expressão Gênica, Instituto Carlos Chagas, Fundação Oswaldo Cruz (Fiocruz), Curitiba, PR, Brazil*

JULIANA CAROLINA AMORIM • *Faculty of Medicine, Catholic University of Cuenca, Cuenca, Azuay, Ecuador*

HIVA AZIZI • *Division of Infectious and Immune Diseases, CHU de Quebec Research Center—Laval University, QuébecQC, Canada*

SABINE BACHMAIER • *Biocenter, Faculty of Biology, Genetics, Ludwig-Maximilians-University Munich (LMU), Martinsried, Germany*

KATHRIN BAJAK • *Deutsche Krebsforschungszentrum (DKF), Heidelberg, Germany*

MICHAEL P. BARRETT • *Wellcome Centre for Integrative Parasitology, Institute of Infection, Immunity & Inflammation, College of Medical, Veterinary & Life Sciences, University of Glasgow, Glasgow, UK*

DANIELLA BARTHOLOMEU • *Departamento de Parasitologia, Universidade Federal de Minas Gerais—Instituto de Ciências Biológicas, Belo Horizonte, Brazil*

MICHEL BATISTA • *Carlos Chagas Institute, Fiocruz Parana, Curitiba, Parana, Brazil*

ASMA BELBELAZI • *Department of Biological and Geographical Sciences, School of Applied Sciences, University of Huddersfield, Huddersfield, UK*

TOM BENEKE • *Sir William Dunn School of Pathology, University of Oxford, Oxford, UK*

CORINNA BENZ • *Division of Biomedical and Life Sciences, Faculty of Health and Medicine, Lancaster University, Lancaster, UK*

JENNIFER BLACK • *Institute of Infection, Immunity and Inflammation, The Wellcome Centre for Integrative Parasitology, University of Glasgow, Glasgow, UK*

MICHAEL BOSHART • *Biocenter, Faculty of Biology, Genetics, Ludwig-Maximilians-University Munich (LMU), Martinsried, Germany*

EMMA M. BRIGGS • *Institute of Infection, Immunity and Inflammation, The Wellcome Centre for Integrative Parasitology, University of Glasgow, Glasgow, UK*

RICHARD BURCHMORE • *Institute of Infection, Immunity and Inflammation and Glasgow Polyomics, College of Medical, Veterinary and Life Sciences, University of Glasgow, Glasgow, UK*

Barbara A. Burleigh • *Department of Immunology and Infectious Diseases, Harvard T.H. Chan School of Public Health, Boston, MA, USA*
Guy Caljon • *Laboratory of Microbiology, Parasitology and Hygiene (LMPH), University of Antwerp, Wilrijk-Antwerp, Belgium*
Samantha Campbell • *Institute of Infection, Immunity and Inflammation, The Wellcome Centre for Integrative Parasitology, University of Glasgow, Glasgow, UK*
Martin Carr • *Department of Biological and Geographical Sciences, School of Applied Sciences, University of Huddersfield, Huddersfield, UK*
Carolina M. C. Catta-Preta • *Centro de Química Medicinal (CQMED)/Structural Genomics Consortium (SGC), Universidade Estadual de Campinas, São Paulo, Brazil*
Mathieu Cayla • *Institute for Immunology and Infection Research, School of Biological Sciences, University of Edinburgh, Edinburgh, UK*
Miguel A. Chiurillo • *Center for Tropical and Emerging Global Diseases, University of Georgia, Athens, GA, USA*
Christine Clayton • *Deutsche Krebsforschungszentrum (DKF), Heidelberg, Germany*
Artur T. Cordeiro • *Brazilian Biosciences National Laboratory, Brazilian Center for Research in Energy and Materials, Campinas, São Paulo, Brazil*
Kathryn Crouch • *Institute of Infection, Immunity and Inflammation, The Wellcome Centre for Integrative Parasitology, University of Glasgow, Glasgow, UK*
Jeziel Damasceno • *Institute of Infection, Immunity and Inflammation, The Wellcome Centre for Integrative Parasitology, University of Glasgow, Glasgow, UK*
Samuel Dean • *Warwick Medical School, University of Warwick, Coventry, UK*
Ricardo Canavate del Pino • *School of Life Sciences, University of Dundee, Dundee, UK*
François Demay • *Sir William Dunn School of Pathology, University of Oxford, Oxford, UK*
Carla Vanessa de Paula Lima • *Molecular Biology Institute of Parana, Curitiba, Parana, Brazil*
Sameer Dixit • *Institute of Parasitology, Biology Centre, Czech Academy of Sciences, České Budějovice (Budweis), Czech Republic; Department of Microbiology, The Ohio State University, Columbus, OH, USA*
Roberto Docampo • *Center for Tropical and Emerging Global Diseases, University of Georgia, Athens, GA, USA*
George Dong • *Infectious Diseases and Immunity in Global Health (IDIGH) Program, Research Institute of the McGill University Health Centre, Montreal, QC, Canada*
Peter C. Dumoulin • *Department of Immunology and Infectious Diseases, Harvard T.H. Chan School of Public Health, Boston, MA, USA*
Markus Engstler • *Lehrstuhl für Zell- und Entwicklungsbiologie, Theodor-Boveri-Institut, Julius-Maximilians-Universität Würzburg, Biozentrum, Am Hubland, Würzburg, Germany*
Esteban D. Erben • *German Cancer Research Center (DKFZ), DKFZ-ZMBH Alliance, Heidelberg, Germany*
Amanda G. Eufrásio • *Brazilian Biosciences National Laboratory, Brazilian Center for Research in Energy and Materials, Campinas, São Paulo, Brazil*
Mark C. Field • *School of Life Sciences, University of Dundee, Dundee, UK; Biology Centre, Faculty of Sciences, Institute of Parasitology, University of South Bohemia, České Budějovice, Czechia*
Alonso Da Silva Lira Filho • *Infectious Diseases and Immunity in Global Health (IDIGH) Program, Research Institute of the McGill University Health Centre, Montreal, QC, Canada*

Wendy Gibson • *Bristol Veterinary School and School of Biological Sciences, University of Bristol, Bristol, UK*
Michael L. Ginger • *School of Applied Sciences, University of Huddersfield, Huddersfield, UK*
Richard Bruno Marcel Moreira Girard • *Laboratory of Biochemistry of Tryps – LaBTryps, Department of Parasitology, Institute of Biomedical Sciences, University of São Paulo, São Paulo, SP, Brazil*
Lucy Glover • *Trypanosome Molecular Biology Group, Institut Pasteur, Paris, France*
Eva Gluenz • *Sir William Dunn School of Pathology, University of Oxford, Oxford, UK*
Samuel Goldenberg • *Laboratório de Regulação da Expressão Gênica, Instituto Carlos Chagas, Fundação Oswaldo Cruz (Fiocruz), Curitiba, PR, Brazil*
Zabdi González-Chávez • *Departamento de Bioquímica, Instituto Nacional de Cardiología Ignacio Chávez, Ciudad de México, Mexico*
Ujwala Gosavi • *Department of Genetics and Genome Sciences, UConn Health, Farmington, CT, USA*
Alessandra A. Guarneri • *Vector Behaviour and Pathogen Interaction Group, Instituto René Rachou, Belo Horizonte, MG, Brazil*
Arthur Günzl • *Department of Genetics and Genome Sciences, UConn Health, Farmington, CT, USA*
Jane Harmer • *Department of Biological and Geographical Sciences, School of Applied Sciences, University of Huddersfield, Huddersfield, UK*
Sarah Hendrickx • *Laboratory of Microbiology, Parasitology and Hygiene (LMPH), University of Antwerp, Wilrijk-Antwerp, Belgium*
Fabiola Barbieri Holetz • *Laboratório de Regulação da Expressão Gênica, Instituto Carlos Chagas, Fiocruz, Curitiba, PR, Brazil*
Guozhong Huang • *Center for Tropical and Emerging Global Diseases, University of Georgia, Athens, GA, USA*
Sebastian Hutchinson • *INSERM, Unit U1201, Paris, France; Trypanosome Cell Biology Unit, Institut Pasteur, Paris, France*
Marcel Kaiser • *Swiss Tropical and Public Health Institute, Basel, Switzerland; University of Basel, Basel, Switzerland*
Daria M. Kania • *Division of Biomedical and Life Sciences, Faculty of Health and Medicine, Lancaster University, Lancaster, UK*
Joachim Kloehn • *Department of Microbiology and Molecular Medicine, CMU, University of Geneva, Geneva, Switzerland; Department of Biochemistry and Molecular Biology, Bio21 Institute of Molecular Science and Biotechnology, University of Melbourne, Parkville, VIC, Australia*
Timothy Krüger • *Lehrstuhl für Zell- und Entwicklungsbiologie, Theodor-Boveri-Institut, Julius-Maximilians-Universität Würzburg, Biozentrum, Würzburg, Germany*
Fernanda Grande Kugeratski • *Department of Cancer Biology, Metastasis Research Center, University of Texas MD Anderson Cancer Center, Houston, TX, USA*
Noelia Lander • *Center for Tropical and Emerging Global Diseases, University of Georgia, Athens, GA, USA*
Kevin Leiss • *Centre for Molecular Biology of Heidelberg University (ZMBH), Heidelberg, Germany*
Aline Castro Rodrigues Lucena • *Carlos Chagas Institute, Fiocruz Parana, Curitiba, Parana, Brazil*

JULIUS LUKEŠ • *Institute of Parasitology, Biology Centre, Czech Academy of Sciences, České Budějovice (Budweis), Czech Republic; Faculty of Science, University of South Bohemia, České Budějovice (Budweis), Czech Republic*
PATRICK LYPACZEWSKI • *Department of Microbiology and Immunology, McGill University, Montreal, QC, Canada*
LOUIS MAES • *Laboratory of Microbiology, Parasitology and Hygiene (LMPH), University of Antwerp, Wilrijk-Antwerp, Belgium*
STEFAN MAGEZ • *Department of Environmental Technology, Food Technology and Molecular Biotechnology, Biomedical Research Centre, Ghent University, Incheon, South Korea; Department of Biochemistry and Microbiology, Ghent University, Ghent, Belgium; Laboratory of Cellular and Molecular Immunology, Vrije Universiteit Brussel, Brussels, Belgium*
FABRICIO KLERYNTON MARCHINI • *Carlos Chagas Institute, Fiocruz Parana, Curitiba, Parana, Brazil*
CATARINA A. MARQUES • *Institute of Infection, Immunity and Inflammation, The Wellcome Centre for Integrative Parasitology, University of Glasgow, Glasgow, UK*
PASCAL MÄSER • *Swiss Tropical and Public Health Institute, Basel, Switzerland; University of Basel, Basel, Switzerland*
GREG MATLASHEWSKI • *Department of Microbiology and Immunology, McGill University, Montreal, QC, Canada*
MALCOLM J. MCCONVILLE • *Department of Biochemistry and Molecular Biology, Bio21 Institute of Molecular Science and Biotechnology, University of Melbourne, Parkville, VIC, Australia*
RICHARD MCCULLOCH • *Institute of Infection, Immunity and Inflammation, The Wellcome Centre for Integrative Parasitology, University of Glasgow, Glasgow, UK*
SANGPHIL MOON • *Department of Environmental Technology, Food Technology and Molecular Biotechnology, Biomedical Research Centre, Ghent University, Incheon, South Korea; Department of Biomedical Molecular Biology, Ghent University, Ghent, Belgium; Laboratory of Cellular and Molecular Immunology, Vrije Universiteit Brussel, Brussels, Belgium*
SILVIA N. J. MORENO • *Center for Tropical and Emerging Global Diseases, University of Georgia, Athens, GA, USA; Department of Cellular Biology, University of Georgia, Athens, GA, USA*
RAFAEL MORENO-SÁNCHEZ • *Departamento de Bioquímica, Instituto Nacional de Cardiología Ignacio Chávez, Ciudad de México, Mexico*
MARIA CRISTINA M. MOTTA • *Laboratório de Ultraestrutura Celular Hertha Meyer, Instituto de Biofísica Carlos Chagas Filho, Centro de Ciências da Saúde, Universidade Federal do Rio de Janeiro, Rio de Janeiro, RJ, Brazil*
JEREMY C. MOTTRAM • *Department of Biology, York Biomedical Research Institute, University of York, York, UK*
ELISHA MUGO • *Department of Biochemistry, Genetics and Microbiology, Institute for Sustainable Malaria Control, University of Pretoria, Hatfield, South Africa*
JULIUS MULINDWA • *Department of Biochemistry, College of Natural Sciences, Makerere University, Kampala, Uganda*
ELMARIE MYBURGH • *York Biomedical Research Institute, Hull York Medical School, University of York, York, UK*

CHRISTINA NAULA • *Institute of Infection, Immunity and Inflammation and Glasgow Polyomics, College of Medical, Veterinary and Life Sciences, University of Glasgow, Glasgow, UK*

HANG THI THU NGUYEN • *Department of Environmental Technology, Food Technology and Molecular Biotechnology, Biomedical Research Centre, Ghent University, Incheon, South Korea; Department of Biochemistry and Microbiology, Ghent University, Ghent, Belgium; Laboratory of Cellular and Molecular Immunology, Vrije Universiteit Brussel, Brussels, Belgium*

MORITZ NIEMANN • *Department of Chemistry and Biochemistry, University of Bern, Bern, Switzerland*

EMMANUEL OBISHAKIN • *Department of Environmental Technology, Food Technology and Molecular Biotechnology, Biomedical Research Centre, Ghent University, Incheon, South Korea; Biotechnology Division, National Veterinary Research Institute, Vom, Plateau, Nigeria*

MARTIN OLIVIER • *Infectious Diseases and Immunity in Global Health (IDIGH) Program, Research Institute of the McGill University Health Centre, Montreal, QC, Canada*

MARITZA PADRÓN-NIEVES • *Laboratorio de Fisiología Molecular, Facultad de Medicina, Instituto de Medicina Experimental, Universidad Central de Venezuela, Caracas, Venezuela*

BARBARA PAPADOPOULOU • *Division of Infectious and Immune Diseases, CHU de Quebec Research Center—Laval University, Québec, QC, Canada; Department of Microbiology, Infectious Disease and Immunology, Faculty of Medicine, Laval University, Québec, QC, Canada*

MILIND S. PATOLE • *National Centre for Microbial Resource, National Centre for Cell Sciences (NCCS), University of Pune, Pune, India*

HARSH PAWAR • *Faculty of Biology, Technion—Israel Institute of Technology, Haifa, Israel*

LORI PEACOCK • *Bristol Veterinary School and School of Biological Sciences, University of Bristol, Bristol, UK*

ALICIA PONTE-SUCRE • *Laboratorio de Fisiología Molecular, Facultad de Medicina, Instituto de Medicina Experimental, Universidad Central de Venezuela, Caracas, Venezuela*

SALOE BISPO POUBEL • *Laboratório de Regulação da Expressão Gênica, Instituto Carlos Chagas, Fiocruz, Curitiba, PR, Brazil*

WILFREDO QUIÑONES • *Laboratorio de Enzimología de Parásitos, Facultad de Ciencias, Universidad de Los Andes, Mérida, Venezuela*

MAGDALENA RADWANSKA • *Department of Environmental Technology, Food Technology and Molecular Biotechnology, Biomedical Research Centre, Ghent University, Incheon, South Korea; Department of Biomedical Molecular Biology, Ghent University, Ghent, Belgium*

JAYNE RAPER • *Hunter College, City University of New York, New York, NY, USA; Ph.D. Program in Biology, The Graduate Center of the City University of New York, New York, NY, USA; Ph.D. Program in Biochemistry, The Graduate Center of the City University of New York, New York, NY, USA*

JOAO REIS-CUNHA • *Departamento de Parasitologia, Universidade Federal de Minas Gerais—Instituto de Ciências Biológicas, Belo Horizonte, Brazil*

RYAN RITCHIE • *Wellcome Centre for Integrative Parasitology, Institute of Infection, Immunity & Inflammation, College of Medical, Veterinary & Life Sciences, University of Glasgow, Glasgow, UK*

BRUNO ACCIOLY ALVES ROMAGNOLI • *Laboratório de Regulação da Expressão Gênica, Instituto Carlos Chagas, Fundação Oswaldo Cruz (Fiocruz), Curitiba, Brazil*

Emma Saavedra • *Departamento de Bioquímica, Instituto Nacional de Cardiología Ignacio Chávez, Ciudad de México, Mexico*
Gajanan Sathe • *Institute of Bioinformatics, Bangalore, India*
Charles Schaub • *Hunter College, City University of New York, New York, NY, USA; Ph. D. Program in Biochemistry, The Graduate Center of the City University of New York, New York, NY, USA*
André Schneider • *Department of Chemistry and Biochemistry, University of Bern, Bern, Switzerland*
Alejandra C. Schoijet • *Laboratorio de Señalización y Mecanismos Adaptativos en Tripanosomátidos, Instituto de Investigaciones en Ingeniería Genética y Biología Molecular "Dr. Héctor N. Torres" (INGEBI), Buenos Aires, Argentina*
Ariel Mariano Silber • *Laboratory of Biochemistry of Tryps – LaBTryps, Department of Parasitology, Institute of Biomedical Sciences, University of São Paulo, São Paulo, SP, Brazil*
Ankita Srivastava • *Department of Genetics and Genome Sciences, UConn Health, Farmington, CT, USA*
Tamara Sternlieb • *Laboratorio de Señalización y Mecanismos Adaptativos en Tripanosomátidos, Instituto de Investigaciones en Ingeniería Genética y Biología Molecular "Dr. Héctor N. Torres" (INGEBI), Buenos Aires, Argentina*
Jack Sunter • *Department of Biological and Medical Sciences, Oxford Brookes University, Oxford, UK*
Balázs Szöőr • *Institute for Immunology and Infection Research, School of Biological Sciences, University of Edinburgh, Edinburgh, UK*
Theresa Thanner • *Biocenter, Faculty of Biology, Genetics, Ludwig-Maximilians-University Munich (LMU), Martinsried, Germany*
Russell Thomson • *Hunter College, City University of New York, New York, NY, USA*
Michael D. Urbaniak • *Division of Biomedical and Life Sciences, Faculty of Health and Medicine, Lancaster University, Lancaster, UK*
Citlali Vázquez • *Departamento de Bioquímica, Instituto Nacional de Cardiología Ignacio Chávez, Ciudad de México, Mexico*
Joseph Verdi • *Hunter College, City University of New York, New York, NY, USA; Ph.D. Program in Biology, The Graduate Center of the City University of New York, New York, NY, USA*
Nick Vereecke • *Department of Environmental Tech, Food Tech, and Molecular Biotechnology, Biomedical Research Center (BMRC), Ghent University, Incheon, South Korea; Department of Biochemistry and Microbiology, Ghent University, Ghent, Belgium; Laboratory of Cellular and Molecular Immunology, Vrije Universiteit Brussel, Brussels, Belgium*
Jan Votýpka • *Institute of Parasitology, Biology Centre, Czech Academy of Sciences, České Budějovice (Budweis), Czech Republic; Faculty of Sciences, Charles University, Prague, Czech Republic*
Andrea Vucetic • *Infectious Diseases and Immunity in Global Health (IDIGH) Program, Research Institute of the McGill University Health Centre, Montreal, QC, Canada*
Richard J. Wheeler • *Sir William Dunn School of Pathology, University of Oxford, Oxford, UK; Peter Medawar Building for Pathogen Research, Nuffield Department of Medicine, University of Oxford, Oxford, UK*
Wen-Wei Zhang • *Department of Microbiology and Immunology, McGill University, Montreal, QC, Canada*

DAN ZILBERSTEIN • *Faculty of Biology, Technion-Israel Institute of Technology, Haifa, Israel*
MARTIN ZOLTNER • *School of Life Sciences, University of Dundee, Dundee, UK; BIOCEV, Department of Parasitology, Faculty of Science, Charles University in Prague, Vestec, Czechia*

Part I

Isolation, Culturing, and Genetic Manipulation of Trypanosomatids

Chapter 1

Field Isolation and Cultivation of Trypanosomatids from Insects

Julius Lukeš and Jan Votýpka

Abstract

Monoxenous (one host) trypanosomatids from insects and other invertebrates can be introduced into axenic culture relatively easily and efficiently, allowing for their transfer from the field into the laboratory. Here we describe simple methods and alternative cultivation protocols, the wider application of which will allow substantial expansion of trypanosomatids available for research.

Key words Trypanosomatids, *Trypanosoma*, Cultivation, Field, Isolation, Axenization, Insects

1 Introduction

Trypanosomatid flagellates belong to the class Kinetoplastea Honigberg, 1963 emend. Vickerman, 1976, order Trypanosomatida Kent, 1880, which is best known for its human parasites responsible for African sleeping sickness (*Trypanosoma brucei*), Chagas disease (*Trypanosoma cruzi*), and diverse leishmaniases (*Leishmania* spp.). Consequently, hundreds of strains belonging to the species of the dixenous genera *Leishmania* and *Trypanosoma* (and to lesser extent *Phytomonas* spp., which are plant pathogens) have so far been isolated from their vertebrate and invertebrate (vector) hosts, introduced into culture and many subjected to extensive research into their morphology, biochemistry, molecular biology, and parasite–host interactions. Indeed, in the databases there are now numerous assembled and annotated genomes for members of these two genera. Consequently, trypanosomes and leishmanias are among the best studied protists [1]. Until recently, we knew very little about parasitic flagellates that constitute their sister groups [2, 3]. However, it turns out that the human-infecting flagellates evolved from species that parasitize exclusively insects [4]. The available data strong point to the fact that the dixenous life cycle (alteration between a vertebrate host and an invertebrate

Paul A. M. Michels et al. (eds.), *Trypanosomatids: Methods and Protocols*, Methods in Molecular Biology, vol. 2116,
https://doi.org/10.1007/978-1-0716-0294-2_1,

vector, almost invariably an insect) of trypanosomes and leishmanias developed from the monoxenous life cycle (a single insect host) retained by the genera *Leptomonas*, *Crithidia*, *Blastocrithidia*, and others [5, 6]. Hence, the study of these neglected parasites of insects (mostly true bugs [Heteroptera] and flies [Diptera]) is more important for our understanding of the evolution of parasitism in vertebrate hosts than appreciated until recently.

Until about a decade ago, globally there were only a dozen or so species and/or strains of insect trypanosomatids available in culture [7, 8]. This has changed after increasing interest in this group of parasites and a protocol was developed that allows relatively straightforward transfer of these flagellates from the field into the culture. As a result of field trips to many tropical, subtropical, and moderate climate countries on all continents [6, 9–12], trypanosomatids were isolated from dissected insect specimens and subjected to limited DNA sequencing. For the purposes of phylogenetic analyses, usually several highly conserved genes have been sequenced. At present, hundreds of species/strains are available in cryobanks around the world; all of them stored potentially indefinitely in liquid nitrogen. With the advent of cheap and large-scale DNA sequencing, this wealth of strains will be useful for insight into the evolution and diversity of trypanosomatid protists.

2 Materials

1. Insect/arthropod traps like funnels, pitfall traps, bottle traps, various modifications of malaise traps, and UV light traps. Different nets, such as aerial, sweep, and aquatic nets and hand (or electrical) aspirators.
2. Various catching traps and instruments must be supplemented by other collecting tools for manipulation with obtained invertebrates. For example, soft forceps, fine-tipped forceps, and aspirators are routinely used; white pan (or white paper) help with invertebrate separation.
3. The captured insects/invertebrates should be kept alive individually in plastic/glass vessels/containers until dissection. For example, 1.5 or 2.0 mL plastic microtubes with perforated lids can be used for smaller specimens; large insect specimens should be kept in 5–10 mL vials.
4. Before dissection, specimens must be anaesthetized/killed in vessels with 70% ethanol and transformed into sterile physiological solution (e.g., saline solution for IV used in hospital). Before their sterilization in ethanol, ethyl acetate (ethyl ethanoate, EtOAc) can be used to anesthetize larger insect specimens or their groups, especially those which survive longer in ethanol.

5. Plate (e.g., glass slides) and tools for dissection (microforceps straight and/or curved, probes blunt and/or sharp, iris scissors, scalpel, needles—for preparation of these tools *see* Subheading 3.3).
6. Optional: Stereomicroscope (dissecting microscope) or some type of watch repair magnifying glasses. However, the basic dissection can be done with just naked eyes.
7. Burner (either Bunsen when gas is available or transportable burner running on 96% ethanol) for dissection tools and coverslip sterilization.
8. Blotting paper (absorbent toilet paper or paper tissue is sufficient).
9. Glass slides (presterilized) and coverslips (optimal size is 20 × 20 mm) for light microscopy.
10. Dissection of insects and any subsequent manipulation with the gut and other organs is done in sterile Insect Ringer's solutions or 0.6–0.86% NaCl solution.
11. Light microscope with ocular lenses of at least 10× magnification and objective lenses of at least 20× magnification. However, an objective of 40× magnification is advantageous, as well as phase contrast. It is also helpful to have a LED diode lighting with the accumulate battery to be independent on the electric current. If necessary, a head torch can be used as a light source.
12. Sterile insulin syringes (up to 1 mL) with permanently attached needle (sterile plastic tips for pipettes).
13. Cultivation is typically just one of several ways how to process the obtained material. Part of the dissected material is regularly used for microscopic slide smears (slides should be air-dried and fixed with methanol). For subsequent DNA extraction, homogenized dissected tissues are stored in plastic 1.5 mL microtubes with ethanol or (preferably) in 1% SDS + 0.1 M EDTA solution. Various standard protocols for DNA extraction are suitable, although "mini" kits are ideal due to the small amount of analyzed material. Isolated DNA is useful not only for parasite (primarily trypanosomatid) detection, but also for any other purposes (host barcoding, microbiome screening, etc.).
14. Primo-culture cultivation can be performed in different types of vials and media (*see* Subheading 3.7). Glass vials with rubber lids supplemented with biphasic media, which consists of the blood agar base and the liquid overlay. This approach provides more feasible conditions for finicky parasite species and is also suitable for isolation of trypanosomes or leishmanias from their vertebrate hosts. On the other hand, monoxenous trypanosomatids are very often able to grow even in much simpler and

nutritionally less rich monophasic media. Various cultivation media can be prepared using of several components (for more details *see* Subheading 3.7): Brain Heart Infusion (BHI), RPMI 1640 (with HEPES), complete Schneider's (Drosophila; Insect) Medium; M 199 Medium; heat-inactivated Fetal Bovine Serum (FBS), rabbit or sheep defibrinated whole blood, agar, neopeptone (or similar), 0.6% NaCl solution and various antibiotics (penicillin, amikacin or gentamicin, streptomycin, chloramphenicol, 5-fluorocytosine).

15. If axenization is required, glass V- or U-shaped tubes are recommended.
16. In case of cloning, a Bürker chamber or cell counter and 96-well plates with F (flat)-bottom are required.
17. For cryopreservation of trypanosomatid cultures, dimethyl sulfoxide (DMSO) and Mr. Frosty™ container (or a similar device) are commonly required.
18. An important aspect of some studies is the preservation of dissected host organisms for subsequent morphological determination, although other methods, such as DNA barcoding, can also be used. It is important to keep not only the insect body but also the genitals that are very often dislodged from the body during dissection. The best way is to store dissected specimens separately in plastic microtubes (1.5 or 2.0 mL) with 70% ethanol and labeled by an ethanol-resistant marker (permanent fine-lined paint marker; e.g., Edding 780). However, simpler and space-saving dry storage methods can be used; a plastic container with sheets of blotting paper for storing dissected specimens will do. In this case, a limited risk of specimen mixing has to be considered.

3 Methods

All methods described below are designed so that they can be performed both inside and outside of the laboratory, in a hotel room, in a porch, or many other locations. In the case of field work, the folding camping table and chair(s) are an important part of the equipment. Electricity is advantageous. However, in the field, use of a microscope (and optional stereomicroscope) with rechargeable batteries means electricity is not a necessity.

3.1 Catching Techniques

We will not describe here all methods used for trapping insects and/or other invertebrates that can be investigated for the presence of trypanosomatids. There is no universal capturing method, and one has to take into consideration the target group of insects/invertebrates, as well as the conditions in the field. Still, some basic methods and principles are mentioned below. Invertebrates are passively caught using funnels, pitfall traps, bottle traps, and various modifications of malaise traps, some of which could be baited with different attractants. Several different types of light traps (ultraviolet lights ["black lights"], mercury vapor, and various others) represent active forms of catching. Physically more demanding but logistically much easier is the usage of different nets: aerial nets are used to collect flying insects; sweep nets (or beat nets) are suitable for sweeping the vegetation; aquatic nets are used to sample in the aquatic environments; litter reducer is designed for extracting soil invertebrates from the forest floor; beat sheets are suitable for collecting insects from branches of trees and shrubs. In specific situations (e.g., thorny forest, shrubs, feces, rooms inside houses) specimens are collected manually or with a hand (or electrical) aspirator.

3.2 Keeping the Hosts

Insects and other invertebrates can be captured by methods such as those described above, with the most applicable being sweep netting, different light trap methods or individual picking. For entomologic purposes, collected insects could be placed into different killing jars with ethyl acetate, the anesthetic we use most frequently. Importantly, for parasitologic purposes, the captured insects/invertebrates are kept alive as long as possible in any suitable plastic/glass vessel or vial prior to dissection. Depending on their size, the captured insects or other invertebrates are placed (preferably individually to prevent contamination by coprophilia or predation) into 1.5–2.0 mL plastic microtubes, or larger plastic or glass containers with pierced lid to allow access of air. In addition to the insect's size, one also has to consider several other aspects. For example, some true bugs (e.g., sting bugs of the superfamily Pentatomoidea) have glands that produce a foul-smelling liquid, which is used defensively to deter potential predators. However, if bugs are kept in a small space, they can kill themselves. Where this is a possibility, the container volume should be at least ten times the volume of the insect.

Insects in microtubes/vials and kept in shade and at room temperature normally survive for 24 h. If long-term storage (up to 1 week) is required, the insect containers should be stored in a refrigerator (4–10 °C). However, cooling of the container may result in precipitation of small droplets of water on its walls, which may lead to insects sticking to the wet walls, followed by aspiration of water into their tracheal system and subsequent drowning on the insect(s). To prevent this situation, adding a piece of blotting paper into vials may improve long-term survival of insects.

3.3 Dissection and Slide Preparation

The selection of dissection tools depends on several aspects: (1) insect size; (2) sclerotization of the cuticle; (3) the used optics (stereomicroscope versus naked eye), and (4) the experience of the person who carries out the dissection and her/his capacity to perform fine work leading to the precise localization of trypanosomatid infection within the insect's organ systems (e.g., infection of digestive tract, hemolymph, or salivary glands). The most universal and preferred way for the dissection of most insects (e.g., hemipterans and dipterans of standard size) is the use of a pair of fine tweezers (microdissecting forceps); the harder and the thinner the spikes are the better. However, tweezer spikes can be easily damaged by careless handling or falling to the ground. Thus, it is advisable to carry several backup tweezers and/or forceps. If the insect's body is too hard (large and/or highly sclerotized specimen) or leather-like (e.g., hippoboscid flies), it is advisable to use for initial opening a small scalpel, which can be substituted by the slanted end of a syringe; this generally pierces and cuts through the body well.

If the investigator is not interested in localizing the infected organ, or is limited by other factors such as time, precise dissection (*see* Subheading 3.3) can be replaced by the following approach. The last one-third of the abdomen can be crushed and teared in a drop of saline solution into small pieces by using a pair of disposable fine-point wooden or bamboo toothpicks. Alternatively, if one wants to perform precise dissection of small insects (few millimeters long), dissection under a stereomicroscope is highly recommended. It is advisable to use special thin needles, such as the entomological pins (stainless steel; 1, 0, 00, or 000) or the minuten pins (stainless steel; 0.15 or 0.20 mm; but not 0.10 mm since these are too thin) set into a wooden (not bamboo) skewer. This tool can be prepared as follows:

1. After one end of the skewer dip has been submerged for a few hours in water, drive a minute pin (by its blunt end) by using a small pliers or forceps into the soft (= wet) end of the skewer.
2. Once the skewer has dried, the bonding can be enhanced by dipping with a glue. The obtained dissecting needles are relatively tough and durable and can be used as such. It is also possible to bend the tip third of the minuten into an "L" shape or into a small hook. These three shapes can be combined during dissection with commercial dissecting needles and tweezers or forceps.

Regardless of the technique and dissecting tools used (except disposable toothpicks), it is necessary to sterilize the tools after each dissection; ideally, clean them mechanically by wiping them into tissue paper to remove any stuck pieces of the dissected insects, shortly dip the tools into $\geq$70% ethanol and sterilize them over a flame from a small portable burner.

When everything is prepared for the dissection, the insect is removed from the container and dropped for a few seconds (or until it stops moving) into a small glass container (preferably transparent) filled with 70% ethanol, where it will quickly drown. This step will kill the insect and sterilize its surface. However, if the specimen remains in ethanol for an extended period of time (more than few minutes), ethanol can penetrate the body and kill intestinal and other endoparasites including trypanosomatids. Next, the dead specimen is taken out, fast-dried on a piece of filter or tissue paper, and dropped into another small glass container with sterile physiological solution. Taking into account the location, date and other "sorting" information, it is possible to perform this operation (ethanol—drying—sterile solution) with several specimens at the same time. The killed insects can stay in the container with physiological solution for several hours; it is even possible to keep them there overnight (e.g., when it is not possible to finish the work). In this case, it is preferable to leave a container with nondissected insects in the refrigerator. The sterile solution and containers can be transported to the laboratory or prepared in situ from a preweighed quantity of salt mixed with water (even drinking water is acceptable). In the field, sterilization can be done, for example, by use of a kettle.

Except for very large insects, a sterile microscopic slide (presterilized from the lab or sterilized over a flame of a small portable burner) is used as a dissecting pad. Before dissection, two or three drops of sterile physiological solution (from a syringe, plastic dropper or, optimally, from a plastic dropping ampulla with sterile NaCl solution) are applied on the slide. Next, the insect kept in a container with sterile physiological solution is transferred onto a slide. It is essential to minimalize the volume of transferred solution from the storage container along with the insect—especially sting bugs release various chemicals (terpenes, etc.) that change the water tension and repel droplets of solution in which the dissection has to take place.

Next, the insect is placed in the supine position. Sometimes it is recommended to remove legs and wings before the dissection. However, since the insects need to be preserved for later morphological determination and also because of the considerable workload of this step, we recommend leaving the legs and wings. A slightly different situation concerns the head. In some insect groups with a bigger head that is loosely connected to the body (e.g., flies and cockroaches), separation of the head is necessary before removal of the intestine. On the other hand, in insects with a relatively small head firmly attached to the body (e.g., true bugs, some beetles, and fleas); separation of the head is unnecessary and, in addition, can be very laborious. After decapitation (optional), the last two or three segments of the abdomen must be removed and gently separated from the rest of the body. Depending on the dissected insect, the digestive tract is more-or-less firmly attached to this abdominal segment and can be pulled out from the body.

Several different situations may occur during the dissection. The ideal situation can be described as follows: together with the separated apical abdominal segments, pull out as one piece the entire digestive system—hindgut (HG), Malpighian tubes (MT), and whole midgut (MG) including cardia (stomodeal valve; stomodeum–mesenteron connection) and diverticules (crop). This is the fastest way and it is highly likely that all parts of the digestive system have been acquired. Moreover, if the intestine remains intact, it is easy to determine its anatomy and distinguish its different parts (HG, MG, crop). Unfortunately, the digestive tract often breaks, most frequently at the hindgut–midgut junction. In such cases, the tweezers or the dissecting needle must be pushed into the abdomen in order to pull out the rest of the digestive system. Sometimes, however, the digestive tract has to be pulled out in several parts. We provide two tips how to improve the dissection and increase the chances of pulling out the entire digestive tract: (1) in case of females, when last abdominal segments are further apart from the body (but still connected with the intestine), remove eggs or developing ovaries from the body cavity because these parts of the insect's tissue block the abdominal opening and make it difficult for the intestinal tract to be pulled out; (2) when pulling out the intestine, it sometimes helps to "massage" the body from the outside in the head-to-abdomen direction.

After removal of the intestine from the body cavity, proceed by separating all other tissues, especially the reproductive organs. Indeed, in females the sclerotized eggs complicate the covering and smashing of the intestine with a coverslip, while the ovaries shadow the microscopic field. In the case of males (or spermatheca in females), the movement of sperm released into the observed sample complicates the detection and observation of the parasitic flagellates. The last two abdominal segments, still attached to the intestine, must be removed as well (exept very small specimens, e.g. flies); otherwise they prevent proper covering and smashing by the coverslip and shadow some parts of the intestine, especially the rectal ampule area. In addition, the male genital organs, such as the aedeagus, are often essential for morphological determination. Removal of these abdominal segments, however, must be done very carefully in order to retain as much of the hindgut as possible, including the rectal ampule.

After removal and careful cleaning, it is recommended to transfer (by tweezer, needle, etc.) the whole intestine to the second (= clean) drop of saline solution on another slide. If the intestine is pulled out in small pieces, it is better to keep it in the "dissecting drop" of the saline solution, from where one shall remove the rest of the body and all the contaminants. The intestine shall be inspected in one piece, as long as it is kept in a stretched-out formation. For bigger specimens, it is better to separate the hindgut + rectal ampule (HG + RA) and midgut + Malpighian tubes

(MG + MT), push these two parts aside and cover them gently by separate coverslips, yet still on the same slide. The slide is large enough to fit three drops: a "dissecting" drop (with insect remnants), a coverslip with HG + RA and a second slip with MG + MT. Afterward, the slide is ready for inspection under the microscope. If the slide is not immediately examined, it should be stored in a humid chamber (food chamber, kitchen dishes, braced plastic bag, etc.) to prevent it from drying out.

For accuracy and completeness, we shall add that the digestive system is not the only tissue that can be infected and henceforth checked for trypanosomatid parasites. For dixenous species (especially trypanosomes and *Phytomonas* spp.), the examination of salivary glands may provide important information about possible vector capacity of the inspected insects. However, dissection of the salivary gland is much more difficult than dissection of the intestine and differs among insect groups. Dissection of the salivary glands is practically impossible with the naked eye and a stereomicroscope, preferably supplemented with transmitted light, is therefore indispensable.

3.4 Light Microscopy

The slide is then inspected under a microscope, preferably using magnification around 100–200× (10× oculars combined with a 10× or 20× objective), which allows for monitoring any moving objects in a relatively large area.

1. First, check for a few minutes the objects under the coverslip without trying to crush the intestine. This will allow precise determination in which part and where inside the intestine the parasites are localized.
2. After the primary examination of the intact intestine, its contents are squeezed by a gentle pressure (e.g., by using tweezers) onto the coverslip, and the homogenate observed again for a few minutes.
3. When the twisting behavior of (usually) slender cells is noticed, switch to 40× objective and eventually use the phase contrast for better observation of the flagellum and other morphological features. This allows for unequivocal distinction of fast-moving sperm cells or elongated bacteria from the trypanosomatids. Once parasitic flagellates have been found in any part of the insect (if this happened before squeezing by the coverslip, it is important to smash the intestine content thoroughly), using tweezers to remove gently the coverslip, add a drop of saline solution or growth medium to the homogenized tissue pieces and carefully mix the content by repeated ingestion and extrusion through the insulin syringe. This will increase the volume of fluid available from the dissected specimen. A sterile insulin syringe (up to 1 mL) with permanently attached needle is

particularly suitable. Using the detachable needle is more laborious and in the case of a very small volume, more material remains in the syringe–needle connection. For some applications, insulin syringes can be replaced by a sterile plastic tip (for pipettes), although the former are more practical. By using a cap, the dissected content can be kept (semi)sterile inside the barrel part of the syringe and tender movement of the plunger will allow homogenizing the content and splitting it up for several application (*see* Subheading 3.5).

3.5 Division of the Sample

It is important to preserve the trypanosomatid morphotypes as they occur within the host. The cultures obtained from the infected samples frequently do not reflect the original situation, either because the morphology changes under specific cultivation conditions, or because only one species prevails from what was originally a mixed infection. Hence, upon detection of a trypanosomatid infection, the infected and homogenized tissue material from the slide is taken up into an insulin syringe and divided into three parts, which are used as follows (for more details also *see* Subheadings 3.6, 3.7 and 3.11): (1) about 1/3 to 1/2 is injected into a vial for primo-culture (start with this step to decrease the chance of contamination); (2) one or two drops are used for a slide smear; (3) the remaining sample is stored for later DNA extraction.

3.6 Preparation of Slides

For morphological inspection, place a small aliquot of the diluted sample on a microscopic slide and using a tilted coverslip (or another slide), make a thin smear (like a blood smear) and allow it to dry. The usage of growth medium (especially if it contains fetal bovine serum) improves the adherence of the parasites to the slide. In a humid environment, the slide may not get dry fast enough. In such case, put the slide for example on the warm part of the microscope and let it dry there. Even dry slides can attract insects (mostly flies) to graze on them and destroy a significant part of the smear. In order to prevent this, describe the slide with an ethanol-resistant marker, place the dry smear into a horizontal position and cover it with a few milliliters of methanol or submerge the slides in vertical position into some container with methanol (can be used repeatedly) for about 5 min. Let the slides dry and afterward place them into a microscopic slide container (with silica gel if there is high humidity) for transportation and further use in the laboratory. There, put the dry slide horizontally onto a rack or vertically into a staining jar and cover it with Giemsa stain (diluted 1:10–20 with water) for 15–30 min, and remove the stain by rinsing the slide under running water. Giemsa is still the golden standard, but several other staining methods (e.g., diff-quick) could be used. Air dried smears are ready for inspection under the microscope. It is practical to later carefully inspect only slides, for which either or both cell culture or DNA sequences are available.

Note: if methanol is not available in the field, dried slides may be kept without fixing for several weeks; however, it is necessary to keep the slides in a dry place to prevent their molding or destruction by any other (micro)organisms.

3.7 Preparation of Vials and Media for Primo-Cultures

In the era of whole genome/transcriptome/proteome sequencing, one should attempt to bring as many trypanosomatid parasites as possible into culture. As they can usually be easily perpetuated in culture as well as cryopreserved, once established the culture can be used for further research and easily shared among laboratories. It will also make possible ultrastructural examination, infection experiments, and other studies.

There are several ways how to transfer parasites inhabiting the gut and/or other organs of their invertebrate hosts into the culture. Some monoxenous trypanosomatids (e.g., species of the genus *Leptomonas*) are very amenable for cultivation and even nutrient-poor and simple media are fully sufficient for their maintenance. Since the cultivation of trypanosomatids from the dissected invertebrate hosts is often plagued by contaminations with various bacteria and/or fungi, the selection of nutritionally poor media has a great advantage in terms of suppressing the growth of these contaminants. On the other hand, some trypanosomatids, mainly belonging to the genus *Blastocrithidia*, grow very slowly and richer and more complex monophasic or biphasic media are required. Finally, it must be mentioned that in some cases (e.g., some species of the "jaculum" group), cultivation is very difficult if at all possible, and thus, so far, all attempts have failed. We have considered the possibility of cultivating these elusive trypanosomatids in insect tissue cultures, but keeping vials with these rather sensitive cultures in proper conditions during the field work is logistically very difficult and also any type of bacterial and fungal contamination can easily overgrow the culture. Taking into account all the above-described limitations and problems, it seems most advantageous to choose a nutrient-rich monophasic medium. Still, several other options will be described below.

In the case of a monophasic medium, sterile plastic 1.5–2.0 mL microtubes are prefilled (max 1.0 mL of medium for a 1.5 mL tube and 1.5 mL of medium for a 2.0 mL tube) in the laboratory and shall be kept at 4 °C before use, preferably within 1 or 2 months. However, if this is not possible, the vials with media keep ready-to-use for a few weeks even in room temperature. The nutrient-rich monophasic growth medium of Brain Heart Infusion (BHI) works most frequently and therefore represents the first choice. Although the liquid form of BHI is also available, powdered medium is the most common form of this commodity. Dissolve 37 g per liter of distilled water, heat it, and stir until completely solubilized. Dispense it into an appropriate container, loosen the cap, and autoclave for 15 min at 121 °C. After cooling, supplement the medium with

10 mg/mL hemin and 10% of heat-inactivated (30 min at 56 °C) fetal bovine serum (FBS). The supplementation with 0–5% FBS represents the less nutrient-rich variation. All media must be supplemented with an antibiotic cocktail (see below). A more nutrient-rich medium shall be prepared by using several commercially available growing cultivation media (Gibco, Sigma-Aldrich, etc.). One option is a mix of RPMI 1640 (with HEPES), Complete Schneider's (Drosophila; Insect) Medium and M 199 Medium (1:1:1) supplemented with 10% FBS and antibiotics (see below).

The preparation of biphasic blood agar media is more complicated. For the blood agar base, 2% agar, 2% neopeptone (or similar), and 0.6% NaCl water solution is prepared and autoclaved (15 min at 121 °C). Being shaken gently, the solution is left to cool to approximately 60 °C. Then, rabbit or ovine (but also other blood sources are usable) defibrinated blood is added to a final 20% concentration, thoroughly mixed and the glass vials are filled as quickly as possible to prevent the solidification of agar in the pipette and/or in the bottle (the bottle with liquid blood agar shall be kept in a thermally insulated tank with hot water). Different types of glass vials can be used. A good choice in terms of storage and ease of handling are narrow 4–5 mL glass vials with a rubber cap (Fig. 1)—different types of capping can be used: the most common is top jaw (requiring sealing jaw capping machine); however, a screw or bayonet cap are also suitable. Open sterile vials are filled with 0.5 mL, agar is poured onto the bottom end and the vial is immediately closed by the sterile rubber lid and placed into a horizontal position where agar is allowed to spread over the side wall to maximize surface coverage (optimally, the agar shall cover one wall from the bottom end of the vial to the cap). To avoid solidification of the agar, it is necessary to work fast and at the same time stay sterile; a heated flow box is a good solution.

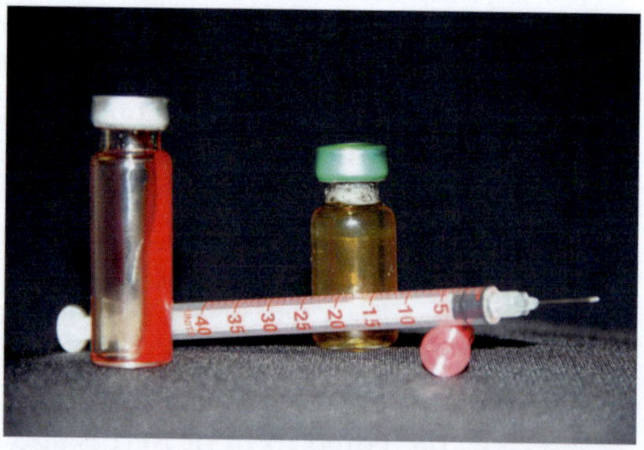

Fig. 1 A biphasic blood agar medium (0.5 mL of blood agar solidified in horizontal position) and liquid phase overlay stored in narrow 5 mL sterile glass vials closed by a rubber cap. A sterile insulin syringe with permanently attached needle is used for injection of the sample by piercing a rubber cover of the glass vial containing the overlay and the solid phase

Agar base represents the solid phase, and various liquid phases (overlays) can be used. The less nutrient-rich overlay consists of 2% neopeptone and 0.6% NaCl water solution (autoclaved). Alternatively, the most complex and nutrient rich medium contains a mix of complete RPMI 1640, Schneider's and M199 (1:1:1) supplemented with 2% human urine (sterile; filtered using 0.2 μm pore filters) and 10–20% heat-inactivated FBS. Do not mix overlay with blood agar before use. Similar to blood agar, the overlay is stored in 4–5 mL vials with a rubber cap (Fig. 1). The vials with blood agar shall be stored at 4 °C until use, preferably within 1 or 2 months.

Crucial and really fundamental for the success of primocultures is the use of antibiotics, regardless of the selected growth media (see above; in case of autoclaving, antibiotics must be added after autoclaving, when the solution already cooled down). In general, potential contaminants (bacteria and fungi) grow faster in nutritionally rich media. In any case, antibiotics need to be used even in less rich growth media. Unlike the cultivation from the more-or-less sterile blood or tissues from vertebrates (for *Trypanosoma* and *Leishmania* species) or tissues from plants (for *Phytomonas* species), the monoxenous trypanosomatids of insects or other invertebrates are mostly derived from the intestinal tract and are therefore contaminated with a large number of microorganisms. It is advisable to use a mix of different antibiotics in a fairly high concentration (higher than is commonly used under laboratory conditions). The following combination is generally suitable: 10,000 IU penicillin, 100 μg/mL amikacin or gentamicin, 100 μg/mL streptomycin, 50 μg/mL chloramphenicol, 1500 μg/mL 5-fluorocytosine.

The use of antibiotics, however, brings one possible limitation. Different obligatory endosymbiotic bacteria have been found in the cytoplasm of monoxenous trypanosomatids belonging to the genera *Strigomonas*, *Angomonas*, and *Kentomonas* [13, 14], as well as in the genus *Novymonas* [15]. Although the abovementioned antibiotics do not affect the endosymbiotic bacteria in these monoxenous trypanosomatids, it cannot be ruled out that in some cases the use of antibiotics may lead to the elimination of endosymbionts and thus either failed cultivation or overgrowth of symbiont-free trypanosomatids, which do not correspond to the natural situation.

In the field, inject about 1/3 to 1/2 of the sample (diluted with a drop of saline solution or growth medium from a sterile insulin syringe) into a vial. This shall be done by opening the microtube with the medium or piercing a rubber cover of the glass vial containing the medium and solid phase. When more types of media are available, using the same syringe to inject roughly equal amounts into each type of medium. At the same time, leave enough sample volume for a slide smear and DNA extraction. After a gentle mix, leave the glass vial with blood agar in horizontal position, while the microtube may be kept in vertical position. All types of media with injected parasites must be kept and transported in shade at room or lower temperature. Especially when in the field, it is really crucial to ensure that the cultivation vials/tubes will never be exposed to high temperature (e.g., when a bag is left in the sunshine, is close to an engine or driveshaft cover in a bus/boat). During prolonged field expeditions, it is advisable to keep the cultivation vials/tubes at lower temperature (10 °C is optimal, but 4 °C is also possible) or passage them each 2 weeks. If the vials/tubes are stored for an extended period of time, it is recommended to shake and mix them occasionally, especially when the microtubes are kept in boxes in vertical position. The surface of the growth media may become covered by fungi, which prevents oxygen from entering the lower part of the liquid column and thus aerobic organisms, trypanosomatids can die from anoxia.

3.8 Axenization

Upon transportation into the laboratory, the next steps depend on whether the cultures have remained sterile or whether they have been contaminated by bacteria and/or yeast (see below). In any case, following the return from the field, attend to the cultivation vials first. Check them for the presence of trypanosomatids as well as contaminants under a microscope with magnification 200–400× (phase contrast is advisable) up to one (two) month after the dissection, in 1-week intervals. In case of glass vials with a rubber lid, which were kept in horizontal position, mix the content thoroughly and using an insulin syringe, transfer a small drop on the slide for inspection. In case of the microtubes, which were kept in vertical position, for the same purpose take carefully a small drop from the surface of the medium.

Although the media contain a mix of antibiotics, at least in some vials a contamination with bacteria and/or fungi will usually occur. There are several ways how to deal with the contaminants and axenize (= separate particular organism from all others) the trypanosomatids growing in the primo-culture. If a given trypanosomatid grows well even in a nutrient-poor medium, fast passages may be sufficient to remove the contaminating yeast. However, this approach is applicable only for yeast contaminants, as it does not work in the more frequent case of bacterial contamination. One possibility is to eliminate bacteria by the addition of another mix of antibiotics.

However, when bacteria become quickly resistant to the newly added antibiotics, which is frequently the case, the next method of choice is the migration technique through a glass V- or U-shaped tube (Fig. 2). A sterile tube is filled with a growth medium about 3 cm above its bottom (V or U bent), and about 500 μL of the contaminated culture is added into one arm. Next, the openings are plugged with cotton wool stoppers (or other type of sterile cover), and the tube is fixed in an upright position. Within a few hours (no later than overnight) a few drops of the medium from the

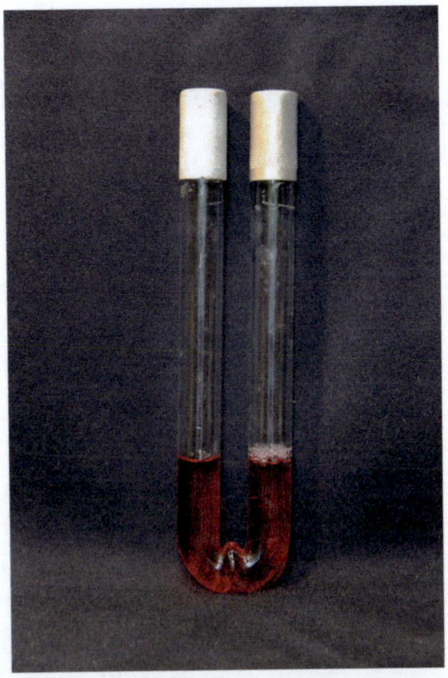

Fig. 2 A U-shaped sterile glass tube filled with a cultivation medium is used for axenization of cell culture contaminated with bacteria or yeast, which is based on migration technique (it utilizes the higher motility of trypanosomes as compared to that of contaminating microorganisms)

surface in the opposite (i.e., noninoculated) arm shall be checked for the presence of trypanosomatids. The motile protists shall actively migrate through the narrow base of the V- or U-shaped tube, while the nonmotile (or by Brownian movement only slowly progressing) contaminants remain behind. It has to be kept in mind that if trypanosomatids grow poorly or do not replicate at all, or if the contaminating microorganisms are also mobile, this method is ineffective. In some very specific cases other axenization techniques can be applied, such as the repetitive purification of trypanosomatids via a Ficoll gradient, cultivation on solid agar media, culture cloning (*see* Subheading 3.9) or different combinations of the abovementioned methods.

3.9 Culture Cloning

A single clone can be obtained from an axenic culture by in vitro cloning. Prior to the initiation of in vitro cloning, several subpassages of the culture are made. This is done by transferring a few drops of the trypanosomatid suspension to a new culture flask (in a ratio 1:10 maximum) at 3- to 10-day intervals (depending on the growth rate). Next, the cell density of an exponentially growing culture has to be established, at least approximately, using a Bürker chamber or cell counter, and the culture is diluted with a fresh preconditioned medium to the density of about 2 cells/mL. It is then pipetted into one to three 96-well plates with F (flat)-bottom (150 μL per well). It is advisable to add into the 96-well plates a preconditioned medium, which is prepared as follows. Cultivation medium from a culture of exponentially growing trypanosomatids is filtered through 0.22 μm filter; the conditioned medium contains undefined secreted growth factors that usually significantly improve the growth rate of the single cloned cells. Using an inverted microscope, in 1-week intervals the plates are screened for the presence of cells. Usually a clonal expansion in at least a few wells occurs within 30 days.

3.10 Cryopreservation

Cryopreservation of trypanosomatids is relatively easy and straightforward. An exponentially (preferably but not necessarily) growing culture is mixed with dimethyl sulfoxide (DMSO) at the final concentration of 5–10%. Due to the inherent toxicity of this cryoprotectant, after defreezing the mix of the cryopreserved culture is diluted with fresh medium at a ratio of at least 1:10. Alternatively, instead of DMSO, glycerol at the final concentration of 30% can also be used. In this case, it is crucial to leave the culture mixed with glycerol for about 15 min before the freezing procedure has been started. This is because glycerol is known to enter the cells significantly less rapidly than DMSO. After mixing with DMSO, the culture must be immediately transferred into the cryopreservation tubes (at least 5 tubes per culture are suggested) and allow gradual decrease of the temperature at a rate of about 1 °C per minute. The simplest way is to use the cheap Mr. Frosty™ container, by placing it along with the tubes into −80 °C deep freezer and leave it there overnight. Next day, the tubes are transferred into a liquid nitrogen tank. When liquid nitrogen is not readily available, trypanosomatids are known to survive cryopreserved for several months even in the deep freezer at about −80 °C. It is advisable to verify the success of the cryopreservation by defreezing one tube next day after the cryopreservation.

3.11 DNA Analysis

Generally, the trypanosomatid flagellates have very few conspicuous morphological characteristics observable by light microscopy that would allow their determination. This makes sequence analysis indispensable [3]. We provide protocols for the PCR amplification of 18S ribosomal RNA (rRNA) [3, 4, 10, 11, 13] and glycosomal glyceraldehyde-3-phosphate dehydrogenase (gGAPDH) genes [16] that are available from hundreds of trypanosomatid species and their sequence will thus allow unambiguous determination to the generic and species level. Another possibility, suitable for taxonomic identification within a genus, is to use the spliced leader (SL) RNA gene sequences [9, 17, 18].

In the field, approximately 1/3 to 1/2 of the dissected intestinal material containing trypanosomatid parasites is preserved for later DNA extraction. Using an insulin syringe, this material is put into a 1.5 mL safe-lock plastic microtube containing 1% SDS and 0.1 M EDTA for tissue lysis and DNA preservation. The volume of SDS + EDTA should be 5–10 times of the volume of the added dissected material and the tube is gently mixed. A labeled tube (by permanent fine-lined paint marker) is ready for transportation.

During transportation, it is advisable to add some tissue paper into the box with tubes, which will absorb the effluent occasionally released from a broken or improperly closed tube. Tubes should be kept in a refrigerator (4 °C) or freezer (−20 °C) whenever possible, and at −20 °C upon delivery to the lab. Still timing is not critical, as in most cases the samples will survive at room temperatures for weeks.

Note: Instead of SDS + EDTA, RNAlater solution can also be used. If none of these solutions is available, sterile physiological solution or PBS can be used instead, but in that case the samples have to be kept frozen for the whole time. Another option is to use ethanol (final concentration 50–100%), but one has to keep in mind that DNA extraction and PCR from ethanol-stored samples may be less efficient.

In the laboratory, briefly vortex the tubes and from the total amount of preserved material, use about 2/3 (to have a backup (1/3) in case the downstream methods failed). Whenever cultures have been successfully established, use about 10^7 cells or less for DNA extraction. Any standard protocols for DNA extraction is suitable; in the case of very small amount of material, various "mini" or "micro" kits shall preferably be used.

To establish taxonomic appurtenance and phylogenetic position, the gene of choice is 18S rRNA with the following primers (forward, AACCTGGTTGATYCTGCCAGTAG and reverse, TGATCCWKCTGCAGGTTCACCTAC) using this PCR program:

94 °C for 3 min.

35 cycles: 94 °C for 30 s, 55 °C for 30 s, 72 °C for 90 s.

72 °C for 10 min.

This protocol is perfectly suitable for DNA samples obtained from cultured flagellates. However, in cases of the environmental sample the application of the nested PCR protocols for 18S rRNA amplification is recommended.

1st PCR: Forward (S763), CATATGCTTGTTTCAAGGAC and reverse (S762), GACTTTTGCTTCCTCTADTG.

94 °C for 3 min.

40 cycles: 94 °C for 30 s, 55 °C for 30 s, 72 °C for 90 s.

72 °C for 10 min.

2nd (nested) PCR: Forward (TRnSSU-F2), GARTCTGCGCATGGCTCATTACATCAGA and reverse primers (TRnSSU-R2), CRCAGTTTGATGAGCTGCGCCT.

94 °C for 3 min.

35 cycles: 94 °C for 30 s, 64 °C for 30 s, 72 °C for 90 s.

72 °C for 10 min.

The second gene of choice is gGAPDH (or other highly conserved genes), amplifiable using one of the below protocols.

gGAPDH protocol I: Forward (M200), ATGGCTCCVVTCAARGTWGGMAT and reverse primers (M201), TAKCCCCACTCRTTRTCRTACCA.

94 °C for 3 min.

35 cycles: 94 °C for 30 s, 55 °C for 45 s, 72 °C for 90 s.

72 °C for 10 min.

gGAPDH protocol II: Forward (GAPDH-F), ATGGCTCCGMTCAAGGTTGGC and reverse primer (GAPDH-R), TTACATCTTCGAGCTCGCGSSGTC.

94 °C for 3 min.

35 cycles: 94 °C for 30 s, 55 °C for 30 s, 72 °C for 90 s.

72 °C for 10 min.

This protocol is perfectly suitable for DNA samples obtained from cultured flagellates; however, it works (with some limitation) also for the environmental samples.

4 Notes

In the last two decades, dozens of new species of monoxenous trypanosomatids have been described and formally named. However, at the same time, a large number of most likely new species were discovered but remain undescribed. We and our collaborators have decided to formally describe (and named) only those trypanosomatids for which either an axenic (cryopreserved) culture is available, or those which frequently parasitize (and/or with high prevalence) widely distributed insect hosts [19], or finally those flagellates that infect hosts kept under laboratory condition.

All other species identified by DNA sequencing and/or other methods remain formally taxonomically undescribed (= unnamed). For that reason, typing units (TUs) are used as proxies of monoxenous trypanosomatid species [3], which are similar to the molecular operational taxonomic units (MOTUs).

Acknowledgments

Support from the Czech Grant Agency 16-18699S, ERC CZ LL1601 and the ERD Funds (project OPVVV 16_019/0000759) is acknowledged.

References

1. del Campo J, Sieracki ME, Molestina R, Keeling P, Massana R, Ruiz-Trillo I (2014) The others: our biased perspective of eukaryotic genomes. Trends Ecol Evol 29:252–259
2. Borghesan TC, Ferreira RC, Takata CSA, Campaner M, Borda CC, Paiva F, Milder RV, Teixeira MMG, Camargo EP (2013) Molecular phylogenetic redefinition of *Herpetomonas* (Kinetoplastea, Trypanosomatidae), a genus of insect parasites associated with flies. Protist 164:129–152
3. Maslov DA, Votýpka J, Yurchenko V, Lukeš J (2013) Diversity and phylogeny of insect trypanosomatids: all that is hidden shall be revealed. Trends Parasitol 29:43–52
4. Lukeš J, Skalický T, Týč J, Votýpka J, Yurchenko V (2014) Evolution of parasitism in kinetoplastid flagellates. Mol Biochem Parasitol 195:115–122
5. Barratt J, Kaufer A, Peters B, Craig D, Lawrence A, Roberts T, Lee R, McAuliffe G, Stark D, Ellis J (2017) Isolation of novel trypanosomatid, *Zelonia australiensis* sp. nov. (Kinetoplastida: Trypanosomatidae) provides support for a Gondwanan origin of dixenous parasitism in the Leishmaniinae. PLoS Negl Trop Dis 11:e0005215
6. Lukeš J, Butenko A, Hashimi H, Maslov DA, Votýpka J, Yuchenko V (2018) Trypanosomatids are much more than just trypanosomes: clues from the expanded family tree. Trends Parasitol 34:466–480
7. Simpson L, Maslov DA (1994) RNA editing and the evolution of parasites. Science 264:1870–1871
8. Podlipaev SA (2001) The more insect trypanosomatids under study—the more diverse trypanosomatidae appears. Int J Parasitol 31:648–652
9. Westenberger SJ, Sturm NR, Yanega D, Podlipaev SA, Zeledon R, Campbell DA, Maslov DA (2004) Trypanosomatid biodiversity in costa rica: genotyping of parasites from Heteroptera using the spliced leader RNA gene. Parasitology 129:537–547
10. Yurchenko VY, Lukeš J, Jirků M, Zeledón R, Maslov DA (2006) *Leptomonas costaricensis* sp. n. (Kinetoplastea: Trypanosomatidae), a member of the novel phylogenetic group of insect trypanosomatids closely related to the genus *Leishmania*. Parasitology 133:537–546
11. Votýpka J, Maslov DA, Yurchenko V, Jirků M, Kment P, Lun Z-R, Lukeš J (2010) Probing into the diversity of trypanosomatid flagellates parasitizing insect hosts in South-West China reveals both endemism and global dispersal. Mol Phylogenet Evol 54:243–253
12. Wilfert L, Longdon B, Ferreira AG, Bayer F, Jiggins FM (2011) Trypanosomatids are common and diverse parasites of *Drosophila*. Parasitology 138:585–865
13. Teixeira MMG, Borghesan TC, Ferreira RC, Santos MA, Takata CS, Campaner M, Nunes VL, Milder RV, de Souza W, Camargo EP (2011) Phylogenetic validation of the genera *Angomonas* and *Strigomonas* of trypanosomatids harboring bacterial endosymbionts with the description of new species of trypanosomatids and of proteobacterial symbionts. Protist 162:503–524
14. Votýpka J, Kostygov AY, Kraeva N, Grybchuk-Ieremenko A, Tesařová M, Grybchuk D, Lukeš J, Yurchenko V (2014) *Kentomonas* gen. g., a new genus of endosymbiont-containing trypanosomatids of Strigomonadinae subfam. n. Protist 165:825–838
15. Kostygov AY, Dobáková E, Grybchuk-Ieremenko A, Váhala D, Maslov DA, Votýpka J, Lukeš J, Yurchenko V (2016) Novel trypanosomatid-bacterium association: evolution of endosymbiosis in action. MBio 7: e01985–e01915
16. Hamilton PB, Gibson WC, Stevens JR (2007) Patterns of co-evolution between trypanosomes and their hosts deduced from ribosomal RNA and protein-coding gene phylogenies. Mol Phylogenet Evol 44:15–25
17. Jirků M, Yurchenko VY, Lukeš J, Maslov DA (2012) New species of insect trypanosomatids from Costa Rica and the proposal for a new subfamily within the Trypanosomatidae. J Eukaryot Microbiol 59:537–547
18. Maslov DA, Westenberger SJ, Xu X, Campbell DA, Sturm NR (2007) Discovery and barcoding by analysis of spliced leader RNA gene sequences of new isolates of Trypanosomatidae from Heteroptera in Costa Rica and Ecuador. J Eukaryot Microbiol 54:57–65
19. Seward EA, Votýpka J, Kment P, Lukeš J, Kelly S (2017) Description of *Phytomonas oxycareni* n. sp. from the salivary glands of *Oxycarenus lavaterae*. Protist 168:71–79

Chapter 2

Culturing and Transfection of Pleomorphic *Trypanosoma brucei*

Sabine Bachmaier, Theresa Thanner, and Michael Boshart

Abstract

Cultivation of pleomorphic *Trypanosoma brucei* strains was introduced in 1996 when matrix dependence of growth of natural isolates was recognized. Semisolid agarose or liquid methylcellulose are currently used and here we provide optimized protocols for these culture methods and for transfection of pleomorphic strains. Although more laborious than standard liquid culture, culture of native pleomorphic strains is important for a number of research questions including differentiation, virulence, tissue tropism, and regulated metabolism. Some subclones of pleomorphic strains have acquired matrix independence upon passage in culture but maintained a pleomorphic phenotype. It appears that matrix dependence and pleomorphism are not tightly linked traits, yet phenotypes have to be verified before choosing one of these subclones for given experiments. Based on direct comparisons, we give recommendations for pleomorphic strain selection and culture conditions that guarantee truly pleomorphic and differentiation competent *Trypanosoma brucei*.

Key words *Trypanosoma brucei*, Pleomorphic, Differentiation, Cultivation, Matrix, Transfection

1 Introduction

The host-triggered developmental program that underlies the life cycle of protozoan parasites is central to our understanding of their adaptation and success during infection and transmission. Growth and differentiation in axenic culture combined with efficient reverse genetic tools is essential for dissection of this developmental program and for identification of the host cues orchestrating it. This chapter presents the current methods to apply these tools as step-by-step protocols. *Trypanosoma brucei* proliferates extracellularly in the bloodstream and tissues (fat, skin) as predominantly slender forms. A quorum sensing mechanism triggers differentiation to a morphologically stumpy, cell cycle-arrested stage that is preadapted to transmission [1]. The simultaneous occurrence of morphologically slender and stumpy trypanosomes in the bloodstream has historically been designated pleomorphism, and trypanosome

Paul A. M. Michels et al. (eds.), *Trypanosomatids: Methods and Protocols*, Methods in Molecular Biology, vol. 2116, https://doi.org/10.1007/978-1-0716-0294-2_2, © Springer Science+Business Media, LLC, part of Springer Nature 2020

isolates from natural hosts and their unadapted derivatives are hence called pleomorphic strains. The ability to differentiate to the quiescent stumpy stage is contributing to parasite population control in the host and is essential for transmission and completion of the life cycle. Serial rapid passage in laboratory rodents and selection for high parasitemia has given rise to variant strains that have lost the ability to differentiate to the stumpy stage. This has been convenient for researchers who needed high yields of parasites from infected animals for biochemical and molecular studies. However, these monomorphic strains have lost important properties of native trypanosomes that are key to understand the infection process. Therefore, there is an increasing need to use pleomorphic strains for reverse genetic experiments and analysis of subtle and complex phenotypes in parasite-specific processes.

Early attempts to culture bloodstream forms of *Trypanosoma brucei* only became successful upon using feeder layers of mammalian cells [2–6]. In these cultures, trypanosomes were mostly observed in tight association with the feeder cells and in spaces between the cells of these monolayers. Duszenko et al. [7] identified one important function of the feeder cells being redox protection and supply of sufficient cysteine, an essential growth factor for trypanosomes. This led to the development of media for axenic culture of bloodstream forms [7–9], and some monomorphic laboratory strains like Lister 427 were successfully adapted to this axenic culture system. The respective strains became the workhorses for molecular research on trypanosomes. While successful axenic culture of native nonadapted pleomorphic strains was not reported, a possible additional mechanism of growth support by the feeder layers remained unnoticed. It was a fortuitous observation that suggested a role of extracellular matrix. To study synchronous differentiation of bloodstream forms to the procyclic stage we had used the pleomorphic strain AnTat 1.1 (grown in mice) [10–12] and attempted a new method to clone on agarose plates. Surprisingly, this strain and all other pleomorphic strains we tested, vigorously grew on agarose plates [10–12]. Agarose could be replaced by a number of additives including methylcellulose in liquid culture [13]. The common denominator was a medium with high viscosity. We reasoned that the extracellular matrix surrounding the feeder cells was a preferred environment for proliferation of native trypanosome strains due to the high viscosity. The severe cell division phenotypes observed upon omission of matrix [11] suggest that the beating flagellum may need the resistance of surrounding medium to generate a force during the process of cytokinesis.

In a previous chapter in this book series we have discussed in detail the culture and gene transfer methods for monomorphic and pleomorphic trypanosomes [14]. Here we provide our updated protocols for culture and gene transfer into pleomorphic strains of

T. brucei. Using optimized protocols, transfection efficiency compares favorably with that obtained for common monomorphic laboratory strains. Therefore, we advocate the use of pleomorphic strains for research questions requiring differentiation competence, fly transmissibility, natural virulence, and host tissue localization. The work with matrix-containing media and low cell densities is more laborious but is worth the effort for biologically significant results. Finally, we discuss the advantage and potential risks of using culture-selected matrix-independent clones of these strains that appear to be more practical.

2 Materials

2.1 Trypanosoma brucei *brucei Strains*

The origin and history of the *T. brucei* strains compared in this chapter is given in Fig. 1.

2.1.1 AnTat 1.1E

The strain AnTat 1.1E was subcloned from a stock collected 1966 in Uganda from a bushbuck and named EATRO 1125 or LUMP 581 as described [15–17]. AnTat 1.1E has been widely used in research requiring pleomorphic trypanosomes [18–21]. We obtained an early passage directly from the Institute of Tropical Medicine Antwerp with written documentation of strain history.

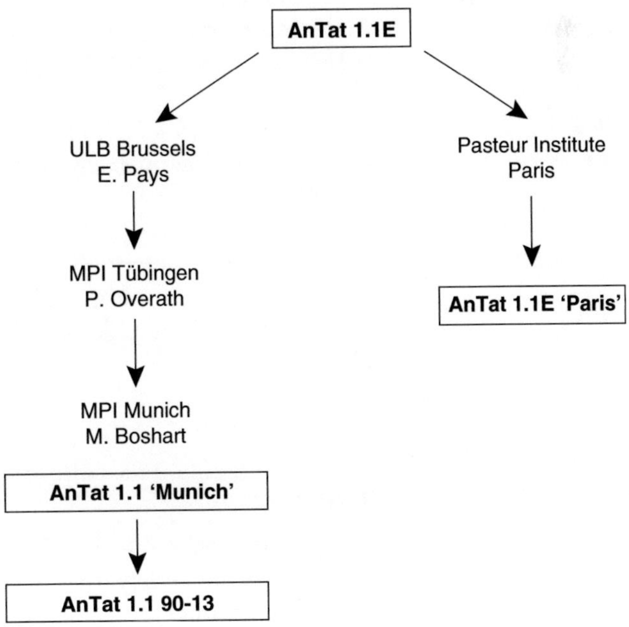

Fig. 1 Pedigree of the *T. brucei* strains compared in this chapter

2.1.2 AnTat 1.1E "Paris"

This strain is derived from strain AnTat 1.1E described above and was used in [22, 23].

2.1.3 AnTat 1.1 "Munich"

This differs from the original AnTat 1.1E described above only by the number of passages and was transferred from the Institute of Tropical Medicine Antwerp via E. Pays, Brussels [18] and P. Overath, Tübingen [24] to the Boshart laboratory in Munich in 1992. It has been further distributed and was used in most studies on trypanosome differentiation [10–13, 25–27].

2.1.4 AnTat 1.1 90-13

This is a transfected clone of AnTat 1.1 "Munich" expressing T7 DNA polymerase (plew13 [28]) and tetracycline repressor (plew90 [28]) and thus suitable for Tet-inducible expression of genes or RNAi. We first reported it in 2004 [25] and have distributed it to several laboratories [29–32].

2.2 T. brucei *Culture Media and Transfection Solutions*

2.2.1 Modified HMI-9

This culture medium contains [per liter]:

840 ml Iscove's modified Dulbecco's medium (IMDM) supplemented with 10 ml of each of the following stock solutions: 100 mM hypoxanthine (in 0.1 N NaOH), 5 mM bathocuproine sulfonate, 20 mM 2-mercaptoethanol, 16 mM thymidine, 10,000 U/ml penicillin, 10 mg/ml streptomycin, 100 mM cysteine (freshly made), and 100 ml heat-inactivated fetal bovine serum (*see* **Note 1**).

2.2.2 HMI-9 with Methylcellulose

HMI-9 including 15% (v/v) fetal bovine serum (*see* **Note 2**) and 1.1% (w/v) methylcellulose (e.g., Sigma-Aldrich Methocel® A4M, Cat. No. 94378) [13, 14].

2.2.3 HMI-9 with Agarose

HMI-9 including 15% (v/v) fetal bovine serum (*see* **Note 2**) and 0.65% (w/v) low melt agarose [11, 14, 33, 34] (*see* **Notes 3** and **4**).

2.2.4 Electroporation Buffer

Transfection buffer described by Schumann Burkard et al. [35]: 90 mM sodium phosphate, 5 mM potassium chloride, 0.15 mM calcium chloride, 50 mM HEPES, pH 7.3 (*see* **Note 5**).

2.3 Equipment for Cultivation of T. brucei

Cell culture incubator (settings: 37 °C, 5% CO_2, >90% humidity).

Plasticware (nonadherent culture flasks with vented caps; petri dishes).

Cell counter (Coulter Z series, Beckman and CASY, OLS OMNI Life Science are widely used in trypanosome labs) or Neubauer counting chambers.

Inverse microscope with 10× and 20× phase-contrast objectives.

2.4 Materials and Equipment for Electroporation of T. brucei

10 μg DNA (linear for most applications, sterile in doubly distilled water).

AMAXA Nucleofector™ II (Lonza, Basel, Switzerland; program CD4+ T cells X-001) (*see* **Note 6**).

Electroporation cuvettes (2 mm gap cuvettes, e.g., BTX Cat. No. 45-0125, Harvard Bioscience or the AMAXA nucleofection cuvettes included in AMAXA Nucleofector™ kits).

Sterilized folded filters (e.g., Macherey-Nagel MN615 1/4, 185 mm diameter).

3 Methods

3.1 Cultivation of Pleomorphic Trypanosoma brucei brucei Strains

Trypanosoma brucei bloodstream forms are cultivated in HMI-9 medium in a humid CO_2 atmosphere at 37 °C. Originally, growth of pleomorphic *T. brucei* strains was described to depend on the presence of a matrix (i.e., feeder cells [8], agarose [11], or methylcellulose [13]). However, some strains emerged that are able to grow in liquid medium comparable to the growth conditions of monomorphic *T. brucei* strains.

3.1.1 Cultivation of T. brucei on Agarose Plates

Preparation of Agarose Plates (Adapted from [33], Modified by [11] and [34])

1. Dissolve 6.5 g low-melting point agarose in 100 ml water and autoclave.
2. Equilibrate agarose solution and HMI-9 medium (including 15% (v/v) FCS) to 50 °C in a water bath.
3. Mix 10 parts of medium with one part of agarose solution (*see* **Note 3**).
4. If needed, add selection antibiotics or tetracycline (for inducible transgene expression) to the final volume (*see* **Note 7**) and mix well.
5. Pipet 20 ml of HMI-9-agarose solution into sterile 10-cm diameter petri dishes and avoid or remove air bubbles.
6. Dry plates for 30 min at room temperature with closed lids.
7. Store plates inverted either at room temperature overnight or sealed with Parafilm at 4 °C for several days to weeks (dependent on the presence of selection drugs in the agar (*see* **Note 7**)).
8. Before use, the sealed plates can be incubated overnight in a 37 °C incubator with a humid 5% CO_2 atmosphere in order to equilibrate pH and temperature.
9. Immediately before plating, dry plate surface with open lids for 30–60 min in a sterile air stream (e.g., a laminar flow cabinet) (*see* **Note 8**).

Spreading of *T. brucei* Bloodstream Forms on Agarose Surface

1. Determine cell density of long slender bloodstream form trypanosomes (from mouse/rat blood, from a blood stabilate (*see* **Note 9**) or from in vitro culture) and dilute to 1×10^5 to 1×10^6 cells/ml in HMI-9.
2. Gently spread 100 μl of cell suspension per plate using a bent Pasteur pipette.
3. Incubate at 37 °C, 5% CO_2, humid atmosphere.
4. Cells can be harvested by two washes with 2–4 ml HMI-9 or phosphate-buffered saline (PBS) containing 10 mM glucose followed by centrifugation (10 min at $1400 \times g$).

The parasites grow in colonies as long slender bloodstream forms and differentiate into cell cycle-arrested short stumpy forms after 3–5 days. The yield in the number of stumpy cells per plate can be increased by (a) higher seeding density (up to 1×10^6 cells/plate; *see* also [10]) and (b) higher humidity of the plate, for example, by shortening the drying period of the open plates or increasing the volume of HMI-9 used for spreading the parasites. The higher humidity allows the parasites to stray over the plate, thus preventing colony formation and supporting a more homogeneous density-dependent differentiation.

3.1.2 Cultivation of T. brucei *in Methylcellulose HMI-9 Medium*

Preparation of Methylcellulose HMI-9 (Adapted from [13])

1. To 11 g methylcellulose (Sigma Methocel) add 366 ml water and a magnetic stirring bar in a 1 l bottle. No stirring or mixing is required at this point. Sterilize methylcellulose by autoclaving. After autoclaving, stir in a cold room until a homogeneous, highly viscous, transparent solution is obtained. This may take several days.
2. Supplement 547.5 ml double concentrated (2×) IMDM basic medium with 15 ml of each of the following stock solutions: 100 mM hypoxanthine (in 0.1 N NaOH), 5 mM bathocuproine sulfonate, 20 mM 2-mercaptoethanol, 16 mM thymidine, 10,000 U/ml penicillin, 10 mg/ml streptomycin, 100 mM cysteine (freshly made), and 225 ml heat-inactivated fetal bovine serum, giving a total volume of 862.5 ml.
3. For 1 l of methylcellulose HMI-9 medium, combine 634 ml of concentrated HMI-9 medium (described in **step 2**) to 366 ml methylcellulose and mix by magnetic stirring. The methylcellulose HMI-9 medium is very viscous and a bit difficult to pipet.

   Trypanosome cultures can be initiated by transferring long slender bloodstream form cells from previous culture, from a stabilate (blood- or culture-derived) (*see* **Note 9**) or from animal blood into methylcellulose HMI-9. In a humidified incubator with 37 °C and 5% CO_2, *T. brucei* AnTat 1.1E and derived strains grow logarithmically with a population doubling time of 5.5–6 h up to a density of ~1×10^6 cells/ml

(Fig. 2a). At higher densities, they undergo density-dependent differentiation to the cell cycle-arrested short stumpy stage (Fig. 2b). In the highly viscous methylcellulose HMI-9 medium, trypanosomes show directed movement (*see* also [36]) and are therefore a bit more difficult to count compared to liquid cultures. To recover trypanosomes from methylcellulose HMI-9, add 5 volumes of PBS containing 10 mM glucose, mix by inverting, and pass through a sterile folded paper filter. Collect the cells that pass the filter by centrifugation (10 min, 1400 × *g*).

3.1.3 Cultivation of Matrix-Independent T. brucei Strains

The *T. brucei* strains AnTat 1.1E "Paris" and AnTat 1.1 90-13 (*see* Fig. 1) can be grown in standard HMI-9 at similar growth rates compared to cultivation in methylcellulose HMI-9 (PDT 5.5–6.8 h; Fig. 2a, b), although a significantly higher number of aberrant cells is seen initially upon transfer from matrix-containing medium (Fig. 2c). After several passages we still note a higher number of aberrant cells, indicating that adaptation to matrix independence is not complete in the two strains. Standard HMI-9 culture of matrix-independent *T. brucei* strains can be started from previous culture, from animal blood or from a stabilate (blood or culture-derived) (*see* **Note 9**). The maximal parasite density for logarithmic growth is 1×10^6 cells/ml, exactly as in methylcellulose HMI-9.

3.2 Transfection of Pleomorphic Trypanosoma brucei brucei Strains

For transfection, trypanosomes need to be collected from their respective growth medium. This is more complicated for matrix-dependent strains compared to strains growing in standard liquid culture.

3.2.1 Preparation of DNA for Transfection

Any type of sterile, column-purified (current kits) DNA (in distilled water) can be used for transfection. Although circular plasmids can be transfected and can theoretically be kept as episomes [37, 38], this has never been reported for pleomorphic trypanosomes. In most cases, linearized plasmids are transfected, for example, for targeted gene deletions or replacements, for expression of double-stranded RNA for RNAi-mediated gene knockdown, for epitope-tagging of proteins, or for expressing transgenes. The linear DNA needs homologous flanks that allow for integration into the trypanosomal genome by homologous recombination. As homologous flanks as short as 50 bp are sufficient for targeted homologous recombination in *T. brucei* [39], transfection of PCR products represents a fast and simple alternative to plasmid-based gene manipulation in trypanosomes [40–42]. In this case, the homologous flanks are part of the primers used for amplification. PCR-based tagging has previously been described for the monomorphic *T. brucei* strain Lister 427 MiTat 1.2 [40, 42], and we have

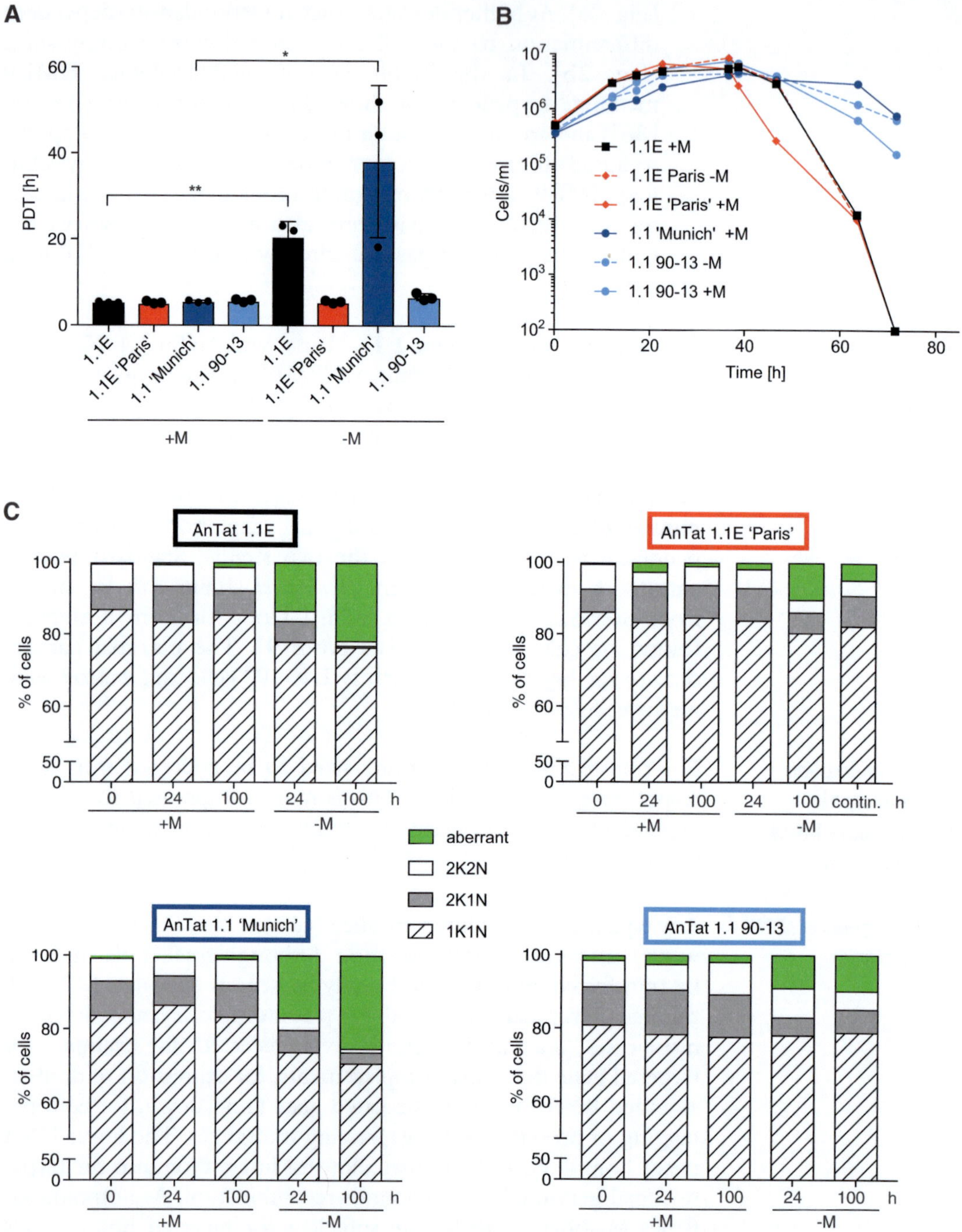

Fig. 2 Comparison of growth and culture characteristics of *T. brucei* AnTat 1.1E and derived strains in liquid (−M) or methylcellulose-containing (+M) HMI-9 medium. (**a**) Population doubling times (PDTs) of logarithmically growing *T. brucei* AnTat 1.1E and derived strains in HMI-9 medium with (+M) or without (−M) methylcellulose. Cultures were counted and diluted daily over 94 h in order to keep the density below 1×10^6 cells/ml (logarithmic growth). PDTs (in hours [h]) are mean ± SD of $n = 3$. Significance between PDTs in liquid (−M) versus methylcellulose (+M) medium was determined using a two-sided Student's *t*-test. ∗Significant ($p < 0.05$); ∗∗highly significant ($p < 0.01$). (**b**) Logarithmic to stationary phase growth of *T. brucei*

successfully used the same protocol for pleomorphic strains. Phenol–chloroform extraction of PCR products significantly improves efficiency ([40], confirmed by our own experience). Length and degree of sequence identity of the homologous flanks show a strong correlation with recombination efficiency [39, 43]. When using plasmids for transfection, homologous flanks of at least 200 bp with 100% sequence identity are recommended [39]. The efficiency of homologous recombination decreases ~10-fold when reducing the homologous flanks to 50 bp and ~3-fold at 1% sequence divergence within the homologous flanks. The amount of DNA needed for *T. brucei* transfection has not been determined systematically. Usually, 5–10 μg of linearized plasmid DNA or PCR product gives optimal results. Critical additional parameters are the purity of the transfected DNA, the fitness of the parasites used for transfection and the transcription of the targeting locus that drives selection marker expression.

Currently, six drug resistance genes have been validated for positive selection in monomorphic *T. brucei* Lister 427 MiTat 1.2 (Table 1). They confer resistance to hygromycin, G418, phleomycin, puromycin, blasticidin, or nourseothricin. We have not tested nourseothricin in pleomorphic bloodstream forms. As these drugs act independently, several drug resistance genes can be selected for at once. The drug concentration required for selection can be dependent on many factors including parasite strain, drug supplier, purity and batch, culture conditions, and serum batch. Suggestions from our experience with pleomorphic AnTat 1.1 are given in Table 1. If problems arise, it is advised to titrate the IC_{50} of the selection drugs under the individual experimental conditions.

The CRISPR-Cas9 technology has started to revolutionize gene and genome editing in various species and recently also in trypanosomes [44–47]. The methods reported for monomorphic bloodstream forms will undoubtedly also be applicable to pleomorphic strains, although suitable cell lines inducibly expressing Cas9 have not yet been reported.

Fig. 2 (continued) AnTat 1.1E and derived strains in liquid (−M) or methylcellulose-containing HMI-9. Cultures were counted at the indicated time points without dilution. The maximal culture density was comparable between all strains and culture conditions (4.5 to 8.8 × 10^6 cells/ml). (**c**) Analysis of kinetoplast/nucleus configurations of *T. brucei* AnTat 1.1E and derived strains. Trypanosomes grown in liquid (−M) or methylcellulose-containing (+M) HMI-9 for the specified time were air-dried, fixed in methanol, and stained with the DNA dye DAPI (1 μM). Since the trypanosome kinetoplast divides prior to the nucleus, three cell cycle phases can be distinguished: cells with one kinetoplast (K) and one nucleus (N) (1K1N; G1 phase of cell cycle), cells with two kinetoplasts and one nucleus (2K1N; S to early M phase of cell cycle) and cells with two kinetoplasts and two nuclei (2K2N; between mitosis and cytokinesis). A logarithmically growing trypanosome population contains around 70% 1K1N cells and around 15% of each 2K1N and 2K2N cells. The number of nuclei (N) and kinetoplasts (K) per cell were determined by fluorescence microscopy and cells were categorized as 1K1N, 2K1N, 2K2N, or aberrant. $n = 400$ cells per cell line

Table 1
Drug resistance markers for positive selection of transformants in *T. brucei* bloodstream forms

Selectable marker[a]	Drug	Concentration monomorphic *T. brucei* MiTat 1.2 (μg/ml)[b,c]	Concentration pleomorphic *T. brucei* AnTat 1.1 (μg/ml)[c,d]
Hygromycin phosphotransferase (HYG)	Hygromycin B	2–5	2
Neomycin phosphotransferase (NEO)	G418 sulfate/ geneticin	1–3	2
Bleomycin resistance gene (BLE)	Phleomycin D1/zeocin	1–2.5	1–2.5
Puromycin acetyltransferase (PAC)	Puromycin HCl	0.1	0.1
Blasticidin deaminase (BSD)	Blasticidin S HCl	2–5	2
Streptothricin acetyltransferase (SAT)	Nourseothricin sulfate	25	n.d.

[a]Commonly used abbreviations of the marker genes are given in parentheses
[b]According to recommendation from G. Cross: http://tryps.rockefeller.edu/trypsru2_genetics.html
[c]The appropriate concentration may be dependent on parasite density as well as on the locus and the promoter and should be titrated individually
[d]Based on our own observations

3.2.2 Transfection of Matrix-Dependent Strains

For transfection of matrix-dependent *T. brucei* strains, we recommend either using trypanosomes from an in vitro culture in methylcellulose HMI-9 or harvesting trypanosomes directly from blood of an infected animal. We have never transfected trypanosomes harvested from an in vitro culture on agarose plates. We think, however, that the population that can be recovered from an agarose plate is probably not optimal for transfection as it contains a substantial fraction of intermediate and stumpy cells due to colony formation.

From In Vitro Culture in Methylcellulose HMI-9 (Adapted from [13])

When cultivating matrix-dependent *T. brucei* strains in methylcellulose HMI-9, the viscous medium needs to be removed prior to transfection.

1. Determine the density of your trypanosome culture (should be lower than 1×10^6 cells/ml) and calculate the volume needed for 2×10^7 cells per transfection. Dilute with 5 volumes of PBS containing 10 mM glucose and pass through a sterile folded paper filter. Count again to exclude loss of cells during filtration.

2. Collect cells by centrifugation (10 min, 1400 × *g*, 37 °C (*see* **Note 10**), pour off supernatant and transfer cells with residual supernatant into a conical-bottom microcentrifuge tube. Collect cells by centrifugation as before.
3. Resuspend cell pellet in 100 μl transfection buffer [35] (*see* Subheading 2.2) equilibrated to 37 °C (*see* **Note 5**). Add 10 μg sterile, linear DNA (1 μg/μl in sterile H_2O), mix briefly, and transfer the mixture into a 2 mm gap electroporation cuvette.
4. Electroporate cells using an AMAXA Nuleofector® IIb machine with program $CD4^+$ T cells X-001 (*see* **Note 6**).
5. Transfer cells into 5 ml liquid HMI-9 and rinse cuvette twice with HMI-9 for complete transfer of transfected cells.
6. Mix briefly and transfer cells to 100 ml methylcellulose HMI-9 (*see* Subheading 2.2). Mix carefully and distribute 5 ml aliquots into the wells of 6-well plates. Usually, you get at least three independent clones by this procedure. Incubate at 37 °C, 5% CO_2, humid atmosphere.
7. After 6–12 h, add selection drugs (*see* Table 1) and continue incubation at 37 °C, 5% CO_2, humid atmosphere.

   After 4–7 days, resistant cells will become visible and can be expanded for freezing stabilates or for downstream analysis.

Transfection of *T. brucei* Derived from Animal Blood

Pleomorphic *T. brucei* bloodstream forms can also be freshly isolated from blood of an infected animal for transfection (see detailed protocol described by MacGregor et al. [30]). They suggest that this method yields the healthiest parasites, thereby resulting in a high transfection efficiency. Moreover, it might reduce the risk of selection for monomorphism. However, when transfecting the pleomorphic AnTat 1.1 "Munich" strain (as well as the derived AnTat 1.1 90-13) from in vitro culture, we have not experienced poor transfection efficiencies or reduced differentiation competence. Transfection from in vitro culture is recommended without reservations, and particularly important for laboratories with limited access to animal facilities or in countries with prohibitive animal welfare legislation.

3.2.3 Transfection of Matrix-Independent Strains

The transfection procedure for *T. brucei* bloodstream forms growing in liquid HMI-9 is much simpler and less time-consuming compared to animal-derived parasites or parasites grown in methylcellulose HMI-9, as the parasites can easily be collected from the medium by centrifugation. We also find a slightly higher transfection efficiency compared to matrix-dependent strains recovered from methylcellulose HMI-9, probably due to a faster transfection procedure.

1. Determine cell density of *T. brucei* bloodstream form culture (should be lower than 1×10^6 cells/ml) and harvest 2×10^7 trypanosomes per transfection by centrifugation (10 min, $1400 \times g$, 37 °C).
2. Resuspend cell pellet in 100 μl transfection buffer [35] (*see* Subheading 2.2) equilibrated to 37 °C (*see* **Note 5**). Add 5–10 μg sterile, linear DNA (1 μg/μl in sterile H_2O) (*see* Subheading 3.2.1), mix briefly, and transfer the mixture into a 2 mm gap electroporation cuvette (e.g., BTX Cat. No. 45-0125).
3. Electroporate cells using an AMAXA Nuleofector® IIb device with program CD4+ T cells X-001 (*see* **Note 6**).
4. Transfer cells into 30 ml HMI-9. Perform two serial dilutions in 27 ml HMI-9 each in order to yield 1:10 and 1:100 dilutions. Distribute 1 ml aliquots into the wells of three 24-well plates. Incubate at 37 °C, 5% CO_2, humid atmosphere.
5. After 6–12 h, add selection antibiotics (*see* Table 1) and continue incubation at 37 °C, 5% CO_2, humid atmosphere.

   After 4–7 days, resistant cells will become visible and can be expanded for freezing stabilates or for downstream analysis.

3.3 Recommendation for Strain Selection

A large part of the molecular and biochemical studies in the past 35 years have used monomorphic clones of stock Lister 427 as the workhorse in trypanosome research. Pleomorphic strains that have been considered difficult to handle and to require laborious culture conditions have been mainly used for work on stage differentiation, fly transmission, virulence, and tissue tropism. With highly efficient tools for reverse genetics in place, we are now analyzing more subtle and complex phenotypes. It is increasingly recognized that using a pleomorphic, fly transmissible strain with many properties close to field isolates adds significance and validity to experiments addressing many of the current research questions. Growth rate and transfection efficiency of the AnTat 1.1E strain is not significantly different from Lister 427, yet the requirement for a highly viscous, matrix containing medium and a strict upper limit of cell density are trade-offs to consider. One reason for wider use of the Antat 1.1 strain was the fortuitous observation that one of its most useful recombinant subclones suitable for Tet-inducible expression, AnTat 1.1 90-13 [25], turned out to be matrix-independent but retained pleomorphic properties. As we show here, matrix independence has been selected for independently at multiple times in AnTat 1.1E derivatives (Fig. 1 and 2a). There seems to be no strict correlation between matrix dependence and pleomorphic phenotype. Matrix-dependent and matrix-independent clones show a comparable growth behavior: (1) logarithmic growth below a density of 1×10^6 cells/ml with a population doubling time between 5 and 6 h (Fig. 2a) and (2) maximal culture density of

4.5–8.8 × 10^6 cells/ml (Fig. 2b). Culture of pleomorphic strains without matrix in standard HMI-9 medium is accompanied by severe cell division problems evidenced by increased aberrant kinetoplast/nucleus configurations [11] (Fig. 2c). Here we show that these phenotypes are also seen to a lesser degree in matrix-independent derived clones. The fraction of aberrant cells decreases upon continuous cultivation of matrix-independent clones in liquid HMI-9 but remain clearly elevated compared to growth in matrix (Fig. 2c). It should be kept in mind that matrix-independent pleomorphic strains went through an ill-defined selection bottleneck in culture. Therefore, we recommend to limit the number of passages in matrix-free medium for all pleomorphic strains. Most importantly, rigorous testing of the biological potential and properties is mandatory prior to use of matrix-independent subclones for a specific research question. Of possible practical value is the observation that AnTat 1.1 "Munich" and the derived clone AnTat 1.1 90-13 show a longer survival period of stumpy forms compared to AnTat 1.1E and AnTat 1.1E "Paris" (Fig. 2b). AnTat 1.1 "Munich" and AnTat 1.1 90-13 have been validated for synchronous stage differentiation (*see* references in Subheading 2.1).

4 Notes

1. The original HMI-9 described by Hirumi and Hirumi (1989) [9] was modified by omission of SerumPlus™ (designated HMI-11 in [9]) and omission of additional sodium pyruvate. We noticed that the benefit of SerumPlus™ is limited to its low content of FCS and trypanosomes excrete pyruvate anyway. To avoid confusion, we continue to name this modified medium HMI-9 in accord with many other laboratories.
2. HMI-9 agarose plates and "methylcellulose HMI-9" are supplemented with 15% (v/v) fetal bovine serum. This increase is a precaution that we maintained and is not evidence-based.
3. The final agarose concentration may be increased to 0.8%, if the agar is too soft for spreading the parasites without damaging the agar surface. This may be caused by differences among agarose brands and batches or by external factors such as humidity and laminar flow.
4. Different brands of low melting point agaroses (e.g., the expensive Seaplaque® GTG agarose (Lonza, Basel, Switzerland) or the cheaper LowMelt agarose from Bio-Budget Technologies (Krefeld, Germany)) performed equally well.
5. Alternatively, Human T Cell Nucleofector™ solution or Basic Parasite Nucleofector Solution 2 (Lonza, Basel, Switzerland) can be used for transfection with comparable transfection efficiency [48].

6. Different versions of the Amaxa Nucleofector™ can be used: Amaxa Nucleofector™ I (program x-001); Amaxa Nucleofector™ II/IIb: program CD4+ T cells X-001; Amaxa Nucleofector™ 4D: program DN-100.
7. Check individual stability of selection antibiotics; blasticidin and hygromycin are less stable compared to puromycin, G418, or phleomycin. Hence, we recommend storing plates containing blasticidin and hygromycin no longer than 1 week. Agarose plates containing tetracycline need to be stored in the dark.
8. The drying period may depend on the laminar flow and should be optimized individually.
9. When thawing a trypanosome stabilate, the cells should be washed with 9 volumes of liquid HMI-9 in order to remove the glycerol used as cryopreservant in freezing media.
10. Harvesting trypanosomes for transfection at 37 °C instead of room temperature results in a slightly higher transfection efficiency.

References

1. Silvester E, McWilliam KR, Matthews KR (2017) The cytological events and molecular control of life cycle development of *Trypanosoma brucei* in the mammalian bloodstream. Pathogens 6(3):E29. https://doi.org/10.3390/pathogens6030029
2. Brun R, Jenni L, Schonenberger M, Schell KF (1981) In vitro cultivation of bloodstream forms of *Trypanosoma brucei*, *T. rhodesiense*, and *T. gambiense*. J Protozool 28(4):470–479
3. Brun R, Jenni L, Tanner M, Schonenberger M, Schell KF (1979) Cultivation of vertebrate infective forms derived from metacyclic forms of pleomorphic *Trypanosoma brucei* stocks. Short communication. Acta Trop 36 (4):387–390
4. Doyle JJ, Hirumi H, Hirumi K, Lupton EN, Cross GA (1980) Antigenic variation in clones of animal-infective *Trypanosoma brucei* derived and maintained in vitro. Parasitology 80 (2):359–369
5. Hirumi H, Doyle JJ, Hirumi K (1977) African trypanosomes: cultivation of animal-infective *Trypanosoma brucei in vitro*. Science (New York, NY) 196(4293):992–994
6. Hirumi H, Hirumi K, Doyle JJ, Cross GA (1980) In vitro cloning of animal-infective bloodstream forms of *Trypanosoma brucei*. Parasitology 80(2):371–382
7. Duszenko M, Ferguson MA, Lamont GS, Rifkin MR, Cross GA (1985) Cysteine eliminates the feeder cell requirement for cultivation of *Trypanosoma brucei* bloodstream forms *in vitro*. J Exp Med 162(4):1256–1263
8. Baltz T, Baltz D, Giroud C, Crockett J (1985) Cultivation in a semi-defined medium of animal infective forms of *Trypanosoma brucei*, *T. equiperdum*, *T. evansi*, *T. rhodesiense* and *T. gambiense*. EMBO J 4(5):1273–1277
9. Hirumi H, Hirumi K (1989) Continuous cultivation of *Trypanosoma brucei* blood stream forms in a medium containing a low concentration of serum protein without feeder cell layers. J Parasitol 75(6):985–989
10. Reuner B, Vassella E, Yutzy B, Boshart M (1997) Cell density triggers slender to stumpy differentiation of *Trypanosoma brucei* bloodstream forms in culture. Mol Biochem Parasitol 90(1):269–280
11. Vassella E, Boshart M (1996) High molecular mass agarose matrix supports growth of bloodstream forms of pleomorphic *Trypanosoma brucei* strains in axenic culture. Mol Biochem Parasitol 82(1):91–105
12. Vassella E, Reuner B, Yutzy B, Boshart M (1997) Differentiation of African trypanosomes is controlled by a density sensing mechanism which signals cell cycle arrest via the cAMP pathway. J Cell Sci 110 (Pt 21):2661–2671
13. Vassella E, Kramer R, Turner CM, Wankell M, Modes C, van den Bogaard M, Boshart M (2001) Deletion of a novel protein kinase with PX and FYVE-related domains increases

the rate of differentiation of *Trypanosoma brucei*. Mol Microbiol 41(1):33–46

14. McCulloch R, Vassella E, Burton P, Boshart M, Barry JD (2004) Transformation of monomorphic and pleomorphic *Trypanosoma brucei*. Methods Mol Biol 262:53–86. https://doi.org/10.1385/1-59259-761-0:053
15. Van Meirvenne N, Janssens PG, Magnus E (1975) Antigenic variation in syringe passaged populations of *Trypanosoma* (Trypanozoon) brucei. 1. Rationalization of the experimental approach. Ann Soc Belg Med Trop 55(1):1–23
16. Le Ray D, Barry JD, Easton C, Vickerman K (1977) First tsetse fly transmission of the "AnTat" serodeme of *Trypanosoma brucei*. Ann Soc Belg Med Trop 57(4-5):369–381
17. Delauw MF, Pays E, Steinert M, Aerts D, Van Meirvenne N, Le Ray D (1985) Inactivation and reactivation of a variant-specific antigen gene in cyclically transmitted *Trypanosoma brucei*. EMBO J 4(4):989–993
18. Rolin S, Paindavoine P, Hanocq-Quertier J, Hanocq F, Claes Y, Le Ray D, Overath P, Pays E (1993) Transient adenylate cyclase activation accompanies differentiation of *Trypanosoma brucei* from bloodstream to procyclic forms. Mol Biochem Parasitol 61(1):115–125
19. Radwanska M, Magez S, Michel A, Stijlemans B, Geuskens M, Pays E (2000) Comparative analysis of antibody responses against HSP60, invariant surface glycoprotein 70, and variant surface glycoprotein reveals a complex antigen-specific pattern of immunoglobulin isotype switching during infection by *Trypanosoma brucei*. Infect Immun 68 (2):848–860
20. Salmon D, Vanwalleghem G, Morias Y, Denoeud J, Krumbholz C, Lhomme F, Bachmaier S, Kador M, Gossmann J, Dias FB, De Muylder G, Uzureau P, Magez S, Moser M, De Baetselier P, Van Den Abbeele J, Beschin A, Boshart M, Pays E (2012) Adenylate cyclases of *Trypanosoma brucei* inhibit the innate immune response of the host. Science (New York, NY) 337(6093):463–466. https://doi.org/10.1126/science.1222753
21. De Muylder G, Daulouède S, Lecordier L, Uzureau P, Morias Y, Van Den Abbeele J, Caljon G, Hérin M, Holzmuller P, Semballa S, Courtois P, Vanhamme L, Stijlemans B, De Baetselier P, Barrett MP, Barlow JL, McKenzie ANJ, Barron L, Wynn TA, Beschin A, Vincendeau P, Pays E (2013) A *Trypanosoma brucei* kinesin heavy chain promotes parasite growth by triggering host arginase activity. PLoS Pathog 9(10):e1003731. https://doi.org/10.1371/journal.ppat.1003731
22. Capewell P, Cren-Travaillé C, Marchesi F, Johnston P, Clucas C, Benson RA, Gorman T-A, Calvo-Alvarez E, Crouzols A, Jouvion G, Jamonneau V, Weir W, Stevenson ML, O'Neill K, Cooper A, Swar NK, Bucheton B, Ngoyi DM, Garside P, Rotureau B, MacLeod A (2016) The skin is a significant but overlooked anatomical reservoir for vector-borne African trypanosomes. elife 5:e17716. https://doi.org/10.7554/eLife.17716
23. Wargnies M, Bertiaux E, Cahoreau E, Ziebart N, Crouzols A, Morand P, Biran M, Allmann S, Hubert J, Villafraz O, Millerioux Y, Plazolles N, Asencio C, Rivière L, Rotureau B, Boshart M, Portais J-C, Bringaud F (2018) Gluconeogenesis is essential for trypanosome development in the tsetse fly vector. PLoS Pathog 14(12):e1007502. https://doi.org/10.1371/journal.ppat.1007502
24. Ziegelbauer K, Quinten M, Schwarz H, Pearson TW, Overath P (1990) Synchronous differentiation of *Trypanosoma brucei* from bloodstream to procyclic forms *in vitro*. Eur J Biochem 192(2):373–378
25. Engstler M, Boshart M (2004) Cold shock and regulation of surface protein trafficking convey sensitization to inducers of stage differentiation in *Trypanosoma brucei*. Genes Dev 18 (22):2798–2811. https://doi.org/10.1101/gad.323404
26. Domenicali Pfister D, Burkard G, Morand S, Renggli CK, Roditi I, Vassella E (2006) A mitogen-activated protein kinase controls differentiation of bloodstream forms of *Trypanosoma brucei*. Eukaryot Cell 5(7):1126–1135. https://doi.org/10.1128/EC.00094-06
27. Engstler M, Pfohl T, Herminghaus S, Boshart M, Wiegertjes G, Heddergott N, Overath P (2007) Hydrodynamic flow-mediated protein sorting on the cell surface of trypanosomes. Cell 131(3):505–515. https://doi.org/10.1016/j.cell.2007.08.046
28. Wirtz E, Leal S, Ochatt C, Cross GA (1999) A tightly regulated inducible expression system for conditional gene knock-outs and dominant-negative genetics in *Trypanosoma brucei*. Mol Biochem Parasitol 99(1):89–101
29. Dean S, Marchetti R, Kirk K, Matthews KR (2009) A surface transporter family conveys the trypanosome differentiation signal. Nature 459(7244):213–217. https://doi.org/10.1038/nature07997
30. MacGregor P, Rojas F, Dean S, Matthews KR (2013) Stable transformation of pleomorphic bloodstream form *Trypanosoma brucei*. Mol Biochem Parasitol 190(2):60–62. https://doi.org/10.1016/j.molbiopara.2013.06.007

31. Mony BM, MacGregor P, Ivens A, Rojas F, Cowton A, Young J, Horn D, Matthews K (2014) Genome-wide dissection of the quorum sensing signalling pathway in *Trypanosoma brucei*. Nature 505(7485):681–685. https://doi.org/10.1038/nature12864
32. Rojas F, Silvester E, Young J, Milne R, Tettey M, Houston DR, Walkinshaw MD, Perez-Pi I, Auer M, Denton H, Smith TK, Thompson J, Matthews KR (2019) Oligopeptide signaling through TbGPR89 drives trypanosome quorum sensing. Cell 176 (1-2):306–317. e316. https://doi.org/10.1016/j.cell.2018.10.041
33. Carruthers VB, Cross GA (1992) High-efficiency clonal growth of bloodstream- and insect-form *Trypanosoma brucei* on agarose plates. Proc Natl Acad Sci U S A 89 (18):8818–8821
34. Tan KS, Leal ST, Cross GA (2002) *Trypanosoma brucei* MRE11 is non-essential but influences growth, homologous recombination and DNA double-strand break repair. Mol Biochem Parasitol 125(1-2):11–21
35. Schumann Burkard G, Jutzi P, Roditi I (2011) Genome-wide RNAi screens in bloodstream form trypanosomes identify drug transporters. Mol Biochem Parasitol 175(1):91–94. https://doi.org/10.1016/j.molbiopara.2010.09.002
36. Heddergott N, Krüger T, Babu SB, Wei A, Stellamanns E, Uppaluri S, Pfohl T, Stark H, Engstler M (2012) Trypanosome motion represents an adaptation to the crowded environment of the vertebrate bloodstream. PLoS Pathog 8(11):e1003023. https://doi.org/10.1371/journal.ppat.1003023
37. Clayton CE (1999) Genetic manipulation of kinetoplastida. Parasitol Today 15(9):372–378
38. Patnaik PK, Kulkarni SK, Cross GA (1993) Autonomously replicating single-copy episomes in *Trypanosoma brucei* show unusual stability. EMBO J 12(6):2529–2538
39. Barnes RL, McCulloch R (2007) *Trypanosoma brucei* homologous recombination is dependent on substrate length and homology, though displays a differential dependence on mismatch repair as substrate length decreases. Nucleic Acids Res 35(10):3478–3493. https://doi.org/10.1093/nar/gkm249
40. Dean S, Sunter J, Wheeler RJ, Hodkinson I, Gluenz E, Gull K (2015) A toolkit enabling efficient, scalable and reproducible gene tagging in trypanosomatids. Open Biol 5 (1):140197. https://doi.org/10.1098/rsob.140197
41. Dyer P, Dean S, Sunter J (2016) High-throughput gene tagging in *Trypanosoma brucei*. J Vis Exp 114. https://doi.org/10.3791/54342
42. Oberholzer M, Morand S, Kunz S, Seebeck T (2006) A vector series for rapid PCR-mediated C-terminal in situ tagging of *Trypanosoma brucei* genes. Mol Biochem Parasitol 145 (1):117–120. https://doi.org/10.1016/j.molbiopara.2005.09.002
43. Bell JS, McCulloch R (2003) Mismatch repair regulates homologous recombination, but has little influence on antigenic variation, in *Trypanosoma brucei*. J Biol Chem 278 (46):45182–45188. https://doi.org/10.1074/jbc.M308123200
44. Beneke T, Madden R, Makin L, Valli J, Sunter J, Gluenz E (2017) A CRISPR Cas9 high-throughput genome editing toolkit for kinetoplastids. R Soc Open Sci 4(5):170095. https://doi.org/10.1098/rsos.170095
45. Rico E, Jeacock L, Kovářová J, Horn D (2018) Inducible high-efficiency CRISPR-Cas9-targeted gene editing and precision base editing in African trypanosomes. Sci Rep 8(1):7960. https://doi.org/10.1038/s41598-018-26303-w
46. Soares Medeiros LC, South L, Peng D, Bustamante JM, Wang W, Bunkofske M, Perumal N, Sanchez-Valdez F, Tarleton RL (2017) Rapid, selection-free, high-efficiency genome editing in protozoan parasites using CRISPR-Cas9 Ribonucleoproteins. MBio 8(6):e01788-01717. https://doi.org/10.1128/mBio.01788-17%JmBio
47. Vasquez JJ, Wedel C, Cosentino RO, Siegel TN (2018) Exploiting CRISPR-Cas9 technology to investigate individual histone modifications. Nucleic Acids Res 46(18):e106. https://doi.org/10.1093/nar/gky517
48. Burkard G, Fragoso CM, Roditi I (2007) Highly efficient stable transformation of bloodstream forms of *Trypanosoma brucei*. Mol Biochem Parasitol 153(2):220–223. https://doi.org/10.1016/j.molbiopara.2007.02.008

Chapter 3

In Vitro Culture for Differentiation Simulation of *Leishmania* spp.

Dan Zilberstein

Abstract

In the 1990s my laboratory discovered that *Leishmania* promastigotes can combine two environmental cues, typical to lysosomes, acidic pH (~5.5) and body temperature (37 °C) into a single signal that induced differentiation. Based on this concept, we modified EARLS-based medium 199 to become an amastigote-specific medium. Shifting promastigotes to this medium followed by incubation in a CO_2 incubator induced differentiation. Axenic amastigotes reach maturation within 5 days, resembling the time it takes in vivo. This chapter provides a complete protocol we developed for *L. donovani* promastigote-to-amastigote differentiation. This protocol should be useful for both old-world and new-world species of *Leishmania*.

Key words *Leishmania*, Development, Phagolysosome, Differentiation, Signaling, Promastigote, Amastigote

1 Introduction

Investigating parasite development inside either host or vector is a difficult mission. Animal models provide excellent tools to study the mature developmental stages (e.g., promastigotes and amastigotes in the case of *Leishmania*). Intermediate developmental forms are not visible; they are part of a black box, hidden inside the animal. A way to open the box is by developing host-free axenic culture that simulates the natural niche, thereby providing parasites the confidence that they have reached their intracellular destination [1]. The outcome of these models can subsequently be validated in vivo. Axenic cultures of promastigotes have been developed long ago, in the 1960s and 1970s [2, 3]. They are well established and accepted for all aspects of *Leishmania* research. Axenic amastigote cultures are more recent and are in the process of being widely used. The aim of this chapter is to propose a unified methodology for host-free *Leishmania* promastigote-to-amastigote differentiation.

Paul A. M. Michels et al. (eds.), *Trypanosomatids: Methods and Protocols*, Methods in Molecular Biology, vol. 2116, https://doi.org/10.1007/978-1-0716-0294-2_3,

During their life, *Leishmania* parasites reside and proliferate in two distinct environments, both of which are hydrolytic. In the vector's midgut, where procyclic promastigotes reside, the pH is slightly alkaline, rich with amino acids and sugar, and the mean temperature is 26 °C [4]. In phagolysosomes, where amastigotes reside, the pH is acidic (~5.5), major nutrients are amino and fatty acids and sugar is scarce (Fischer Weinberger, R. et al., in preparation) [5]. Hence, in order for *Leishmania* to successfully develop in both host and vector, they established tools to rapidly adjust to each of these environments [6]. Investigating each life stage is possible but requires isolation of parasites from either vector or model animal. However, in order to investigate the process of development inside the host an in vitro model system that enables time course analysis of promastigote-to-amastigote differentiation was required.

In the early 1990s we hypothesized that macrophage-invading promastigotes identify their lysosome target by merging two physical cues, the lysosome acidic environment and high temperature of the host body [7]. Growing promastigotes at pH 5 and 26 °C induced expression of amastigote-specific genes but their morphology did not change [8]. Interestingly, growing promastigotes of *L. donovani* at 37 °C and pH 7 in a 100% fetal calf serum medium resulted in amastigote-shaped cells [9]. These cells grew at the same rate as promastigotes and released amastigote-type acid phosphatase. This experiment suggested that amastigote medium should contain serum at a concentration higher than in the promastigotes' media. Elevating the growth temperature of *L. donovani* promastigotes to 37 °C in a medium that contained 25% fetal calf serum, without changing the pH, resulted in growth arrest and cell aggregation, but without morphological change [10]. Interestingly, shifting this culture from pH 7 to 5.5 released promastigotes from growth arrest, they immediately doubled and subsequently started to differentiate into amastigote-shaped cells [10]. The analyses indicated that *Leishmania* promastigotes process the two distinct signals, 37 °C and pH 5.5 into a single signal that initiated promastigote differentiation into amastigotes [7, 11].

Over two decades ago Paul Bates and colleagues established the first axenic host-free culture for *L. mexicana* amastigotes [12]. A few years later our laboratory established the first method for axenic *L. donovani* amastigote culture [11]. Both employed the same principle that exposing promastigotes to a lysosome-like environment induces promastigote transformation into amastigotes-like parasites. Other laboratories used the same principles to design their own *L. donovani* amastigote culture [13, 14]. These studies used stage-specific markers to show that their axenic amastigotes resembled animal-derived amastigotes.

To date, the axenic experimental system is widely used in our field, helping to understand and predict in vivo processes. According to PubMed (www.pubmed.com), to date (mid of 2019), 421 research papers that used axenic amastigotes have been published. These describe the use of both old-world and new-world species. On the one hand, it is a great benefit to being able to use this system to investigate many processes in the amastigotes that are free of host molecules. But on the other hand, many laboratories developed their own protocol and culture conditions. Lack of a consensus method for in vitro cultivation of axenic *Leishmania* culture is problematic as it makes it difficult to repeat experiments that use diverse in vitro axenic amastigote protocols. Being the leading laboratory in characterizing the process of promastigote-to-amastigote differentiation, we decided to provide an in-depth description of the method and quality control assays for axenic amastigote culture. The aim of this chapter is to describe, in detail, the method we use to differentiate in culture *L. donovani* promastigotes into amastigotes. To date, literature indicates that the protocol for all old-world species resembles that of new-world species. Furthermore, visceral species differentiate best at 37 °C in a CO_2 environment, whereas cutaneous species differentiate best at 33 °C without CO_2 [1].

2 Materials

2.1 Promastigote Growth Medium

1. Earls based medium 199 (M4530, Sigma-Aldrich Ltd. MO) supplemented with 10% heat inactivated fetal bovine serum, 0.1 mg/ml streptomycin, and 100 U/ml penicillin.
2. In many cultures hemin, adenine, and biotin are added, as in many species and strains they are essential for growth.
3. We recommend that each laboratory use its own protocol for axenic growth of promastigotes.

2.2 Amastigote Growth Medium

1. Earls based medium 199 supplemented with 10 mM succinic acid, 25% fetal bovine serum (**not** heat inactivated), 0.1 mg/ml streptomycin, 100 U/ml penicillin. Titrate to pH 5.5 with HCl and finally filter to sterilize.
2. Additional supplements such as hemin, adenine, and biotin should be added according to local protocols.

2.3 Serum for Amastigote Media

1. When purchasing a new batch of serum we recommend that you check aggregate formation at 5–8 h of differentiation. As indicated below, aggregation is essential for successful differentiation. The factor that induces cell aggregation is sensitive to heat (Zilberstein, D. unpublished).
2. We recommend purchase and use of *non–heat-inactivated serum*.

3 Methods

3.1 Protocol for Axenic Promastigote-to-Amastigote Differentiation

1. The following protocol was designed for *L. donovani* (*see* **Note 1**). However, it should work equally well for all old-world species such as *L. infantum* and *L. tropica*. Interestingly, efforts to differentiate axenic *L. major* promastigotes into amastigotes failed. They do differentiate inside macrophage cell lines but not in axenic culture [1].
2. Spin down late log phase promastigotes (2-day-old culture, 10^7 cells/ml) at 1200 × *g* in a swing out rotor (10 min, room temperature).
3. Discard supernatant and then suspend pellet in a room temperature prewarmed amastigote medium to the same cell density.
4. Transfer the cell suspension into sterile plastic flasks and subsequently incubate at 37 °C in a 5% CO_2 incubator for 24 h.
5. On the second day, dilute the culture 1:10 by adding a 37 °C prewarmed amastigote medium and then transfer to larger flasks (Note, do not exceed the recommended volume indicated on each flask).
6. Continue incubation in the CO_2 incubator for additional 4 days. Amastigotes should mature by 5 days (120 h) after exposure to amastigote differentiation conditions (Fig. 1).
7. We highly recommend following morphological progression of differentiation using microscopy at 40× magnification (see details below).

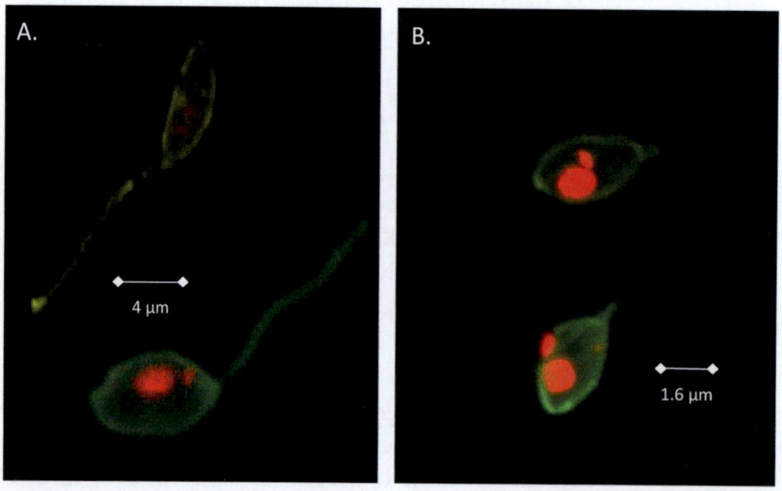

Fig. 1 Axenic amastigotes (**a**) and promastigotes (**b**) of *L. donovani*. Immunofluorescence of mature parasites of each stage. Cells were stained with anti-membrane antibodies kindly provided by Dr. Dennis M. Dwyer [11] and DNA with propidium iodide

8. In our experience, growth rate of mature axenic amastigotes is 24 h per generation. For experimental use, we recommend diluting the cell culture 1:3 at the fourth day (96 h) of differentiation. If parasites are used later than the time of maturation (i.e., longer than 5 days), we recommend diluting them 1:3 once every 3 days, using prewarmed amastigote medium.
9. In our hands, the axenic amastigotes are at their best as soon as they mature (120 h). They will stay amastigotes for a few additional days, sometimes a few weeks. In many cases they become unstable; amino acid transport is less effective and RNA and DNA extraction less efficient (*see* **Notes 1** and **3**) .

3.2 Morphological Assessment of Differentiation

1. Our analyses over two decades indicated that *L. donovani* promastigote-to-amastigote differentiation is a highly regulated process [15]. Barak et al. (2005) [10] determined a time course for morphological development. They divided differentiation into four phases (Table 1). Phase 1 ($t = 0$–4 h) was defined as the signal perception and processing period; during this time, parasites undergo cell cycle arrest at G1 [10]. In phase 2 ($t = 5$–9 h) cells cease movement, aggregate and start rounding. In phase 3 ($t = 10$–23 h) parasites undergo morphogenesis, they round and subsequently lose their flagella. In phase 4 ($t = 24$–120 h) parasites become mature amastigotes.
2. To make sure axenic differentiation is successful, we look at the culture under the microscope at three time points: first at 5–7 h to make sure parasites cease movement and start to aggregate.
3. Next, at 24 h, where most cells should be in large aggregates that have a deep brown-gray color. If cells are not viable the aggregates will look clear inside and transparent.
4. The third point at which we assess differentiating parasites is at the end of maturation, at 120 h. Cells should be in large aggregates, no single cells in the field should be visible (Fig. 2). If the latter is checked positively, axenic amastigotes are ready to use.

3.3 Cell Aggregation Is Essential for Differentiation Progression

1. We found that in the second phase of axenic differentiation the parasites start to aggregate. In an unpublished study we observed that at around 5–7 h after differentiation initiated, parasites release an adhesion molecule that induces aggregation.
2. We observed that the serum contains a heat sensitive factor that induces parasites to release an adhesion factor. We found that heating the serum at 70 °C for 30 min inactivates this factor and as a result parasite do not aggregate. The same happens if heat inactivation at 60 °C is longer than 60 min. These

Table 1
Morphological time course of *L. donovani* promastigote-to-amastigote differentiation

Time in differentiation (hours)	Description	Picture
Phase 1: 0–4	Signal perception	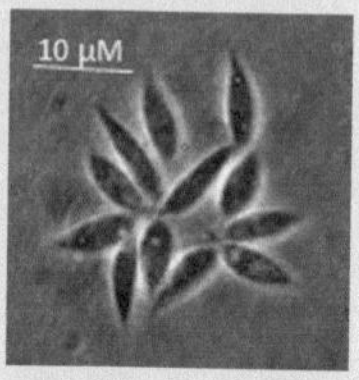
Phase 2: 5–9	Movement secession and aggregation	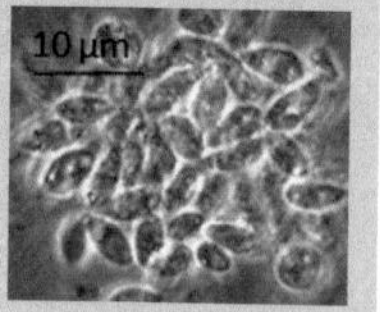
Phase 3: 10–23	Morphogenesis	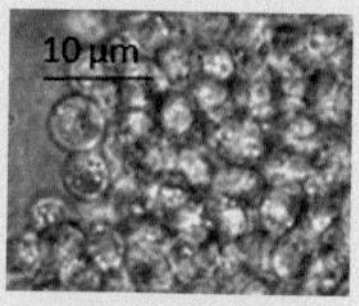
Phase 4: 24–120	Amastigote maturation	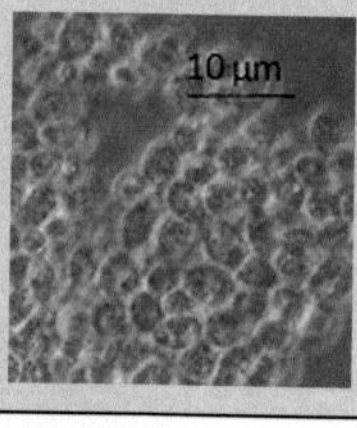

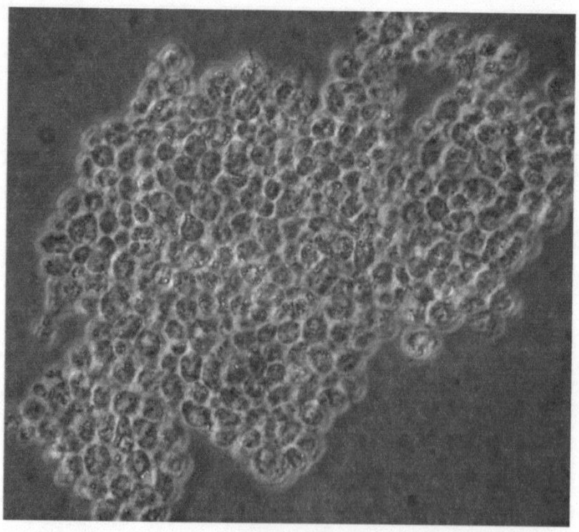

Fig. 2 Axenic amastigotes aggregate during differentiation in culture. Phase microscopy of mature amastigote aggregate

parasites do not differentiate and die after a few days if they remain in amastigote medium at 37 °C. Hence, to avoid any difficulty, the amastigote medium should contain non-heat-inactivated serum.

3.4 Quality Control

1. *Differentiating axenic amastigotes back to promastigotes*: Following a blood meal from an infected mammal, amastigotes encounter the slightly alkaline environment in the sand fly gut and subsequently differentiate to procyclic promastigotes. Similarly, axenic amastigotes should be able to differentiate back to promastigotes by subjecting them to promastigote growth conditions. We recently demonstrated that shifting axenic amastigotes to promastigote medium followed by incubation at 26 °C resulted in parasite differentiation into promastigotes [16]. It takes almost 48 h for axenic amastigotes to complete differentiation into mature promastigotes. Furthermore, we observed that at any time point during promastigote differentiation into amastigotes, parasites can be shifted to promastigote growth conditions and they will differentiate back to promastigotes [10] (unpublished results). Hence, this phenomenon is a great tool to assess parasite viability and quality during and at the end of axenic differentiation. The protocol is very simple; take an aliquot of the axenic amastigotes and dilute 1:20 into promastigote medium and then incubate at 26 °C [16].
2. *2,3-Trans-enoyl CoA isomerase*: We propose this protein as a reliable marker of differentiation progression. The putative 2,3-*trans*-enoyl CoA isomerase, mitochondrial precursor (LdteCi, LinJ.31.2400) abundance increases seven-fold at late stages of promastigote-to-amastigote differentiation [15, 17]. The *L. donovani* genome contains two genes encoding isoforms of this protein: LdteCi.2 (LinJ.31.2320) is 89% identical to LdteCi.1, but lacks 7 amino acids near its N-terminus and has a divergent C-terminal region. Antibodies that we raised against LdteCi.1 detect both isoforms. As shown in Fig. 3, axenic promastigotes express predominantly LdteCi.1. The level of expression decreases gradually until 15 h of differentiation. LdteCi.2 starts to appear 2.5 h after differentiation initiated and stays unchanged until amastigotes mature (Fig. 3). Following LdteCi.1 expression provides reliable information on differentiation progression. Interestingly, using LdteCi expression for the reverse process of amastigote-to-promastigote differentiation provides the point where amastigotes turn into promastigotes [16]. Polyclonal antiserum against LdteCi is available to the public. We will send this upon request.

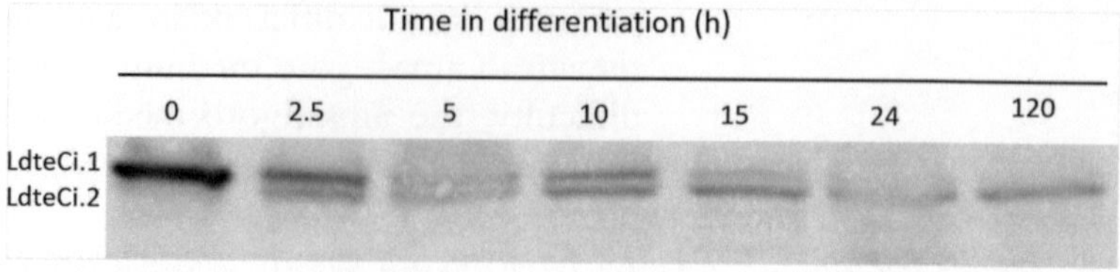

Fig. 3 Expression of LdteCi during *L. donovani* promastigote-to-amastigote differentiation. Western blot of *L. donovani* at indicated time point of differentiation. Cell lysate proteins were subjected to Western blot and then interacted with anti-LdreCi that we raised [16]

3. *LPG expression*. Lipophosphoglycan (LPG) forms a thin layer that covers *Leishmania* promastigote cells. Saar et al. [11] showed that like the in vivo situation, axenic promastigotes shed this layer. Hence, we propose that LPG expression in axenic parasites be assessed at least once when you establish the method. A protocol for quantitative assessment of LPG can be found in [11, 18].

4 Notes

1. Over the years we learned that short-passage, animal-derived promastigotes (e.g., that have recently been recovered from mice or hamster) are difficult to differentiate in culture. We recommend passaging these parasites a few weeks in culture before your next attempt.
2. Counting axenic amastigotes in culture might be difficult because they are in large aggregates. We recommend breaking the aggregates using a 25G needle and then counting.
3. To differentiate a small aliquot of promastigote culture you may dilute promastigotes into amastigote medium at 1:20 and then incubate at 37 °C without further dilution. Amastigotes will mature by day 5.

References

1. Zilberstein D (2008) Physiological and biochemical aspects of *Leishmania* develpment. In: Myler PJ, Fasel N (eds) *Leishmania* after the genome: biology and control. Horizon Scientific Press and Caiser Academic Press, New York, pp 107–122
2. Lemma A, Schiller EL (1964) Extracellular sultivation of *Leishmanial* bodies of species belonging to the protozoan genus Leishmania. Exp Parasitol 15:503–513
3. Steiger RF, Steiger E (1977) Cultivation of *Leishmania donovani* and *Leishmania braziliensis* in defined media: nutritional requirements. J Protozool 24(3):437–441
4. Zilberstein D (2018) Nutrient transport and sensing as pharmacological targets for Leishmaniasis. In: Rivas L, Carmen G (eds) Drug discovery for Leishmaniasis. Drug discovery, vol 60. The Royal Society of Chemistry, London, pp 282–296
5. Harms E, Gochman N, Schneider JA (1981) Lysosomal pool of free-amino acids. Biochem Biophys Res Commun 99(3):830–836

6. Burchmore RJ, Barrett MP (2001) Life in vacuoles—nutrient acquisition by *Leishmania* amastigotes. Int J Parasitol 31(12):1311–1320
7. Zilberstein D, Shapira M (1994) The role of pH and temperature in the development of *Leishmania* parasites. Annu Rev Microbiol 48:449–470
8. Zilberstein D, Blumenfeld N, Liveanu V, Gepstein A, Jaffe CL (1991) Growth at acidic pH induces an amastigote stage-specific protein in *Leishmania* promastigotes. Mol Biochem Parasitol 45(1):175–178
9. Doyle PS, Engel JC, Pimenta PF, da Silva PP, Dwyer DM (1991) *Leishmania donovani*: long-term culture of axenic amastigotes at 37 °C. Exp Parasitol 73(3):326–334
10. Barak E, Amin-Spector S, Gerliak E, Goyard S, Holland N, Zilberstein D (2005) Differentiation of *Leishmania donovani* in host-free system: analysis of signal perception and response. Mol Biochem Parasitol 141(1):99–108
11. Saar Y, Ransford A, Waldman E, Mazareb S, Amin-Spector S, Plumblee J, Turco SJ, Zilberstein D (1998) Characterization of developmentally-regulated activities in axenic amastigotes of *Leishmania donovani*. Mol Biochem Parasitol 95(1):9–20
12. Bates PA, Robertson CD, Tetley L, Coombs GH (1992) Axenic cultivation and characterization of *Leishmania mexicana* amastigote-like forms. Parasitology 105:193–202
13. Debrabant A, Joshi MB, Pimenta PF, Dwyer DM (2004) Generation of *Leishmania donovani* axenic amastigotes: their growth and biological characteristics. Int J Parasitol 34:205–217
14. Goyard S, Segawa H, Gordon J, Showalter M, Duncan R, Turco SJ, Beverley SM (2003) An in vitro system for developmental and genetic studies of *Leishmania donovani* phosphoglycans. Mol Biochem Parasitol 130:31–42
15. Rosenzweig D, Smith D, Opperdoes F, Stern S, Olafson RW, Zilberstein D (2008) Retooling *Leishmania* metabolism: from sand fly gut to human macrophage. FASEB J 22 (2):590–602
16. Bachmaier S, Witztum R, Tsigankov P, Koren R, Boshart M, Zilberstein D (2016) Protein kinase A signaling during bidirectional axenic differentiation in *Leishmania*. Int J Parasitol 46:75–82
17. Saxena A, Lahav T, Holland N, Aggarwal G, Anupama A, Huang Y, Volpin H, Myler PJ, Zilberstein D (2007) Analysis of the *Leishmania donovani* transcriptome reveals an ordered progression of transient and permanent changes in gene expression during differentiation. Mol Biochem Parasitol 152:53–65
18. Mengeling BJ, Zilberstein D, Turco SJ (1997) Biosynthesis of *Leishmania* lipophosphoglycan: solubilization and partial characterization of the initiating mannosylphosphoryltransferase. Glycobiology 7:847–853

Chapter 4

Tsetse Fly Transmission Studies of African Trypanosomes

Lori Peacock and Wendy Gibson

Abstract

African trypanosomes are naturally transmitted by bloodsucking tsetse flies in sub-Saharan Africa and these transmission cycles can be reproduced in the laboratory if clean tsetse flies and suitable trypanosomes are available for experiments. Tsetse transmission gives access to more trypanosome developmental stages than are available from in vitro culture, albeit in very small numbers; for example, the sexual stages of *Trypanosoma brucei* have been isolated from infected tsetse salivary glands, but have not yet been reported from culture. Tsetse transmission also allows for the natural transition between different developmental stages to be studied.

Both wild-type and genetically modified trypanosomes have been successfully fly transmitted, and it is possible to manipulate the trypanosome environment inside the fly to some extent, for example, the induction of expression of genes controlled by the Tet repressor by feeding flies with tetracycline.

Key words Tsetse, *Glossina*, *Trypanosoma brucei*, *Trypanosoma congolense*, Salivary glands, Proventriculus, Cibarium, Proboscis

1 Introduction

African trypanosomes such as *Trypanosoma brucei* and *T. congolense* are naturally transmitted by bloodsucking tsetse flies (genus *Glossina*) in sub-Saharan Africa. Inside the insect, trypanosomes undergo complex cycles of development, involving repeated rounds of differentiation and proliferation. For example, when a fly imbibes a bloodmeal containing *T. brucei* or *T. congolense*, the parasites first differentiate from bloodstream forms (BSF) to procyclics and then proliferate within the bloodmeal; note that although BSF and procyclics are both trypomastigotes by morphology (kinetoplast posterior to the nucleus), they differ markedly in metabolism and surface molecules. Midgut procyclics subsequently cross the peritrophic matrix (PM), the thin sheath enclosing the bloodmeal, and

Electronic supplementary material: The online version of this chapter (https://doi.org/10.1007/978-1-0716-0294-2_4) contains supplementary material, which is available to authorized users.

Paul A. M. Michels et al. (eds.), *Trypanosomatids: Methods and Protocols*, Methods in Molecular Biology, vol. 2116, https://doi.org/10.1007/978-1-0716-0294-2_4, © Springer Science+Business Media, LLC, part of Springer Nature 2020

invade the ectoperitrophic space before migrating anteriorly to the proventriculus, the valve that separates the midgut from the foregut; proventricular forms (long trypomastigotes) re-cross the PM and migrate via the foregut to the mouthparts of the fly. For *T. congolense*, proventricular forms attach to the walls of the proboscis and the cibarium, a widening of the alimentary tract in the head that acts as a pump [1–4]. Here they proliferate as epimastigotes (kinetoplast anterior to the nucleus) and eventually invade the hypopharynx, the narrow tube that delivers saliva to the tip of the proboscis, where they differentiate into infective metacyclics; morphologically the metacyclics are trypomastigotes and, like BSF, now have a variant surface glycoprotein (VSG) coat. In contrast, proventricular forms of *T. brucei* undergo an asymmetric division en route to the mouthparts and the short epimastigotes that are produced go on to colonize the salivary glands and subsequently differentiate into metacyclics [5–7]. For both species, the final differentiation step is to infective metacyclics that cease proliferation until they are inoculated via the saliva into a new animal when the fly next takes a bloodmeal. In *T. brucei* sexual reproduction, involving a meiotic division and the production of haploid gametes, takes place in the salivary glands [8–10], and likewise *T. congolense* hybrids are formed in the fly mouthparts [11].

We routinely use the methods described below for investigations of life cycle stages and transmission dynamics of *T. brucei* and *T. congolense* (savannah subgroup). The methods are also applicable to transmission experiments on other African trypanosomes that develop in the fly gut such as *T. simiae*, *T. godfreyi*, and *T. grayi*, as infections are initiated and flies dissected in the same way. For *T. vivax* transmission, tsetse infection is by bloodstream forms and the relevant fly organs for examination are the cibarium and proboscis.

Our general methods for maintaining tsetse flies in the lab are derived from procedures developed by the Bristol Tsetse Research Laboratory for maintaining tsetse flies by in vitro feeding [12] and are not described in detail here.

2 Materials

Solutions are made up in distilled water, unless stated otherwise.

2.1 Tsetse Infection

1. Tsetse flies (*see* **Note 1**).
2. Trypanosomes—procyclic cultures of *T. brucei* or *T. congolense* (*see* **Note 2**).
3. Sterile defibrinated horse blood. Aliquot aseptically and store at 4 °C for up to 3 weeks.

4. Hanks Balanced Salt Solution (HBSS) with $CaCl_2$, $MgCl_2$ and phenol red. Store at 4 °C.
5. Washed horse red blood cells resuspended in HBSS. To prepare, centrifuge 50 mL whole defibrinated horse blood at 3000 × *g* for 10 min at 4 °C. Remove serum and resuspend cells in HBSS and centrifuge again. Remove the supernatant and repeat this wash step. Finally resuspend the cells in HBSS to make up to 50 mL. Store at 4 °C until use; OK for a month.
6. ATP, 100 mM stock solution. Aliquot and store frozen at −20 °C (*see* **Note 3**).
7. L-Glutathione, 500 mM stock solution. Store frozen at −20 °C (*see* **Note 4**).
8. Tsetse feeding plates—plastic or metal trays covered by silicone rubber membranes.
9. Heating plate at 37 °C.
10. Household bleach for disinfection.

2.2 Tsetse Dissection

1. Glass petri dish with lid.
2. Ice bucket.
3. Waste pot containing 70% ethanol.
4. 70% ethanol spray for disinfection.
5. Paper towels.
6. Phosphate buffered saline (PBS) pH 8.
7. Microscope slides and coverslips (18 × 18 or 22 × 22 mm).
8. Fine forceps (watchmaker's forceps), 2 pairs with straight and curved tips.
9. Dissecting microscope.
10. Compound microscope, phase contrast.

2.3 Isolation of Trypanosomes

1. Cunningham's medium (*see* **Note 5**).
2. Anticontamination cocktail, ACC [13]. For 100× stock: 6 mg/mL penicillin G sodium salt, 10 mg/mL kanamycin sulfate, 5 mg/mL flucytosine (5-fluorocytosine), 1% v/v chloramphenicol (100 mg/mL stock in ethanol). Store at 4 °C for a month; long-term storage at −20 °C (*see* **Note 6**).
3. Phosphate buffered saline (PBS) pH 8 with 20% v/v fetal calf serum (FCS).
4. 24-Well tissue culture plates with flat bottom wells.
5. 96-Well tissue culture plates with flat bottom wells.
6. T25 tissue culture flasks.
7. 1.5 mL microcentrifuge tubes.

8. Round coverslips (10–13 mm diameter), sterile.
9. Incubator 28 °C.
10. Inverted microscope.

2.4 Tsetse Salivary Exudate Sampling

1. Microscope slides.
2. 70% ethanol.
3. Coplin jar.
4. Phosphate buffered saline (PBS) pH 8.

3 Methods

3.1 Infecting Tsetse with Trypanosomes

Tsetse flies may be obtained as pupae from a laboratory-maintained colony (*see* **Note 1**). The pupae are kept on sand at 25 °C and 70% relative humidity until the flies emerge, typically around 30 days after larval deposition.

1. Prepare flies the day before infection (*see* **Note 7**). Cold anesthetize the flies by placing them in a chiller at just below 4 °C to immobilize them; sort into males and females (Fig. 1a) and de-wing as a safety precaution to prevent escape; each fly has one wing removed at the base with sharp scissors. Place the prepared flies in escape-proof cages; the number per cage varies with tsetse species and cage size (*see* **Note 8**). Secure the cage with a cork held firmly in place with flexible tape (electrical insulating tape); the tape should go right round the cage and overlap; fix a second cork opposite the first for handling (Fig. 1b).

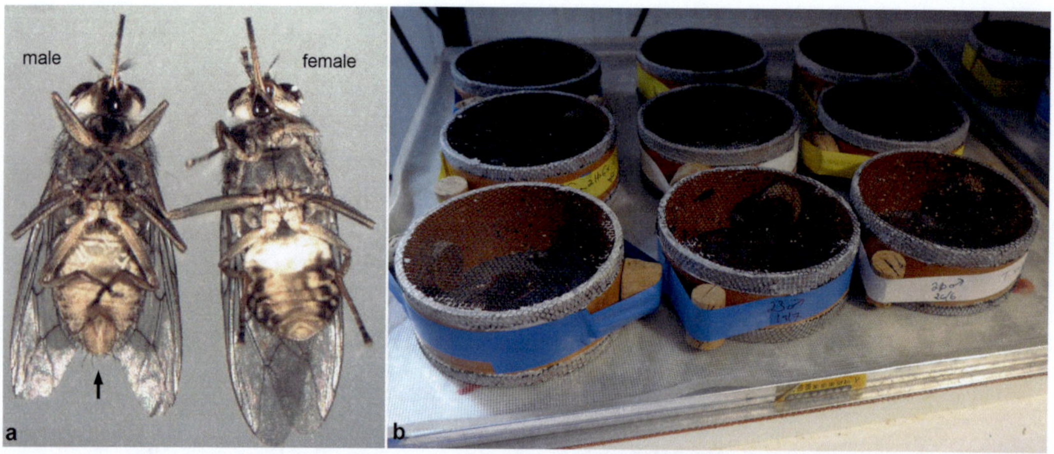

Fig. 1 Tsetse flies. Panel (**a**) shows ventral views of male and female flies, *Glossina morsitans morsitans*. Males are easily distinguished by the prominent hypopygium at the hind end of the abdomen (arrowed). Panel (**b**) shows cages of infected flies feeding on blood underneath a silicone membrane on a heating plate at 37 °C. The cages are secured with tape and are handled using the corks at either side

2. Allow the flies to recover overnight in the insectary. For *Glossina morsitans* and *G. pallidipes*, insectary conditions are 25 °C and 70% relative humidity.
3. Prepare the infective bloodmeal using aseptic conditions in a laminar flow hood. Typically we infect flies with procyclic trypanosomes, but also occasionally use bloodstream form trypanosomes, usually from a cryopreserved stabilate (*see* **Note 9**). Pellet the procyclics from the culture medium by centrifugation at 3000 × *g* for 5–10 min at 4 °C; additionally, wash once in PBS if the medium contains antibiotics such as hygromycin that are potentially harmful to flies. Mix the trypanosome pellet with washed red blood cells in HBSS; allow 10^6–10^7 trypanosomes per mL of blood per cage of flies. Supplement with 10 mM L-glutathione (20 μL of 0.5 M stock solution per mL of blood, *see* **Note 4**).
4. Label the cage of prepared flies with date and details of infective feed. Spread the infective bloodmeal under a sterile silicone rubber membrane on a ribbed acrylic plastic tray and allow flies to feed for up to 30 min; hungry flies start to feed immediately, so check whether all flies have fed—indicated by red abdomen filled with blood—every 5 min or so. Once all flies have fed, transfer cage to a tray lined with paper towel to absorb fly excreta.
5. Immerse the used feeding membrane and tray in a solution of 0.1% (1:1000 dilution) household bleach to disinfect and rinse well in several changes of tap water to remove all traces of bleach. Heat-sterilize the feeding membrane and tray (12 h at 100 °C).
6. To allow flies time to digest the infective feed, start routine feeding a day or two later. Feed the flies on sterile defibrinated horse blood, supplemented with 1 mM ATP (10 μL of 100 mM stock solution per mL of blood, *see* **Note 3**) four or five times a week until dissection. During this period the cages must never be opened.

3.2 Dissection of Infected Tsetse

3.2.1 Examining the Gut and Salivary Glands

This dissection is shown in Movie S1 and Fig. 2 shows the critical steps. We prefer to work without gloves, unless dissecting flies containing human infective trypanosomes. Have a 70% alcohol spray bottle and paper towels at the ready to disinfect forceps between flies, and use a waste pot containing 70% alcohol for fly debris.

1. Use a glass petri dish with a lid to hold the flies securely before dissection. Cool the petri dish on ice while you cold anesthetize the flies to be dissected.
2. Place the whole cage of flies in a −20 °C freezer for a couple of minutes, just until the flies are no longer able to move; do not

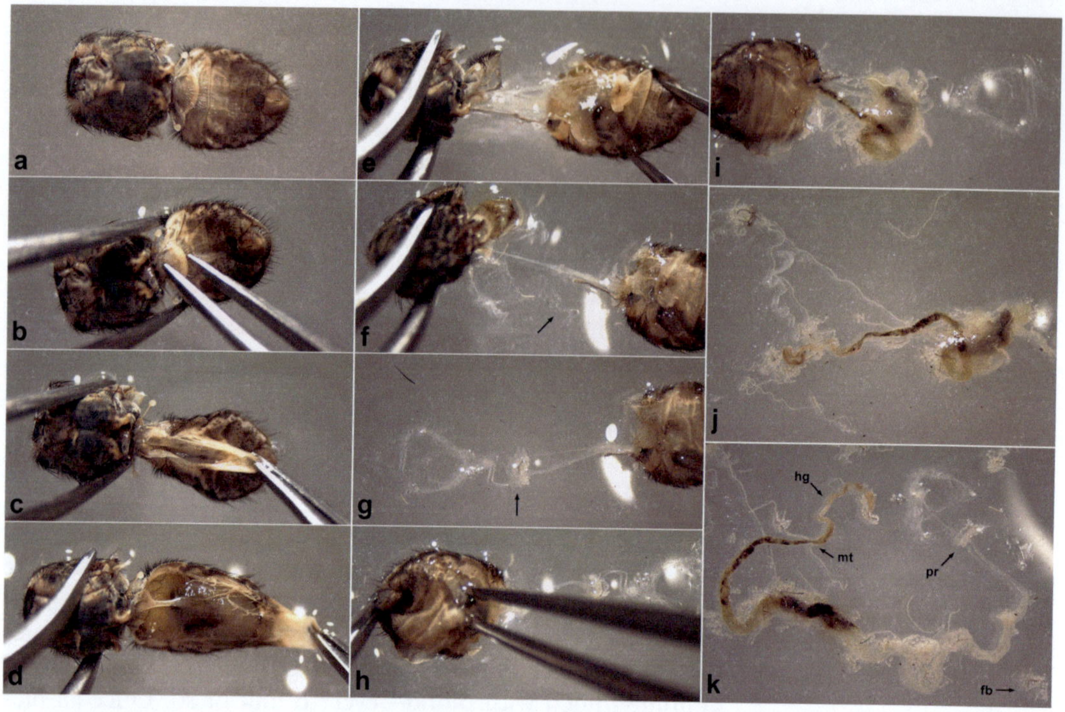

Fig. 2 Dissection of the tsetse gut and salivary glands. Sequential steps during dissection of the midgut and salivary glands of *Glossina pallidipes* (**a**–**k**). Movie S1 shows the whole sequence. In panel (**a**) the head, wings, and legs have been removed and the fly is ready for dissection; this is the ventral view of a male fly. In panel (**f**) one of the salivary glands is clearly seen (arrowed). In panel (**g**) the proventriculus (arrowed) is still attached to the foregut and crop on the left and the anterior midgut on the right. In panel (**k**) the whole gut is spread out, with the hindgut (hg, arrowed) on the left and the anterior organs on the right. The Malpighian tubules (mt, arrowed) arise at the junction of the midgut and hindgut. The proventriculus (pr, arrowed) is attached to the anterior end of the midgut; the membranous structure above it is the collapsed crop. The remains of a previous bloodmeal (dark brown matter) are in the posterior midgut and hindgut, while most of the midgut is empty. Small bobbles of fat body (fb, arrowed) can be seen, some still surrounding the gut

let them freeze! Quickly open the cage and shake the flies out into the petri dish on ice and cover immediately with the lid to prevent escape. Flies will remain immobile for an hour or so until dissected.

3. Dissect the flies one at a time as follows, using sterile PBS and forceps disinfected with 70% alcohol between flies.
4. Place the fly on a paper towel and remove the head with a scalpel. Keep the head if you want to dissect the proboscis or cibarium (*see* Subheading 3.2.2); otherwise discard into the waste pot. Pull off the legs and wings, either with your fingers or forceps, and discard.
5. Place the fly on its back in a drop of PBS on a microscope slide under a dissecting microscope (Fig. 2a). While holding the thorax with one pair of forceps, grasp the top segment of the

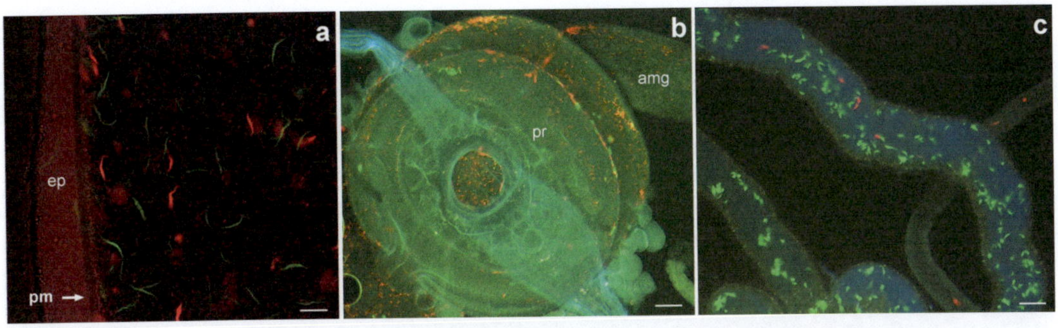

Fig. 3 Trypanosomes in tsetse organs. Green and red fluorescent trypanosomes (*Trypanosoma brucei*) imaged in the midgut (**a**), the proventriculus (**b**), and the salivary glands (**c**). Panel (**a**) shows an early stage of midgut infection when trypanosomes have not yet crossed the peritrophic matrix (pm, arrowed) and invaded the ectoperitrophic space (ep). Scale bar = 25 μm. In panel (**b**) trypanosomes are present in the anterior midgut (amg, top right) and the proventriculus (pr); the membranous tubes over the proventriculus are the foregut and the duct to the crop. Scale bar = 100 μm. Panel (**c**) shows several sections of the same salivary gland; this is an early infection and the density of trypanosomes is low, particularly in the narrower portion of the gland. Scale bar = 50 μm

abdomen (a triangular flap) with forceps held in the other hand and pull steadily to peel back the ventral wall of the abdomen (Fig. 2b). Keeping hold of the thorax with one pair of forceps, use the other pair of forceps to nick the sides of the abdomen to separate it from the thorax. Then grasp the top of the abdomen and pull steadily to expose the anterior part of the midgut and the paired salivary glands (Fig. 2c–f). Make sure to keep these organs immersed in PBS as they dry out quickly.

6. If the salivary glands are required, pick them up with forceps and transfer to another drop of PBS to minimize contamination with midgut contents; if the salivary glands are not visible, they can sometimes be retrieved by probing the thorax or abdomen with forceps. Cover with a coverslip and view using a compound microscope (200–400×); *see* Fig. 3c.
7. Still holding the thorax, grasp the anterior midgut and pull gently until the proventriculus pops out of the thorax (Fig. 2g); if the midgut breaks, the proventriculus can sometimes be retrieved by probing the thorax cavity with forceps.
8. Discard the thorax and turn the abdomen around. Holding the tip of the abdomen with one pair of forceps, grasp the gut with the other pair of forceps and pull steadily to remove the whole gut from the abdomen, keeping the gut immersed in PBS (Fig. 2h, i).
9. Discard the abdomen, severing any remaining connection to the hindgut. Keeping the gut immersed in PBS, tease out the midgut, hindgut, and proventriculus, without rupturing the gut (Fig. 2j, k). The proventriculus can be severed and transferred to another drop of PBS if required. Similarly, different

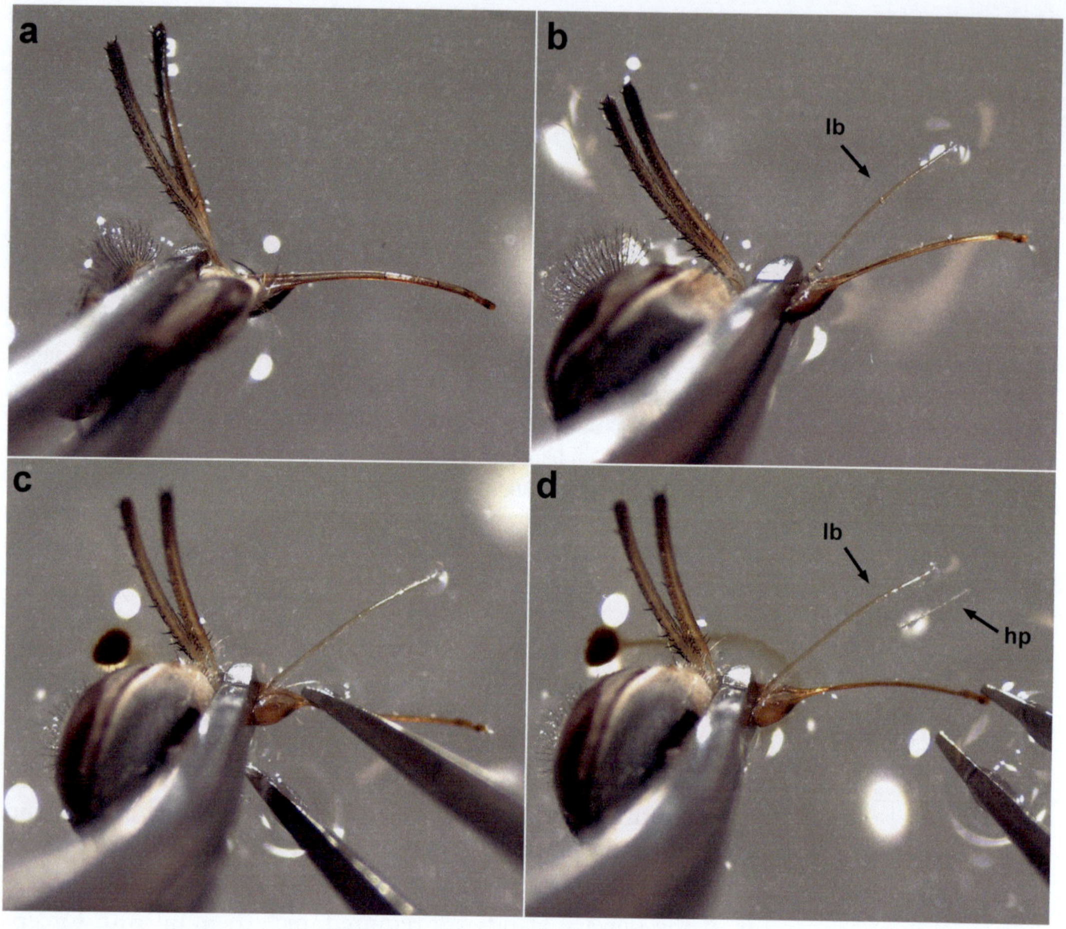

Fig. 4 Dissection of the tsetse proboscis. Sequential steps during dissection of the proboscis of *Glossina pallidipes* (**a–d**). Movie S2 shows the whole sequence. In panel (**a**) the intact proboscis is horizontal, while the palps, that normally protect the proboscis except during feeding, are vertical. Squeezing the bulb of the proboscis springs the labrum (lb, arrowed) apart from the labium (**b**). In panel (**c**) the hypopharynx is gently released from the labial groove with the tip of the forceps, revealing the three separate parts of the proboscis (**d**): labrum (lb), hypopharynx (hp), and the darkly pigmented labium with the bulb at the proximal end

parts of the gut can be isolated into separate drops of PBS. Cover specimens with a coverslip and view using a compound microscope (200–400×); *see* Fig. 3a, b, gut and proventriculus.

10. Freeze any remaining flies to kill them before discarding as waste. To make absolutely sure the flies are dead, cut the heads off before freezing.

3.2.2 Examining the Proboscis and Cibarium

These dissections are shown in Movies S2 and S3, and Figs. 4 and 6 show the critical steps.

1. To examine the proboscis and cibarium for trypanosome infection, proceed as **steps 1–4** in Subheading 3.2.1.

2. Place the head in a drop of PBS on a microscope slide. Grasp the head with one pair of forceps and spring the proboscis into its component parts (labrum and labium) by squeezing the bulb of the proboscis with forceps (Fig. 4b and Movie S2). If the labrum does not immediately spring apart, insert the tip of one arm of the forceps between the labrum and labium close to the bulb and slide towards the tip of the proboscis.
3. Use the same technique to remove the hypopharynx from the groove within the labium (Fig. 4c). Keep the specimen immersed in PBS.
4. Grip the proboscis at the bulb to remove from the head; discard this into the waste pot unless you intend to dissect the cibarium. Check that the component parts of the proboscis remain separate; if not, gently tease apart again with forceps before covering with a coverslip. View under a compound microscope (200–400×); *see* Fig. 5 (*see* **Note 10**).
5. To remove the cibarium, holding the head firmly with one set of forceps, dislodge the dark-colored plate at the back of the head, where it was joined onto the thorax, and grasp the cibarium with forceps to remove it (Fig. 6 and Movie S3). Flatten the cibarium under a coverslip and view using a compound microscope (200–400×); *see* Movie S4 (*see* **Note 11**). Discard the head into the waste pot.

3.3 Isolation of Trypanosomes

3.3.1 Isolating Trypanosomes from the Midgut

1. To procyclic growth medium (*see* **Note 5**), add 5× anticontamination cocktail (ACC, [13]) (*see* **Note 6**). Pipet 100 μL wells of this medium into a 96-well tissue culture plate with flat bottom wells—set up sufficient wells for the number of flies to be dissected.
2. Follow **steps 1–9** of Subheading 3.2.1, but do not place a coverslip over the midgut. Using forceps, quickly transfer each midgut to one well of medium in the 96-well plate; keep the plate in the laminar flow hood, or keep covered with its lid as much as possible if working on the open bench. Continue until all flies have been dissected.
3. View the plate under an inverted microscope and mark the wells that contain trypanosomes. Incubate the plate overnight at 28 °C in a humid box to minimize evaporation.
4. Examine the plate the following day and check for growth of trypanosomes in all wells—some wells containing trypanosomes may not have been noticed immediately after dissection (*see* **Note 12**). Wells with dense populations of trypanosomes and vigorous growth need to be subpassaged by transferring 50 μL from the original to a new well containing 50 μL of fresh medium (procyclic growth medium with 5× anticontamination

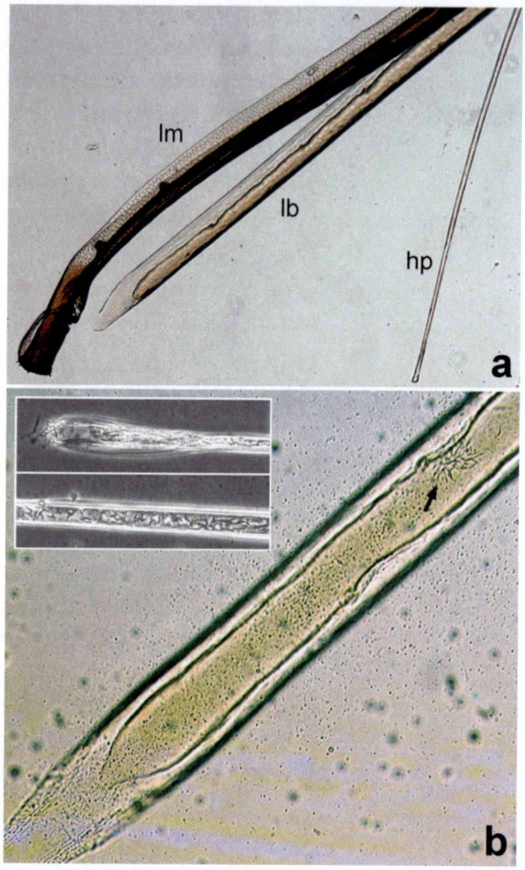

Fig. 5 Component parts of the tsetse proboscis. In panel (**a**) the three parts of the proboscis have been split apart: labium (lm), labrum (lb), and hypopharynx (hp). Panel (**b**) shows a higher power phase contrast image of the labrum with a cluster of attached *Trypanosoma congolense* epimastigotes (arrowed). The inset shows two sections of a hypopharynx infected with *T. congolense*; the upper panel shows the distal tip of the hypopharynx with a single trypanosome at the tip and others visible within; the infection is denser in the lower panel with a mixture of long and short trypanosomes, probably metacyclics

cocktail as in **step 1**); avoid carryover of gut tissue into the new well. Replace 50 μL of medium in the original well to maintain growth.

5. Continue to monitor growth and subpassage as necessary to obtain a dense culture free of bacterial and fungal contamination. The volume of medium can be expanded as the trypanosomes proliferate, subculturing first to 1 mL wells of medium in a 24-well tissue culture plate, and subsequently to 5 mL of medium in a T25 tissue culture flask. The ACC can be omitted once the culture is free from contamination. Pure cultures of procyclic trypanosomes may be cryopreserved for long-term storage.

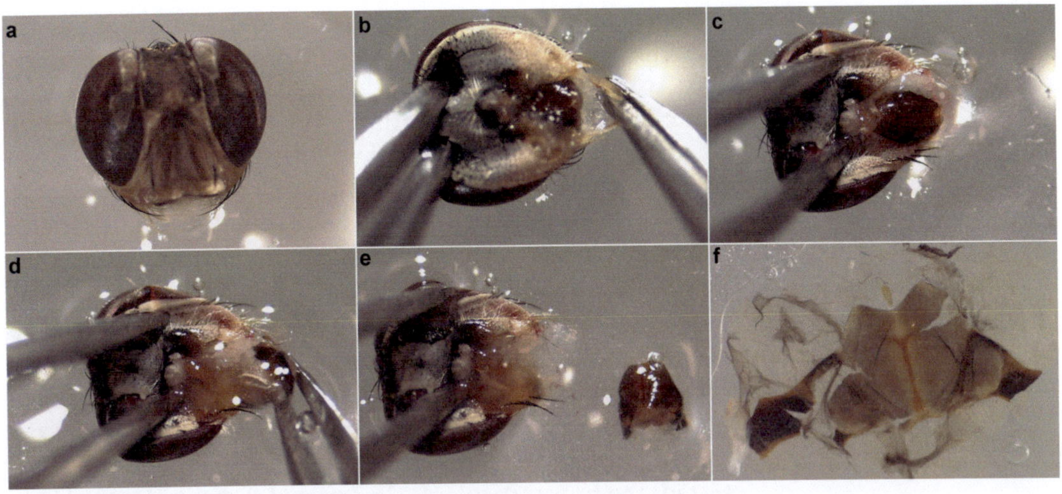

Fig. 6 Dissection of the tsetse cibarium. Sequential steps during dissection of the cibarium of *Glossina pallidipes* (**a**–**f**). Movie S3 shows the whole sequence. The head, seen in front view (**a**), is turned over for dissection (**b**). The dark-colored plate protecting the cibarium is first exposed (**c**) and then removed (**d**, **e**). The characteristic Y-shaped feature of the internal cibarium is seen in this enlarged view (**f**)

3.3.2 Isolating Trypanosomes from the Salivary Glands

We use this method for the recovery of unattached trypanosomes (including metacyclics, meiotic dividers, and gametes) from pooled salivary glands (e.g., characterization of gametes of *T. brucei*) [10].

1. Using aseptic technique, pipet 30 μL of CM into a 1.5 mL microcentrifuge tube. This is sufficient for around 10 pairs of salivary glands.
2. Follow **steps 1–5** of Subheading 3.2.1. Using forceps, quickly transfer both salivary glands to the tube by immersing the tips of the forceps in the culture medium; if the glands remain stuck to the forceps, wiggle the forceps in the medium until they are dislodged. Continue until all flies have been dissected.
3. Tap the tube gently to mix and leave on the bench at room temperature for about 10 min to allow the trypanosomes to emerge into the medium.
4. Tap the tube gently to mix and, avoiding the salivary glands, remove a small aliquot of medium (~3 μL) to a microscope slide to check the density and life cycle stage(s) present (*see* **Note 13**).
5. The trypanosome suspension can then be used for experiments, either on living or fixed trypanosomes.

3.3.3 Isolating Trypanosomes from the Proventriculus

We use this method for the recovery of proventricular trypanosomes of *T. congolense*, (e.g., analysis of development of proventricular forms in vitro) [14].

1. Using aseptic technique, prepare ~5 mL procyclic growth medium (*see* **Note 5**) containing 1× anticontamination cocktail (ACC, [13]) (*see* **Note 6**). Pipet 30 μL of this medium into a sterile 1.5 mL microcentrifuge tube and set up a 24-well tissue culture plate with the same medium as follows: pipet 500 μL medium into five 1 mL wells and place a sterile, round (10–13 mm diameter) glass coverslip in each well with sterile forceps, so that it lies flat on the bottom of the well; gently tap with forceps if necessary.
2. Follow **steps 1–7** of Subheading 2.3, **step 1**. Using a needle or a forceps, cut the proventriculus from the adjoining foregut and midgut as close as possible to the proventriculus, and quickly transfer each proventriculus to the medium in the microcentrifuge tube. Continue until all flies have been dissected; the proventriculi of ~15 infected flies may be pooled in the same tube.
3. Tap the tube gently to mix and leave on the bench at RT for 10 min to allow the proventricular trypanosomes to emerge into the medium.
4. Tap the tube gently to mix and remove a small aliquot of medium (~3 μL) to a microscope slide to check the density; the trypanosome density will depend on how many flies had an infected proventriculus (*see* **Note 14**).
5. In the laminar flow hood, tap the tube to mix and pipet 5 μL of the trypanosome suspension into each well containing a coverslip. This volume may need to be adjusted depending on the density of trypanosomes observed in **step 4** (*see* **Note 14**).
6. Inspect each well using an inverted microscope focused on the upper surface of the coverslip. Several attached trypanosomes should be visible in each field.
7. Incubate the plate at 28 °C overnight in a humid box to minimize evaporation.
8. The following day, remove most of the medium (~450 μL) and replace with PBS containing 20% v/v FCS (*see* **Note 15**). By this time, trypanosomes will have shortened and started to proliferate. Incubate as before.
9. In a few days, small rosettes of dividing epimastigotes should be seen, attached to the glass coverslip. Trypanosomes can be harvested at any time point during incubation by removing the coverslip, along with the attached cells, with sterile forceps.

3.3.4 Isolating Trypanosomes from the Foregut Via Salivary Exudate

This method was originally described by Burtt [15] to identify infected tsetse and we use it to obtain foregut developmental stages of *T. brucei* or *T. congolense* [4, 16]. The salivary exudate is produced as hungry flies probe a glass microscope slide with the proboscis and is a mixture of saliva and fluid regurgitated from the foregut.

1. Cage flies individually in plastic universal bottles closed with netting (*see* **Note 16**). Infect with trypanosomes as described in Subheading 3.1. Do not feed for ~48 h prior to the experiment, so the flies are hungry.
2. Clean glass microscope slides before use with 70% ethanol and tissues. Use a permanent marker to draw two circles the size of the bottle cap on each slide. Place the slides on a 37 °C heating plate and invert two individual bottles on the circles on each slide, so that flies can probe through the netting onto the slide (Fig. 7). The circles help to locate where the flies have deposited saliva on the slide.
3. Leave flies to probe for a maximum of 30 min, checking progress periodically. Once a fly has probed, remove the cage; stop flies resting on the sides of the cage by tapping the bottle to encourage them to move to the bottom. When all flies have probed, transfer the cages to a feeding membrane and give them a blood feed.
4. This cycle of starvation, probing and feeding can be repeated to provide saliva samples for as long as required.
5. The salivary exudate dries almost immediately it is deposited on the warmed slide. Check for the presence of trypanosomes under phase contrast (100–200× magnification) and fix and stain slides as required; *see* Fig. 8.
6. For viewing fluorescent trypanosomes (e.g., GFP), rehydrate slides in PBS in a Coplin jar for ~20 min. Remove slides and fix with 2% PFA for 20 min, followed by three PBS washes to remove the PFA. Add mounting medium with DAPI and view using a fluorescence microscope (200–400×).

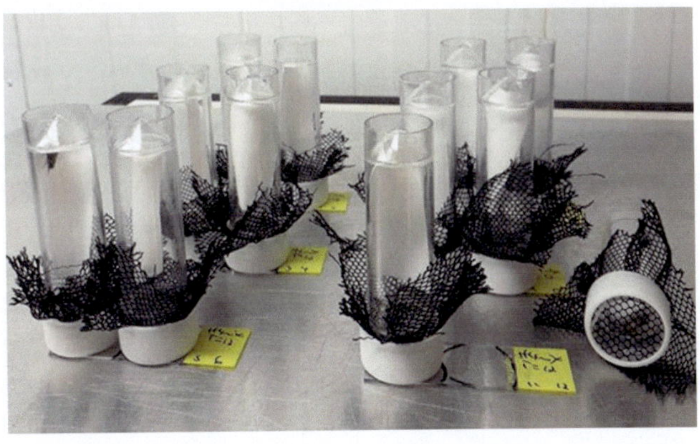

Fig. 7 Collection of tsetse saliva samples. Tsetse flies held in individual cages are allowed to probe through the netting onto glass microscope slides on a heating plate at 37 °C. The cage on the right is lying horizontally to show how the top opening is closed with netting

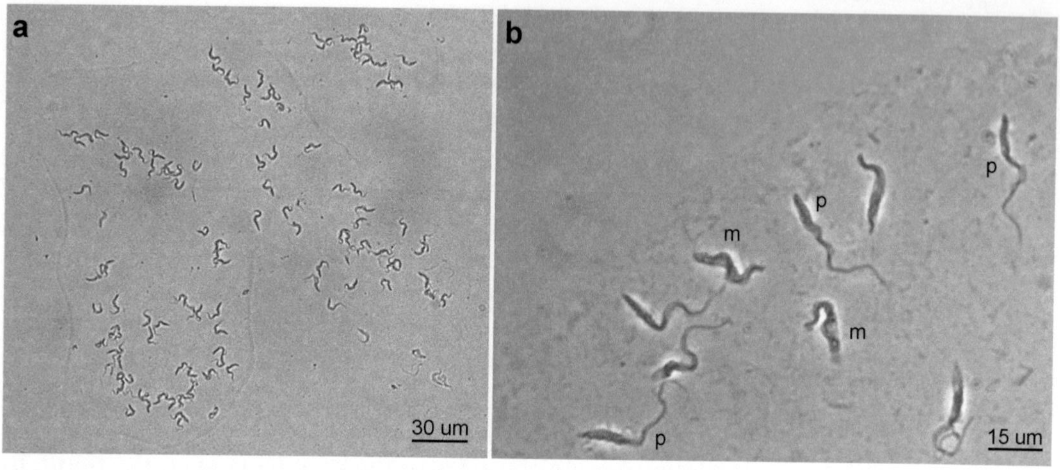

Fig. 8 Trypanosomes in samples of tsetse salivary exudate. Phase contrast images. In panel (**a**) the majority of trypanosomes (*Trypanosoma brucei*) are metacyclics, while in panel (**b**) different developmental stages of *T. congolense* are present including long proventricular forms (p) and shorter metacyclics (m)

4 Notes

1. At the time of writing, there are a handful of laboratories worldwide that maintain colonies of tsetse flies, but most are willing to supply small numbers of pupae either free or for a small charge. Several colony-reared tsetse species are available, but subspecies of *Glossina morsitans* are commonly used for experimental infection with *Trypanosoma brucei* or *T. congolense*. We keep tsetse (*G. m. morsitans* and *G. pallidipes*) in a secure insectary at 25 °C and 70% relative humidity. Experimental tsetse flies infected with pathogenic trypanosomes are a potential safety hazard and in the UK our experiments are regulated and licensed by the Health and Safety Executive (HSE) of the UK government, as well as being subject to local safety rules.
2. Pathogenic trypanosomes such as *Trypanosoma brucei* and *T. congolense* pose a safety hazard and are classified as Category 2 pathogens by the UK Advisory Committee on Dangerous Pathogens (ACDP) and Specified Animal Pathogens Order (SAPO), which both come under HSE. Our experiments are regulated and licensed by these authorities, as well as being subject to local safety rules.
3. The addition of 1 mM ATP to the bloodmeal stimulates feeding [17] and we routinely add it to the blood just before feeding.

4. The antioxidant L-glutathione significantly increases midgut infection rates by neutralizing oxygen radicals [18]. In the past we have also used the lectin-inhibitory sugars D-glucosamine and *N*-acetyl glucosamine to enhance midgut infection rates [19], but now we solely use L-glutathione.
5. We routinely use a modified version of Cunningham's medium (CM, [20]) to grow procyclics of *T. brucei*, *T. congolense*, and related trypanosomes. The recipe is given below.
   (a) *Cunningham's Medium (CM).*

   For 1 L of medium, combine the 5 solutions listed below and add 0.2× BME vitamin mixture (2 mL of 100× stock) and phenol red (10 mg/L). Adjust the pH to 7.5 using 5 M NaOH and then make up to 1 L with distilled water. Aliquot the medium into 100 mL Duran bottles and store frozen at −20 °C for up to ~1 month. To use, thaw in a 37 °C water bath, swirling the liquid occasionally to dissolve any precipitate. Add 0.2× hemin (100× stock: 2.5 mg/mL hemin dissolved in 50 mM NaOH), gentamycin (0.01 mg/mL) and 15% v/v heat-inactivated fetal calf serum and filter sterilize using a 0.2 μm syringe filter. Store at 4 °C for up to 2 weeks.

   (b) Salts 100 mL.

   4.42 mM NaH_2PO_4.

   14.95 mM $MgCl_2$.

   15.01 mM $MgSO_4$.

   40.00 mM KCl.

   (c) $CaCl_2$ 50 mL.

   1.02 mM $CaCl_2$.

   (d) Sugars 100 mL.

   3.89 mM glucose.

   2.22 mM fructose.

   1.17 mM sucrose.

   (e) TCA intermediates 50 mL.

   5.00 mM L-malic acid.

   2.53 mM α-ketoglutaric acid.

   0.47 mM fumaric acid.

   0.51 mM succinic acid.

   (f) Amino acids 600 mL.

   6.12 mM L-alanine.

   22.47 mM beta-alanine.

   2.53 mM L-arginine.

1.82 mM L-asparagine.

0.83 mM L-aspartic acid.

0.57 mM L-cysteine.

0.13 mM L-cystine.

1.70 mM L-glutamic acid.

11.23 mM L-glutamine.

1.60 mM L-glycine.

1.03 mM L-histidine.

0.69 mM L-isoleucine.

0.69 mM L-leucine.

1.03 mM L-lysine.

1.34 mM L-methionine.

1.21 mM L-phenylalanine.

60.00 mM L-proline.

1.90 mM L-serine.

0.84 mM L-threonine.

0.49 mM L-tryptophan.

1.10 mM L-tyrosine.

1.79 mM L-valine.

20.00 mM HEPES.

6. Bacterial and/or fungal contamination of tsetse-derived tissues is often unavoidable, so we routinely add anticontamination cocktail—a mixture of three antibiotics and an antifungal [13]—to the medium and maintain this concentration as the culture is expanded. However, even this cocktail sometimes fails to prevent microbial overgrowth, so we routinely set up replicate cultures from individual tsetse midguts and select the least contaminated. Fortunately, cultures derived from other tissues, such as the proventriculus, are less prone to contamination. The concentration of ACC can be reduced to 1× and finally omitted once the culture is free of contamination.
7. Flies can be starved longer before infection if needed (e.g., 48–72 h). Flies become refractory to trypanosome infection (*T. brucei*, *T. congolense*) after their first bloodmeal, so best to use newly emerged flies (tenerals) for infection. This rule does not apply to *T. vivax* though, as this species develops in the proboscis and cibarium, and not in the midgut. The immune system of the fly ramps up after the first bloodmeal, making the midgut very inhospitable for trypanosomes.
8. Cages are made of ~4.5 cm sections of plastic drainage pipe 10 cm internal diameter, with a single 2.5 cm hole drilled in the

side, which is secured with a cork (Fig. 1b). The cut section of pipe is covered on both sides with black nylon netting (~2 mm hole diameter) secured with plastic weld glue. Typically we put single-sex groups of 15–20 flies (*G. pallidipes*) or 25–30 flies (*G. m. morsitans*) per cage. Cages for individual flies are described in **Note 16**.

9. If bloodstream form (BSF) trypanosomes are used for infection, whole blood can be used instead of washed red blood cells; the serum is removed to protect procyclic trypanosomes from complement lysis. It is convenient to use a single batch of cryopreserved aliquots of BSF trypanosomes for consistency of infection; we typically infect with ~10^6 to 10^7 BSF trypanosomes per mL of bloodmeal. If flies are to be dissected less than 3 days after infection, the red blood cells in the feed will obscure observation, so fetal calf serum, culture medium or HBSS can be used in place of blood.

10. Typically, the highest densities of trypanosomes are found in the labrum closest to the bulb, though they may be scattered throughout [4, 21]. The dark pigment of the bulb and labium tends to obscure any trypanosomes present.

11. Trypanosomes in the cibarium tend to be concentrated around the arms of the distinctive Y-shaped structure [4] (Movie S4). The same methods for dissecting the proboscis and cibarium will work for flies infected with other trypanosomes of subgenus *Nannomonas* and *T. vivax.*

12. 10^5 to 10^6 trypanosomes of *T. brucei* or *T. congolense* may be found in a single infected midgut, so starting density of midgut cultures can be quite high.

13. The life cycle stages recovered by this method are those that are not firmly attached to the salivary gland epithelium. After the glands are removed, saliva continues to be forced out of the broken ends by peristaltic action for some minutes, carrying unattached trypanosomes with it. The number of trypanosomes present and the life cycle stages present depend on the length of infection: colonization of the glands starts about 14 days after flies take the infective bloodfeed; around 21 days there are many meiotic dividers and gametes but relatively few metacyclics [10], whereas later metacyclics predominate.

14. The number of proventricular trypanosomes recovered depends on the percentage of infected proventriculi and the number of trypanosomes per proventriculus, which varies from a few hundred to several thousands. An ideal seeding density is >30 attached trypanosomes per field of view. Examining an aliquot of the suspension before dispensing into the 24-well

plate gives a good guide to the amount to be seeded into each well.

15. In our first attempts to initiate epimastigote cultures from proventricular trypanosomes, we found that trypanosomes ceased proliferating and died after a few days if left in growth medium, whereas diluting the medium tenfold with PBS with 20% v/v FCS prolonged survival; replacing the medium after 24 h had the added advantage of reducing microbial contamination.
16. Individual cages are made using clear plastic universals, with the center of the screw cap drilled out. The top of the bottle is covered with black nylon netting (~2 mm hole diameter) held in place by the drilled-out screw cap (Fig. 7). These cages can be used to house single flies or 2–3 individuals. Inserting a length of filter paper provides the flies with a rough surface to rest on, other than the netting.

Acknowledgments

We acknowledge current support from the UK Biotechnology and Biological Sciences Research Council (BBSRC) for our work on tsetse–trypanosome interactions. We are ever grateful to the staff who run the tsetse colonies at the International Atomic Energy Agency in Vienna for their generous supply of tsetse pupae, and thank the many colleagues who have developed and shared the methods compiled in this chapter. We are indebted to Chris Kay and Sue Holwell for guidance and assistance on the video microscopy.

References

1. Buxton PA (1955) The natural history of tsetse flies. Memoir 10 London School of hygiene and tropical medicine. HK Lewis, London
2. Hoare CA (1972) The trypanosomes of mammals. Blackwell Scientific Publications Oxford, Hoboken, New Jersey
3. Jefferies D, Helfrich MP, Molyneux DH (1987) Cibarial infections of Trypanosoma vivax and T. congolense in Glossina. Parasitol Res 73:289–292
4. Peacock L, Cook S, Ferris V, Bailey M, Gibson W (2012) The life cycle of Trypanosoma (Nannomonas) congolense in the tsetse fly. Parasit Vectors 5:109
5. Sharma R, Peacock L, Gluenz E, Gull K, Gibson W, Carrington M (2008) Asymmetric cell division as a route to reduction in cell length and change in cell morphology in trypanosomes. Protist 159:137–151
6. Van den Abbeele J, Claes Y, Van Bockstaele D, Le Ray D, Coosemans M (1999) Trypanosoma brucei spp. development in the tsetse fly: characterization of the post-mesocyclic stages in the foregut and proboscis. Parasitology 118:469–478
7. Lewis EA, Langridge WP (1947) Developmental forms of Trypanosoma brucei in the "saliva" of Glossina pallidipes and *G. austeni*. Ann Trop Med Parasitol 41:6–13
8. Gibson W, Peacock L, Ferris V, Williams K, Bailey M (2008) The use of yellow fluorescent hybrids to indicate mating in Trypanosoma brucei. Parasit Vectors 1:4
9. Peacock L, Ferris V, Sharma R, Sunter J, Bailey M, Carrington M, Gibson W (2011) Identification of the meiotic life cycle stage of Trypanosoma brucei in the tsetse fly. Proc Natl Acad Sci U S A 108:3671–3676

10. Peacock L, Bailey M, Carrington M, Gibson W (2014) Meiosis and haploid gametes in the pathogen Trypanosoma brucei. Curr Biol 24:1–6
11. Gibson W, Kay C, Peacock L (2017) Trypanosoma congolense: molecular toolkit and resources for studying a major livestock pathogen and model trypanosome. Adv Parasitol 98:283–309
12. Mews AR, Langley PA, Pimley RW, Flood MET (1977) Large-scale rearing of tsetse flies (Glossina spp.) in the absence of a living host. Bull Entomol Res 67:119–128
13. Maser P, Grether-Buhler Y, Kaminsky R, Brun R (2002) An anti-contamination cocktail for the in vitro isolation and cultivation of parasitic protozoa. Parasitol Res 88:172–174
14. Peacock L, Kay C, Bailey M, Gibson W (2018) Shape-shifting trypanosomes: Flagellar shortening followed by asymmetric division in Trypanosoma congolense from the tsetse proventriculus. PLoS Pathog 14:e1007043
15. Burtt E (1946) Salivation by Glossina morsitans onto glass slides: a technique for isolating infected flies. Ann Trop Med Parasitol 40:141–144
16. Peacock L, Ferris V, Bailey M, Gibson W (2007) Dynamics of infection and competition between two strains of Trypanosoma brucei brucei in the tsetse fly observed using fluorescent markers. Kinetoplastid Biol Dis 6:4
17. Galun R, Margalit J (1969) Adenine nucleotides as feeding stimulants of tsetse fly Glossina austeni Newst. Nature 222:583–584
18. Macleod ET, Maudlin I, Darby AC, Welburn SC (2007) Antioxidants promote establishment of trypanosome infections in tsetse. Parasitology 134:827–831
19. Peacock L, Ferris V, Bailey M, Gibson W (2006) Multiple effects of the lectin-inhibitory sugars D-glucosamine and N-acetyl-glucosamine on tsetse-trypanosome interactions. Parasitology 132:651–658
20. Cunningham I (1977) New culture medium for maintenance of tsetse tissues and growth of trypanosomatids. J Protozool 24:325–329
21. Gibson W, Peacock L, Hutchinson R (2017) Microarchitecture of the tsetse fly proboscis. Parasit Vectors 10:430

Chapter 5

Infecting Triatomines with Trypanosomes

Alessandra A. Guarneri

Abstract

The infection of triatomines with trypanosomes can be performed with different forms of the parasite, and the procedure is important not only for vector–parasite interaction studies but also for maintaining the infectivity of parasite strains, which guarantees more realistic biological and molecular investigations. Here, I describe how to infect the vector *Rhodnius prolixus*, a model species, with two different species of *Trypanosoma*.

Key words *Rhodnius prolixus*, *Trypanosoma cruzi*, *Trypanosoma rangeli*, Infection, Artificial feeding

1 Introduction

The study of the interaction between trypanosomes and their invertebrate hosts is an important topic in the area of parasitology, but unfortunately, it has not received the same attention as parasite development in mammalian hosts. Even though several studies have tried to understand the processes involved in the development of trypanosomes inside their vectors, only in the last few years have the molecular mechanisms involved in parasite development begun to be understood [1]. Triatomines (Reduviidae: Triatomine) are hemimetabolous insects whose development includes eggs, five nymphal instars, and adults. The ingestion of blood is obligatory for all developmental phases in the majority of species. In *Rhodnius prolixus*, each nymphal instar needs at least one complete blood meal to molt to the next instar. For this species, the development from egg to adult takes 3–4 months under laboratory conditions. Triatomines can be infected by two species of trypanosomes, *Trypanosoma cruzi* and *Trypanosoma rangeli*. *Trypanosoma cruzi* is the causative agent of Chagas disease and is ingested by triatomines when they blood-feed on infected mammals. This parasite colonizes the intestinal tract of the insect and differentiates into metacyclic trypomastigote forms in the rectum. Parasite transmission by the vector can occur when triatomine feces are deposited onto the

Paul A. M. Michels et al. (eds.), *Trypanosomatids: Methods and Protocols*, Methods in Molecular Biology, vol. 2116, https://doi.org/10.1007/978-1-0716-0294-2_5,

mucous tissues of the vertebrate host, or areas injured by the insect bite; or when the vector is predated by insectivorous mammals, or accidentally ingested by humans. *Trypanosoma rangeli* shares the same hosts as *T. cruzi*, and is also ingested by the vector during a bloodmeal on infected mammals. However, unlike *T. cruzi*, *T. rangeli* is able to cross the intestinal barrier and colonizes the hemolymph and salivary glands, where metacyclogenesis occurs. The latter parasite species is then injected with saliva into the host skin during blood-feeding. As mentioned, for both trypanosome species, the parasite form that first enters in contact with vector tissues is the blood-stage trypomastigote. It has been shown that more than 80% of the *T. cruzi* parasites are killed in the *R. prolixus* anterior midgut during the first 24 h after ingestion [2, 3]. Apparently, only parasites that differentiate into intermediary forms, and reach the posterior midgut, can survive and differentiate into epimastigotes (the multiplicative form) and thus initiate infection in this vector [3]. This information is relevant, as cultured epimastigotes are usually used to start experimental *T. cruzi* infections in *R. prolixus*. This is problematic for studying molecular interactions in the anterior midgut, as in this location epimastigotes are not naturally found. In the case of *T. rangeli*, epimastigogenesis occurs in the anterior midgut, and the parasite is able to colonize all the intestinal portions of the vector [4]. In this chapter, I will describe the methodologies we routinely use to infect *R. prolixus* with *T. cruzi* and *T. rangeli*, using either cultured epimastigotes or blood-stage trypomastigotes.

2 Materials

2.1 Culture Media and Solutions

2.1.1 Liver Infusion Tryptose (LIT) Medium [5]

1. 10% LIB (liver infusion broth): Prepare a 10% solution dissolving the liver infusion broth in distilled water. Aliquot the solution in volumes of 50 mL/flask (screw cap flasks). Autoclave at 121 °C for 20 min. Allow the solution to cool to room temperature. Store protected from light at −20 °C.
2. Hemin solution: Mix 2.5 mL of triethanolamine and 2.5 mL of distilled water in a glass beaker; add 125 mg of hemin, vortexing until it is completely dissolved (20–30 min). Prepare the solution just before the use. Do not store.
3. Salt solution: Measure 1 L of distilled water; warm approximately 900 mL (~30 °C) in a glass beaker; weigh 20 g of NaCl, 2 g of KCl, 40 g of Na_2HPO_4, and 25 g of tryptose and transfer each, one by one, to the beaker, stirring until completely dissolved; then add the hemin solution while continuously stirring the mixture. Adjust the pH to 7.4 with NaOH or H_3PO_4; do not use HCl. Add distilled water to make a final volume of 1 L. Aliquot the solution in volumes of 250 mL/flask (screw cap

flasks). Sterilize by autoclaving at 121 °C for 20 min. Allow the solution to cool to room temperature. Store protected from light at 4 °C.

4. 40% Glucose solution: Prepare the solution by dissolving the glucose in distilled water. Aliquot the solution in volumes of 10 mL/flask (screw cap flasks). Sterilize by autoclaving at 121 °C for 20 min. Allow the solution to cool to room temperature. Store protected from light at −20 °C.
5. Fetal bovine serum (FBS): Allow serum to warm to room temperature for a minimum of 10 min; place the serum into a 56 °C water bath. Gently stir the bottle every 3–5 min to facilitate uniform heating throughout the serum. Remove the heat-inactivated serum after 30 min. Aliquot the solution in volumes of 150 mL/flask (screw cap flasks). Allow the solution to cool to room temperature. Store at −20 °C (*see* **Note 1**).
6. Antibiotics: Prepare a solution of 100 U/mL penicillin G potassium and 100 μg/mL streptomycin sulfate with a final volume of 10 mL (*see* **Note 2**).
7. Preparation of the complete medium: add 50 mL of 10% LIB, 250 mL of salt solution, 10 mL of 40% glucose solution, 150 mL of FBS, and complete to 1 L with distilled water (*see* **Note 3**). Sterilize the mixture by filtration (0.22 μm). Add the antibiotic solution. Separate a 5 mL aliquot and incubate at 37 °C for 24–48 h to test the sterility before use. Store protected from light at 4 °C.

2.1.2 Novy, McNeal, and Nicolle (NNN) Medium

This medium is biphasic and consists of blood agar and LIT medium.

1. Weigh 1.4 g of agar and 0.6 g of NaCl and transfer to a beaker with 85 mL of distilled water. Heat until completely dissolved. Sterilize by autoclaving at 121 °C for 20 min.
2. Allow the agar solution to cool to 45–50 °C and aseptically add 15 mL of defibrinated rabbit or human blood. Mix well and dispense in 5 mL amounts in screw caps tubes. Allow tubes to cool in a slanted position.
3. Add approximately 3 mL of LIT medium over the solidified blood agar. Store protected from light at 4 °C, for no more than 30 days. Warm to room temperature immediately before parasite inoculation.

2.1.3 Hemolymph Anticoagulant Solution [6]

Solution: 0.01 M ethylenediamine tetraacetate (EDTA), 0.1 M glucose, 0.062 M NaCl, 0.03 M trisodium citrate, 0.026 M citric acid. Measure 50 mL of distilled water and transfer approximately 40 mL to a glass beaker. Weigh 0.186 g of EDTA, 0.9 g of glucose, 0.181 g of NaCl, 0.441 g of trisodium citrate, and 0.273 g of citric acid, and transfer one by one to the beaker, stirring until completely

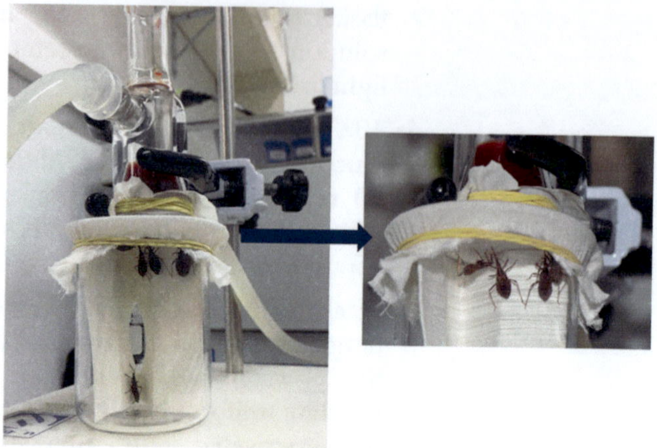

Fig. 1 Artificial blood-feeder used to infect *Rhodnius prolixus*. The glass feeder contains an internal cone where the blood is kept, surrounded by a water-filled cylindrical container which presents a lower inlet and an upper outlet with silicone hoses connected to a circulating water bath. A piece of a latex glove is used as a membrane

dissolved. Adjust the pH to 4.6. Add distilled water to make a final volume of 50 mL. Aliquot the solution in microtubes in volumes of 1.5 mL. Store at −20 °C.

2.2 Insect Feeding

1. Artificial feeder: There are several different models of artificial blood-feeders for hematophagous insects [7–9]. In general, they comprise a chamber for containing the blood, a covering membrane, and a system to maintain blood temperature at 36–38 °C (Fig. 1) (*see* **Note 4**).
2. Blood: Different blood sources can be used for feeding triatomines, each with approximately similar efficiencies [10]; the most commonly used are from rabbits, humans, sheep, and cattle (*see* **Note 5**).
3. Anticoagulants: Sodium citrate solution (2%; 0.055 M glucose, 0.561 M sodium citrate, 0.06 g/mL citric acid), sodium heparin (0.2 mg or 20 units/mL blood), or EDTA (1.2–2.0 mg/mL blood) (*see* **Note 6**).
4. Mammalian hosts: Swiss mice, maintained according to ethical rules for animal care (*see* **Note 7**).
5. Neubauer chamber.

2.3 Insect Inoculum

1. Microliter syringe 50 μL (*see* **Note 8**).
2. Disposable needle (13 × 3·30 G, 1/2″) (*see* **Note 9**).
3. Sterile phosphate buffered saline (PBS; 0.15 M sodium chloride, 0.01 M sodium phosphate, pH 7.4).
4. Neubauer chamber.

3 Methods

3.1 Parasite Culture Techniques

T. cruzi and *T. rangeli* epimastigotes can be maintained in LIT medium by two weekly passages (*see* **Note 10**). The ideal initial concentration of parasites is 1×10^6 parasites/mL in 3 mL of medium (*see* **Note 11**). The temperature can range from 25 to 27 °C, as temperatures above 27 °C can impair the development of *T. rangeli* [11]. NNN medium can be used whenever cultures have a decreased growth rate.

3.2 Infection of R. prolixus with Trypanosomes

The infection of *R. prolixus* can be done either using cultured epimastigotes or trypomastigotes. In the first case, it is possible to standardize the inoculum, but the infection will be initiated with a form of the parasite that does not occur at this location in naturally acquired infections. Trypomastigotes should be used in the study of acute infections, as these are the first forms with which the insect enters into contact in the context of natural transmission.

3.2.1 Infection with Cultured Epimastigotes

1. Centrifuge the whole blood (612 × *g* for 10 min at 10 °C) and transfer the plasma to another tube. Incubate the plasma (56 °C for 30 min) and wash the blood cells three times in sterile PBS (612 × *g* for 10 min at 10 °C). Reconstitute the whole blood, by mixing the heat-inactivated plasma with the washed blood cells.
2. Calculate the number of parasites taking into account the quantity of blood ingested by the insects (*see* **Note 12**). Separate the respective volume of culture and wash it with sterile PBS (958 × *g* for 10 min at 13 °C). Remove the supernatant and resuspend the parasites in 50 μL of PBS. Add the parasite solution to the blood, mixing well, and transfer the parasite-containing blood to the artificial feeder. Mix the blood every 3–5 min to maintain parasites and blood cells in suspension.
3. For the uninfected control group add the same amount of PBS to the blood. Use blood from the same lot, and feed infected and control groups simultaneously.

3.2.2 Infection with Blood Trypomastigotes

Trypanosoma cruzi

1. Blood-feed infected fourth or fifth instar nymphs (nymphs which were fed on infected mice as second instar) and immediately transfer each insect to separate microcentrifuge tubes (1.5 mL). Leave the insects in the tubes for 1–2 h, until the products of diuresis are excreted.
2. Prepare a pool of the excreted diuretic material, and estimate the number of parasites (*see* **Note 11**). Inoculate a mouse intraperitoneally with a concentration of 1×10^6 parasites/mL (*see* **Note 13**).

3. At the peak parasitemia (which varies depending on the *T. cruzi* strain), anesthetize the mouse with an intraperitoneal injection of a mixture of ketamine (150 mg/kg) and xylazine (10 mg/kg), and allow starved nymphs (from 7 days after the molt) to feed on the mouse (*see* **Note 14**).

Trypanosoma rangeli

1. Anesthetize a mouse with an intraperitoneal injection of a mixture of ketamine (150 mg/kg) and xylazine (10 mg/kg). Expose the mouse to starved salivary gland-infected fifth instar nymphs for 10 min (nymphs which were inoculated with culture epimastigotes as fourth instar, as described in **step 4**). Interrupt feeding at regular intervals to guarantee that the insects salivate several times (*see* **Note 15**).
2. Seven-to-fourteen days after infection, anesthetize the mouse and offer it to starved third instar nymphs (from 7 days after the molt) (*see* **Note 16**). For control groups of triatomines, use uninfected mice from the same cohort as the blood source.
3. Since the rates of *T. rangeli* migration across the intestine are highly variable in *R. prolixus* (2–50%), it is necessary to inoculate parasites directly into the coelomic cavity, in order to guarantee the production of metacyclic forms and standardize parasite densities across different experimental groups of triatomines. Calculate the number of cultured epimastigotes required for a dose of $1–5 \times 10^4$ parasites/mL of PBS. At this concentration, using a volume of 1 μL for each injection will give 10–50 parasites per inoculum.
4. Use the previously infected nymphs (**step 2**) 7–10 days after they have molted to fourth instar. For the inoculation, hold the nymph so that the side portion of the insect is perpendicular to the index finger and thumb. Insert the needle in the insertion of the right leg of the third pair, in a position parallel to the insect body (Fig. 2) (*see* **Note 17**). Inject 1 μL of the solution and wait for a few seconds before removing the needle (*see* **Note 18**). For the control groups, inoculate the same volume of sterile PBS.
5. Twenty-four hours after injection, blood-feed the insects to repletion.

3.3 Confirming the Infection

3.3.1 Trypanosoma cruzi

Infection can be confirmed by either collecting the products of diuresis as described before, or by dissecting the intestinal tract of the insect. The first option is recommended in instances when it is necessary for the insects to be kept alive.

1. For dissecting the intestinal tract, cut the final portion of the ninth abdominal segment of the nymph.
2. Press the abdomen until some of the intestine appears. With the aid of forceps, pull the intestine out and transfer it to a microtube with 100–200 μL of PBS.

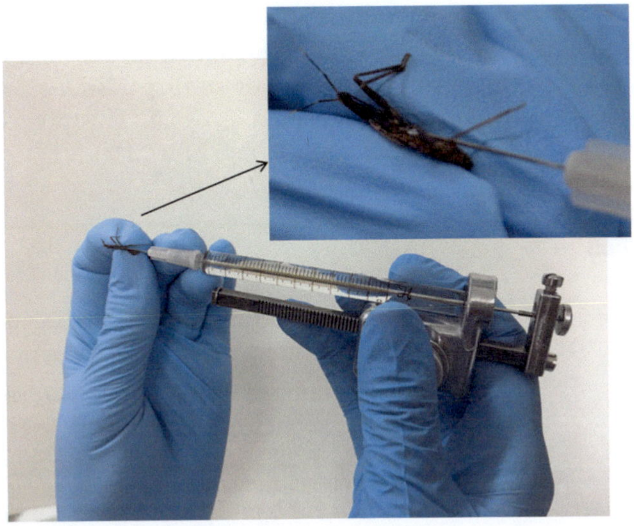

Fig. 2 Inoculation of *Rhodnius prolixus* nymphs

3. Disrupt the tissues with a pestle and examine a sample under a light microscope (*see* **Note 11**).

3.3.2 Trypanosoma rangeli

1. Intestine: Intestinal infections can be confirmed by dissecting the intestinal tract of the insect as described for *T. cruzi* infections.
2. Hemolymph: cut off the terminal segment of a hind leg and collect a drop of hemolymph on a microscope slide. Examine under a light microscope without the use of coverslips (100×). For parasite or cell counting, collect the hemolymph with a micropipette and transfer to a microtube with anticoagulant solution. Use in a ratio of 1:10 hemolymph–anticoagulant.
3. Salivary glands: separate the head from the thorax with the aid of forceps; salivary glands usually stay attached to the head. Examine the glands on a drop of saline solution under a light microscope.

3.4 Maintaining Trypanosome Infectivity

1. *Trypanosoma cruzi*: Infect a mouse as described in Subheading 3.2.2. At the peak parasitemia (which varies depending on the *T. cruzi* strain), anesthetize and bleed the mouse by cardiac puncture after cleaning the area with 70% alcohol. In a laminar flow hood transfer the blood to a tube containing 3 mL of LIT. Maintain at 25–27 °C for 15 days, or until parasite growth is measurable. Proceed to cultivation as usual. This procedure should be repeated every 3–6 months (*see* **Note 19**).
2. *Trypanosoma rangeli*: Infect a mouse as described in Subheading 3.2.2. Three-to-ten days after infection, anesthetize and bleed the mouse by cardiac puncture after cleaning the area

with 70% alcohol. In a laminar flow hood transfer the blood to a tube containing 3 mL of LIT. Maintain at 25–27 °C for 15 days, or until parasite growth is measurable. Proceed to cultivation as usual. This procedure should be repeated every 3 months (*see* **Note 19**).

4 Notes

1. Prefer serum tested against endotoxins and mycoplasma, as they can interfere with parasite growth.
2. Do not use antifungal agents, such as amphotericin B or nystatin, as these compounds have trypanocidal activity.
3. For *T. rangeli* cultures, 20% FBS can be used.
4. *Rhodnius prolixus* is a species easily artificially fed, but this is not the rule for the other triatomine species. Latex gloves (previously boiled to remove substances that can confer taste) or Parafilm M® work well as membranes for the artificial feeders.
5. It is important to have control of the maintenance of the vertebrate animal from which blood will be used; the use of antibiotics and anthelmintics for treating these animals, as well as pesticides in the animal food, can be toxic to triatomines. Blood should preferentially be used fresh; when collected in sterile conditions, it can be kept refrigerated for 7–10 days.
6. Sodium citrate is the most common anticoagulant used, but the other options can also be used. A recent work tested different anticoagulants on *R. prolixus* artificial blood-feeding and recommended heparin as the anticoagulant of choice for feeding and infection experiments [12].
7. Knockout interferon gamma (INF-γ) mice can be used when a high blood parasitemia is needed [3].
8. We use a dispenser (Repeating Dispenser; PB600-1; Hamilton®) coupled to the syringe (80501; Hamilton®) to increase the precision of the inoculum. It is worth mentioning that only species from the *Rhodnius* genus can produce metacyclic forms of *T. rangeli*.
9. These needle measurements are suitable for *R. prolixus* nymphs from the fourth instar onward; for smaller individuals, it is recommended to use thinner needles.
10. *T. rangeli* kept for long periods in culture can lose its capacity to invade the salivary glands of *R. prolixus* [11]. Additionally, one should be careful when choosing the combination of *T. rangeli* strain and *Rhodnius* species, since the KP1(+) strains are restricted to *R. robustus* lineage, while the KP1(−) strains complete the developmental cycle only in the *R. pictipes* lineage [13]. Regarding *T. cruzi*, although no studies have been published, we observed such a decrease in *R. prolixus* infection

rates when our strains are maintained for long periods in culture. *See* Subheading 3.4 for details on maintaining trypanosome infectivity.

11. Parasite numbers can be determined by using either a Neubauer chamber or Brener's method [14].
12. Different numbers of parasites can be fed to the insects; usually a high concentration is used to guarantee the infection (we normally use 10^6 to 10^7 parasites/mL for *T. cruzi* and 10^5 parasites/mL for *T. rangeli* infections). In our conditions, *T. cruzi* metacyclic forms can be found in the insect rectum in 21–30 days after the infective feeding. The infection rates will depend on the strain characteristics as well as its maintenance conditions. For the Dm28c strain, for example, we usually get rates close to 100%. Regarding *T. rangeli*, almost 100% of *R. prolixus* will present positive salivary glands in ~25 days after the parasites of the Choachi strain reach the hemolymph. For both parasites, infections last throughout the insect life, as long as they are not exposed to nutritional stress conditions. Nevertheless, it is important to mention that in nature the infection is normally started with a small number of parasites. It is recommended to test which would be the smallest parasite concentration necessary to start the infection for each strain and triatomine species used. The average amount of blood consumed by the different instars of *R. prolixus* is 4.9, 15.3, 45.0, 109.0, and 277 mg for first, second, third, fourth, and fifth instar nymphs, respectively [15].
13. The concentration of parasites can vary depending on the strain virulence; 1×10^6 parasites/mL works well for CL and Dm28c strains. Give preference to older mice, as they would be heavier and provide large amounts of blood.
14. Twenty-to-thirty mg of blood is sufficient to infect a *R. prolixus* fourth instar nymph with CL and Dm28c strains. We usually weigh some nymphs before and immediately after feeding to get an idea of the enlargement of the abdomen that this volume of blood represents. Insects can be fed artificially to repletion when the period of observation exceeds 15 days; this methodology reduces the use of mice, as well as increasing the number of insects infected with the same batch of parasites.
15. Triatomines do not need to ingest blood to infect a mouse, as they also release the parasites together with the saliva while searching for a blood vessel; preventing individual triatomines from having a complete blood meal allows them to feed upon multiple hosts, enabling the same source of parasites to be used to infect several mice.

16. A *R. prolixus* third instar takes approximately 45 mg of blood; an infected mouse (40 g) should be sufficient to infect 35–40 nymphs.
17. The position of the needle will prevent the rupture of the intestinal tract.
18. As some hemolymph can escape through the hole left by the needle, waiting for a period with the needle inserted into the coelomic cavity will guarantee the dispersion of the solution throughout the insect. It is important to prepare the solution of epimastigotes in PBS immediately before inoculation, as *T. rangeli* can lose its infectivity when maintained in PBS.
19. Make sure to have samples of the culture kept in liquid nitrogen.

Acknowledgments

A.A.G. was supported by CNPq productivity grants. This work received financial support from Fundação de Amparo à Pesquisa do Estado de Minas Gerais (FAPEMIG), Conselho Nacional de Desenvolvimento Científico e Tecnológico (CNPq), and the Instituto Nacional de Ciência e Tecnologia em Entomologia Molecular (INCT-EM/CNPq).

References

1. Guarneri AA, Lorenzo MG (2017) Triatomine physiology in the context of trypanosome infection. J Insect Physiol 97:66–76
2. Dias FA, Guerra B, Vieira LR, Perdomo HD, Gandara ACP, do Amaral RJV, Vollu RE, Gomes SAO, Lara FA, Sorgine MHF, Medei E, Oliveira PL, Salmon D (2015) Monitoring of the parasite load in the digestive tract of *Rhodnius prolixus* by combined qPCR analysis and imaging techniques provides new insights into the trypanosome life cycle. PLoS Negl Trop Dis 9(10):e0004186
3. Ferreira RC, Kessler RL, Lorenzo MG, Paim RMM, Ferreira LL, Probst CM, Alves-Silva J, Guarneri AA (2016) Colonization of *Rhodnius prolixus* gut by *Trypanosoma cruzi* involves an extensive parasite killing. Parasitology 143:434–443
4. Ferreira RC, Teixeira CF, de Sousa VFA, Guarneri AA (2018) Effect of temperature and vector nutrition on the development and multiplication of *Trypanosoma rangeli* in *Rhodnius prolixus*. Parasitol Res 117:1737–1744
5. Camargo EP (1964) Growth and differentiation in *Trypanosoma cruzi*. I. Origin of metacyclic trypanosomes in liquid media. Rev Inst Med Trop Sao Paulo 6:93–100
6. Mello CB, Garcia ES, Ratcliffe NA, Azambuja P (1995) *Trypanosoma cruzi* and *Trypanosoma rangeli*: interplay with hemolymph components of *Rhodnius prolixus*. J Invertebr Pathol 65:261–268
7. Garcia ES, Azambuja PD, Contreras VT (1984) Large scale rearing of *Rhodnius prolixus* and preparation of metacyclic trypomastigotes of *Trypanosoma cruzi*. In: Morel CM (ed) Genes and antigens of parasites: a laboratory manual. Fundação Oswaldo Cruz, FINEP, CNPq, World Health Organization, Rio de Janeiro, pp 43–46
8. Huebner E, Harrison R, Yeow K (1994) A new feeding technique for experimental and routine culturing of the insect *Rhodnius prolixus*. Can J Zool 72:2244–2247
9. Romano D, Stefanini C, Canale A, Benelli G (2018) Artificial blood feeders for mosquitoes and ticks—where from, where to? Acta Trop 183:43–56
10. Gomes JEPL, Azambuja P, Garcia ES (1990) Comparative studies on the growth and reproductive performances of *Rhodnius prolixus*

reared on different blood sources. Mem Inst Oswaldo Cruz 85:299–304

11. Rodrigues JDO, Lorenzo MG, Martins-Filho OA, Elliot SL, Guarneri AA (2016) Temperature and parasite life-history are important modulators of the outcome of *Trypanosoma rangeli–Rhodnius prolixus* interactions. Parasitology 143:1459–1468
12. Silva-Cardoso L, Dias FA, Fampa P, Pereira MG, Atella GC (2018) Evaluating the effects of anticoagulants on *Rhodnius prolixus* artificial blood feeding. PLoS One 13(11):e0206979
13. Vallejo GA, Guhl F, Carranza JC, Triana O, Perez G, Ortiz PA, Marin DH, Villa M, Suarez J, Sanchez IP, Pulido X, Rodriguez IB, Lozano LE, Urrea DA, Rivera FA, Cuba CC, Clavijo JA (2007) Interaccion tripanosoma-vector-vertebrado y su relacion con la sistematica y la epidemiologia de La tripanosomiasis americana. Biomedica 27:110–118
14. Brener Z (1962) Therapeutic activity and criterion of cure on mice experimentally infected with *Trypanosoma cruzi*. Rev Inst Med Trop Sao Paulo 4:389–396
15. Friend WG, Choy CTH, Cartwright E (1965) The effect of nutrient intake on the development and the egg production of *Rhodnius prolixus* Ståhl (Hemiptera: Reduviidae). Can J Zool 43:891–904

Part II

Trypanosomatid Genome-Wide Analyses

Chapter 6

High-Throughput Sequencing for Trypanosome Transcriptome Characterization

Julius Mulindwa, Kevin Leiss, and Christine Clayton

Abstract

High-throughput sequencing of cDNA (RNASeq) is now the method of choice for analysis of transcriptomes. This chapter details important considerations in the design of RNASeq experiments for kinetoplastids grown in culture or experimental animals. It contains protocols for obtaining parasites from rodents, and for removal of rRNA from total RNA. In addition, custom pipelines for sequence alignment, and for data analysis and visualization, are described.

Key words RNASeq, Rodent, Rat, Mouse; *Trypanosoma*, Gene expression, rRNA depletion, Transcriptome, Gene regulation

1 Introduction

1.1 General Considerations

High-throughput sequencing is the method of choice for gene expression analysis. In this chapter we supply protocols that can be used to measure *Trypanosoma brucei* transcriptomes, but most of the special considerations are the same for other kinetoplastids. Once the RNA of interest has been obtained, sequencing methods are the same as for preparation from other biological sources.

When designing an experiment, the critical choices to be made concern the following:

1. The growth conditions.
2. Cell harvesting and if necessary, parasite purification.
3. RNA preparation.
4. Removal of rRNA.
5. Time points after experimental manipulations.

After the sequence reads have been obtained, bioinformatic analysis has to be adapted to take account of the very unusual structure of kinetoplastid genomes relative to other eukaryotes,

Paul A. M. Michels et al. (eds.), *Trypanosomatids: Methods and Protocols*, Methods in Molecular Biology, vol. 2116, https://doi.org/10.1007/978-1-0716-0294-2_6,

especially the presence of many genes in several (almost) identical copies.

The results obtained are affected by all of the different steps. Ideally, for transcriptome comparisons every parameter, except the one to be analyzed, should be exactly the same.

1.2 Transcriptomes of Cultured Trypanosomes

Many factors can affect trypanosome transcriptomes. For cultures these are the culture medium, the temperature, the culture history, and the cell density. When different cultures are compared, unless one of these is the variable parameter, it is absolutely essential that all four conditions be identical (*see* **Note 1**).

Often, parasites are compared with and without induced depletion or expression of a particular protein. If this is done, the time point should be chosen to be the earliest time at which the chance of secondary effects is minimal (*see* **Note 2**).

1.3 Preparing RNA from Trypanosomes in Animals

When isolating trypanosomes from rodents it is important to consider the cell density and growth history. Comparisons of different strains or populations should be done with conditions and differentiation states as similar as possible (*see* **Note 3**). When analyzing different growth phases or tissue sources the population is likely to be mixed. For all animal samples, smears must be made and assessed for stumpy differentiation both by morphology and by staining for a suitable marker such as PAD1.

To obtain sufficient reads from trypanosome RNA, it is helpful to decrease contamination with leukocytes. Otherwise the majority of reads will come from the host animal. For human samples, a leukocyte has approximately ten times as much mRNA as a trypanosome [1]. For *T. rhodesiense* and *T. brucei* in rodents, satisfactory samples can usually be obtained by taking the buffy coat. If the parasitemia is very low, bloodstream-form trypanosomes can be purified away from the red blood cells by passing through a DEAE cellulose column [2]. Even if the method is truncated to the minimum, however, this takes at least 20 min, which can affect the transcriptome [1, 3].

Ruminants with salivarian trypanosome infections often have very low parasitemias ($<10^3$ parasites/ml) which means that obtaining transcriptomes is not practical. However cryopreserved stabilates can be made from this low parasitemia blood. Later the trypanosomes can be propagated in mice or rats (*see* **Note 4**).

To choose an appropriate time to take samples, do preliminary experiments in order to determine the time course of infection.

1.4 Trypanosomes from Clinical Samples

Human clinical samples are extremely challenging to analyze: they are very valuable, samples are small, and the previous parasite parasitemia history is not known. Under field conditions it is not possible to standardize the time needed in order to purify the parasites. Therefore, whole samples must be used. Moreover, we found it impossible to get intact RNA from patient CSF and blood [1] unless we used stabilizing medium in blood Paxgene tubes.

Ethical approval must be obtained for use of human samples, and a consent form must be signed by the patient or a patient representative. This is equally true if the samples are "left over" from normal diagnostic procedures. Ethical approval must also be obtained for the use of rodents in experimental infections.

1.5 Selecting RNA for Sequencing

90% of cellular RNA is rRNA, but for the vast majority of experiments, investigators are interested only in the mRNA and do not to waste money generating unwanted sequences. A variety of methods are available to remove the rRNA.

1. Purification of poly(A) + RNA by hybridization to an oligo-d (T) or oligo(U) matrix. This was initially the method of choice, but it has later been found to affect transcriptomes significantly [1, 4] (*see* **Note 5**).
2. Depletion of rRNA by hybridization to a matrix containing oligonucleotides complementary to rRNA (*see* **Note 6**). Currently this can be done only using homemade affinity beads (*see* **Note 7**).
3. Digestion of the RNA with Terminator 5′-phosphate-dependent exonuclease followed by RNase-free DNase I [5].
4. Depletion of rRNA using oligonucleotide hybridization (*see* **Note 7**) followed by RNase H treatment. This method is in routine use in our laboratory. We recently compared a transcriptome made using this method with one of total RNA without any depletion and the number of significantly changed mRNAs was no higher than would be expected by chance (*see* **Note 8**).
5. For patient samples, human rRNA must be depleted using a standard Illumina kit. For blood it is also necessary to deplete globin mRNAs. Without this depletion parasite read depth will be inadequate.

1.6 Sequence Analysis: Aligning and Counting Reads

To align the sequences and obtain read counts, we use our own custom pipeline which is called TrypRNAseq. Instructions for using this are below. A commonly used alternative is available from the Galaxy project (https://usegalaxy.org). Briefly, the necessary steps are always as follows:

1. Quality check.
2. Trimming of primers, poly(A) tail, and spliced leaders (*see* **Note 9**).
3. Aligning to the chosen genome.
4. Counting the numbers of reads aligned to each open reading frame or transcript.

Because of the unique features of kinetoplastid genomes, you should never use a standard alignment pipeline without checking the parameters. For example, most abundant kinetoplastid mRNAs are encoded by at least two, and sometimes up to twenty, virtually identical gene copies—but many standard RNAseq quantification pipelines ignore all sequence reads that align to the genome more than once. This will leave you with almost no reads for the mRNAs that should really have the most. You must also decide whether to include untranslated regions (*see* **Note 10**).

1.7 Differential Gene Expression Analysis: Comparing Conditions

Differential expression (DE) analyses are used to identify differences between transcriptomes of cells grown under different conditions. The R-package DEseq2 is well established in the field and is able to model gene expression based on only two replicates [6]. EdgeR is a good alternative [7], and the two approaches can also be combined [8]. Our R-shiny app, DESeqUI [9] is a very easy-to-use interface to apply DEseq2 to trypanosome RNA-seq experiments. The app is designed to work seamlessly with the output of the TrypRNAseq pipeline but can also be used to analyze any other trypanosome RNA-seq datasets. All you need is a .csv file: the first column is the gene ID list and the remaining columns are the corresponding raw read counts. (Note that this must be the original read counts, *not* reads per million reads.) The program is currently set to use the TREU927 reference genome.

1.8 Visualizing Relationships Between Datasets and Finding Coregulated Genes

It is often important to be able to find RNAs that show similar patterns when different conditions are compared, such as mRNAs whose expression changes in a similar way over time. To do this we use the app "ClusterViewer" [1], which produces such information both in graph format and as heat maps.

2 Materials

2.1 Trypanosomes from Culture

1. Trypanosomes as desired.
2. Your favorite RNA preparation reagents. (We use TRIzol.)

2.2 Trypanosomes from Blood and Clinical Samples

2.2.1 Growing Parasites in Rodents

1. Mice (*Mus musculus*)—2-weeks-old white Swiss mice.
2. Rats (*Rattus rattus*)—4- to 6-week-old white inbred rats.
3. Blood stabilates, *T. brucei* infected whole blood (1 ml) in 40% glycerol PSG.
4. Phosphate saline glucose (PSG): 44 mM NaCl, 57 mM Na_2HPO_4, 3 mM KH_2PO_4, 55 mM glucose.
5. Bright field Microscope with 40–100× objectives, Microscope slides.

6. Giemsa stain; DAPI (Diamino pimelic acid) stain (300 μM stock).
7. Syringes and hypodermic needles.
8. Dissection kit.
9. EDTA tubes (BD-VAcutainer®).
10. Microfuge (e.g., Eppendorf 5424R).
11. Clinical/cell culture centrifuge (e.g., HERMLE Z306).
12. Hemocytometer.

2.2.2 Purification Using DEAE Cellulose

1. DEAE-Cellulose (Sigma D6418, D0909, D3764).
2. Phosphate saline glucose (PSG): 44 mM NaCl, 57 mM Na_2HPO_4, 3 mM KH_2PO_4, 55 mM glucose.

2.2.3 Trypanosomes from Clinical Samples

1. Syringes 21G.
2. PAXgene Blood RNA Tubes (PreAnalytiX).
3. Bright field Microscope with 40–100× objectives, microscope slides.
4. For counting: Phosphate saline glucose (PSG): 44 mM NaCl, 57 mM Na_2HPO_4, 3 mM KH_2PO_4, 55 mM glucose; hemocytometer.
5. RNA preparation reagents (TRIzol or the Qiagen RNeasy kit).
6. Clinical centrifuge.

2.2.4 Trypanosomes from CSF

1. Bright field Microscope with 40–100× objectives, Microscope slides.
2. For counting: Phosphate saline glucose (PSG): 44 mM NaCl, 57 mM Na_2HPO_4, 3 mM KH_2PO_4, 55 mM glucose; hemocytometer.
3. RNA preparation reagents (TRIzol or the Qiagen RNeasy kit).
4. Clinical centrifuge.
5. RNA preparation reagents (TRIzol or the Qiagen RNeasy kit).

2.3 Removal of rRNA by RNase H Digestion

Autoclaved Millipore water is used. Solution and media are stored at 4 °C if not mentioned otherwise.

1. 5× hybridization buffer: 500 mM Tris–HCl, pH 7.5, 1 M NaCl. Mix 500 μl Tris–HCl, pH 7.5, 250 μl 4 M NaCl, and 250 μl H_2O.
2. Anti-rRNA oligo mix (131 oligos ~50b, in 3275 μl of the mix—0.5 μM conc. of each oligo) (*see* **Note 7**).
3. PCR tubes.
4. PCR machine.

5. 5 U/μl RNase H (e.g., Thermo Fisher), stored at −20 °C.
6. 10× RNase H buffer (e.g., Thermo Fisher), stored at −20 °C.
7. Heat-block.
8. Turbo DNase I (Ambion), stored at −20 °C.
9. 10× Turbo DNase I buffer (Ambion), stored at −20 °C.
10. RNA clean-up & concentrator columns (Zymo Research).

2.4 Sequence Data Analysis

1. As raw input for the pipeline the sequenced reads, a Bowtie2 indexed reference genome and its annotation (modified GTF file) is needed.
2. We recommend running TrypRNAseq on MacOS (the platform on which the pipeline was developed) or a Linux machine. There is an interactive user guide. A minimum of 16 GB of RAM, a disc capacity of roughly 400 GB, and a processor with 2.7 GHz are recommended. Machines with lower specifications might be able to run the pipeline, but at a considerably slower speed.

3 Methods

3.1 Trypanosomes from Culture

1. Centrifuge the trypanosomes to pellet them and remove the supernatant. Washing should be avoided but you may wish to give a brief second spin and remove the remaining medium.
2. Resuspend in your chosen RNA preparation reagent. At this point a few weeks' storage at −70 °C is possible.

   Purify RNA according to the manufacturer's instructions.

3.2 Trypanosomes from Blood and Clinical Samples

3.2.1 Growing Parasites in Rats

1. Thaw a cryopreserved blood stabilate at room temperature and immediately inoculate the 2 mice intraperitoneally with 0.5 ml (each mouse) of the stabilate at 3 different sites (*see* **Note 11**).
2. Monitor the growth of the parasites every 24 h following inoculation, by microscopically observing blood collected from the lateral tail vein. Tail bleeding is carried out by slight cut on the lateral tail vein using a scalpel blade. To simply detect parasites, release a drop of blood onto the microscope slide for a wet smear preparation. Add a coverslip. To count the cells, take up 5 μl with a micropipette directly from the tail, dilute it into 500 μl PSG, and count with a hemocytometer.
3. As soon as enough long slender parasites are available, the mouse is bled out. To bleed, the mouse is sedated in a chloroform chamber, dissected to expose the heart and blood drawn by cardiac puncture using a 21G syringe and released into an EDTA Vacutainer. 500 μl aliquots of this blood can be used to make at least two blood stabilates and also used to infect rats to propagate parasites for RNA preparation.

4. For RNA preparation, rats are infected as in [1] with 5000 (*see* **Note 12**) parasites per rat, using the blood obtained from infected mice.
5. Once parasites are detectable, monitor every day until the desired density or parasitemia stage is attained (*see* **Note 13**). Count the cell density daily using a hemocytometer since good documentation is essential. In addition, make thin smears every day.
6. Before harvesting, also, assess parasitemia using a hemocytometer and make at least two dry thin smears for later morphological characterization.
7. To bleed: the rat is sedated (in a chloroform chamber or alternative permitted method), dissected to expose the heart, and blood drawn by cardiac puncture using a 21G syringe and released into an EDTA Vacutainer.
8. Centrifuge the EDTA rat blood at 1490 × *g* (3000 rpm in the HERMLE Z306) for 10 min at room temperature to differentially separate the blood cells, buffy coat and plasma fractions. The buffy coat layer is located above the erythrocyte and leucocyte layers and contains the trypanosomes.
9. Draw off the plasma using a Pasteur pipette. Carefully pipette the buffy coat (approximately 500 μl) into an microfuge tube without agitating the erythrocyte fraction below.
10. Centrifuge at 3381 × *g* (6000 rpm in the Eppendorf 5424R) for 2 min.
11. Carefully take off the supernatant and add 1 ml TRIzol (or alternative reagent).
12. Purify RNA according to the manufacturer's instructions.

3.2.2 Purification of Trypanosomes from Blood by DEAE-Cellulose Chromatography

1. Prepare the DEAE-Cellulose resin by suspending in 5 volumes of distilled water and allow settling for 30–45 min.
2. Pack 20 ml of slurry volume of the DEAE-Cellulose in a 30 ml Syringe and equilibrate it with 4 column volumes of phosphate saline glucose (PSG), pH 8, for approximately 45 min, at room temperature.
3. Load the column with 4 ml rat blood from the EDTA tube (**step** 7) and elute the trypanosomes with PSG into a 15 ml tube. Centrifuge the tube for 10 min at 1030 × *g* (2500 rpm in the HERMLE Z306) and then suspend the trypanosome pellet in TRIzol reagent for RNA extraction.

3.2.3 Infected Human Blood

Trypanosoma brucei rhodesiense often presents with relatively high parasitemias in blood, which are readily diagnosed by microscopy of a wet smear.

1. Following diagnosis, phlebotomy is carried out on the patient where approximately 5 ml of peripheral blood is drawn using syringe with 21G needle.
2. Immediately, insert the syringe into a Paxgene tube. By suction, the syringe will release approximately 2 ml into it; then insert the syringe into a second tube and release another 2 ml.
3. Mix by inverting the Paxgene tube several times and then leave at room temperature for at least 2 h.
4. Meanwhile, use the rest of the blood from the syringe to make thin smears and (if feasible) to measure the parasitemia: dilute 100× into PSG and use a hemocytometer. If desired, also make frozen trypanosome stabilates.
5. Place the Paxgene tubes at −20 °C (or −80 °C) for storage.
6. The Paxgene samples can be transported back to the lab for RNA extraction.

3.2.4 Human CSF

1. Second stage patients are diagnosed by drawing CSF (2–4 ml) in a 15 ml tube via lumbar puncture, preparing a wet smear, and observing trypanosomes and white blood cells (>5 cells) under the microscope.
2. Take a small sample into a hemocytometer for counting.
3. Spin the CSF volume at 1490 × *g* for 10 min. Meanwhile, count the cells and trypanosomes in a hemocytometer.
4. Aspirate off the supernatant leaving 250–500 μl.
5. Resuspend and take a small sample (20 μl) to make a smear to test trypanosome morphology.
6. Transfer the remainder to a 1.5 ml tube and centrifuge at 6000 rpm for 2 min in a cold centrifuge. Meanwhile, make the smear.
7. Resuspend the pellet fraction in 1 ml TRIzol reagent and transfer to a cryotube.
8. Freeze immediately in liquid nitrogen. Transfer to the lab for RNA preparation according to the manufacturer's instructions.

3.3 rRNA Depletion Using Oligonucleotides and RNase H

1. Mix 5 μl 5× hybridization buffer, 10 μg RNA, 3.275 μl anti-rRNA oligo mix and fill up with H_2O to 25 μl in a PCR tube.
2. Hybridize for 2 min at 95 °C.
3. Cool to 37 °C in steps of 0.1 °C per second using a PCR machine.
4. Add 1 μl RNase H, 3 μl 10× RNase H buffer, and 1 μl H_2O to the tube and mix.
5. Incubate for 20 min at 37 °C.

6. Add 5 μl 10× DNase I buffer, 1 μl Turbo DNase I, and 14 μl H_2O.
7. Incubate for 20 min at 37 °C.
8. Purify RNA using RNA purification columns (e.g., RNA cleanup & concentrator columns) according to the manufacturer's protocol.
9. For quality control run about 1/10 of the purified RNA on a denaturing agarose gel, along with a similar amount of the input RNA, and blot. Check that the rRNA bands are reduced in the depleted sample (methylene blue stain of the blot). Probe for an abundant RNA such as alpha- or beta-tubulin. A degree of degradation is expected but the full-length band should also be visible.

3.4 Sequence Analysis

3.4.1 Sequence Alignment

1. Retrieve the newest version of TrypRNAseq from GitHub (https://github.com/agclayton/TrypRNAseq) [10].
2. Unpack the downloaded archive into a folder where you want to install the pipeline.
3. Place the read-containing FASTQ files (the ones you obtained from the sequencing facility) in a folder.
4. Start the pipeline by navigating within the terminal to the TrypRNAseq installation directory and enter the following into a terminal session: python3 tryprnaseq.py.
5. Make sure that the dependencies, which are listed on the GitHub page, are installed and available via the terminal, without the need to enter the full path of each tool: Add the paths to the different dependencies to your $PATH global variable before starting the pipeline.
6. The interactive user guide will help you to enter the desired set of parameters for alignment and readcount extraction. The standard parameters are set as follows: All overrepresented sequences are removed and all reads longer and equal to 30 bases in length are used for alignment.

   The pipeline will automatically run through the following steps:

   (a) In the pipeline we have set Bowtie2 so that it aligns each read against the indexed genome up to 20 times. (At present only single-end sequencing is formally possible within the pipeline but for simple gene expression analyses we find that linked paired end files give essentially identical results.)

   (b) Samtools generates .bam files (samtools view command) of the alignments (.sam-format) and indexes them (samtools index command). The bam files are only machine-readable but can be processed and indexed much faster than .sam files. The .bam files can also be used as input for various applications including visualization in Artemis (*see* **Note 14**).

(c) The read-counts for each gene are counted using a custom script. Briefly, the script uses the genome annotation and counts the reads per listed feature using samtools. The output of this is saved in a tab-separated file.

7. To update the indexed reference genome, simply replace the file that you have with the new version. You can also change to a different genome.
8. To obtain reads from all genes (not just open reading frames) or from 3′-UTRs, you need to change which features you wish to examine (*see* **Note 15**).

3.4.2 Differential Expression Analysis

1. Get the app from GitHub (https://github.com/agclayton/DESeqUI) and unpack the archive.
2. In RStudio, open the file: DESeqUI/app.R.
3. Click in RStudio the "Run App" button which will open the app in a browser window.
4. Within the app, the raw readcount matrix can be loaded from a file, where columns equal to experiments (treatments, conditions) and rows to GeneIDs.
5. We therefore use a manually curated gene list that includes only one representative of each repeated gene. This is called the "unique" gene list (see file DEseqUI/unique_list_transcLength.txt.).
6. For each column, the user specifies the group the experiment belongs to (i.e., control or treatment) and then specifies which groups should be tested against each other for differential gene expression and the accepted significance level.
7. After clicking "Update," the app will run. This can be followed by watching the script in RStudio. At the end, a principal component analysis is displayed (tab "PCA") and can be downloaded as a pdf file. A list of relative log expression values can also be downloaded (tab "content") to input into our third app, ClusterViewer (see below).
8. DESeqU1 analyses your results for mRNA length bias. Results for mRNAs whose full lengths have not been annotated are not included. This is toward the bottom of the "DeSeq" tab.
9. An additional feature of DESeqUI is the analysis of differentially expressed mRNAs according to the functions of the encoded proteins. The file "DEseqUI/unique_list_transcLength.txt" includes not only the transcript length but also annotation of the protein function ("Annotation") and a single

keyword that assigns the protein to a particular functional class ("Class"). The classes were manually assigned. Both they and the annotations can be updated either within the text file or after importing them into a spreadsheet.

10. To assess enrichment of functional groups, apply the cutoffs you wish to use on the side-panel, then examine the results in the "Classes" tab. At the bottom, this will also display enrichment according to the cell-cycle stage at which the mRNAs are maximally expressed.
11. The complete result table can also be downloaded for further analysis.
12. Note that DeSeq2 is suitable only for comparisons of datasets in which expression of most genes does not change (*see* **Note 16**).

3.4.3 Visualizing the Differences Between Samples Using ClusterViewer

ClusterViewer uses the same unique gene list as DESeqU1, but without the mRNA lengths; it is called "UniqueList.txt". ClusterViewer is available as a supplementary file called "S1 app" for the paper [1]. After downloading the zip file, unpack it, then follow the instructions: "How to set up a sequence comparison."

3.4.4 Calculating the Average Number of mRNAs per Cell

1. Select the raw read numbers for all genes on the "Unique" gene list from DeSeqU1 "DEseqUI/unique_list_transcLength.txt" or from ClusterViewer "UniqueList.txt" (*see* **Note 17**).
2. Delete the data for the remaining genes (*see* **Note 18**).
3. For each column of reads, calculate the reads per million reads. To simplify viewing the data, round the results to remove everything after the decimal point.
4. For Lister 427 bloodstream-form and procyclic-form trypanosomes there are approximately 22,000 and 44,000 mRNAs per cell, respectively [11]. Therefore, to work out the average numbers of each mRNA, the RPM value is multiplied by either 0.022 or 0.044.

4 Notes

1. Ideally—unless you specifically wish to look at stumpy forms or mixed populations—cells should be in mid-log phase. Beyond mid-log, translation inhibition sets in and levels of some mRNAs are considerably diminished [12]. Moreover bloodstream-form cells might start to express some stumpy-form characteristics, even if they are not completely differentiation-competent. To obtain cells in mid-log phase, take care to split the cells in the days before harvest to ensure

optimal growth kinetics. Mid-log phase is at least five times lower than the maximal (stationary phase) density. This depends on both the life-cycle stage, strain, and parasite passage history. For example, our monomorphic Lister 427 bloodstream forms have a maximal density of 5–6 $\times$ 10^6 cells/ml, so the ideal harvest density is 8–1.0 $\times$ 10^6 cells/ml; but our pleomorphic EATRO1125 bloodstream forms reach stationary phase at about 2 $\times$ 10^6 cells/ml. Appropriate densities must be determined individually for each cell line. Even a twofold difference in cell density can make a difference.

2. For RNAi experiments, choose the earliest time at which the *protein* is at least tenfold depleted. (This is likely to be later than disappearance of the mRNA.) Ideally, cells should still be dividing with no evident phenotypic effects. If the protein is required for growth, and the cells are taken at a time beyond which no further growth occurs, secondary effects due to growth arrest will probably be present.
3. For example, when comparing two different strains it would be ideal to take cells during the first rising phase of parasitemia, at a density that is too low to promote stumpy formation.
4. By cardiac puncture, an adult mouse gives approximately 2 ml of blood whereas a rat can give up to 5 ml of blood. All animal experiments should be done by appropriately qualified personnel and with ethical approval.
5. In principle, poly(A) selection might result in the following:
    (a) Loss of 5′-ends if mRNAs are not intact.
    (b) Loss of mRNAs that have very short poly(A) tails at steady state, of mRNA degradation intermediates that lack poly (A) tails, and of other RNAs which may be of interest such as snoRNAs, tRNAs, and snRNAs.
    (c) Preferential selection of mRNAs with very long poly (A) tails, or with oligo(A) tracts within the mRNA body.
    (d) Loss of mRNAs that are preferentially trapped in the matrix.
    (e) In the case of trypanosomes, poly(A) selection results in loss of longer mRNAs [1].
6. This is the basis of commercially available kits for rRNA depletion. Up until about 2014, the RiboMinus Eukaryote kit successfully removed trypanosome rRNA [13]. However, the manufacturers have since "optimized" the kit and as a consequence, it no longer works for kinetoplastids. It is therefore necessary to make the column matrix using your own oligonucleotides.

7. These should span the entire sequence of the mature mRNAs. Check suppliers carefully to work out which format and length will work out most economical. The oligos do not need to be quality-controlled and the most economical version is usually to buy as a batch on microtiter plates. It is not necessary to by modified oligonucleotides, since the biotinylation can be done afterward [14].
8. Incubation of total RNA with the oligonucleotide mix and RNase H results in digestion of the rRNA into fragments of less than 50 bases. Prior to library building, the RNA mix is fragmented and pieces of about 300 bases will be selected; this step removes the rRNA fragments. For details concerning the oligonucleotides (*see* **Note 6**).

   Disadvantages of this method are:

   (a) Some degradation of the mRNA also occurs. For this reason it is essential to check the RNA quality by Northern blotting prior to sequencing.

   (b) Bioanalyzer output reveals a large peak of degraded RNA, while the longer RNA that you are interested in is no longer visible. If you are using a library-building facility or company you will have to convince them that the RNA is actually OK (using the Northern results) and explain the reason for the abnormal profile.

   (c) The method cannot be used if you want to analyze RNAs that are less than 100 bases long, because the rRNA fragments will be included during library construction.
9. All pipelines include removal of sequencing adapters and poly (A) tails. For kinetoplastids, it is also necessary to remove spliced leaders present at the 5′-ends of mRNAs. TrypRNAseq uses the tool Cutadapt to do this. However we have also included an extra step that removes reads from rRNAs—which is particularly important if the input RNA was not poly (A) selected. The easiest and most straightforward approach is doing quality control using FastQC, with subsequent removal of all overrepresented sequences which the tool identified. Another approach, which ensures only the removal of rRNA reads, is to provide a FASTA file of ribosomal sequences, which are then used to trim the sequenced reads. Our pipeline does this.
10. TrypRNASeq is customized in order to allow each read to align 20 times. But Cufflinks, which is used to map RNA reads across *cis*-splice junctions and is included as a standard part of the Galaxy pipeline, removes multicopy sequences by default. Since almost no *cis*-splicing occurs in kinetoplastids, identification of splice junctions is unnecessary, so this step should be removed. The standard settings of TrypRNAseq give a final output of

reads mapping to open reading frames. This was done because for many genes, the 3′-untranslated region has not been annotated. These regions also include low-complexity and repeated sequences which may result in inaccurate counts. For any other pipeline it is essential to decide how to proceed. If you wish to look at gene families with differing untranslated regions, these can be examined separately [15].

11. The viability of cryopreserved stabilates varies. In order to get highly reproducible rat infections, it is therefore best to infect with fresh infected blood from a mouse. The parasites should be in the rising phase of parasitemia in order to be certain that they are mostly infective long slender forms.

12. The number of parasites will vary depending on isolate virulence and the desired infection characteristics. This number is for *T. brucei brucei* or *T. brucei rhodesiense* that have been isolated from natural infections and have not subsequently undergone extensive syringe passage or culture.

13. The duration of infection will also depend on the parasites, the animals and the stage which you wish to investigate.

14. If disk space is limiting, the SAM files can be deleted as soon as the BAM file generation is completed. Using samtools view, the human readable SAM file can be regenerated from BAM files. Aligning just one dataset at a time will help, since only one SAM file will be made at a time.

15. TrypRNAseq uses its own genome annotation format, based on the widely used GTF/GFF3 format. The annotation is a simple tab separated table, where each row contains information about a single feature. The columns are ordered as follows: Feature identifier, chromosome identifier (needs to be the same as the identifier used in the indexed FASTA genome file), feature start, feature end nucleotide, and the feature length. Using commonly used scripting languages like BASH or Python, such a table can easily be generated from a GTF file, or manually curated if the number of features is short.

16. When analyzing pull-down experiments (e.g., immunoprecipitation of an RNA-binding protein and looking for bound RNAs), this criterion may well not be fulfilled—and other comparison algorithms work on the same assumption. For pull-downs it is better to calculate RPMs using the "unique" gene list, and then to divide the eluted (bound) RNA RPM by the input or unbound RPM. Reproducibly enriched RNAs can then be found. If the RNA was digested before the pull-down was done you will need to use completely different software to find the peaks.

17. Use of the unique genes list, and extraction of reads only from open reading frames, has one big disadvantage: it ignores genes that have similar open reading frames but different regulation and also eliminates results for families of similar but nonidentical genes (*see* [16] for the cutoff criteria). The 3′-untranslated regions (3′-UTRs) of such genes are, however, usually different and, indeed, responsible for the differing expression. It is therefore possible detect this by counting 3′-UTR reads instead of coding sequences [15].
18. Since each read was allowed to align up to 20 times on the reference genome, the raw data in the complete list cannot be used to determine mRNA abundance. Multiple gene copies genes therefore have to be removed.

References

1. Mulindwa J, Leiss K, Ibberson D, Kamanyi Marucha K, Helbig C, Melo do Nascimento L, Silvester E, Matthews K, Matovu E, Enyaru J et al (2018) Transcriptomes of Trypanosoma brucei rhodesiense from sleeping sickness patients, rodents and culture: effects of strain, growth conditions and RNA preparation methods. PLoS Negl Trop Dis 12:e0006280
2. Lanham S, Godfrey D (1970) Isolation of salivarian trypanosomes from man and other mammals using DEAE-cellulose. Exp Parasitol 28:521–534
3. Mulindwa J, Fadda A, Merce C, Matovu E, Enyaru J, Clayton C (2014) Methods to determine the transcriptomes of trypanosomes in mixtures with mammalian cells: the effects of parasite purification and selective cDNA amplification. PLoS Negl Trop Dis 8:e2806
4. Sultan M, Amstislavskiy V, Risch T, Schuette M, Dokel S, Ralser M, Balzereit D, Lehrach H, Yaspo ML (2014) Influence of RNA extraction methods and library selection schemes on RNA-seq data. BMC Genomics 15:675
5. Kolev N, Franklin J, Carmi S, Shi H, Michaeli S, Tschudi C (2010) The transcriptome of the human pathogen Trypanosoma brucei at single-nucleotide resolution. PLoS Pathog 6:e1001090
6. Love M, Huber W, Anders S (2014) Moderated estimation of fold change and dispersion for RNA-Seq data with DESeq2. Genome Biol 15:550
7. Schurch NJ, Schofield P, Gierliński M, Cole C, Sherstnev A, Singh V, Wrobel N, Gharbi K, Simpson G, Owen-Hughes T et al (2016) How many biological replicates are needed in an RNA-seq experiment and which differential expression tool should you use? RNA 22:839–851
8. Varet H, Brillet-Gueguen L, Coppee JY, Dillies MA (2016) SARTools: a DESeq2- and EdgeR-based R pipeline for comprehensive differential analysis of RNA-Seq data. PLoS One 11: e0157022
9. Leiss K, Clayton C (2016) DESeqUI—trypanosome RNAseq analysis made easy. Zenodo. https://doi.org/10.5281/zenodo.165132
10. Leiss K, Merce C, Muchunga E, Clayton C (2016) TrypRNAseq—A easy to use pipeline for Trypanosoma RNAseq data. Zenodo. https://doi.org/10.5281/zenodo.158920
11. Haanstra J, Stewart M, Luu V-D, van Tuijl A, Westerhoff H, Clayton C, Bakker B (2008) Control and regulation of gene expression: quantitative analysis of the expression of phosphoglycerate kinase in bloodstream form Trypanosoma brucei. J Biol Chem 283:2495–2507
12. Häusler T, Clayton CE (1996) Post-transcriptional control of HSP70 mRNA in Trypanosoma brucei. Mol Biochem Parasitol 76:57–72
13. Fadda A, Ryten M, Droll D, Rojas F, Färber V, Haanstra J, Bakker B, Matthews K, Clayton C (2014) Transcriptome-wide analysis of mRNA decay reveals complex degradation kinetics and suggests a role for co-transcriptional degradation in determining mRNA levels. Mol Microbiol 94:307–326
14. Gaspar I, Wippich F, Ephrussi A (2017) Enzymatic production of single-molecule FISH and RNA capture probes. RNA 23:1582–1591

15. Naguleswaran A, Doiron N, Roditi I (2018) RNA-Seq analysis validates the use of culture-derived Trypanosoma brucei and provides new markers for mammalian and insect life-cycle stages. BMC Genomics 19:227

16. Siegel T, Hekstra D, Wang X, Dewell S, Cross G (2010) Genome-wide analysis of mRNA abundance in two life-cycle stages of Trypanosoma brucei and identification of splicing and polyadenylation sites. Nucleic Acids Res 38:4946–4957

Chapter 7

Polysome Profiling and Metabolic Labeling Methods to Measure Translation in *Trypanosoma brucei*

Kathrin Bajak and Christine Clayton

Abstract

The amount of a protein that is made in a cell is determined not only by the corresponding mRNA level but also by the efficiency with which the mRNA is translated. Very powerful transcriptome-wide methods are available to analyze both the density of ribosomes on each mRNA and the rate at which polypeptides are elongated. However, for many research questions, simpler, less expensive methods are more suitable. Here we describe two methods to assess the general translation status of cells: polysome profiling by sucrose density gradient centrifugation and metabolic labeling using radioactive amino acids. Both methods can also be used to examine translation of individual mRNAs.

Key words Translation, Ribosome, Polysome, Pulse labeling, Sucrose gradient, Metabolic labeling

1 Introduction

The amount of a protein that is made in a cell is determined not only by the corresponding mRNA level but also by the efficiency with which the mRNA is translated. Translation efficiency can be divided into two states: initiation and elongation. The current gold-standard method for translation measurement is ribosome profiling, which measures the average number of ribosomes on each mRNA [1]. Ribosome profiling can reveal extensive translation regulation and is invaluable for defining functional open reading frames. This method is evolving, but for descriptions of its use in kinetoplastids *see* [2–4].

Ribosome profiling not only demands a lot of material but is also very expensive. A more economical way to find out whether mRNAs are being translated or not is to separate polysomes on a sucrose gradient, then to characterize RNA from different fractions. For individual mRNAs, this can be done by RT-PCR or northern blotting, and transcriptome-wide results can be obtained by sending fractions for RNA sequencing (for examples *see* [5–7]).

Paul A. M. Michels et al. (eds.), *Trypanosomatids: Methods and Protocols*, Methods in Molecular Biology, vol. 2116, https://doi.org/10.1007/978-1-0716-0294-2_7,

A method for examining polysomes by sucrose gradient centrifugation, based on [8], is given below.

Neither ribosome nor polysome profiling measures the translation rate. Two opposite artifacts could give misleading results: very fast elongation following initiation could lead to sparse dispersal of ribosomes on a coding region, whereas blocks in elongation can result in a pileup of ribosomes [9]. To measure transcriptome-wide translation rates in animal cells, ribosome profiling is performed at various times after addition of the initiation inhibitor Harringtonine [10]. It is not yet clear whether Harringtonine inhibits translation initiation in kinetoplastids, although it is toxic for *Trypanosoma brucei* [11]. In order to avoid counting stalled ribosomes, only the actively translating ones can be selected [12].

If one is interested in the general status of protein synthesis under particular conditions, or in the translation of a few specific mRNAs, pulse labeling is the most appropriate approach: it is economical and is completed within 2 days. Metabolic labeling is also useful for measuring protein half-life [13]. Below we describe metabolic labeling using [^{35}S]-labeled amino acids as tracers (*see*, e.g., [14–16]). This can be done only if appropriate facilities for working with, and disposal of, radioactive materials are available. Alternative nonradioactive methods are also available in kit form (e.g., [17]) (*see* **Note 1**). Overall protein synthesis rates can also be measured by assaying puromycin-mediated chain termination, although in that case, the polypeptides will not be full length [18, 19].

The highest translation rates are seen when the parasites are in mid-log phase, with at least two cell cycles possible before attaining stationary phase. The required density will depend on the trypanosome line and developmental stage and must be determined individually. When comparing genetically different cultures (or, e.g., cells with and without RNAi induction) it is imperative, if possible, to use cultures that are growing similarly.

2 Materials

2.1 Polysome Gradients

Autoclaved high-quality filtered water is used. Solutions and media are stored at 4 °C, unless otherwise mentioned.

1. Ice.
2. Dry ice.
3. Serum-free medium: HMI-9 medium without FCS.
4. 1× PBS: Mix 100 ml 10× PBS, pH 7.4, with 900 ml H_2O.
5. Lysis buffer: 20 mM Tris–HCl, pH 7.5, 20 mM KCl, 2 mM $MgCl_2$, 2 mM dithiothreitol (DTT), 1000 U RNasin, 10 μg/ml Leupeptin, 0.2% IGEPAL, 200 mM sucrose, 100 μg/ml

cycloheximide. Mix 40 µl 1 M Tris–HCl, pH 7.5, 40 µl 1 M KCl, 4 µl 1 M $MgCl_2$, 4 µl 1 M DTT, 25 µl RNasin, 2 µl 10 mg/ml leupeptin (*see* **Note 2**), 40 µl 10% IGEPAL, 400 µl 1 M sucrose (analytical grade) (*see* **Note 3**), and 2 µl 100 mg/ ml cycloheximide in ethanol (*see* **Note 4**), and fill up with H_2O to 2 ml. Place on ice.

6. Polysome buffer: 20 mM Tris–HCl, pH 7.5, 120 mM KCl, 2 mM $MgCl_2$, 1 mM DTT, 10 µg/ml Leupeptin, 65 µl 100 µg/ml cycloheximide. Mix 1.3 ml 1 M Tris–HCl, pH 7.5, 7.8 ml 1 M KCl, 130 µl 1 M $MgCl_2$, 65 µl 1 M DTT, 65 µl 10 mg/ml leupeptin, 65 µl 100 mg/ml cycloheximide, and 55.6 ml H_2O.
7. Sucrose solutions for the gradients. These are made using polysome buffer. For example, to prepare 15% (w/v) sucrose, put 4.5 g sucrose into a 50 ml sterile conical tube or bottle with volume markers. Fill up with polysome buffer to 30 ml. You need 15%, 50% and 60% sucrose.
8. Chloroform.
9. Isopropanol.
10. 10 mg/ ml glycogen (stored at −20 °C).
11. 70% (v/v) ethanol.
12. peqGOLD TriFast FL (VWR) or other denaturing RNA preparation reagent.
13. Analytical grade sucrose.
14. 1 ml syringe.
15. 21G × 1½″ syringe needles.
16. 27G × 4/5″ syringe needles.
17. Centrifuge for cell cultures.
18. Microfuge.
19. Ultracentrifuge.
20. Swing-out rotor for ultracentrifuge, 5 ml tubes, rated to 50,000 rpm.
21. 5 ml thin wall polypropylene tubes for use in ultracentrifuge rotors.
22. Heating block.
23. Ideally, a gradient fraction collector setup. We use a combination from Teledyne Isco: a BRANDEL tube piercer, a Foxy R1 fraction collector, a TRIS peristaltic pump, a FOXYR1 fraction collector, and a UV/VIS detector. It is possible to manage without all of this but it is more laborious and the continuous profile will not be obtained.
24. 5×10^8 trypanosomes per gradient, in mid-log phase unless you are specifically investigating other conditions.

2.2 Metabolic Labeling to Measure Protein Synthesis

1. Commercial methionine-free tissue culture medium (we use methionine-free DMEM). If working with procyclic forms, add proline (final concentration: 0.6 mg/ml). You need about 2 ml medium per sample.
2. If your plan includes an incubation of more than 60 min, dialyzed heat-inactivated fetal or newborn calf serum should also be included (10% in the methionine-free medium). Dialyze the FCS against HEPES buffer (7.14 g/l, pH 7.4) with 3 changes. Keep at −20 °C in aliquots, filter-sterilize if there will subsequently be a longer incubations. Longer incubations are needed only if you wish to label all proteins to steady state, or you want to assay protein half-life.
3. 1× PBS + 0.5% glucose: Mix 100 ml 10× PBS, pH 7.4, with 10 ml 50% glucose and 890 ml H_2O.
4. L-[^{35}S]-methionine, 10 μCi per sample/assay (*see* **Note 5**).
5. 1 M KCl.
6. SDS-PAGE gel materials and equipment.
7. Gel dryer.
8. Equipment to detect [^{35}S] (autoradiography film and developer, or phosphorimager with appropriate cassettes for exposure).
9. Live trypanosomes. To analyze total protein synthesis use ~5 × 10^6 cells per sample.

3 Methods

3.1 Polysome Analysis Using Sucrose Gradients

3.1.1 Preparation of Sucrose Gradients

1. If you have a gradient pourer: Make a 4.0 ml 15–50% sucrose gradient according to the instructions on the machine. Proceed to Subheading 3.1.2.
2. If you do not have a gradient pourer, use the freezing method [20] (*see* **Note 6**). First place the polypropylene tubes in a box filled with dry ice. If you do not have dry ice, put the tube at −80 °C for 30 min instead.
3. Pour 790 μl 50% sucrose in the polypropylene tubes and wait until the sucrose is frozen.
4. Mix 7.5 ml 50% sucrose with 2.5 ml 15% sucrose (enough for 12 gradients) and pour 790 μl of the sucrose solution in the polypropylene tubes and wait until the sucrose is frozen.
5. Mix 5 ml 50% sucrose with 5 ml 15% sucrose (enough for 12 gradients) and pour 790 μl of the sucrose solution in the polypropylene tubes and wait until the sucrose is frozen.

6. Mix 2.5 ml 50% sucrose with 7.5 ml 15% sucrose (enough for 12 gradients) and pour 790 μl of the sucrose solution in the polypropylene tubes and wait until the sucrose is frozen.
7. Pour 790 μl 15% sucrose in the polypropylene tubes and wait until the sucrose is frozen. The gradients can be stored at −80 °C for some weeks.
8. Transfer gradients to 4 °C overnight for thawing. Choose a place that is free of vibration!

3.1.2 Lysate Preparation and Gradient Loading

1. Prepare 2 ml lysis buffer. Place on ice.
2. Collect 5 × 10^8 cells per gradient by centrifugation at (2000 × *g*, 4 °C) for 15 min and remove supernatant.
3. Resuspend cell pellet in 50 ml serum-free medium and transfer to a 50 ml conical tube.
4. Pellet cells by centrifugation at (1000 × *g*, 4 °C) for 7 min and remove supernatant.
5. Resuspend cell pellet in 1 ml ice-cold 1× PBS and transfer to an Eppendorf tube. Centrifuge.
6. Resuspend cells in 350 μl lysis buffer.
7. Pass cells 15 times through the 21 gauge needle using a 1 ml syringe.
8. Pass cells 15 times through the 27 gauge needle using a 1 ml syringe.
9. Clear lysate by centrifugation at 15,000 × *g* (top speed) for 10 min at 4 °C in a microfuge.
10. Adjust salt concentration to 120 mM KCl by adding 35 μl 1 M KCl to the lysate.
11. Load the lysate slowly on the 4 ml continuous linear 15–50% sucrose gradient.
12. Ultracentrifuge the gradients at 164,326 × *g* (this is 40,000 rpm in the Beckman SW60) for 2 h at 4 °C using the swinging bucket rotor.
13. Take out the rotor first, then the tubes extremely carefully. Place the buckets on ice with the tubes inside.

3.1.3 Fractionation (See **Note 7**)

1. Switch on the UV light.
2. Clean the tubing with H_2O.
3. Pump air through the tubing to remove water.
4. Assemble the gradient holder and needle.
5. Pump 60% sucrose through the tubing until it comes out of the needle.
6. Clean the tubing between the UV detector and fractionator with H_2O and afterwards with air using a syringe with a needle.

7. Set the velocity to 50% and the sensitivity to 1.
8. Set the baseline to 20–40 (or as appropriate) using the record off-set button (*see* **Note 8**).
9. Switch the computer on and open Peak Trak.
10. Take out the first tube using forceps. Assemble the first gradient in the fractionator according to the manufacturer's instructions.
11. Pump 60% sucrose through the needle to pump the gradient up.
12. Stop pumping as soon as the absorption is detected by the UV detector.
13. Start collecting 16 fractions with a volume of 250 μl in Eppendorf tubes and follow absorption with Peak Trak.
14. RNA or protein can be purified from the single fractions (see below).
15. Pump back the sucrose until the tubing of UV detector is empty.
16. Remove tube and assemble next gradient in the fractionator.
17. Repeat procedure until you are done with all gradients.
18. Cleaning of the fractionator: Wash the tubing with H_2O first by pumping it through the tubing.
19. Wash the tubing with ethanol.
20. Pump through with air.
21. Disassemble the gradient holder and needle and clean with H_2O.
22. Open each chromatogram with the Peak Trak software.
23. Chromatogram can be saved as .pdf-file for printing.
24. .pks-file can be opened and processed in Excel.

3.1.4 RNA Analysis

1. If you wish to include a control for the purification efficiency, "spike" each fraction with a synthetic RNA which is absent in trypanosomes.
2. To obtain RNA: add 750 μl PeqGOLD TriFast FL, or the correct amount of your favored alternative, to each fraction and mix. At this point samples can be stored at −80 °C.
3. Follow the manufacturer's instructions to purify the RNA.
4. To quantify all mRNAs in each fraction, use northern blotting, with an oligonucleotide probe complementary to the spliced leader. Quantify the whole smear but omit the spliced leader donor RNA. A transcript of interest can be measured by northern blotting using with a specific probe, or by quantitative reverse transcription followed by PCR.

5. For RNA-Seq: Pool the fractions as desired. One option is to take soluble + subunits, monosomes, disomes, and trisomes, and heavier polysomes. Save at least a tenth of each pool in order to quantitate all mRNAs using the spliced leader probe as in step 4: This is essential in order to normalize the RNA-Seq results [5–7].

3.1.5 Proteins from the Fractions

1. Add 6 μl 6× Laemmli to 30 μl solution from each fraction and mix.
2. Boil for 5 min at 95 °C on a heating block.
3. Analyze samples by western blotting.

3.2 Pulse Labeling

1. Centrifuge ~5×10^6 cells at 2000 × *g* (about 3000 rpm in a cell centrifuge) for 10 min at room temperature.
2. Take off the supernatant, resuspend in 1 ml PBS containing 0.5% glucose, and transfer to a microfuge tube. Centrifuge at 1000 × *g* for 5 min.
3. Take off the supernatant, resuspend in 1 ml PBS containing 0.5% glucose, and transfer to a microfuge tube. Centrifuge at 1000 × *g* for 5 min.
4. Take off the supernatant and resuspend in 500 μl methionine-free medium. Incubate at the appropriate temperature (depending on the life cycle stage) for 15 min.
5. Add ^{35}S-methionine (10 μCi at about 800 Ci/mmol; if the solution is 10 mCi/ml this is 1 μl). Incubate for 30 min (*see* **Note 9**) at the appropriate temperature (depending on the life cycle stage).
6. Pellet the cells in a microfuge at 1000 × *g* for 5 min (this is 3000 rpm in a tabletop centrifuge). If measuring protein half-life, skip to **step 11**.
7. Take off the supernatant, resuspend in 1 ml PBS containing 0.5% glucose, and transfer to a microfuge tube. Centrifuge at 1000 × *g* for 5 min.
8. Take off the supernatant, resuspend in 1 ml PBS containing 0.5% glucose, and transfer to a microfuge tube. Centrifuge at 1000 × *g* for 5 min.
9. To examine the total protein synthesis pattern: resuspend in Laemmli buffer, heat, then separate by SDS-PAGE. The Coomassie-stained gel is dried down before [^{35}S] detection.
10. To examine individual proteins: resuspend in a lysis buffer appropriate for immunoprecipitation.
11. To measure protein half-life, resuspend the cells in an appropriate volume of full medium including serum (*see* **Note 10**).

4 Notes

1. For example, incorporation of L-azidohomoalanine, azido-modification by click chemistry followed by fluorescence-based detection [21]. This is the basis of the "Click-IT" kit from ThermoFisher.
2. You can also add a commercial EDTA-free protease inhibitor cocktail. However, kinetoplastids vary quite a lot in their protease content, and money can be saved by choosing a few appropriate inhibitors. For bloodstream-form trypanosomes we have found it is usually sufficient to include only leupeptin. Procyclic-form trypanosomes and *Leishmania* require more inhibitors. For *Leishmania tarentolae*, 200 μM TPCK (N-p-Tosyl-l-phenylalanine chloromethyl ketone), 200 μM TLCK (Nα-Tosyl-l-lysine chloromethyl ketone), and 200 μg/ml o-phenanthroline were effective [22] during protein purification.
3. Do not make this solution up in advance and autoclave it, you will get a syrup!
4. This solution has to be stored at −20 °C. Cycloheximide is a poison, so weigh under the fume hood and wear gloves. Cycloheximide is added to "freeze" the polysomes and prevent ribosome runoff during centrifugation and the initial phase of the lysis procedure. It is also possible to do 5-min incubation with cycloheximide before harvest: this will usually yield slightly more ribosomes per mRNA, but it can give misleading results, since it is known to cause a pileup of ribosomes near the initiation codon.
5. This is available from PerkinElmer; a mix of [^{35}S]-methionine and cysteine is also sold. The half-life is 87 days, so the reagent can be used for at least 3 months before you need to order a new batch. It is, nevertheless, a good idea to plan all the experiments that you want to do before ordering the label because it is expensive.
6. If you have very steady hands it is also possible to omit the freezing step. For this, put the 15% sucrose in first. Then, using a long Pasteur pipette, take up the next densest layer. Without any bubbles, place the pipette into this layer and gently expel the denser sucrose. It should drop to the bottom. Repeat until all the layers have been made. You should be able to see the layers by holding the tube up to the light.
7. If you do not have a fractionator: Using a 1 ml micropipette, carefully take off successive 250 μl fractions from the top meniscus of the gradient. Do not measure the optical density using cuvettes because of the risk of RNase contamination.

8. The baseline has to be set individually. Usually a baseline between 20 and 40 is fine. If you expect a high monosomal peak, for example, you have to set it to a lower value (e.g., 10). If the baseline is too low, you will lose the low signals.
9. For pulse-chase measurements the labeling time can be extended to 1 h.
10. Full medium contains a considerable excess of amino acids, so it is not necessary to add more. Ideally, the radioactive culture should be diluted directly into full medium, since this results in minimal disturbance to the cells: centrifugation is in itself stressful. However, this does increase the volume of radioactive waste. Prolonged incubation of the cells in microfuge tubes will result in anaerobic conditions, which impair growth of both bloodstream and procyclic forms.

Acknowledgments

Work by Kathryn Bajak is supported by the Deutsche Forschungsgemeinschaft (DFG), grant Cl112/24 to C. Clayton.

References

1. McGlincy N, Ingolia N (2017) Transcriptome-wide measurement of translation by ribosome profiling. Methods 126:112–129
2. Vasquez JJ, Hon CC, Vanselow JT, Schlosser A, Siegel TN (2014) Comparative ribosome profiling reveals extensive translational complexity in different *Trypanosoma brucei* life cycle stages. Nucleic Acids Res 42:3623–3637
3. Jensen BC, Ramasamy G, Vasconcelos EJ, Ingolia NT, Myler PJ, Parsons M (2014) Extensive stage-regulation of translation revealed by ribosome profiling of *Trypanosoma brucei*. BMC Genomics 15:911
4. Antwi E, Haanstra J, Ramasamy G, Jensen B, Droll D, Rojas F, Minia I, Terrao M, Mercé C, Matthews K et al (2016) Integrative analysis of the *Trypanosoma brucei* gene expression cascade predicts differential regulation of mRNA processing and unusual control of ribosomal protein expression. BMC Genomics 17:306
5. Schott J, Reitter S, Philipp J, Haneke K, Schafer H, Stoecklin G (2014) Translational regulation of specific mRNAs controls feedback inhibition and survival during macrophage activation. PLoS Genet 10:e1004368
6. Mugo E, Clayton C (2017) Expression of the RNA-binding protein RBP10 promotes the bloodstream-form differentiation state in *Trypanosoma brucei*. PLoS Pathog 13:e1006560
7. Minia I, Merce C, Terrao M, Clayton C (2016) Translation regulation and RNA granule formation after heat shock of procyclic form *Trypanosoma brucei*: many heat-induced mRNAs are increased during differentiation to mammalian-infective forms. PLoS Negl Trop Dis 10:e0004982
8. Djikeng A, Shi H, Tschudi C, Shen S, Ullu E (2003) An siRNA ribonucleoprotein is found associated with polyribosomes in Trypanosoma brucei. RNA 9:802–808
9. Richter JD, Coller J (2015) Pausing on polyribosomes: make way for elongation in translational control. Cell 163:292–300
10. Ingolia N, Lareau L, Weissman J (2011) Ribosome profiling of mouse embryonic stem cells reveals the complexity and dynamics of mammalian proteomes. Cell 147:789–802
11. Krstin S, Peixoto HS, Wink M (2015) Combinations of alkaloids affecting different molecular targets with the saponin digitonin can synergistically enhance trypanocidal activity against Trypanosoma brucei brucei. Antimicrob Agents Chemother 59:7011–7017
12. Clamer M, Tebaldi T, Lauria F, Bernabo P, Gomez-Biagi RF, Marchioretto M, Kandala DT, Minati L, Perenthaler E, Gubert D et al

(2018) Active ribosome profiling with RiboLace. Cell Rep 25:1097–1108. e1095

13. Minia I, Clayton C (2016) Regulating a post-transcriptional regulator: protein phosphorylation, degradation and translational blockage in control of the trypanosome stress-response RNA-binding protein ZC3H11. PLoS Pathog 12:e1005514
14. Gale M Jr, Carter V, Parsons M (1994) Translational control mediates the developmental regulation of the Trypanosoma brucei Nrk protein kinase. J Biol Chem 269:31659–31665
15. Begolo D, Vincent I, Giordani F, Pöhner I, Witty M, Rowan T, Bengaly Z, Gillingwater K, Freund Y, Wade R et al (2018) The trypanocidal benzoxaborole AN7973 inhibits trypanosome mRNA processing. PLoS Pathog 14:e1007315
16. Terrao M, Kamanyi Marucha K, Mugo E, Droll D, Minia I, Egler F, Braun J, Clayton C (2018) The suppressive cap-binding-complex factor 4EIP is required for normal differentiation. Nucleic Acids Res 46:8993–9010
17. Kuo T, Lew MJ, Mayba O, Harris CA, Speed TP, Wang JC (2012) Genome-wide analysis of glucocorticoid receptor-binding sites in myotubes identifies gene networks modulating insulin signaling. Proc Natl Acad Sci U S A 109:11160–11165
18. Schmidt EK, Clavarino G, Ceppi M, Pierre P (2009) SUnSET, a nonradioactive method to monitor protein synthesis. Nat Methods 6:275–277
19. Aviner R, Geiger T, Elroy-Stein O (2014) Genome-wide identification and quantification of protein synthesis in cultured cells and whole tissues by puromycin-associated nascent chain proteomics (PUNCH-P). Nat Protoc 9:751–760
20. Luthe DS (1983) A simple technique for the preparation and storage of sucrose gradients. Anal Biochem 135:230–232
21. Dieterich DC, Hodas JJ, Gouzer G, Shadrin IY, Ngo JT, Triller A, Tirrell DA, Schuman EM (2010) In situ visualization and dynamics of newly synthesized proteins in rat hippocampal neurons. Nat Neurosci 13:897–905
22. Cristodero M, Böttcher B, Diepholz M, Scheffzeck K, Clayton C (2008) The exosome of *Leishmania tarentolae*: purification and structural analysis by electron microscopy. Mol Biochem Parasitol 159:24–29

Chapter 8

Immunoprecipitation for the Analysis of Macromolecular Complexes in *Trypanosoma cruzi*

Bruno Accioly Alves Romagnoli, Samuel Goldenberg, and Lysangela Ronalte Alves

Abstract

Immunoprecipitation is a helpful tool to assess interactions between proteins and proteins or nucleic acids (DNA or RNA). Its principle consists in capturing and enriching one or multiple target proteins from a complex sample with a specific antibody conjugated to a solid matrix and isolating the RNA and/or protein molecules associated to those target(s) group of proteins that can be further identified by advanced techniques such as RNA-seq and/or mass spectrometry. Since this technique allows for identifying, mapping, and checking new protein–protein and protein–RNA interactions, its use is very convenient in situations where many proteins remain with their functions uncharacterized, as is the case of the protozoan *Trypanosoma cruzi*. Here we describe a protocol that is based on the cryogrinding method for cell lysis and the use of antibodies conjugated to magnetic beads to capture and purify protein complexes in a robust and efficient way.

Key words Immunoprecipitation, Cryogrinding, Magnetic beads, *Trypanosoma cruzi*, Protein complexes

1 Introduction

Immunoprecipitation is a technique that relies on the interaction between a specific antibody and its antigen (e.g., a protein of interest) to find and recover proteins from complex samples, such as a cell lysate. Since proteins establish interactions and can form a great variety of complexes with other molecules (e.g., proteins and/or RNAs), when immunoprecipitated, the target protein can serve as a bait for capturing subsets of proteins and/or RNAs that are interacting (in a direct or indirect manner) with it.

Briefly, this technique can be divided into the following steps: cell lysis and extraction of proteins/RNAs; purification/enrichment of the target proteins from a pool sample; and elution of the associated proteins/RNAs candidates.

Paul A. M. Michels et al. (eds.), *Trypanosomatids: Methods and Protocols*, Methods in Molecular Biology, vol. 2116, https://doi.org/10.1007/978-1-0716-0294-2_8,

Since many of these interactions can be highly dynamic (especially the ones involving RNAs) it is essential to optimize the cell lysis and extraction conditions to preserve these associations. The rupture of the cellular membrane and release of its internal content can be achieved by either mechanical or nonmechanical ways [1]. An example of a nonmechanical method for cell rupture prior to immunoprecipitation is the use of buffers containing a nonionic detergent (e.g., Nonidet® P40, Triton® X-100, Tween® 20) to permeabilize the cell membrane. Despite the ability of this nonionic component to break lipid–lipid interactions efficiently, its action can also disrupt interactions between proteins and RNAs and result in release of components from complexes. On the other hand, the mechanical lysis approach lacks the chemical-associated interference and uses only shear force to rupture the cell membrane. One of the mechanical lysis methods, bead mill, consists in using small beads (dense spheres made of glass, steel, or ceramic) and make them roll over the cells at high speed to provoke complete membrane disruption and subsequent cell content release. Since there is a lot of friction from these collisions between beads and cells, high heat can be generated in this process which may lead to disruption of molecular interactions and eventually protein and RNA degradation [1].

To preserve the complexes from heat damage, a more recently developed mechanical method called cryogrinding is being efficiently used in immunoprecipitations approaches, including for *Trypanosoma cruzi* [2–4]. The cryogrinding approach for trypanosomes was first described as a highly efficient method to isolate protein complexes from the nuclear envelope [4]. Briefly, this method is based on the bead mill strategy but, instead of letting the friction lead to heat, it maintains the sample temperature very low by the presence of liquid nitrogen during the cell lysis process. This milling processing at low temperature coupled with a frozen sample preparation (also with liquid nitrogen) maximizes the maintenance of the macromolecular complexes and increases the protection against potential destabilizing factors such as proteases and nucleases at the time of harvest [4, 5]. At the end of this processing, a freeze cell powder is generated that can be promptly thawed in a desirable buffer for protein extract preparation and afterward the protein purification/enrichment step [6].

Immunoprecipitation can be performed with antibodies linked to different sets of columns, resins, or beads. Here we describe the method that uses antibodies conjugated to magnetic beads due to the benefits presented by this approach. Accordingly, conjugation with magnetic beads allows one to effortlessly and efficiently capture the beads and its ligands (antibodies and their target molecules) using a simple magnetic field device like a magnetic separation stand [7]. This magnetic separation also renders easiest the rinsing procedures and does not require columns or centrifugation steps. After washing out the contaminants, the purified complexes can be eluted and used for further applications. Another advantage of using magnetic beads includes its large surface area-to-volume ratio as consequence of their small size (2.8 μm) and, since the antibody binding occurs on the bead surface, there is no theoretical limitation regarding the size of bound complexes [6, 8].

2 Materials

Important: Please be aware of the safety procedures for each equipment and potentially dangerous materials and reagents used in the described protocol. Keep yourself always updated with the Material Safety Data Sheets and your institute's health regulations to prevent accidents.

All solutions should be prepared using ultrapure water (resistivity of 18.2 MΩ·cm at 25 °C). We highly recommend using nuclease-free reagents and materials (e.g., tubes and tips), especially when RNAs associated candidates are being studied.

2.1 Materials

Cryoprotective gloves.

Dry ice.

Microcentrifuge tubes.

Falcon 50 mL conical centrifuge tubes.

Ice.

Insulated container.

Large tweezers.

Liquid nitrogen.

Magnetic separation stand.

Pipette with 1000-μL tips.

Pipette with 200-μL tips.

Retsch grinding jars.

Safety goggles.

Spatula.

Steel milling balls.

Sterile culture flasks.

Styrofoam rack.

2.2 Reagents

3 M ammonium sulfate solution

Antibody*.

Bead resuspension buffer: 0.1 M sodium phosphate buffer, pH 7.4.

Table 1
Extraction buffer composition (suggestion as a starting point)

20 mM HEPES, pH 7.4, 50 mM sodium citrate, 0.1% CHAPS or 0.5% Triton X-100
20 mM HEPES, pH 7.4, 150 mM sodium citrate, 0.1% CHAPS or 0.5% Triton X-100
20 mM HEPES, pH 7.4, 250 mM sodium citrate, 0.1% CHAPS or 0.5% Triton X-100
20 mM HEPES, pH 7.4, 50 mM sodium chloride, 0.1% CHAPS or 0.5% Triton X-100
20 mM HEPES, pH 7.4, 150 mM sodium chloride, 0.1% CHAPS or 0.5% Triton X-100
20 mM HEPES, pH 7.4, 250 mM sodium chloride, 0.1% CHAPS or 0.5% Triton X-100
Salt concentration will define buffer stringency from low (≤50 mM) to high (≥150 mM)
All buffers should be supplemented with protease and RNase inhibitors to prevent protein and RNA degradation

Elution buffer: 2% SDS and 20 mM Tris–HCl, pH 8.0.

Extraction buffer (*see* Table 1 for suggestions).

LIT (liver infusion tryptose) medium supplemented with 10% heat-inactivated FBS (fetal bovine serum).

Magnetic beads.

Protease and RNase inhibitors.

Sterile PBS (Phosphate buffered saline) 1×.

*Each antibody will depend on a specific approach, but this immunoprecipitation methodology is compatible with mono or polyclonal antibodies against native proteins and epitope/fusion tags (e.g., FLAG, GFP, HA, and Myc).

2.3 Equipment

Cryogenic grinding equipment (Retsch mixer mill MM 400).

Rotating shaker.

Thermomixer.

Microtip sonicator.

3 Methods

3.1 Cell Preparation

1. Cultivate *T. cruzi* epimastigotes forms to a density of 2–3 × 10^7 parasites mL^{-1} in culture flasks containing LIT medium supplemented with 10% FBS at 28 °C. (For suggested volumes *see* **Note 1**).
2. Harvest the parasites at 5000 × *g* for 5 min in a precooled centrifuge at 4 °C.
3. Wash cells twice with sterile PBS 1×.

4. Resuspend cells in 15 mL of PBS 1× plus protease inhibitors cocktail.
5. Transfer cells to a 50 mL Falcon tube and centrifuge at 3000 × *g* for 10 min.
6. While centrifuging, place another 50 mL Falcon tube in a Styrofoam rack and fill it with liquid nitrogen approximately half of its capacity (20–30 mL) and wait for the temperature stabilization. Keep it open to prevent tube explosion due to high nitrogen pressure.
7. Discard the supernatant from centrifuged cells (**step 5**) and resuspend them in the residual PBS solution and drip the cell pellet using a 200 μL micropipette into the liquid nitrogen-containing Falcon tube (*see* **Note 2**).
8. After completely dripping the cells, close the Falcon tube with a predrilled cap and place it on dry ice to allow for complete liquid nitrogen evaporation.
9. Store the frozen cells at −80 °C until needed for cryogrinding.

3.2 Cell Lysis

The protocol of cryogrinding in trypanosomes was adapted by Obado et al. [4] from yeast [6] and mammalian cells [9]. Here we briefly describe it with few modifications:

1. Precool the disassembled Retsch grinding jars and the steel milling balls with liquid nitrogen within an insulated container.
2. Once cooled, remove all components from the liquid nitrogen using tweezers.
3. Put the frozen cells into the assembled and cooled grinding jar.
4. Clamp down the grinding jar following the manufacturer's instructions. (For more detailed instructions see the equipment manual at https://www.retsch.com/products/milling/ball-mills/mixer-mill-mm-400/information-downloads/.)
5. Set the mixer mill MM 400 to mill the frozen material at a frequency of 30 Hz for 2 min.
6. Repeat **step 5** five times, cooling the assembled grinding jar in liquid nitrogen between each cycle.
7. Unclamp and remove the grinding jar from the equipment and carefully open it and transfer the grindate into a precooled 50 mL Falcon tube using a spatula.
8. Store milled powder until needed at −80 °C.

3.3 Bead Preparation

The following protocol is designed to use with the Dynabeads ™ M-270 Epoxy (Invitrogen), but it can also be adapted for other magnetic beads, respecting the respective manufacturer's specifications. Here we suggest using Dynabeads ™ M-270 Epoxy, based on the feedback from our colleagues and our own experience.

1. In a microcentrifuge tube weight out and resuspend 5 mg of lyophilized beads in 1 mL bead resuspension buffer.
2. Vortex the bead-containing solution for 30 s and incubate in a rotating shaker for 10 min.
3. Place the tube in a magnetic separation stand for 1 min (or until solution total clearance, what happens first) and discard the supernatant.
4. Remove the tube from the magnetic stand and resuspend the beads in 1 mL bead resuspension buffer.
5. Repeat the **steps 2** and **3** and proceed to the antibody conjugation step.

For antibody conjugation, 5 mg of beads (~3.3×10^8) can couple up to 100 μg of ligand. Calculate the ligand volume based on its concentration to maintain the proportion 1:1:1 of ligand volume, the beads in resuspension buffer and the 3 M ammonium sulfate solution. As recommended by the manufacturer, the final ammonium sulfate concentration for a conventional reaction is 1 M.

1. Resuspend the captured beads from the last step in the same volume of the bead resuspension buffer as calculated for the antibody volume and mix or vortex.
2. Add the antibody-containing solution (maintaining the volume proportion) and mix or vortex.
3. Slowly add the same volume of the 3 M ammonium sulfate solution (should correspond to 1/3 of total final volume). Do it slowly to avoid protein precipitation.
4. Incubate for at least 16 h at 30 °C on a rotation shaker.
5. Place the tube on the magnetic stand for 1 min (or until solution total clearance, what happens first) and remove the supernatant.
6. Wash the antibody-conjugated beads with 1 mL of PBS resuspending the beads, capturing them with the magnetic stand and removing the supernatant as performed in previously steps.
7. Repeat **step 6** four times and then resuspend the coated beads to the desired concentration. For instance, starting this procedure with 5 mg (~3.3×10^8) and resuspended it in a volume of 100 μL should result in a bead concentration of ~3.3×10^9 beads mL^{-1}.
8. Store the coupled beads at −20 °C or proceed directly to the immunoprecipitation step.

3.4 Immunoprecipitation

Here we describe a generic protocol based on already published protocols [3, 4, 10]. We will not get into further details since our intention is only to provide a starting point. Since every protein–protein and protein–RNA complex may interact and stabilize with different affinities and under different conditions, we strongly recommend testing different immunoprecipitation conditions to determine an optimized protocol setting. It is important to have in mind when designing your experiment that efficient isolation of target protein complexes depends on bead concentration, target concentration, antibody affinity, and time.

1. Remove the Falcon tube with the cell powder (Subheading 3.2, **step 8**) from the −80 °C freezer and place it in an insulated container containing liquid nitrogen. Use a support (e.g., Styrofoam rack) to maintain the Falcon standing still.
2. Weight out 50 mg of cell powder into a prechilled microcentrifuge tube and incubate on ice until it gets close to thawing (*see* **Note 3**).
3. Resuspend the grindate by vortexing and/or pipetting up and down in 1 mL extraction buffer containing protease and RNase inhibitors at room temperature.
4. After resuspending the cell powder, sonicate on ice with a microtip sonicator to guarantee complete resuspension. One pulse at 30% is sufficient to break apart remaining aggregates.
5. Centrifuge at 20,000 × *g* for 10 min at 4 °C to obtain a clarified cell lysate.
6. Recover the supernatant and incubate with the magnetic beads (previously coupled) for 1 h at 4 °C under constant stirring.
7. Wash the magnetic beads three times with the extraction buffer, always capturing the magnetic beads with the magnetic stand and removing the supernatant between each wash.
8. Transfer the magnetic beads to an identified new microcentrifuge tube and place it on the magnetic stand again to remove the supernatant.
9. Elute the ligands from the antibody-conjugated beads with the elution buffer and place it on a thermomixer device at 72 °C for 20 min.

4 Notes

1. According to the cryogrinding protocol first established for trypanosomes by Obado et al. [4], the authors recommend an amount of cells in the magnitude order of 10^{10} to perform the cryomilling procedure as a way to guarantee a good-sized

cell pellet, since during the processing there are losses of material. To achieve that with a 2×10^7 parasites mL^{-1} density, one should prepare a culture of at least 500 mL.

2. In this condition, cells are quickly frozen as soon as they got near the liquid nitrogen so beware not to get to close from it with the tip, otherwise it will also freeze. Remember to do this procedure within a safe distance.
3. Up to 1 g of cell powder can be used according to the expression level of your target protein. As suggested by Obado et al. [4], 50 mg of cell power corresponds to a good amount of material to perform the protocol optimization (e.g., buffers compositions, proportion of cell powder and conjugated beads, and binding conditions.)

References

1. Islam MS, Aryasomayajula A, Selvaganapathy PR (2017) A review on macroscale and microscale cell lysis methods. Micromachines (Basel) 8(3):83
2. Kalb LC, Frederico YCA, Boehm C, Moreira CMDN, Soares MJ, Field MC (2016) Conservation and divergence within the clathrin interactome of *Trypanosoma cruzi*. Sci Rep 6:31212. https://doi.org/10.1038/srep31212
3. Wippel HH, Inoue AH, Vidal NM, da Costa JF, Marcon BH, Romagnoli BAA, Santos MDM, Carvalho PC, Goldenberg S, Alves LR (2018) Assessing the partners of the RBP9-mRNP complex in Trypanosoma cruzi using shotgun proteomics and RNA-seq. RNA Biol 15(8):1106–1118
4. Obado SO, Field MC, Chait BT, Rout MP (2016) High-efficiency isolation of nuclear envelope protein complexes from trypanosomes. In: Shackleton S, Collas P, Schirmer EC (eds) The nuclear envelope: methods and protocols, methods in molecular biology, vol 1411. Springer, New York, NY, pp 67–80
5. Field MC, Adung'A V, Obado S, Chait BT, Rout MP (2012) Proteomics on the rims: insights into the biology of the nuclear envelope and flagellar pocket of trypanosomes. Parasitology 139(9):1158–1167
6. Oeffinger M, Wei KE, Rogers R, DeGrasse JA, Chait BT, Aitchison JD, Rout MP (2007) Comprehensive analysis of diverse ribonucleoprotein complexes. Nat Methods 4 (11):951–956
7. Safarik I, Safarikova M (2004) Magnetic techniques for the isolation and purification of proteins and peptides. Biomagn Res Technol 2 (1):7
8. LaCava J, Molloy KR, Taylor MS, Domanski M, Chait BT, Rout MP (2015) Affinity proteomics to study endogenous protein complexes: pointers, pitfalls, preferences and perspectives. BioTechniques 58 (3):103–119
9. Domanski M, Molloy K, Jiang H, Chait B, Rout M, Jensen T, LaCava J (2012) Improved methodology for the affinity isolation of human protein complexes expressed at near endogenous levels. BioTechniques 109 (10):4580–4595
10. Kalb LC, Frederico YCA, Batista CM, Eger I, Fragoso SP, Soares MJ (2014) Clathrin expression in Trypanosoma cruzi. BMC Cell Biol 15:23. https://doi.org/10.1186/1471-2121-15-23

Chapter 9

Analysis of the In Vivo Translation Process in *Trypanosoma cruzi* Using Ribosome Profiling

Saloe Bispo Poubel, Fabiola Barbieri Holetz, Bruno Accioly Alves Romagnoli, Samuel Goldenberg, and Lysangela Ronalte Alves

Abstract

The technique of ribosome profiling is based on the isolation of sequences around 30 nucleotides in size protected by mRNA-associated ribosomes, following digestion with specific nucleases, generating a footprint. After isolation and purification, these 30-nucleotide sequences are converted to a cDNA library and analyzed by deep sequencing, providing a high-precision picture of the translation process in vivo. In addition, this powerful technique allows for the study of several biological phenomena such as alternative splicing, alternative codon usage and initiation of translation by non-AUG codons. Furthermore, the ribosome footprinting technique has proved to be very efficient for studies of ribosome pause sites on mRNAs, which could act as key regulators in the translation process. Here we describe a modified protocol of the ribosome footprinting technique for translation efficiency analysis in *Trypanosoma cruzi*.

Key words Ribosome profiling, *Trypanosoma cruzi*, Translatome

1 Introduction

The ability to detect changes in gene expression is essential for understanding the genetic determinants and molecular responses of the cell to different conditions. For several years, many studies have been carried out to identify the mechanisms involved in the regulation of gene expression in *Trypanosoma cruzi*. It is nowadays clear that posttranscriptional mechanisms play a major role in all steps of the parasite's life cycle. In this regard, the processes related to the storage, degradation, and mobilization of mRNAs to the translation machinery are key players in differential gene expression [1–6].

Although the isolation of polyribosomes was established several years ago, the capacity to identify and quantify the mRNAs actively engaged in translation was possible only recently, by the technique

Paul A. M. Michels et al. (eds.), *Trypanosomatids: Methods and Protocols*, Methods in Molecular Biology, vol. 2116, https://doi.org/10.1007/978-1-0716-0294-2_9,

of "ribosome footprinting" developed by Ingolia and collaborators in 2009 [7]. This technique relies on the generation of a profile of mRNAs associated to the translation machinery, by capturing the position of the ribosomes on the mRNA molecules. The mapping of the transcripts effectively associated with ribosomes provides a high-precision measurement of the translation process in vivo [7–9]. It allows for, for example, the study of alternative splicing [10], investigation of alternative initiation codons usage [11–13], and internal ribosome entry sites [14]. In addition, the ribosome footprinting technique is very efficient for studies of ribosome pause sites on mRNAs that could act as key regulators in the translation process [8].

2 Materials

Important. Please stay always updated with the Material Safety Data Sheets and the safety procedures of your facility. Always use protection equipment when manipulating biologicals and potentially dangerous materials or reagents used in this protocol.

All reactions should be prepared using ultrapure nuclease-free water (resistivity of 18.2 MΩ·cm at 25 °C), and we highly recommend using nuclease-free reagents and materials (e.g., tubes and tips) to avoid contamination with nucleases. These precautions significantly reduce the risk of RNA degradation.

2.1 Materials

Microcentrifuge 0.2 mL tubes.

Microcentrifuge 1.7 mL tubes.

Centrifuge 15 mL tubes.

Ice.

Pipette with 10-μL tips.

Pipette with 1000-μL tips.

Pipette with 200-μL tips.

Ultracentrifuge tubes.

0.22 μm micron filter column.

2.2 Reagents

Hypotonic buffer (NKM): 140 mM NaCl, 5 mM KCl, and 1.5 mM $MgCl_2$, to be chilled to 4 °C before use ethanol (EtOH).

LIT (liver infusion tryptose) medium supplemented with 10% heat-inactivated fetal bovine serum (FBS).

2 M sucrose in NKM buffer, supplemented with 5 mM β-mercaptoethanol (final concentration) and 10 μg/mL heparin.

UltraPure™ TBE Buffer, 10× (Invitrogen™).

300 mM sodium acetate (NaOAc).

TRIzol® Reagent (*see* **Note 1**).

10% Nonidet™ (NP-40).

10 mg/mL cycloheximide.

14.7 M β-mercaptoethanol (pure liquid).

20 U/μL SUPERase In™ RNase Inhibitor.

Chloroform (*see* **Note 2**).

RNase I 10 U/μL.

GlycoBlue™ (Ambion®) 15 mg/mL.

10 mg/mL heparin.

2.3 Equipment

Microcentrifuge.

Optical microscope.

Ultracentrifuge.

NanoDrop 2000/2000c Spectrophotometer or similar apparatus.

Agilent 2100 Bioanalyzer system.

3 Methods

3.1 Cell Culture

1. Culture *T. cruzi* epimastigote forms to the late exponential phase, at a density of 2–3 × 10^7 parasites mL^{-1}, with less than 0.1% of metacyclic cells, in culture flasks containing 100 mL of LIT medium supplemented with 10% FBS, grown at 28 °C.
2. Add cycloheximide to a final concentration of 100 μg/mL to the LIT culture flask containing 2.5 × 10^9 cells and incubate for 10 min at 28 °C.
3. Collect the cells by centrifugation at 7000 × *g* at 4 °C for 5 min.
4. Aspirate the culture medium, rinse the cells twice with 5 mL NKM buffer, supplemented with 100 μg/mL cycloheximide.

3.2 Cell Lysis

1. Resuspend the cells in 9 mL of NKM to which is added 1% NP-40 from the 10% stock solution, β-mercaptoethanol to an 8% final concentration and 10 μg/mL heparin. Pipet up and down to aid lysis.
2. Lysis must be followed by optical microscopy (the nucleus remains intact). Stop lysis by the addition of 2 M sucrose to a 0.25 mM final concentration.

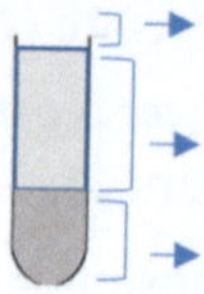

Fig. 1 Lysate sample is layered gently on the top of the sucrose cushion. Under centrifugal force, heavy polysomes move through the sucrose cushion and are pelleted at the bottom of the tubes, while cell constituents with a lighter mass remain on top of the cushion

3. Centrifuge at 10,000 × *g*, at 4 °C for 30 min for cell debris removal.
4. Transfer the lysate to a 15 mL chilled centrifuge tube.

3.3 Polysome Isolation

1. Add 2 mL of the 2 M sucrose solution, remembering that β-mercaptoethanol and heparin must be added at the time of use (*see* Subheading 2.2), into RNase-free Open-Top Thickwall tubes on ice, to form a cushion for centrifugation (Fig. 1) (*see* **Note 3**).
2. Load gently 9 mL of the lysate onto the sucrose cushion. Polysomes are obtained by centrifugation for 2 h at 365,000 × *g*, 4 °C.

3.4 Digestion

Carefully remove the tubes from the ultracentrifuge, to avoid disturbing the pellet.

1. Aspirate the supernatant and the sucrose cushion carefully not to remove the pellet.
2. Leave the tube upside down for 3 min at room temperature, to remove all remaining sucrose that could interfere with enzymatic activity.
3. Resuspend the pellet in 400 μL NKM buffer, transfer the suspension to a new microcentrifuge tube and add 60 U RNase I. Incubate for 45 min at 25 °C. Stop the digestion by the addition of 10 μL SUPERase In, or immediate extract RNA fragments with TRIzol.

3.5 Ribosome Footprinting Isolation

We strongly recommend the extraction of the RNA fragments with TRIzol immediately after the digestion.

1. Add an equal volume of TRIzol to the digested lysate.
2. Vortex samples and incubate for 5 min to permit dissociation of the nucleoprotein complex.
3. Add 100 μL of chloroform, cap the tube, and incubate for 2 min.
4. Centrifuge the sample for 15 min at 12,000 × *g* at 4 °C and transfer the aqueous phase to a fresh tube.

5. Precipitate the RNA with 1 μL GlycoBlue, 1/10 volume 3 M NaOAc pH 5.2, and 2 volumes of chilled 100% EtOH; keep at −80 °C overnight.
6. After precipitation, pellet the fragmented RNA in a microcentrifuge for 30 min at 4 °C by full-speed centrifugation.
7. Wash the pellet twice using 1 mL of 80% EtOH and centrifuge the sample for 15 min at 4 °C by full-speed centrifugation and air-dry it.
8. Resuspend the pellet in 25 μL nuclease-free water and measure the RNA concentration using a NanoDrop Spectrophotometer.

3.6 RNA Size Selection

Samples are size-separated by gel electrophoresis on a 10% denaturing polyacrylamide gel.

1. Add 6% urea, 10 mL water, 9.8 mL 40% polyacrylamide solution, 4 mL 10× TBE, 20 μL TEMED and 1 mL 10% ammonium persulfate (APS) to a large gel plate of 20 cm × 22 cm × 1.0 mm.
2. We use oligonucleotides with different sizes (30, 35 nt) and a 25 bp RNA Ladder, to facilitate the precise determination of the ribosome protected mRNA fragments (RPF) fraction in the gel.
3. After electrophoresis, excise from the gel the sample region corresponding to the 30 nt position, corresponding to the size of the ribosome protection onto the mRNA molecule (Fig. 2).

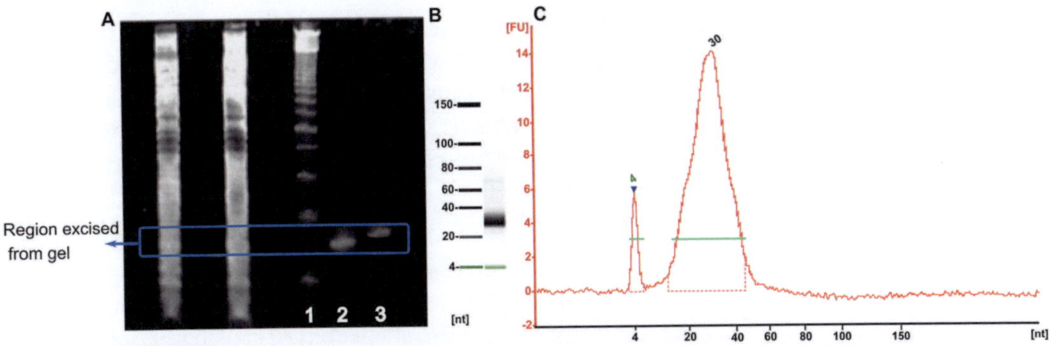

Fig. 2 Size selection and gel extraction of ribosome-protected mRNA fragments (RPF). (**a**) The RNA obtained through the ribosome profiling protocol was subjected to polyacrylamide–urea gel electrophoresis (6%) (180 V, 320 mA). Oligonucleotides and RNA Ladder with sizes close to the RPF fraction are used to determine the exact position in the gel to be excised (~30 nts). We used a 25 bp RNA Ladder (Invitrogen) (A, column 1), oligonucleotides with 25 nucleotides (A, column 2), and oligonucleotides with 30 nucleotides (A, column 3). The RPF was purified and analyzed on an Agilent 2100 Bioanalyzer, Small RNA electrophoresis with the 2100 Bioanalyzer System (**b** and **c**) and corresponds to fragments of approximately 30 nucleotides

4. Put the excised sample in a 0.2 mL microtube with a hole (puncture the bottom of a sterile, nuclease-free, 0.2 mL microcentrifuge tube 1–2 times with a 21-gauge needle), assemble this tube in a 1.7 mL microcentrifuge tube and centrifuge at 1500 × *g* for 10 min or until the entire gel fragment has passed into a 1.7 mL microcentrifuge tube.
5. Add 100 μL of nuclease-free water and heat the sample at 70 °C for 10 min.
6. Filter the sample containing RNA/acrylamide in 0.22 μm Microcon filter and spin it at 8000 × *g* for 2 min to collect the eluted RNA sample.
7. Precipitate the RNA with 1 μL GlycoBlue, 1/10 volume 3 M NaOAc pH 5.2, and 2 volumes of 100% EtOH, and keep it at −80 °C overnight.
8. After precipitation, pellet the RNA corresponding to the RPF in a microcentrifuge for 60 min at 4 °C by full-speed centrifugation.
9. Discard the supernatant carefully and wash the pellet once using 1 mL of 80% EtOH.
10. Centrifuge the sample at full speed for 15 min at 4 °C and air-dry the pellet.
11. Dissolve the pellet into 20 μL nuclease-free water and analyze the size of the RNA fragments using the Agilent 2100 Bioanalyzer system, small RNA kit (Part Number: 5067-1548).

4 Notes

1. Caution: TRIzol™ Reagent is harmful if swallowed or in contact with the skin. It causes severe skin burns and eye damage, is fatal if inhaled, may cause respiratory irritation, suspected of causing genetic defects and may cause damage to organs through prolonged or repeated exposure. It should be used with appropriate safety measures, such as latex gloves and sufficient ventilation.
2. Caution: Chloroform is harmful if swallowed or in contact skin, causes severe skin burns and eye damage, is fatal if inhaled, may cause respiratory irritation, suspected of causing genetic defects and may cause damage to organs through prolonged or repeated exposure. It should be used with appropriate safety measures, such as latex gloves and sufficient ventilation.

   All waste should be handled according to hazardous waste regulations.

3. For polysomes purification through a sucrose cushion, we advise using of RNase-free Open-Top Thickwall tubes and maintaining the rotor buckets in a refrigerator prior to centrifugation, to prevent heating of the lysate, in order to avoid RNase action.

References

1. Avila AR, Dallagiovanna B, Yamada-Ogatta SF, Monteiro-Goes V, Fragoso SP, Krieger MA, Goldenberg S (2003) Stage-specific gene expression during *Trypanosoma cruzi* metacyclogenesis. Genet Mol Res 2(1):159–168. Review
2. Fragoso SP, Plazanet-Menut C, Carreira MA, Motta MC, Dallagiovana B, Krieger MA, Goldenberg S (2003) Cloning and characterization of a gene encoding a putative protein associated with U3 small nucleolar ribonucleoprotein in *Trypanosoma cruzi*. Mol Biochem Parasitol 126(1):113–117
3. Nardelli SC, Avila AR, Freund A, Motta MC, Manhães L, de Jesus TC, Schenkman S, Fragoso SP, Krieger MA, Goldenberg S, Dallagiovanna B (2007) Small subunit rRNA processome proteins are translationally regulated during differentiation of *Trypanosoma cruzi*. Eukaryot Cell 6(2):337–345
4. Holetz FB, Correa A, Ávila AR, Nakamura CV, Krieger MA, Goldenberg S (2007) Evidence of P-body-like structures in *Trypanosoma cruzi*. Biochem Biophys Res Commun 356:1062–1067
5. Holetz FB, Alves LR, Probst CM, Dallagiovanna B, Marchini FK, Manque P, Buck G, Krieger MA, Correa A, Goldenberg S (2010) Protein and mRNA content of TcDHH1-containing mRNPs in *Trypanosoma cruzi*. FEBS J 277:3415–3426
6. Costa JF, Ferrarini MG, Nardelli SC, Goldenberg S, Avila AR, Holetz FB (2018) *Trypanosoma cruzi* XRNA granules colocalise with distinct mRNP granules at the nuclear periphery. Mem Inst Oswaldo Cruz 113: e1705317
7. Ingolia NT, Ghaemmaghami S, Newman JR, Weissman JS (2009) Genome-wide analysis in vivo of translation with nucleotide resolution using ribosome profiling. Science 324:218–223
8. Ingolia NT, Lareau LF, Weissman JS (2011) Ribosome profiling of mouse embryonic stem cells reveals the complexity and dynamics of mammalian proteomes. Cell 147:789–802
9. Smircich P, Eastman G, Poubel S, Duhagon MA, Guerra-Slompo E, Garat B, Goldenberg S, Munroe DJ, Dallagiovanna B, Holetz F, Sotelo-Silveira JR (2015) Ribosome profiling reveals translation control as a key mechanism generating differential gene expression in *Trypanosoma cruzi*. BMC Genomics 16:443
10. Nilsen TW, Graveley BR (2010) Expansion of the eukaryotic proteome by alternative splicing. Nature 463(7280):457–463
11. Plotkin JB (2010) Transcriptional regulation is only half the story. Mol Syst Biol 6:406
12. Kolev NG, Franklin JB, Carmi S, Shi H, Michael S, Tschudi C (2010) The transcriptome of the human pathogen Trypanosoma brucei at single-nucleotide resolution. PLoS Pathog 6(9):1001090
13. Touriol C, Bornes S, Bonnal S, Audigier S, Prats H, Prats AC, Vagner S (2003) Generation of protein isoform diversity by alternative initiation of translation at non-AUG codons. Biol Cell 95(3–4):168–178
14. Vagner S, Galy B, Pyronnet S (2001) Irresistible IRES. Attracting the translation machinery to internal ribosome entry sites. EMBO Rep 2 (10):893–898

Chapter 10

Proteome-Wide Quantitative Phosphoproteomic Analysis of *Trypanosoma brucei* Insect and Mammalian Life Cycle Stages

Corinna Benz and Michael D. Urbaniak

Abstract

Mass spectrometry based proteomics allows for the identification and quantification of protein and phosphorylation site abundance on a proteome wide scale. Here we describe the metabolic labeling of cultured *Trypanosoma brucei* cells in either the bloodstream or procyclic life cycle stage using stable isotope labeling of amino acids in cell culture (SILAC), and the production of samples suitable for analysis by liquid chromatography tandem mass spectrometry. The protocols require little specialist equipment, and they typically enable quantification of over 4500 proteins and 9000 phosphorylation sites.

Key words *Trypanosoma brucei*, SILAC, High pH reverse phase, Proteomics, Phosphoproteomics

1 Introduction

The identification and quantification of phosphorylation site dynamics is a crucial component in the elucidation of signaling pathways and may also improve drug discovery efforts through improved candidate selection and detailed mode-of-action studies [1]. Recent advances in the field of mass spectrometry based phosphoproteomics have resulted in the routine identification and quantification of thousands of in vitro phosphorylation sites, generating evidence of dynamic phosphorylation in an unbiased, system-wide approach [2]. The increasing availability of commercial analytical services has allowed for the technique to be applied outside of specialist mass spectrometry laboratories.

Global phosphoproteomic experiments involve digesting proteins into peptides (typically with trypsin), enrichment of phosphopeptides, and fractionation before analysis by liquid chromatography–mass spectrometry (Fig. 1). The peptides and phosphopeptides are identified and quantified from the mass spectra and mapped to the intact protein by automated database

Paul A. M. Michels et al. (eds.), *Trypanosomatids: Methods and Protocols*, Methods in Molecular Biology, vol. 2116, https://doi.org/10.1007/978-1-0716-0294-2_10,

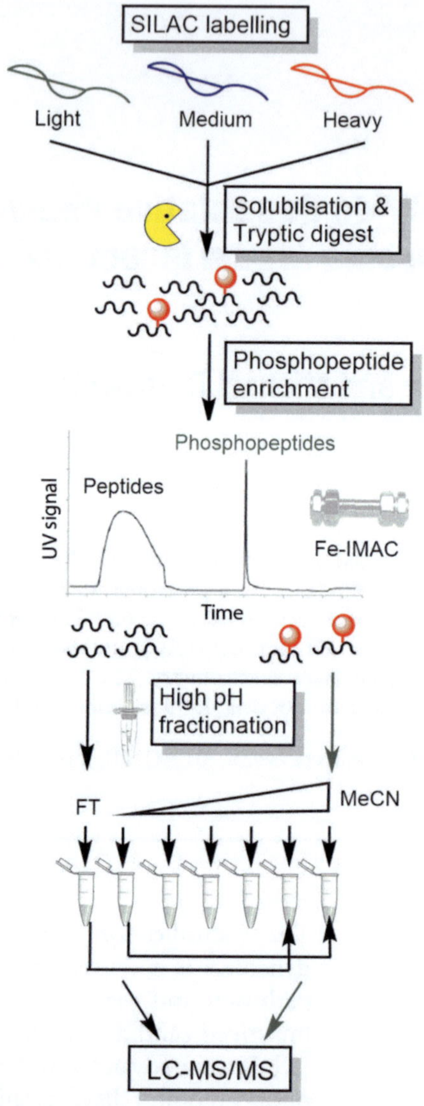

Fig. 1 Quantitative global proteomic and phosphoproteomic analysis of *T. brucei*. SILAC labeled cells are treated according to the experimental regimen, combined, and the proteins solubilized and subjected to tryptic digest. Phosphopeptides are enriched by Fe-IMAC, and recovered peptides and phosphopeptides processed in parallel using high pH fractionation to reduce sample complexity prior to analysis by liquid chromatography–tandem mass spectrometry

searching [3]. It is essential to enrich for phosphopeptides prior to analysis due to the low stoichiometry of phosphorylation and the poor ionization of phosphopeptides in the mass spectrometer. Measurement of both peptide and phosphopeptide abundance is important to distinguish whether changes occur at the level of protein or through a change in phosphorylation site occupancy.

Fractionation is required to reduce the sample complexity and ensure that low-abundance peptides and phosphopeptides can be detected, and results in improved depth of coverage. Although quantitation can be achieved in several ways [4], metabolic labeling achieved through stable isotope labeling of amino acids in cell culture (SILAC) provides high accuracy and reproducibility. SILAC has been applied to both the mammalian and insect form of *Trypanosoma brucei* [5–7], and to the insect forms of *Trypanosoma cruzi* [8] and *Leishmania* species [9]. If direct labeling of samples is unfeasible then spike-in SILAC may be used, where a heavy isotope labeled standard may be used to compare ex vivo or clinical samples [10].

2 Materials

For best results, all chemicals must be of the highest grade available, and ideally solvents should be of LC-MS grade. Where solutions must be made freshly, this is indicated in the text.

2.1 SILAC Labeling of Cultures and Cell Lysis

1. SILAC HMI-11T [6] (*see* **Note 1**): To 450 ml Iscove's Modified Dulbecco's Medium (IMDM) without L-arginine and L-lysine (Pierce) add the following ingredients in order with stirring: 55 mg Pyruvic acid (Na salt), 19.5 mg Thymidine, 14 mg Bathocuproinedisulphonic acid, 2.5 ml Hypoxanthine solution (1.36 g in 100 ml of 0.1 M NaOH, warm to dissolve, store at −20 °C), 50 ml dialyzed fetal calf serum (*see* **Note 2**), 5 ml 100× L-alanyl-L-glutamine. Adjust to pH 7.3–7.4 as required, filter-sterilize and incubate at 37 °C for >24 h prior to use to check for absence of microbial growth.
2. SILAC SDM-79 [5] (*see* **Note 3**): To 425 ml SDM-79 without L-arginine and L-lysine (custom synthesis) add the following ingredients in order with stirring: 375 μl Hemin stock (10 mg/ml in 0.1 M NaOH), 1 g Sodium bicarbonate, 75 ml dialyzed heat-inactivated fetal calf serum (*see* **Note 2**), 5 ml 100× L-alanyl-L-glutamine. Adjust to pH 7.3–7.4 as required, filter-sterilize and incubate at 37 °C for >24 h prior to use to check for absence of microbial growth.
3. SILAC medium that has been stability approved must be supplemented with either normal isotopic concentration of L-arginine and L-lysine (R0K0, light label), $^{13}C_6$ L-arginine and $^{2}H_4$ L-lysine (R6K4, medium label), or $^{13}C_6{}^{15}N_4$ L-arginine and $^{13}C_6{}^{15}N_2$ L-lysine (R10K8, heavy label) under sterile conditions. The heavy, medium, and light labels are used at 30% of standard concentrations as given in Table 1 (*see* **Note 4**).
4. Culture flasks (25 and 150 cm^2 surface area), nontreated.

Table 1
Quantities of stable isotope labeled L-arginine and L-lysine

Label (100 mg/ml, −20 °C)	Mw	HMI-11 (mg/L)	SDM-79 (mg/L)
L-Arg.HCl (R0)	210.6	25.3	64.5
L-Arg.HCl (R6-$^{13}C_6$)	216.6	25.8	66.3
L-Arg.HCl (R10-$^{13}C_6$,$^{15}N_4$)	220.6	26.2	67.5
L-Lys.HCl (K0)	182.6	43.8	21.6
L-Lys.2HCl (K4-$^{2}H_4$)	223.1	53.5	26.7
L-Lys.2HCl (K8-$^{13}C_4$,$^{15}N_4$)	227.1	54.5	27.3

5. Phosphate buffered saline (PBS): 137 mM NaCl, 2.7 mM KCl, 10 mM Na_2HPO_4, 1.5 mM KH_2PO_4.
6. Cell lysis buffer: 0.1 μM Tosyl phenylalanyl chloromethyl ketone (TLCK), 1 μg/ml leupeptin, 1× phosphatase inhibitor cocktail II (Calbiochem), 1 mM phenyl methyl sulfonyl fluoride (PMSF), 1 mM Benzamidine. Prepare fresh just prior to use; stocks of TLCK and leupeptin can be prepared and stored at −20 °C, but Benzamidine and PMSF (in dry isopropanol) must be freshly prepared each time.

2.2 Protein Solubilization and Tryptic Digest

1. Solubilisation buffer: 8% sodium dodecyl sulfate (SDS), 200 mM Tris pH 8.5, 200 mM dithiothreitol (DDT). Add DTT immediately before use.
2. Centrifugal filter devices: Vivaspin 20, 30 kDa molecular weight cutoff (Sartorius).
3. UA buffer: 8 M urea, 0.1 M Tris pH 8.5, prepared fresh on the day.
4. Iodoacetamide solution (IAA): 50 mM iodoacetamide in UA buffer, prepared immediately before use.
5. Ammonium bicarbonate (ABC): 50 mM ammonium bicarbonate, prepared fresh on the day.
6. Trypsin stock solution: MS grade Trypsin (Promega) at a concentration of 1 μg/μl in 50 mM acetic acid, store at −80 °C for up to a month.
7. Optional: SDS-PAGE gels, sample loading buffer, running buffer, and rapid Coomassie stain.

2.3 Desalting Using a C18 Column

1. Methanol.
2. C18 columns: Discovery DSC-18, 3 ml tubes (Supelco) or Micro Spin Columns (Harvard Apparatus).
3. C18 wash buffer: 0.1% trifluoroacetic acid (TFA).
4. C18 elution buffer: 0.1% TFA, 60% acetonitrile.

2.4 Fe-Immobilized Metal Ion Affinity Chromatography (Fe-IMAC)

All solutions should be filtered through a 0.2 μM membrane and degassed before use.

1. HPLC column: ProPac, IMAC-10, BioLC Guard, 4 × 50 mm (Thermo Scientific).
2. HPLC or FPLC capable of maintaining a flow rate of 1–200 μl/min, injecting 100 μl samples and UV monitoring at 280 nm, and collecting fractions every 2 min.
3. 20 mM formic acid (FA).
4. Iron charging solution: 25 mM $FeCl_3$ in 100 mM acetic acid.
5. 50 mM EDTA.
6. IMAC loading solvent: 30% acetonitrile, 0.07% TFA.
7. IMAC elution solvent: 30% acetonitrile, 0.5% NH_4OH.
8. LoBind protein 1.5 ml microcentrifuge tubes (Eppendorf).

2.5 High pH Fractionation

1. High pH Reversed-Phase Peptide Fractionation Kit (Pierce).
2. Elution buffers: 2%, 3%, 4%, 6%, 10%, and 50% acetonitrile in 5 mM NH_4OH. 1 ml of each is sufficient per peptide/phosphopeptide sample pair.
3. LoBind protein 1.5 ml microcentrifuge tubes (Eppendorf).

2.6 Liquid Chromatography–Tandem Mass Spectrometry (LC-MS/MS)

1. LC-MS/MS system: Ultimate U3000 Nano LC System (Dionex) coupled to an LTQ Orbitrap Velos Pro mass spectrometer (Thermo Scientific) equipped with a Proxeon nanospray ion source (*see* **Note 5**).
2. LC columns: 1 × 5 mm C_{18} trap column and a 75 μm × 15 cm reverse phase C_{18} nanocolumn.

2.7 Data Analysis

1. Proteomic processing software: MaxQuant [11], freeware available from the Max Plank Institute of Biochemistry.
2. Statistical software: Perseus [12], freeware available at from the Max Plank Institute of Biochemistry.

3 Methods

3.1 SILAC Labeling of Cultures and Cell Lysis

1. Culture bloodstream form (Bsf) in SILAC-HMI11-T at 37 °C, 5% CO_2, 100% humidity or procyclic form (Pcf) in SILAC-SDM-79 at 28 °C. Grow for more than seven cell divisions in the appropriate label before harvest of log-linear culture (*see* **Note 6**). *Optional—apply treatment as dictated by the experimental regimen* (*see* **Note 7**).
2. Harvest cells by centrifugation at 1000 × *g* for 10 min at 4 °C.
3. Remove the supernatant and resuspend the cell pellet in PBS.

4. Transfer cells to microfuge tube and harvest at full speed for 15 s.
5. Remove the supernatant, lyse cells at 1×10^9 cells/ml in freshly prepared ice-cold lysis buffer and incubate at room temperature for 5 min (*see* **Note 8**).
6. Divide into suitable aliquots and store at −80 °C.

3.2 Protein Solubilization and Digestion

1. Thaw cell lysates and combine according to the experimental design (i.e., equal number of light and heavy cells, or light, medium, and heavy cells) (*see* **Note 9**).
2. Add an equal volume of 2× solubilization buffer.
3. Vortex for 30 s, boil at 95 °C for 3 min, vortex again for 30 s, and sonicate for 3 min in a sonic bath. Repeat these steps if sample still viscous (*see* **Note 10**).
4. Spin at 16,000 × g for 10 min and discard the pellet. *Optional—Save a small sample of the supernatant for SDS-PAGE analysis (start sample).*
5. Dilute the remaining supernatant 1:6.6 with UA buffer and mix well by pipetting.
6. Transfer to a Vivaspin 6 column (30 kDa MWCO) and spin at 4000 × g for 60 min at RT or until the volume is ≤0.5 ml (*see* **Note 11**).
7. Add 6 ml UA and spin at 4000 × g for 60 min at RT until volume is ≤0.5 ml.
8. Add 3 ml IAA solution and mix for 1 min.
9. Incubate 20 min at RT in the dark without mixing. *Optional—Take a small sample for SDS-PAGE analysis (after IAA sample).*
10. Spin at 4000 × g for 45 min at RT until volume is ≤0.3 ml.
11. Add 3 ml UA and spin at 4000 × g for 45 min at RT until volume is ≤0.3 ml. Repeat twice.
12. Add 1.5 ml ABC and spin at 4000 × g for 30 min at RT until volume is about 0.3 ml. Repeat twice (*see* **Note 12**). *Optional—Save a small sample before tryptic digest for SDS-PAGE analysis (before trypsin sample).*
13. Add 600 μl ABC + 1:50 approximate ratio trypsin to protein.
14. Seal the filter tube with Parafilm and incubate for more than 18 h at 37 °C in an oven. *Optional—Following overnight digestion, take a small sample for SDS-PAGE analysis (after trypsin sample). Run all four protein samples on an SDS-PAGE gel and stain the gel with Coomassie to confirm that the amount of trypsin used is sufficient* (*see* **Note 13**).

15. If sample is completely digested, dilute it to a final volume of 3 ml with ABC buffer and remove from the spin column (*see* **Note 14**).
16. Add TFA to a final concentration of 0.1% and proceed with desalting.

3.3 Desalting Using a C18 Cartridge

1. Wash a 3 ml C18 column with 3 ml of 100% methanol (*see* **Note 15**). Repeat twice.
2. Wash column with 3 ml of C18 elution buffer. Repeat twice.
3. Wash column with 3 ml of C18 wash buffer. Repeat twice.
4. Apply sample to column.
5. Wash column with 3 ml of C18 wash buffer. Repeat twice.
6. Elute sample with 3 ml of C18 elution buffer.
7. Add 2 ml of milliQ water and lyophilize overnight (*see* **Note 16**).

3.4 Fe-IMAC to Separate Peptides from Phosphopeptides

1. To charge the column with iron, first rinse with 3 column volumes (CVs) of FA at 100 μl/min, charge the column with 3 CVs of Fe charging solution at 100 μl/min, then flush out unbound Iron with at least 20 CVs of FA at 100 μl/min (*see* **Note 17**).
2. Remove column from system and store. Flush the HPLC lines (without a column) at 200 μl/min with ≥20 ml ddH_2O at 200 μl/min, then ≥20 ml 50 mM EDTA at 200 μl/min and finally with ≥10 ml ddH_2O at 200 μl/min.
3. Reconnect the column to system. Wash the column at 100 μl/min with 5 ml Fe IMAC elution solvent, then equilibrate with ≥20 ml Fe IMAC loading solvent until the absorbance at 280 nm is stable.
4. Dissolve the lyophilized sample in 100 μl of Fe IMAC loading solvent, spin at 16,000 × *g* for 1 min to remove insoluble material (*see* **Note 18**). Prepare a 100 μl blank sample (Fe-IMAC loading solvent only) as well.
5. Run the blank followed by the sample on the following gradient:

   0–3 min—Fe IMAC loading solvent at 50 μl/min.

   3–4 min—Fe IMAC loading solvent at 150 μl/min.

   4–15 min—Fe IMAC loading solvent at 100 μl/min.

   15–76 min—0–45% Fe IMAC elution solvent at 100 μl/min.

   76–77 min—100% Fe IMAC elution solvent at 100 μl/min.

   77–82 min—100% Fe IMAC elution solvent at 100 μl/min.

   82–85 min—100–0% Fe IMAC elution solvent at 200 μl/min.

85–115 min—Fe IMAC loading solvent at 200 μl/min.

6. Monitor the UV absorption at 280 nm and collect fractions of the sample every 2 min in protein LoBind tubes (*see* **Note 19**). Peptides that do not bind to the column will generally elute immediately in fraction 2 (after 2–4 min) while phosphopeptides will elute at a concentration of approximately 11% Fe-IMAC elution solvent in fraction 15 (after 28–30 min) (*see* **Note 20**).
7. Lyophilize the appropriate fractions overnight.
8. To strip the Fe IMAC column, flush at 200 μl/min with 30 CVs of 50 mM EDTA, then with ≥10 ml of FA. Recharge and equilibrate (**steps 1–3**) before next run (*see* **Note 17**).

3.5 High pH Fractionation

1. Peptide and phosphopeptide fractions should be processed in parallel, but only 10% of the total peptide fraction should be processed further due to its higher abundance. Redissolve lyophilized combined peptide fraction in 1 ml 5 mM NH_4OH and the combined phosphopeptide fraction in 100 μl 5 mM NH_4OH.
2. Wash the spin column with 300 μl acetonitrile (5000 × *g*, 2 min), discard the flow through.
3. Wash the spin column with 300 μl 0.1% TFA (5000 × *g*, 2 min), discard the flow through.
4. Wash the spin column twice with 300 μl 5 mM NH_4OH (5000 × *g*, 2 min), discard the flow through.
5. Apply 100 μl sample to column, collect, and reapply the flow-through (3000 × *g*, 2 min).
6. Collect flow-through for desalting (using C18 spin tips) before combining with other fractions (*see* **Note 21**).
7. Wash column 3× with 300 μl 5 mM NH_4OH (3000 × *g*, 2 min), discard the flow through.
8. Elute with 300 μl of 2%, 3%, 4%, 6%, 10%, and 50% acetonitrile in 5 mM NH_4OH, saving each elution in separate protein LoBind tubes (*see* **Note 19**).
9. Concatenate the eluates into five fractions in protein LoBind tubes (*see* **Note 19**) using the following scheme: F1 = 2% and 50%, F2 = 3%, F3 = 4%, F4 = 6%, F5 = desalted FT and 10% (*see* **Note 22**). Lyophilize overnight.

3.6 Liquid Chromatography–Tandem Mass Spectrometry (LC-MS/MS)

1. Resuspend samples in 0.1% formic acid (buffer A), inject onto a 1 × 5 mm C_{18} trap column, wash onto a 75 μm × 15 cm reverse phase PepMap C_{18} nanocolumn (LC Packings, Dionex), and elute with a linear gradient from 5% to 40% buffer B

over 65 min into an LTQ Orbitrap Velos Pro mass spectrometer (Thermo Scientific) (*see* **Note 5**).

2. For phosphoproteomic analysis, operate in data dependent mode to perform a survey scan over a range 335–1800 m/z in the Orbitrap analyzer ($R = 60{,}000$), with each MS scan triggering 15 MS^2 acquisitions of the 15 most intense ions using multistage activation on the neutral loss of 98 and 49 Thomsons in the LTQ ion trap [13] (*see* **Note 23**). It is recommended to acquire two technical replicates of each fraction to improve the coverage of the phosphoproteome.
3. For proteomic analysis, operate in data dependent mode with each MS scan triggering 15 MS^2 acquisitions of the 15 most intense ions in the LTQ ion trap. Calibrate the Orbitrap mass analyzer on the fly using the lock mass of polydimethylcyclosiloxane at m/z 445.120025.

3.7 Data Analysis

1. Process data using MaxQuant [11] to search against a protein sequence database containing T. brucei *brucei* 927 annotated proteins (obtained from TriTrypDB [14] http://www.tritrypdb.org/) supplemented with frequently observed contaminants (*see* **Note 24**).
2. Use the experimental design to appropriately group samples to experimental groups, allowing for matching between runs for the concatenated fractions in each experiment and group two technical replicates of the phosphoproteomic samples together (*see* **Note 25**).
3. Set carbamidomethylation of cysteine as a fixed modification and oxidation of methionine, N-terminal protein acetylation and N-pyroglutamate as variable modifications. For phosphoproteomic data only use phosphorylation of serine, threonine, and tyrosine residues as variable modifications. Set the false discovery rates (FDRs) of 0.01 at the levels of peptides, proteins, and modification sites. Allow SILAC ratios to be calculated only where at least one peptide could be uniquely mapped to a given protein group and there is a minimum of two SILAC pairs.
4. Import the data into Perseus for visualization and statistical analysis. Filter to remove known contaminants and reverse sequences, and any phosphorylation sites with a <0.75 localization probability. Log_2 transform ratio data and perform further analysis as appropriate for the experiment.

4 Notes

1. SILAC HMI-11T is a modification of original HMI11 [15] (HMI9 without serum plus) based on IMDM without L-arginine and L-lysine (Pierce), and substituting 1-Thioglycerol for

β-mercaptoethanol and L-alanyl-L-glutamine for L-glutamine to improve stability.

2. Fetal calf serum dialyzed against PBS with a 1000 molecular weight cutoff membrane (1 K MWCO) is recommended in preference to 3 or 10 K MWCO. It is critical to batch test dialyzed FCS for growth with the specific T. brucei cell line, as the quality of the serum is critical to successful cell culture and may lead to slower growth rates and lower final cell densities. Often, this is more critical for Bsf cells than Pcf cells. Occasionally poor growth may improve on prolonged passage in dialyzed serum, particularly when genetically altered cell lines are used.

3. At the time of writing SILAC SDM-79 is not commercially available, and must be purchased as a custom synthesis made to the original SDM-79 formulation [16] but without L-arginine and L-lysine for SILAC labeling and with sodium bicarbonate and L-glutamine removed to improve the shelf life. The SILAC SDM-79 medium has also been used to SILAC label *Leishmania* [9] and *Trypanosoma cruzi* [8] for quantitative proteomics, and the sample processing protocols described here are applicable to these species.

4. We have found that reducing the quantity of L-arginine and L-lysine in the media to 30% of the original concentration has no effect on the cell growth or efficiency of SILAC labeling, and substantially reduces the cost of the media.

5. It is not essential to have access to a suitable LC-MS/MS system in-house, as analysis is increasingly available as a commercial service. Alternative instruments with high mass accuracy and resolution will yield similar coverage.

6. Greater than seven cell divisions is required to ensure >98% incorporation of isotopic label. The culture can be expanded while this is ongoing to save media and time.

7. Once labeling is complete, the samples can be treated according to the experimental regimen, that is, addition of external stimulus, induction of RNAi etc. Careful consideration must be given to experimental design to ensure that suitable control experiments are performed (i.e., swapping label in replicates) and that sufficient biological replicates are employed to ensure effects are reproducible.

8. Cells lysis can be verified by microscopy during this incubation step. The final cell lysate is 0.5×10^9 cells/ml or approximately 5 mg/ml total protein content.

9. The total number of cells recommended for a combined proteomic and phosphoproteomic experiment is approximately 5×10^8 combined over the different labels used, allowing for quantification of over 4500 proteins and 9000 phosphorylation sites. Lower amounts of starting material will yield a reduced coverage

of lower abundance proteins and phosphorylation sites. If only proteomic analysis is required, a total of 5×10^7 cells is sufficient.

10. A minimum of two cycles of boiling and sonication is needed to solubilize structural and membrane proteins and shear DNA. Viscosity can be checked by pipetting the sample up and down. It is crucial to completely solubilize the sample and reduce its viscosity at this point, otherwise the filter might become clogged later on and centrifugation times will increase disproportionately.
11. Centrifugation times can vary from run to run, and it is therefore recommended to check how fast or slow the current sample is flowing through the filter, thus the times stated are an indication only. The sample must be reduced to $\leq$0.5 ml before dilution to ensure efficient removal of SDS which interferes with downstream MS analysis.
12. The required centrifuge running times increase a lot during the ABC washes. If the flow rate becomes close to zero, dilute the sample in ABC buffer until the concentration of urea is below 1 M, and proceed to tryptic digest according to protocol but with a larger total reaction volume.
13. Analysis of success of the solubilization and digestion by SDS-PAGE is optional but recommended, as it may identify any problems before the expense of LC-MS/MS analysis. Take care to stop the gel well before the dye front runs out or you will lose your peptide band. Alternatively use a gradient gel, which helps in clearly visualizing the digested peptides.
14. While the original FASP procedure [17] allows for the digested peptides to elute through the centrifugal filter device, this led to variable results in our hands with peptides being retained within the column and even persisting there following the high salt washes. To avoid this we simply removed the digested peptide solution from the column and proceeded directly with desalting.
15. Washes, loading and elution are by gravity flow, but can be accelerated by applying a gentle pressure to the column (e.g., by using a customized syringe or a vacuum manifold).
16. Dilution is required to reduce the organic content sufficiently to allow for lyophilization. Aliquot samples out into 1.5 ml tubes for lyophilization to allow for faster freezing and more efficient drying.
17. A new Fe-IMAC column can be charged directly; strip column first if it has not been used for over a week or in between samples of different origin.
18. The sample usually dissolves completely but can be sonicated if any insoluble residue is apparent.

19. Protein LoBind tubes are essential to avoid loss of peptides and phosphopeptides on untreated plastic surfaces.
20. The phosphopeptide peak usually appears when the pH changes from acidic to basic during the run; this corresponds roughly to 11% of freshly prepared Fe-IMAC elution solution. This might differ depending on the age/storage conditions of the buffers and it is recommended to collect all fractions (every 2 min) to avoid losing the important one.
21. Desalting using C18 spin tips follows the same principle as the 3 ml C18 columns with reduced volumes. All washing and elution steps are in 100 μl volumes and centrifugation is at 200 × *g* for 1 min per step. Final elution is in 3 × 100 μl.
22. Concatenation of the seven high pH fractions reduces the number of sample analyzed by MS, and hence reduces the cost, without sacrificing coverage as the combined sample have complementary LC-MS/MS profiles.
23. In our experience, using collision-induced decay (CID) with multistage acquisition (MSA) outperforms the use of high-energy C-trap dissociation (HCD) for the complex samples required for global phosphoproteomic studies.
24. Alternative data processing programs are available. The computational resources required can be considerable for larger data sets, but MaxQuant is scalable and can be run on a standard desktop machine albeit with long analysis times. As a rough guide, processing 120 LC-MS/MS phosphoproteomic data files requires ~600 Gb storage and currently takes approximately 48 h to run on 24 fast CPU cores with ≥2 Gb RAM per core.
25. Instructions for use of MaxQuant are beyond the scope of this protocol, but help and tutorials are available online and there are annual residential training courses.

References

1. Urbaniak MD (2014) Trypanosomatid phosphoproteomics. In: Doerig C, Spath G, Wiese M (eds) Protein phosphorylation in parasites: novel targets for antiparasitic intervention, vol 5. Drug discovery in infectious diseases. Wiley-VCH, Weinheim, pp 63–77
2. Grimsrud PA, Swaney DL, Wenger CD, Beauchene NA, Coon JJ (2010) Phosphoproteomics for the masses. ACS Chem Biol 5 (1):105–119. https://doi.org/10.1021/cb900277e
3. Perkins DN, Pappin DJ, Creasy DM, Cottrell JS (1999) Probibility-based protein identification by searching sequence databases using mass spectrometry data. Electrophoresis 20:3551–3567
4. Bantscheff M, Schirle M, Sweetman G, Rick J, Kuster B (2007) Quantitative mass spectrometry in proteomics: a critical review. Anal Bioanal Chem 389(4):1017–1031. https://doi.org/10.1007/s00216-007-1486-6
5. Urbaniak MD, Guther MLS, Ferguson MAJ (2012) Comparative SILAC proteomic analysis of *Trypanosoma brucei* bloodstream and procyclic lifecycle stages. PLoS One 7(5):e36619. https://doi.org/10.1371/journal.pone.0036619.g001

6. Urbaniak MD, Martin DM, Ferguson MA (2013) Global quantitative SILAC phosphoproteomics reveals differential phosphorylation is widespread between the procyclic and bloodstream form lifecycle stages of *Trypanosoma brucei*. J Proteome Res 12(5):2233–2244. https://doi.org/10.1021/pr400086y
7. Domingo-Sananes MR, Szoor B, Ferguson MA, Urbaniak MD, Matthews KR (2015) Molecular control of irreversible bistability during trypanosome developmental commitment. J Cell Biol 211(2):455–468. https://doi.org/10.1083/jcb.201506114
8. Roberts AJ, Fairlamb AH (2016) The N-myristoylome of *Trypanosoma cruzi*. Sci Rep 6:31078. https://doi.org/10.1038/srep31078
9. Wyllie S, Thomas M, Patterson S et al (2018) Cyclin-dependent kinase 12 is a drug target for visceral leishmaniasis. Nature 560 (7717):192–197. https://doi.org/10.1038/s41586-018-0356-z
10. Ishihama Y, Sato T, Tabata T, Miyamoto N, Sagane K, Nagasu T, Oda Y (2005) Quantitative mouse brain proteomics using culture-derived isotope tags as internal standards. Nat Biotechnol 23(5):617–621. https://doi.org/10.1038/nbt1086
11. Cox J, Mann M (2008) MaxQuant enables high peptide identification rates, individualized p.p.b.-range mass accuracies and proteome-wide protein quantification. Nat Biotechnol 26(12):1367–1372. https://doi.org/10.1038/nbt.1511
12. Tyanova S, Temu T, Sinitcyn P, Carlson A, Hein MY, Geiger T, Mann M, Cox J (2016) The Perseus computational platform for comprehensive analysis of (prote)omics data. Nat Methods 13(9):731–740. https://doi.org/10.1038/nmeth.3901
13. Schroeder MJ, Shabanowitz J, Schwartz JC, Hunt DF, Coon JJ (2004) A neutral loss activation method for improved phosphopeptide sequence analysis by quadrupole ion trap mass spectrometry. Anal Chem 76(13):3590–3598. https://doi.org/10.1021/ac0497104
14. Aslett M, Aurrecoechea C, Berriman M et al (2010) TriTrypDB: a functional genomic resource for the Trypanosomatidae. Nucleic Acids Res 38(Database issue):D457–D462. https://doi.org/10.1093/nar/gkp851
15. Hirumi H, Hirumi K (1989) Continous cultivation of *Trypanosoma brucei* bloodstream forms in a medium containing a low concentration of serum protein without feeder cell layers. J Parasitol 75:985–989
16. Brun R, Schonenberger M (1979) Cultivation and in vivo cloning of procyclic culture forms of *Trypanosoma brucei* in a semi-defined medium. Acta Trop 36:289–292
17. Wisniewski JR, Zougman A, Nagaraj N, Mann M (2009) Universal sample preparation method for proteome analysis. Nat Methods 6 (5):359–362. https://doi.org/10.1038/nmeth.1322

Chapter 11

Genome-Wide Proteomics and Phosphoproteomics Analysis of *Trypanosoma cruzi* During Differentiation

Michel Batista, Juliana Carolina Amorim, Aline Castro Rodrigues Lucena, Fernanda Grande Kugeratski, Carla Vanessa de Paula Lima, and Fabricio Klerynton Marchini

Abstract

Trypanosoma cruzi is a pathogenic protozoan that still has an impact on public health, despite the decrease in the number of infection cases along the years. *T. cruzi* possesses an heteroxenic life cycle in which it differentiates in at least four forms. Among the differentiation processes, metacyclogenesis has been exploited in different views by researchers. An intriguing question that rises is how metacyclogenesis is triggered and controlled by cell signaling and which are the differentially expressed proteins and posttranslational modifications involved in this process. An important cell signaling pathway is the protein phosphorylation, and it is reinforced in *T. cruzi* in which the gene expression control occurs almost exclusively posttranscriptionally. Additionally, the number of protein kinases in *T. cruzi* is relatively high compared to other organisms. A way to approach these questions is evaluating the cells through phosphoproteomics and proteomics. In this chapter, we will describe the steps from the cell protein extraction, digestion and fractionation, phosphopeptide enrichment, to LC-MS/MS analysis as well as a brief overview on peptide identification. In addition, a published method for in vitro metacyclogenesis will be detailed.

Key words *Trypanosoma cruzi*, Metacyclogenesis, Proteomics, Phosphoproteomics, Mass spectrometry, LC-MS/MS

1 Introduction

Trypanosoma cruzi has a medical relevance and presents several biological aspects uncommon to other eukaryotic cells, making it an important biological model. During its life cycle, *T. cruzi* differentiates into four developmental forms: epimastigote, metacyclic trypomastigote (MT), amastigote, and blood trypomastigote. The trypomastigote forms are infective, and the study of the differentiation to these forms can provide insights regarding the traits responsible for the acquisition of infectivity and general biological properties of *T. cruzi*. The differentiation to MT, named metacyclogenesis, takes place inside the insect host and can be mimicked

Paul A. M. Michels et al. (eds.), *Trypanosomatids: Methods and Protocols*, Methods in Molecular Biology, vol. 2116, https://doi.org/10.1007/978-1-0716-0294-2_11,

in vitro under controlled laboratory conditions through different methods [1–4]. Metacyclogenesis varies in the number of MT obtained according to *T. cruzi* strain [5] and the differentiation method. The method described by Contreras et al. [2], later improved by Bonaldo et al. [3], allows for studies along the entire process. The method can mimic metacyclogenesis steps, that in vivo takes place in the insect's rectum, such as the phases of nutritional stress, adherence and differentiation to MT. This method consists in submitting epimastigotes to a nutritional stress in a chemically poorly defined medium, followed by the incubation in the same medium supplemented with specific amino acids and glucose. During this incubation, the cells adhere to the flask's surface through the flagellum and after 48–96 h, a fraction is released in the supernatant. The cells adhered and released represent distinct populations, which include nondifferentiated cells (epimastigotes and intermediate forms) and MT [6]. The latter can be purified from the cellular pool by its differential surface characteristics [7].

Throughout the years, metacyclogenesis has been studied through different approaches [8–11]. By the sequencing of the *T. cruzi* genome [12] combined with technological advances, it became possible to apply different high-throughput analyses, such as RNA-Seq and proteomics to study this model. Proteomics using liquid chromatography coupled to mass spectrometry (LC-MS/MS) allows for the identification and quantification of thousands of proteins, including posttranslational modifications (PTMs) such as phosphorylation at specific sites (phosphoproteomics). This technology can be applied to a variety of experimental designs aiming to understand, for example, the cell response to different experimental conditions, such as gene silencing, addition of drugs, stress, or cellular differentiation [13–15]. The importance of studying protein phosphorylation is reinforced in *T. cruzi* in which the gene expression control occurs almost exclusively posttranscriptionally [16, 17] and the number of protein kinases is relatively high compared to other organisms [18]. During metacyclogenesis, the proteome and phosphoproteome of cells have been investigated at distinct time points, such as prestress, stress, adhered forms, and MT [10, 11, 15]. These studies showed several proteins and phosphosites modulated along metacyclogenesis. These modulations are associated to cellular processes potentially related to metacyclogenesis, among them cytoskeleton remodeling, intaking of nutrients, and protein translation and turnover.

Shotgun proteomics and phosphoproteomics comprise a variety of protocols along to several methodological steps, starting from protein extraction, protein fractionation and digestion, peptide fractionation, phosphopeptide enrichment until LC-MS/MS configuration. The choice of workflow depends on the aim of the investigation (experimental design), the expertise of the researcher in such techniques and the availability of technologies, mainly related to the type of mass spectrometer. The choice of experimental design exerts direct impact on the coverage of the proteome and phosphoproteome and on the quality of the data. Figure 1 depicts an option of workflow that can be used to study metacyclogenesis. In the following paragraphs, we will present an overview of general proteomics and phosphoproteomics protocols, which can be applied not only to *T. cruzi* but also to other species.

Depending on the cell type, the lysis step should be adapted. *T. cruzi* lysis for protein extraction is a relatively easy procedure; a buffer comprising a strong detergent (for example SDS) and a reducing agent under high temperature can solubilize most of the proteins as well as inactivate proteases and phosphatases satisfactorily. While SDS allows for a good protein extraction, it must be removed from the sample after lysis because of its incompatibility with the downstream steps. An efficient protocol to remove SDS from micrograms to milligrams of protein extracts is through washing the extract with 8 M urea in a centrifugal filter device. This filter contains a porous cellulose membrane with a 30 kDa mass cutoff. Besides removing SDS, this wash is directly coupled to the protein digestion step in a method known as filter-aided sample preparation—FASP [19, 20]. FASP has the advantage of combining the removal of SDS and digestion interfering substances with an efficient recovery of peptides, supporting the digestion of up to milligrams of protein.

After recovering the peptides from FASP, there is an optional step of peptide offline fractionation (or prefractionation, since another fractionation will be done at the nano-LC). High pH reversed-phase (HPRP) chromatography [21, 22] provides a good orthogonality to the traditional low pH reversed-phase nano-LC and may be considered if a deeper proteome coverage is aimed; however, this step increases the LC-MS time of acquisition and initial protein input. For proteomics analysis, after desalting in C18 stage-tips or cartridges, peptides are ready for injection in the LC-MS system. For phosphoproteomics, due to the low stoichiometry in the sample, phosphopeptides require enrichment prior to the analysis. Several phosphopeptide enrichment methods are available, varying in efficiency and specificity toward single or multiphosphorylated peptides [23]. The majority of phosphoenrichment strategies are based on the affinity of the phosphate group to a metal, such as iron, gallium, and titanium, among others [24–27]. Titanium dioxide beads have high affinity to phosphopeptides and support the enrichment in batch. In the reaction, a competitor agent (phthalic acid or dihydroxybenzoic acid) with an intermediate affinity to titanium can be added to diminish the binding of acidic peptides, such as the ones rich in aspartic or glutamic acid. The titanium dioxide-based method has been improved, allowing for less peptide input and high-throughput screening [27].

Another crucial step to obtain good proteomics data is the chromatography prior to MS analysis. Through the combination

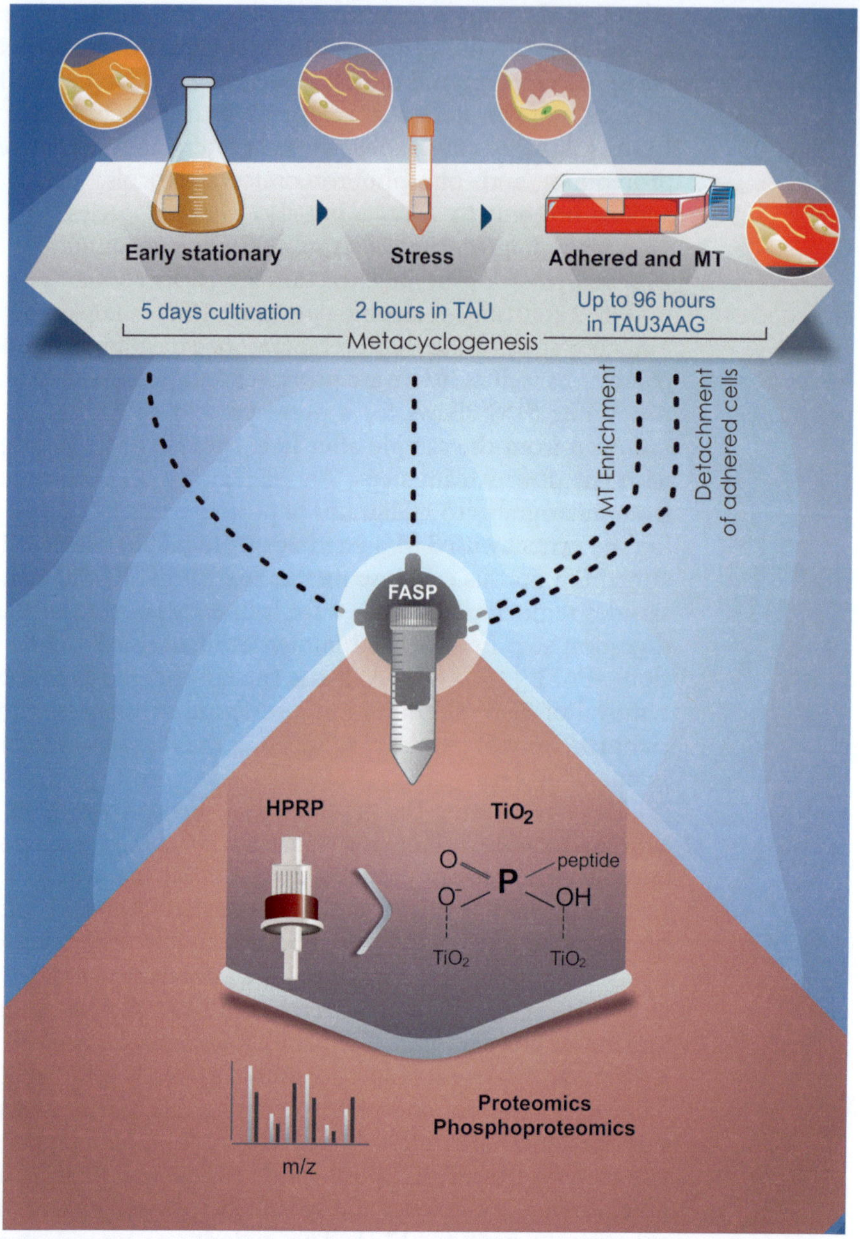

Fig. 1 Metacyclogenesis proteomics and phosphoproteomics workflow. After 5 days cultivation in LIT medium, *T. cruzi* epimastigotes are subjected to nutritional stress in TAU medium for 2 h, and then incubated in TAU3AAG up to 96 h. The cells can be collected and the proteome and phosphoproteome evaluated at any point of metacyclogenesis, from the early stationary phase up to 96 h. The adhered phase is composed of a cell mixture containing epimastigotes, intermediate forms, and metacyclic trypomastigotes (MT); the latter are gradually released in the supernatant. Collected cells are lysed and the protein extract is processed by filter-aided sample preparation (FASP), the peptides can be fractionated by high pH reversed-phase (HPRP) chromatography and analyzed by LC-MS/MS (proteomics) or first enriched for phosphopeptides based on titanium dioxide affinity (phosphoproteomics)

of sub-2 micron C18 particles-containing columns (particles preferably packaged directly into the emitter) and ultrahigh-performance liquid chromatography (UHPLC) systems it is possible to reach a high-resolution chromatographic separation. Indeed, the analytical columns can be packed in-house and customized accordingly to the user's requirements at a relatively low cost [28]. The parameters of UHPLC, such as length and inclination of the gradient will depend on the nature of the sample, the column features and the mass spectrometer speed. For example, we recommend a 4 h gradient for proteomics analysis when combining UHPLC with a high resolution, relative low speed mass spectrometer (e.g., LTQ Orbitrap XL). In fact, UHPLC can be coupled not only to new generation mass spectrometers (e.g., high field orbitraps), but also to older models, improving significantly the data acquisition. The spectra acquisition method will depend on the mass spectrometer model, for example, in a data-dependent acquisition (DDA), the number of ions selected to MS/MS varies according to the speed of mass analyzer. Despite differences between mass spectrometers, the acquisition method setup is similar for proteomics and phosphoproteomics, the main exception being the need of neutral loss parameters for the latter. The neutral loss of phosphate groups occurs during the fragmentation by both collision-induced dissociation (CID) and higher-energy collisional dissociation (HCD). The energy applied to phosphopeptide fragmentation is partially directed to the phosphate group, which may affect the fragmentation of peptidic bonds. To circumvent this, in linear trap quadrupole mass analyzers it is possible to combine the neutral loss detection with refragmentation of the poorly fragmented phosphopeptide. After suffering neutral loss, the peptide can be refragmented in a pseudo MS3 method called multistage activation (MSA) [29].

The data generated by MS are used as input to peptide and phosphorylation site identification by peptide spectrum match (PSM) in an algorithm against a protein database. There are many algorithms for this purpose, each one with its own specificity [30–32]. One of the most used algorithms and freely available is MaxQuant—MQ [32, 33]. MQ uses a probabilistic score model for peptide identification and generates an intensity for each protein or phosphorylation site calculated from the tridimensional area (time to m/z to intensity) of eluted peptides acquired in the full scan (MS1). MQ is amenable to label-free and label-based quantification strategies, generating protein intensity values or protein normalized ratios, respectivelly. The output of MQ can be further analyzed in the Perseus platform [34], which offers several options for data treatment, such as protein intensity normalization, statistical analysis, and functional annotation, among others. The downstream analysis depends on the aim of the project and can include both qualitative and quantitative analysis.

In this chapter, we will describe methods for proteomics and phosphoproteomics analysis of *T. cruzi* during metacyclogenesis. The cells may be analyzed at virtually any point along metacyclogenesis, from the nutritional stress up to 96 h of adhesion or more if desired. Both the nonadhered cell populations and the adhered ones may be evaluated, the latter obtained by mechanical detachment from the cultivation flask's surface.

2 Materials

The reagents used in the protocols should have high analytical grade and it is suggested that the buffers, media, and solutions should be prepared using ultrapure water (resistivity of 18.2 MΩ-cm at 25 °C). All culture media after the preparation must be sterilized through filtration (0.2 μm filter) and then tested for contamination at 37 °C for 48 h.

1. Epimastigote-stage form of *T. cruzi Dm*28c.
2. Liver infusion tryptose (LIT) medium: 5.4 mM KCl, 150 mM NaCl, 24 mM glucose, 5% (v/v) liver extract, 0.025% (w/v) hemin, 2% (w/v) yeast extract, and 1.5% (w/v) tryptose, with 10% heat-inactivated FBS.
3. Phosphate buffered saline (PBS): 137 mM NaCl, 4.3 mM Na_2HPO_4, 2.7 mM KCl, 1.5 mM KH_2HPO_4, adjust solution to pH 7.2.
4. Triatomine artificial urine (TAU) medium: 190 mM NaCl, 17 mM KCl, 2 mM $MgCl_2$, 3 mM $CaCl_2$, and 8 mM phosphate buffer, adjust to pH 6.0.
5. Triatomine artificial urine medium supplemented with three amino acids and glucose (TAU3AAG): TAU medium supplemented with 10 mM L-proline, 50 mM L-sodium glutamate, 2 mM L-sodium aspartate, and 10 mM D-glucose.
6. Purification of the metacyclic form of *T. cruzi*: Phosphate saline glucose buffer (PSG): 47.47 mM $Na_2HPO_4 \cdot 12H_2O$, 2.5 mM $NaH_2PO_4 \cdot H_2O$, 36.76 mM NaCl, and 55.5 mM D-glucose, adjust to pH 8.0, and a chromatographic column containing 2-(diethylamino) ethyl ether cellulose (DEAE-cellulose) resin equilibrated with PSG (*see* **Note 1**).
7. SDS lysis buffer: 0.1 M Tris–HCl, pH 7.6, 0.1 M DTT and 4% (v/v) SDS.
8. FASP solutions: UA solution (8 M urea, 0.1 M Tris–HCl, pH 8.5), UA-DTT solution (UA solution + 0.01 M DTT), UA-IAA (UA solution + 0.05 M iodoacetamide), ABC solution (0.05 M ammonium bicarbonate), trypsin 1:100 (w/w enzyme-to-substrate ratio) and 0.5 M NaCl.

9. High pH reversed-phase fractionation solutions: Methanol, equilibrium solution (ammonium formate (AF): 0.08% (v/v) ammonium hydroxide with 0.016% (v/v) formic acid, at pH 10), 20 mM AF with 10, 14, 18, or 60% (v/v) of acetonitrile (MeCN), 0.5% (v/v) trifluoroacetic acid (TFA).
10. Phosphopeptide enrichment solutions: Loading solution (2.5% (v/v) TFA, 80% (v/v) MeCN, 70 mg/mL phthalic acid), wash buffer A (80% (v/v) MeCN, 0.1% (v/v) TFA), wash buffer B (0.1% (v/v) TFA), elution solution (0.3 M ammonium hydroxide).
11. Solutions for proteomics and phosphoproteomics runs: Mobile phase A (0.1% (v/v) formic acid, 5% (v/v) DMSO), mobile phase B (0.1% (v/v) formic acid, 5% (v/v) DMSO in MeCN), injection solution: 0.1% (v/v) formic acid and 5% (v/v) DMSO.
12. Suggested materials: Filter with porous cellulose membrane with a 30 kDa mass cutoff [e.g., Amicon Ultra-0.5 centrifugal filter unit 30K (Merck-Millipore, Darmstadt, Germany)], microbeads of TiO_2 [e.g., 10 μm TiO_2 microbeads (GL Science, Saitama, Japan)], reversed-phase silica column [e.g., 130-mg Sep-Pak C18 Plus Light Cartridge (Waters, Milford, USA)], chromatographic nanoLC C18 column and C18 stage-tips.
13. General equipment: Temperature-controlled incubators, cell counter equipment, inverted microscope, laminar flow cabinets, general plasticware for cultivation of parasites, centrifuge, spectrophotometer, ultrasonic homogenizer, freezer for storage at −80 °C, ultrahigh-performance liquid chromatography (UHPLC) connected to a nanoelectrospray ionization source coupled to a high-resolution mass spectrometer.

3 Methods

3.1 T. cruzi *Cultivation*

We recommend to use an automatic cell counter to improve experimental accuracy at all stages of parasite counting, including after each wash. To avoid temperature stress on parasites, we suggest to warm at 28 °C the required amount of media used to grow or differentiate parasites before use. Under all conditions, the volume of cultures should be maintained at a ratio of 1: 5 (v/v) to the total volume of the culture flasks.

1. The first step in conducting *T. cruzi* experiments is to condition the newly thawed culture in the LIT medium (*see* **Note 2**). This procedure is performed by constant culture renewal every 3 days with an initial inoculum of 1×10^6 parasites/mL maintained at 28 °C in the LIT medium supplemented with 10%

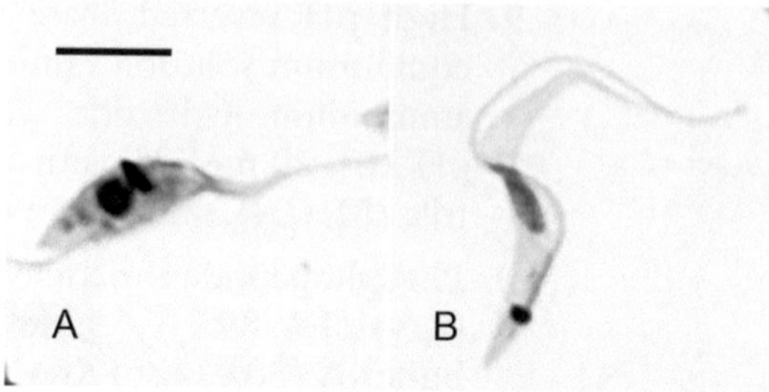

Fig. 2 Microscopy visualization of *T. cruzi*. Epimastigote (**a**) and metacyclic trypomastigote (**b**) forms of *T. cruzi* were stained with Romanowsky stain according to Kessler et al. [35]. The images were acquired with 1000× magnification. Scale bar represents 5 μm

FBS. Figure 2, prepared according to Kessler et al. [35], shows the typical shape of epimastigote form (*see* **Note 3**).

2. After the conditioning procedure, the growth in the LIT medium should be performed from 1×10^6 parasites/mL (initial inoculum) (*see* **Note 4**).

3.2 T. cruzi Metacyclogenesis and Purification of the Metacyclic Form

1. For the in vitro metacyclogenesis of *T. cruzi*, the epimastigotes, after reaching a density of 5×10^7 parasites/mL (late exponential phase, approximately 5 days of culture), should be collected by centrifugation at $3000 \times g$ for 10 min at 20 °C.
2. Wash once in TAU medium to decrease the concentration of LIT medium.
3. For the nutritional stress process, incubate 5×10^8 parasites/mL at 28 °C in TAU medium for 2 h. Samples of the culture may be collected at intermediate time points of the nutritional stress period.
4. To stimulate adhesion of parasites, after 2 h of nutritional stress, dilute the cultures to 5×10^6 parasites/mL in TAU3AAG medium, transfer to culture flasks and incubate for 96 h at 28 °C. Samples of the culture may be collected at intermediate time points of the adhesion phase (*see* **Note 5**).
5. To collect adhered parasites during metacyclogenesis, remove the supernatant (to be saved for the next step (**step 7** below) of parasite harvesting) and add fresh TAU3AAG, shake the flasks vigorously to release the adhered parasites (*see* **Note 6**).
6. Purification of metacyclic trypomastigote forms of *T. cruzi* from the supernatant of differentiation involves using an in-house prepared ion-exchange chromatography system with DEAE-cellulose resin. To that end, assemble first the

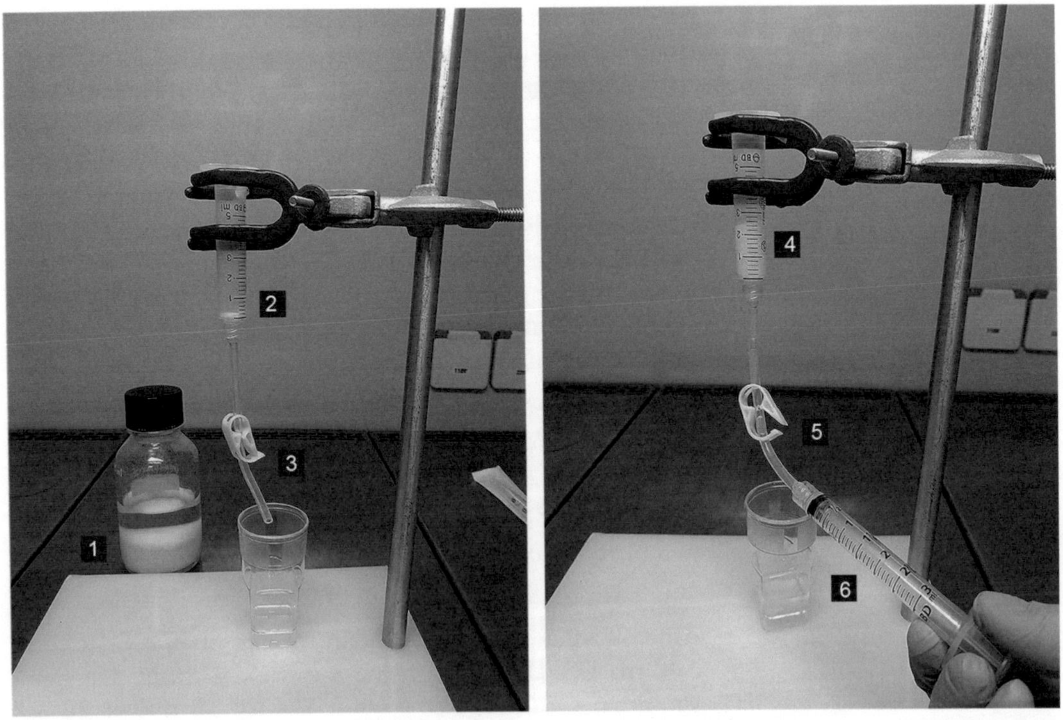

Fig. 3 Schematic representation of DEAE-cellulose chromatographic column preparation. Required materials: DEAE-cellulose resin resuspended in PSG solution (1); 5 mL or 10 mL syringe with glass wool at the bottom (2) and a flexible tube of approximated 10 cm at the end of the syringe with a clamp (3) to open and close the liquid flow. To pack the DEAE-cellulose in the column (4), attach a syringe at the end of the flexible tube (6), open the clamp (5) and extract 1 mL of solution, the resin volume will compact. Remove the syringe and count the flow rate (drops/min); repeat this process until a flow rate of 20–25 drops/min is obtained

chromatographic column and adjust it to a PSG flow of 25 drops/min (Fig. 3) (*see* **Note 7**).

7. Collect the cells from the supernatants of the flasks cultures after 96 h incubation (obtained in **step 5**) by centrifugation at 7000 × *g*, 10 min at 10 °C, resuspend them in PSG and pass them through the column, always completing the layer of solvent on top with PSG to avoid flow interruption and resin dryness. MT cells will pass through the resin at first, making the eluent material turbid. Collect the eluent while it is still turbid (MT cells) and stop the chromatography when the eluent starts to clear. An extended collection time may cause the elution of intermediate and epimastigote forms. To ensure that the metacyclic form of *T. cruzi* is collected with a high degree of purity, a constant microscopic examination should be conducted. Figure 2 shows epimastigote and MT forms (*see* **Notes 6** and **8**).

3.3 Sample Preparation for Proteomics and Phosphoproteomics

3.3.1 Filter-Aided Sample Preparation (FASP)

1. Harvest cells and wash twice in PBS at 4 °C. To obtain 1 mg of protein, use 3×10^8 *T. cruzi* epimastigotes (the same cultures from Subheading 3.2, **steps 1** or **3**) or intermediate forms (collect cells as described in Subheading 3.2, **step 5**), or 6×10^8 MT (collect cells as described in Subheading 3.2, **step 7**).
2. Lyse the cell pellet in SDS lysis buffer, mix using a pipette and vortex for 30 s (*see* **Note 9**). Boil the sample at 95 °C for 3 min. Sonicate in a sonicator bath for 1 h to remove the viscosity of the sample. Centrifuge at 20,000 × *g* for 5 min at 20 °C. Transfer supernatant to a clean tube (*see* **Notes 10** and **11**).
3. Selecting the appropriate filter size:
   - Use Amicon® 0.5 mL for up to 50 μL of sample volume and maximum of 200 μg of protein.
   - Use Amicon® 15 mL for sample volume higher than 100 μL and protein content range from 400 μg to 5 mg.
4. Washing out SDS and reduction of protein disulfide bonds:
   - Amicon® 0.5 mL: Add protein sample on the filter. Add 200 μL UA-DTT. Mix using a pipette without damaging the filter. Centrifuge at 14,000 × *g* for 15 min at 20 °C. Discard the flow-through. Repeat wash with 200 μL UA-DTT twice (*see* **Notes 12** and **13**).
   - Amicon® 15 mL: Add protein sample on the filter. Add 8 mL UA-DTT. Mix using a pipette without damaging the filter. Centrifuge at 4000 × *g* during 30–40 min at 20 °C. Discard the flow-through. Repeat wash twice (*see* **Notes 12** and **13**).
5. Alkylation of cysteines:
   - Alkylation steps are performed protected from light.
   - Amicon® 0.5 mL: Add 100 μL UA-IAA. Mix in thermomixer at 600 rpm for 1 min, 20 °C. Incubate for 20 min. Centrifuge at 14,000 × *g* for 10 min at 20 °C. Discard the flow-through (*see* **Note 13**).
   - Amicon® 15 mL: Add 2 mL UA-IAA. Mix using pipette without damaging the filter. Incubate 30 min. Centrifuge at 4000 × *g* for 20 min at 20 °C. Discard the flow-through (*see* **Note 13**).
6. Wash:
   - Amicon® 0.5 mL: Add 100 μL UA. Mix using a pipette. Centrifuge at 14,000 × *g* for 15 min at 20 °C. Discard the flow-through. Repeat step once (*see* **Note 13**).
   - Amicon® 15 mL: Add 10 mL UA. Mix using a pipette. Centrifuge at 4000 × *g* for 30–40 min at 20 °C. Discard the flow-through. Repeat step once (*see* **Note 13**).

7. Exchange urea by ABC:
   - Amicon® 0.5 mL: Add 100 μL of 50 mM ABC. Mix using a pipette. Centrifuge at 14,000 × *g* for 15 min at 20 °C. Discard the flow-through. Repeat step once (*see* **Note 13**).
   - Amicon® 15 mL: Add 10 mL of 50 mM ABC. Mix using a pipette. Centrifuge at 4000 × *g* for 30–40 min at 20 °C. Discard the flow-through. Repeat step once (*see* **Note 13**).
8. Protein digestion:
   - Amicon® 0.5 mL: Add 1 μg of trypsin per 100 μg of protein in 40 μL of 0.05 M ABC. Incubate for 16–18 h at 37 °C in humidified chamber.
   - Amicon® 15 mL: Add 1 μg of trypsin per 100 μg of protein in 1–2 mL of 0.05 M ABC. Incubate for 16–18 h at 37 °C.
9. Peptide elution:
   - Keep filter in the same orientation; do not invert.
   - Amicon® 0.5 mL: transfer filter containing the peptides to a clean tube. Centrifuge at 14,000 × *g* for 10 min at 20 °C. Add 40 μL of 0.05 M ABC on the filter and centrifuge at 14,000 × *g* for 10 min at 20 °C. Add 50 μL of 0.5 M NaCl and centrifuge at 14,000 × *g* for 10 min at 20 °C. Collect everything in the same tube.
   - Amicon® 15 mL: transfer filter containing the peptides to a clean tube. Centrifuge at 4000 × *g* for 15 min at 20 °C. Add 1 mL 0.05 M ABC and centrifuge at 4000 × *g* for 10 min at 20 °C. Add 1 mL of 0.5 M NaCl and centrifuge at 4000 × *g* for 10 min at 20 °C. Collect everything in the same tube.
10. The determination of the peptide yield can be performed using Nanodrop at 280 nm, Qubit or tryptophan fluorescence [36].
11. Acidify sample to pH 2.5.
12. Desalt and concentrate peptides using C18 stage-tips [37, 38] or cartridge depending on the amount of the sample (*see* **Note 14**).

3.3.2 High pH Reversed-Phase Fractionation

1. Use at least 100 μg (300–500 μg for phosphoproteomics) of peptides eluted from FASP.
2. Purify the peptides using C18 stage-tips and a centrifuge at 1000 × *g* or cartridges with syringe or vacuum manifold (*see* **Note 14**).
3. Dilute the volume of eluted peptides in 19 volumes of 20 mM ammonium formate (FA) pH 10, diluted 1:10 from FA 200 mM (0.8%, ammonium hydroxide, 0.16% formic acid).

4. Activate stage-tips with 100 μL or cartridges with 5 mL of methanol, and subsequently equilibrate with 100 μL or 10 mL of 20 mM FA, respectively.
5. Distribute the peptides in the stage-tips or cartridges, centrifuge for the required time until the full volume passes through the stage-tips. For cartridges use a syringe or vacuum manifold.
6. Wash the stage-tips with 100 μL or the cartridges with 10 mL of 20 mM FA.
7. Elute in four sequential steps using 40 μL (1 mL for cartridges) of the following solutions: 20 mM FA in 10%, 14%, 18% and 60% of acetonitrile.
8. Use stage-tips to desalt and concentrate samples for proteomics analysis (*see* **Note 14**).

3.3.3 Phosphopeptide Enrichment

The method of enrichment of phosphopeptides is based on Bodenmiller et al. [23] with modifications by Amorim et al. [15].

1. Dry in a vacuum centrifuge 0.5 mg of desalted peptides from FASP or from HPRP fractionation.
2. Resuspend the peptides in 900 μL of loading solution.
3. Add 2 mg of TiO_2 microbeads preequilibrated in the loading solution (20 mg TiO_2 per mL loading solution) and incubate with end-over-end rotation for 60 min (*see* **Note 15**).
4. Centrifuge 1000 × *g* for 1 min to spin-down beads and remove the supernatant.
5. Add 500 μL of loading solution, mix with the pipette and centrifuge 1000 × *g* for 1 min. Repeat this step.
6. Add 500 μL of wash buffer A, mix with the pipette and centrifuge 1000 × *g* for 1 min. Repeat this step.
7. Add 500 μL of wash buffer B, mix with the pipette and centrifuge 1000 × *g* for 1 min. Repeat this step.
8. To elute the peptides, add 25 μL of elution solution, mix with the pipette and centrifuge 1000 × *g* for 1 min. Store the supernatant. Repeat this step three times.
9. Dry the peptides in a vacuum centrifuge, desalt in C18 stage-tips and store at 4 °C until LC-MS/MS analysis.

3.4 Proteomics and Phospho-proteomics Analysis by LC-MS/MS

1. Peptides are eluted from stage-tips with 0.1% formic acid, 40% MeCN, dried and resuspended in 0.1% formic acid, 5% DMSO in a volume enough for 2–3 runs (phosphopeptides) or set to 0.2–0.4 μg/μL for proteomics analysis (*see* **Note 16**).
2. For the chromatography, in pipetting step, the autosampler captures 5 μL of peptides solution and puts it into the sample loop.

3. The sample is then loaded into the analytical column at a flow rate of 250 nL/min followed by a linear gradient from 5% to 40% MeCN in 0.1% formic acid, 5% DMSO for 240 min (proteomics) or 120 min (phosphoproteomics). If available, enable the LSP (Load Speed Protection) option in the UHPLC, to pause the race if there is an increase in pressure, indicating that there has been clogging in the analytical column.
4. After the end of the gradient, increase to 100% MeCN for 20 min, to clean the analytical column.
5. Decrease to 5% MeCN for 20 min, to reequilibrate the analytical column.
6. The analytical column is maintained at 60 °C during the entire process.
7. It is recommended to carry out the LC-MS/MS analysis in an UHPLC coupled to a high-resolution mass spectrometer. The method depends on the characteristics of the system, but in general a data-dependent acquisition (DDA) is used. When using ion traps for MS2 acquisition, the neutral loss parameter should be configured and MSA enabled for phosphoproteomics (*see* **Note 16**).

3.5 Proteomics and Phosphoproteomics Data Analysis

For data analysis, an option is the MaxQuant computational platform, which is freely available for download. First, the .raw MS files are processed in the MaxQuant software, coupled to Andromeda search engine [32, 33]. Then, the statistical analysis and graphical visualization of the data are performed using Perseus [34]. For additional information about this platform, refer to [39–41].

3.5.1 Processing MS Data with MaxQuant

1. Place all .raw files in a folder. The processed data will be saved inside the same folder once the run is complete.
2. Load the .raw MS files in MaxQuant.
3. Generate the experimental design template, in which the information related to fractions and experimental names are included.
4. Quantification:
   - For label-free: keep multiplicity 1. The quantification is provided as LFQ intensity.
   - For SILAC (*see* **Note 2**): define multiplicity 2 and select the heavy amino acids labels used in the study (e.g., Arg10 and Lys8). When working with triple SILAC select multiplicity 3 and add the medium and heavy labels. Enable "re-quantify." The quantification is provided as SILAC ratios.
5. PTMs: In variable modifications, add the PTMs of interest. For phosphoproteomics select Phospho(STY).

6. Load the FASTA file containing the protein sequences of reference. This can be downloaded from UniProt or another data bank for the organism of interest (for example, TriTrypDB for *T. cruzi*).
7. The option "match between runs" can be enabled to increase the peptide identification. The missing spectra in one run can be complemented by the data from another run in a specific chromatographic time window.
8. For the remaining parameters, we recommend the default settings.

3.5.2 Analyzing MS Data Using Perseus

Total Proteome Analysis

1. In Perseus, load the "ProteinGroups.txt" file generated by MaxQuant (Load → Generic matrix upload).
2. Add each element of the file in the appropriate option. For example, the expression values will be placed in the main column option: for SILAC, the expression values are the Ratio H/L normalized, and for label-free the LFQ intensity. Add the IDs and FASTA headers in Text. Add the numerical values in Numerical and so on. Note that a data analysis matrix can be saved at any time (Export → Generic matrix export) and reimported (Load → Generic matrix upload). Moreover, the entire Perseus session can be saved and reopened, only make sure to use the same version of Perseus software to create and reopen the session. Finally, the figures generated by each analysis can be exported in various formats.
3. Using the filter option, remove: "common contaminants," "reverse," and "only identified by site" (Processing → Filter rows → Filter rows based on categorical column).
4. Using filter option, filter for the number of unique peptides required in the identification of the proteins (e.g., at least 1 or 2 unique peptides).
5. For SILAC, invert the SILAC ratios if necessary using the transform option and the formula "$1/x$" (Processing → Basic → Transform).
6. Logarithmize the expression values using the log2 formula ("log2(x)") in Processing → Basic → Transform.
7. Logarithmize the intensity using the log10 formula ("log10 (x)") in Processing → Basic → Transform.
8. Define the number of valid values required for your study [e.g., when working with three biological replicates, for a robust quantitative information, one can require that at least two out three values are valid, or even three out of three (Processing → Filter rows → Filter rows based on valid values)].

9. Add annotations of interest (e.g., GOBP, GOCC, GOMF, KEGG, and Pfam, in Processing → Annot. columns → Add annotation).
10. Verify the data distribution using histograms (Analysis → Visualization → Histogram). If distribution is not normal or not centered in zero, normalization strategies should be employed.
11. Verify the reproducibility across replicates and the similarities and differences induced by treatment or life cycle stages by looking at correlation coefficients (Analysis → Visualization → Multi scatter plot).
12. For hierarchical clustering, use Analysis → Clustering/PCA → Hierarchical clustering. Here, one can identify groups of coregulated proteins, verify whether the biological replicates cluster together, how the time points of different stages of differentiation cluster, and so on.
13. For principal component analysis, use Analysis → Clustering/PCA → PCA. Before doing the PCA analysis make sure all values are valid.
14. For determination of differentially regulated proteins across the experimental conditions, use t-test when comparing two samples or ANOVA for multiple samples (Processing → Tests → select desired test).
15. For visualization of samples (how replicates compare to each other, plotting averaged expression values against intensity, etc.) add scatter plot (Analysis → Visualization → Scatter plot).
16. For grouping of replicates, use Processing → Annot. rows → Categorical annotation rows and then create the groups according to the replicates. Then, average the SILAC ratios (or LFQ intensities) of the replicates to work with a single value per condition (Processing → Annot. rows → Average groups).
17. For Venn diagram: to determine the number of proteins present/absent in the distinct treatment groups go to Analysis → Misc. → Numeric Venn diagram.
18. To identify significantly enriched functional categories (GOBP, GOCC, GOMF, KEGG, Pfam) in a subset of proteins of interest (e.g., among upregulated, downregulated or a cluster of coregulated proteins from the hierarchical clustering analysis) use Fisher's test (Processing → Annot. columns → Fisher exact test).

Phosphoproteome Analysis

MaxQuant software generates an output file called "Phospho(STY) sites.txt", which contains the information related to the phosphorylated residues and their quantitative information. In Perseus, the analysis of the phosphoproteomics data, for the most part, follows the steps described above for the proteomics data. However, there are distinct and additional steps that should be performed:

1. In Perseus, load the "Phospho(STY)sites.txt" file (Load → Generic matrix upload).
2. Using the filter option, remove: "common contaminants" and "reverse" (Processing → Filter rows → Filter rows based on categorical column).
3. Filter for Class I phosphosites: localization probability >0.75 and score difference >5 Processing → Filter rows → Filter rows based on numerical/expression column).
4. Use the option expand site table to obtain the information of phosphorylations in the peptide (single or multiple phosphorylations). For this, use Processing → Modifications → Expand site table.
5. Add the following:
   (a) Site-specific sequence features (Processing → Modifications → Add sequence features).
   (b) Linear motifs using the sequence window of the modification (Processing → Modifications → Add linear motifs).
6. After the quantitative values for the phosphosites are obtained, normalize them to the total levels of the protein (*see* **Note 17**).

4 Notes

1. The column used to purify MT cells is a regular 10 mL plastic syringe with glass wool at the bottom to contain the resin, the syringe should be attached to a flexible tube of 10 cm at the end with a clamp, to open and close the flow easily and securely.
2. LIT medium is a complex, high nutritive medium, commonly used to cultivate epimastigote forms of *T. cruzi*. Most of the proteomic experiments can be performed using the traditional *T. cruzi* cultivation protocol, but if using quantitative protocols based on metabolic labeling of proteins, such as SILAC, it is indispensable to use chemically defined conditions of cultivation. In this case, an alternative option of defined medium is LM14B [42] or SDM-79 with modifications [43, 44].
3. The growth of *T. cruzi* should be monitored at each culture renewal through cell counting and microscopic observation. Parasites are considered adapted to in vitro cultivation when the growth rate reaches approximately 3×10^7 parasites/mL in 3 days of cultivation at an initial inoculum of 1×10^6 parasites/mL. Another crucial characteristic to be monitored is the cell

shape, activity, and proportion of dead cells: epimastigotes with less than 3 days of cultivation (exponential growth phase) have an elongated egg shape, with high activity of the flagellum, and the cultures do not have apparent dead cells (Fig. 2). Cultures at the exponential growth phase do not have cell sediments. It is recommended to determine a growth curve of epimastigotes after the adaptation to your laboratory conditions to determine the late exponential/early stationary growth phase (around 5×10^7 parasites/mL); this provides essential data to perform in vitro metacyclogenesis.

4. Do not open the culture flasks after starting the experiment (initial inoculum). The manipulation of culture may interfere with the growth rate of the parasites.
5. The culture volume during metacyclogenesis depends on the size of the culture flasks, for example 100 mL of TAU3AAG culture for 175 cm^2 flasks and 200 mL of TAU3AAG culture for 300 cm^2 flasks.
6. The entire *T. cruzi* cultivation protocol requires security procedures, because the supernatant of all stages of differentiation contains MT forms. MT forms are potentially infective, therefore extra care must be taken during culture manipulation: all procedures performed with live MT forms must be conducted in laminar flow cabinets, using personal protective equipment (gloves, eyeglasses, lab coat).
7. The DEAE-cellulose resin is packed in an adapted 10-mL plastic syringe (*see* **Note 1**), with a 4 cm resin column. The resin must be packed to obtain an eluent flow of 20–25 drops/min: start adding approximately 10 mL of activated resin/PSG mix in the column, let the resin decant (it should remain around 5 mL of resin). To pack the resin, attach a syringe at the end of plugged flexible tube and extract 1 mL of diluent, then verify the flow rate and repeat the process until reaching the ideal flow rate.
8. Approximately ten flasks of 300 cm^2 culture (containing 200 mL of culture volume) are concentrated in 1 mL of PSG and passed through the column. After the purification, approximately 98% of the cells are metacyclic trypomastigotes.
9. The cell lysate will be very viscous, mix by pipetting immediately after buffer addition while carefully avoiding foaming.
10. Depending on the amount of starting material available, we recommend distinct methods for sample preparation for proteomics. For situations when the amount of starting material is limited, the cells can be lysed in urea lysis buffer and the proteins digested into peptides using in-solution digestion. The in-solution digestion method is very straightforward, it requires only 2–10 μg of starting material and without further

fractionation protocols yields the identification of approximately 4000 proteins in single runs [14]. When the amount of starting material is not a limiting factor, we recommend to use FASP, where cells are lysed in buffer with SDS and subsequently the SDS is exchanged by urea and ABC on-filter [15]. FASP has the advantage of providing a better solubilization of membrane proteins [19].

11. Avoid to store cell pellets (even in ultrafreezers −80 °C). Protein extract can be stored at −80 °C.
12. SDS buffer is not compatible with most protein determination methods. The determination of a SDS protein extract can be performed by measuring tryptophan fluorescence [36].
13. In the FASP procedure, the step of mixing with a pipette is crucial to have a satisfactory sample preparation. A longer centrifugation time may be necessary depending on the amount of protein or the efficiency of viscosity removal from the protein extract; make sure the protein extract is completely nonviscous before starting the filtration. To avoid longer centrifugation time, turn around the filter between the washes to use both sides of the filter membranes.
14. Use one stage-tip for up to 10 μg of peptide, for greater amounts use more stage-tips or C18 cartridges, for example, up to 500 μg of peptide use a 130-mg Sep-Pak C18 Plus Light Cartridge (Waters, Milford, USA). For cartridges use a syringe or vacuum manifold. After desalting, the peptides can be stored in C18 stage-tips or cartridges, at 4 °C.
15. It is recommended to use 1.5 mL microtubes instead of 2.0 mL. The format of the second one makes difficult to manipulate the supernatant and beads.
16. When using label-free samples, perform at least two runs per sample for phosphoproteomics and three runs for proteomics. For labeled samples, the number of runs per sample may be lower. The use of 5% DMSO in the LC mobile phase enhances the electrospray ionization of peptides considerably [45, 46]. In the MS1 acquisition, when internal calibration is not available, enable the lock mass option at 401.922718 m/z to reach a sub-ppm mass error [47].
17. The use of quantitative proteomics has two aims in the experiment. The first one is to identify protein modulations under experimental conditions, and the second one is the possibility of normalizing each phosphorylation site intensity by the respective protein intensity. In this way, the protein modulation effect is separated from the phosphorylation site quantification. The limitation using this approach is the necessity of having both protein and phosphorylation site intensities. Perseus offers the option "matching rows by name" for combining

the "proteinGroups" and "Phospho (STY)Sites" matrixes, always using the late as matrix base.

Acknowledgments

The authors are very grateful to Dr. Rafael Luis Kessler for kindly providing the microscopy images of *T. cruzi* and to MSc Wagner Nagib de Souza Birbeire for assistance in artwork design.

References

1. Sullivan JJ (1982) Metacyclogenesis of Trypanosoma cruzi in vitro: a simplified procedure. Trans R Soc Trop Med Hyg 76(3):300–303
2. Contreras VT, Salles JM, Thomas N, Morel CM, Goldenberg S (1985) In vitro differentiation of Trypanosoma cruzi under chemically defined conditions. Mol Biochem Parasitol 16 (3):315–327. 0166-6851(85)90073-8 [pii]
3. Bonaldo MC, Souto-Padron T, de Souza W, Goldenberg S (1988) Cell-substrate adhesion during Trypanosoma cruzi differentiation. J Cell Biol 106(4):1349–1358
4. de Camara Mde L, Bouvier LA, Miranda MR, Reigada C, Pereira CA (2013) Laboratory techniques to obtain different forms of Trypanosoma cruzi: applications to wild-type and genetically modified parasites. Folia Parasitol (Praha) 60(5):406–410
5. Martinez-Diaz RA, Escario JA, Nogal-Ruiz JJ, Gomez-Barrio A (2001) Biological characterization of Trypanosoma cruzi strains. Mem Inst Oswaldo Cruz 96(1):53–59
6. Goncalves CS, Avila AR, de Souza W, Motta MCM, Cavalcanti DP (2018) Revisiting the Trypanosoma cruzi metacyclogenesis: morphological and ultrastructural analyses during cell differentiation. Parasit Vectors 11(1):83. https://doi.org/10.1186/s13071-018-2664-4
7. de Sousa MA (1983) A simple method to purify biologically and antigenically preserved bloodstream trypomastigotes of Trypanosoma cruzi using DEAE-cellulose columns. Mem Inst Oswaldo Cruz 78(3):317–333
8. Contreras VT, Morel CM, Goldenberg S (1985) Stage specific gene expression precedes morphological changes during Trypanosoma cruzi metacyclogenesis. Mol Biochem Parasitol 14(1):83–96. 0166-6851(85)90108-2 [pii]
9. Krieger MA, Avila AR, Ogatta SF, Plazanet-Menut C, Goldenberg S (1999) Differential gene expression during Trypanosoma cruzi metacyclogenesis. Mem Inst Oswaldo Cruz 94(Suppl 1):165–168
10. Marchini FK, de Godoy LM, Rampazzo RC, Pavoni DP, Probst CM, Gnad F, Mann M, Krieger MA (2011) Profiling the Trypanosoma cruzi phosphoproteome. PLoS One 6(9): e25381. https://doi.org/10.1371/journal.pone.0025381. PONE-D-11-10301 [pii]
11. de Godoy LM, Marchini FK, Pavoni DP, Rampazzo Rde C, Probst CM, Goldenberg S, Krieger MA (2012) Quantitative proteomics of Trypanosoma cruzi during metacyclogenesis. Proteomics 12(17):2694–2703. https://doi.org/10.1002/pmic.201200078
12. El-Sayed NM, Myler PJ, Bartholomeu DC, Nilsson D, Aggarwal G, Tran AN, Ghedin E, Worthey EA, Delcher AL, Blandin G, Westenberger SJ, Caler E, Cerqueira GC, Branche C, Haas B, Anupama A, Arner E, Aslund L, Attipoe P, Bontempi E, Bringaud F, Burton P, Cadag E, Campbell DA, Carrington M, Crabtree J, Darban H, da Silveira JF, de Jong P, Edwards K, Englund PT, Fazelina G, Feldblyum T, Ferella M, Frasch AC, Gull K, Horn D, Hou L, Huang Y, Kindlund E, Klingbeil M, Kluge S, Koo H, Lacerda D, Levin MJ, Lorenzi H, Louie T, Machado CR, McCulloch R, McKenna A, Mizuno Y, Mottram JC, Nelson S, Ochaya S, Osoegawa K, Pai G, Parsons M, Pentony M, Pettersson U, Pop M, Ramirez JL, Rinta J, Robertson L, Salzberg SL, Sanchez DO, Seyler A, Sharma R, Shetty J, Simpson AJ, Sisk E, Tammi MT, Tarleton R, Teixeira S, Van Aken S, Vogt C, Ward PN, Wickstead B, Wortman J, White O, Fraser CM, Stuart KD, Andersson B (2005) The genome sequence of Trypanosoma cruzi, etiologic agent of Chagas disease. Science 309(5733):409–415. 309/5733/409 [pii]. https://doi.org/10.1126/science.1112631
13. Batista M, Kugeratski FG, de Paula Lima CV, Probst CM, Kessler RL, de Godoy LM, Krieger

MA, Marchini FK (2017) The MAP kinase MAPKLK1 is essential to Trypanosoma brucei proliferation and regulates proteins involved in mRNA metabolism. J Proteomics 154:118–127. S1874-3919(16)30527-9 [pii]. https://doi.org/10.1016/j.jprot.2016.12.011

14. Kugeratski FG, Batista M, Lima CVP, Neilson LJ, da Cunha ES, de Godoy LM, Zanivan S, Krieger MA, Marchini FK (2018) Mitogen-activated protein kinase kinase 5 regulates proliferation and biosynthetic processes in procyclic forms of Trypanosoma brucei. J Proteome Res 17(1):108–118. https://doi.org/10.1021/acs.jproteome.7b00415

15. Amorim JC, Batista M, da Cunha ES, Lucena ACR, Lima CVP, Sousa K, Krieger MA, Marchini FK (2017) Quantitative proteome and phosphoproteome analyses highlight the adherent population during Trypanosoma cruzi metacyclogenesis. Sci Rep 7(1):9899. https://doi.org/10.1038/s41598-017-10292-3

16. Clayton CE (2002) Life without transcriptional control? From fly to man and back again. EMBO J 21(8):1881–1888. https://doi.org/10.1093/emboj/21.8.1881

17. Kramer S (2012) Developmental regulation of gene expression in the absence of transcriptional control: the case of kinetoplastids. Mol Biochem Parasitol 181(2):61–72. S0166-6851(11)00225-8 [pii]. https://doi.org/10.1016/j.molbiopara.2011.10.002

18. Parsons M, Worthey EA, Ward PN, Mottram JC (2005) Comparative analysis of the kinomes of three pathogenic trypanosomatids: Leishmania major, Trypanosoma brucei and Trypanosoma cruzi. BMC Genomics 6:127. . 1471-2164-6-127 [pii]. https://doi.org/10.1186/1471-2164-6-127

19. Wisniewski JR, Zougman A, Nagaraj N, Mann M (2009) Universal sample preparation method for proteome analysis. Nat Methods 6 (5):359–362. . nmeth.1322 [pii]. https://doi.org/10.1038/nmeth.1322

20. Wisniewski JR (2018) Filter-aided sample preparation for proteome analysis. Methods Mol Biol 1841:3–10. https://doi.org/10.1007/978-1-4939-8695-8_1

21. Gilar M, Olivova P, Daly AE, Gebler JC (2005) Two-dimensional separation of peptides using RP-RP-HPLC system with different pH in first and second separation dimensions. J Sep Sci 28 (14):1694–1703

22. Yang F, Shen Y, Camp DG 2nd, Smith RD (2012) High-pH reversed-phase chromatography with fraction concatenation for 2D proteomic analysis. Expert Rev Proteomics 9 (2):129–134. https://doi.org/10.1586/epr.12.15

23. Bodenmiller B, Mueller LN, Mueller M, Domon B, Aebersold R (2007) Reproducible isolation of distinct, overlapping segments of the phosphoproteome. Nat Methods 4 (3):231–237. . nmeth1005 [pii]. https://doi.org/10.1038/nmeth1005

24. Andersson L, Porath J (1986) Isolation of phosphoproteins by immobilized metal (Fe^{3+}) affinity chromatography. Anal Biochem 154(1):250–254. 0003-2697(86)90523-3 [pii]

25. Posewitz MC, Tempst P (1999) Immobilized gallium(III) affinity chromatography of phosphopeptides. Anal Chem 71(14):2883–2892

26. Pinkse MW, Uitto PM, Hilhorst MJ, Ooms B, Heck AJ (2004) Selective isolation at the femtomole level of phosphopeptides from proteolytic digests using 2D-NanoLC-ESI-MS/MS and titanium oxide precolumns. Anal Chem 76(14):3935–3943. https://doi.org/10.1021/ac0498617

27. Humphrey SJ, Karayel O, James DE, Mann M (2018) High-throughput and high-sensitivity phosphoproteomics with the EasyPhos platform. Nat Protoc 13(9):1897–1916. https://doi.org/10.1038/s41596-018-0014-9

28. Kim MS, Choie W-S, Shin YS, Yu MH, Lee SW (2004) Development of ultra-high pressure capillary reverse-phase liquid chromatography/tandem mass spectrometry for high-sensitive and high-throughput proteomics. Bull Kor Chem Soc 25(12):1833–1839

29. Schroeder MJ, Shabanowitz J, Schwartz JC, Hunt DF, Coon JJ (2004) A neutral loss activation method for improved phosphopeptide sequence analysis by quadrupole ion trap mass spectrometry. Anal Chem 76(13):3590–3598. https://doi.org/10.1021/ac0497104

30. Eng JK, McCormack AL, Yates JR (1994) An approach to correlate tandem mass spectral data of peptides with amino acid sequences in a protein database. J Am Soc Mass Spectrom 5 (11):976–989. https://doi.org/10.1016/1044-0305(94)80016-2

31. Perkins DN, Pappin DJ, Creasy DM, Cottrell JS (1999) Probability-based protein identification by searching sequence databases using mass spectrometry data. Electrophoresis 20 (18):3551–3567. https://doi.org/10.1002/(SICI)1522-2683(19991201)20:18<3551::AID-ELPS3551>3.0.CO;2-2

32. Cox J, Mann M (2008) MaxQuant enables high peptide identification rates, individualized p.p.b.-range mass accuracies and proteome-wide protein quantification. Nat Biotechnol

26(12):1367–1372. . nbt.1511 [pii]. https://doi.org/10.1038/nbt.1511

33. Cox J, Neuhauser N, Michalski A, Scheltema RA, Olsen JV, Mann M (2011) Andromeda: a peptide search engine integrated into the MaxQuant environment. J Proteome Res 10 (4):1794–1805. https://doi.org/10.1021/pr101065j
34. Tyanova S, Temu T, Sinitcyn P, Carlson A, Hein MY, Geiger T, Mann M, Cox J (2016) The Perseus computational platform for comprehensive analysis of (prote)omics data. Nat Methods 13(9):731–740. nmeth.3901 [pii]. https://doi.org/10.1038/nmeth.3901
35. Kessler RL, Soares MJ, Probst CM, Krieger MA (2013) Trypanosoma cruzi response to sterol biosynthesis inhibitors: morphophysiological alterations leading to cell death. PLoS One 8(1):e55497. https://doi.org/10.1371/journal.pone.0055497. PONE-D-12-29152 [pii]
36. Wisniewski JR, Gaugaz FZ (2015) Fast and sensitive total protein and Peptide assays for proteomic analysis. Anal Chem 87 (8):4110–4116. https://doi.org/10.1021/ac504689z
37. Rappsilber J, Ishihama Y, Mann M (2003) Stop and go extraction tips for matrix-assisted laser desorption/ionization, nanoelectrospray, and LC/MS sample pretreatment in proteomics. Anal Chem 75(3):663–670
38. Rappsilber J, Mann M, Ishihama Y (2007) Protocol for micro-purification, enrichment, pre-fractionation and storage of peptides for proteomics using StageTips. Nat Protoc 2 (8):1896–1906. . nprot.2007.261 [pii]. https://doi.org/10.1038/nprot.2007.261
39. Schaab C, Geiger T, Stoehr G, Cox J, Mann M (2012) Analysis of high accuracy, quantitative proteomics data in the MaxQB database. Mol Cell Proteomics 11(3):M111.014068. M111.014068 [pii]. https://doi.org/10.1074/mcp.M111.014068
40. Tyanova S, Temu T, Carlson A, Sinitcyn P, Mann M, Cox J (2015) Visualization of LC-MS/MS proteomics data in MaxQuant. Proteomics 15(8):1453–1456. https://doi.org/10.1002/pmic.201400449
41. Tyanova S, Cox J (2018) Perseus: a bioinformatics platform for integrative analysis of proteomics data in cancer research. Methods Mol Biol 1711:133–148. https://doi.org/10.1007/978-1-4939-7493-1_7
42. De Paula Lima CV, Batista M, Kugeratski FG, Vincent IM, Soares MJ, Probst CM, Krieger MA, Marchini FK (2014) LM14 defined medium enables continuous growth of Trypanosoma cruzi. BMC Microbiol 14:238. . s12866-014-0238-y [pii]. https://doi.org/10.1186/s12866-014-0238-y
43. Greig N, Wyllie S, Patterson S, Fairlamb AH (2009) A comparative study of methylglyoxal metabolism in trypanosomatids. FEBS J 276 (2):376–386. . EJB6788 [pii]. https://doi.org/10.1111/j.1742-4658.2008.06788.x
44. Roberts AJ, Fairlamb AH (2016) The N-myristoylome of Trypanosoma cruzi. Sci Rep 6:31078. srep31078 [pii]. https://doi.org/10.1038/srep31078
45. Meyer JG, A Komives E (2012) Charge state coalescence during electrospray ionization improves peptide identification by tandem mass spectrometry. J Am Soc Mass Spectrom 23(8):1390–1399. https://doi.org/10.1007/s13361-012-0404-0
46. Hahne H, Pachl F, Ruprecht B, Maier SK, Klaeger S, Helm D, Medard G, Wilm M, Lemeer S, Kuster B (2013) DMSO enhances electrospray response, boosting sensitivity of proteomic experiments. Nat Methods 10 (10):989–991. nmeth.2610 [pii]. https://doi.org/10.1038/nmeth.2610
47. Olsen JV, de Godoy LM, Li G, Macek B, Mortensen P, Pesch R, Makarov A, Lange O, Horning S, Mann M (2005) Parts per million mass accuracy on an Orbitrap mass spectrometer via lock mass injection into a C-trap. Mol Cell Proteomics 4(12):2010–2021. . T500030-MCP200 [pii]. https://doi.org/10.1074/mcp.T500030-MCP200

Chapter 12

Genome-Wide Proteomics and Phosphoproteomics Analysis of *Leishmania* spp. During Differentiation

Harsh Pawar, Gajanan Sathe, and Milind S. Patole

Abstract

Determining variations in protein abundance and/or posttranslational modification as a function of time or upon induction by a signal in a particular cell type is central to quantitative proteomics. Isobaric labeling methodologies now allow for parallel quantification of proteins at various conditions concurrently or multiplexing in relatively quantitative proteomics workflows. Hence, mapping the protein expression profiles of various developmental stages of *Leishmania* parasites is possible with high-resolution mass spectrometry. To analyze global changes in protein expression and cellular signaling pathways during *Leishmania* differentiation and development is possible with a quantitative proteomics approach. The tandem mass tags (TMT) approach provides a chemical labeling method based on the principle of amine reactive tags; the maximum number of conditions that can be multiplexed is 10-plex. We describe herein a detailed method for sample preparation, TMT-labeling, mass spectrometry and data analysis of different developmental stages of *Leishmania donovani* parasites. This quantitative proteomic approach is useful to study dynamic changes in protein expression levels during *L. donovani* differentiation, and also allows in-depth analysis of signaling pathways via phosphoproteomics.

Key words Tandem mass tag (TMT), *Leishmania* development, Parasite differentiation, Signaling, Promastigote, Amastigote, Proteogenomics

1 Introduction

The kinetoplastid *Leishmania* parasite has a digenetic life cycle where extracellular promastigotes replicate in the midgut of the phlebotomine insect vector and the intracellular amastigotes replicate within mammalian macrophage cells. The physiological and physical milieus of the two environments in which the leishmanial parasite survives and proliferates are very much dissimilar. Both environments are rich in hydrolytic enzymes. The parasite has evolved to adjust to the two different niches by differentiating into two morphotypes. The process of differentiation of the leishmanial parasite is not merely a change in cell volume, morphology or loss of flagellar appendage. Rather, it is a complex progression that involves a number of changes at the level of gene expression

Paul A. M. Michels et al. (eds.), *Trypanosomatids: Methods and Protocols*, Methods in Molecular Biology, vol. 2116, https://doi.org/10.1007/978-1-0716-0294-2_12, © Springer Science+Business Media, LLC, part of Springer Nature 2020

leading to the synthesis of new soluble and membrane proteins. This results in changes of the metabolism and immunogenicity of the parasite. The changes in gene expression can be monitored by microarray-based expression profiling [1, 2] or transcriptome profiling using RNA-seq [3].

In the midgut of the phlebotomine sand fly the parasite exists as the motile flagellated procyclic promastigote form. The midgut milieu is rich in amino acids and sugars with a mild alkaline pH and the vector has a mean body temperature of approximately 26 °C [4]. In contrast, in the host macrophages, the parasite lodges in phagolysosomes, replicating as nonmotile amastigote forms. The *Leishmania* parasite encounters a higher temperature of 37 °C within the host macrophages. Amastigote cellular volume is much smaller than promastigote cell volume [5]. The pH of phagolysosomes is acidic (~5.5), and major nutrients are amino acids and fatty acids, while sugars are scarce [6, 7]. The *Leishmania* amastigotes are auxotrophic for most nutrients such as purines, amino acids, vitamins, and heme [8]. Nonetheless, a recent study with *L. mexicana* indicates that intracellular amastigotes in activated macrophages rely preferentially on sugars as the primary energy source [9]. Thus the *Leishmania* parasite, in order to survive and proliferate within the vector and the macrophage, has developed mechanisms involving rapid changes in gene and protein expression profiles [10]. These two life stages can be studied from the vector and vertebrate host but it requires extensive expertise and also there are issues relating to contaminations from these systems. A much cleaner system is required for analyzing differentiation and development of parasites of the promastigotes to amastigote life stages of parasites. Here in vitro differentiation model systems developed for *Leishmania* by various research groups across the world, including our own group, are useful to study the time course of parasite differentiation [11]. *Leishmania* parasites when axenically grown at 26 °C at pH 5 express amastigote-specific genes with no change in parasite morphology [12]. However, when *L. donovani* is grown at 37 °C at pH 7 there is a change in the parasite morphology to the amastigote oval shape while the growth kinetics are similar to those of promastigotes [13]. Thus *L. donovani* recognizes two specific signals (37 °C and pH 5.5) which results in differentiation of individual promastigotes into amastigotes [11, 14].

Global proteomic analysis of *Leishmania* parasites can be broadly categorized into two major types: qualitative (profiling) and quantitative analysis. Qualitative proteomic analysis of *Leishmania* parasites results in cataloguing of stage-specific expressed proteins [15, 16]. Additionally, when high-resolution mass spectrometry is coupled with a proteogenomic approach, not only can we create detailed proteomic maps of different life stages of *Leishmania* parasites [17, 18], but we can also identify new life-stage specific genes previously not annotated during the genome sequence analysis [19–21]. Cataloguing studies can also be used to map in-depth subcellular proteomes such as in the case of glycosomes [22] and other organelles [23]. However, protein cataloguing using qualitative proteomic approaches has serious limitations, especially when studying global proteome changes during parasite development or differentiation in a time-dependent manner. This is especially important for studying proteins associated with parasite differentiation, which are either upregulated or downregulated depending on the environmental cues the parasite encounters during its development. Toward this end, quantitative proteomics approaches are highly useful.

Currently there are various quantitative proteomics techniques available and each of them being applied dependent on the question to be addressed. The majority of studies use relative quantitation to identify differentially expressed proteins between two or more conditions. These are either label-free or labeling-based methods. Among the label-based methods there are two types of metabolic labeling methods such as stable isotopic labeling of amino acids in cell culture (SILAC) [24, 25]. The other types are the chemical labeling methods such as isobaric tags for relative and absolute quantitation (iTRAQ) and tandem mass tags (TMT). These two techniques are based on a similar principle of using amine reactive tags but the maximum number of conditions that can be multiplexed is different in both of these iTRAQ (8-plex) and TMT (10-plex). In recent years, Professor Steve Gygi's research group combined SILAC and TMT to increase the number of conditions that can be compared simultaneously to 18-plex [26] and 54-plex [27]. This approach of multiplexing is referred to as Hyperplexing. The iTRAQ-based quantitative proteomic approach has been used previously to study differentiation and signaling in *L. donovani* [10, 28–30]. The various approaches for proteomic analysis of *Leishmania* parasites used so far by various groups are outlined in Fig. 1.

Here we describe the standard protocol for quantitative global proteomics and phosphoproteomics using the TMT-labeling approach to analyze stage-specific differentiation of *L. donovani* parasites.

2 Materials

2.1 Promastigote Growth Medium

EARLs based medium 199 (M199) supplemented with 10% heat-inactivated fetal bovine serum, 0.1 mg/ml streptomycin and 100 U/ml penicillin.

2.2 Amastigote Growth Medium

EARLs based medium 199 supplemented with 25% fetal bovine serum (non-heat inactivated), 0.1 mg/ml streptomycin, and

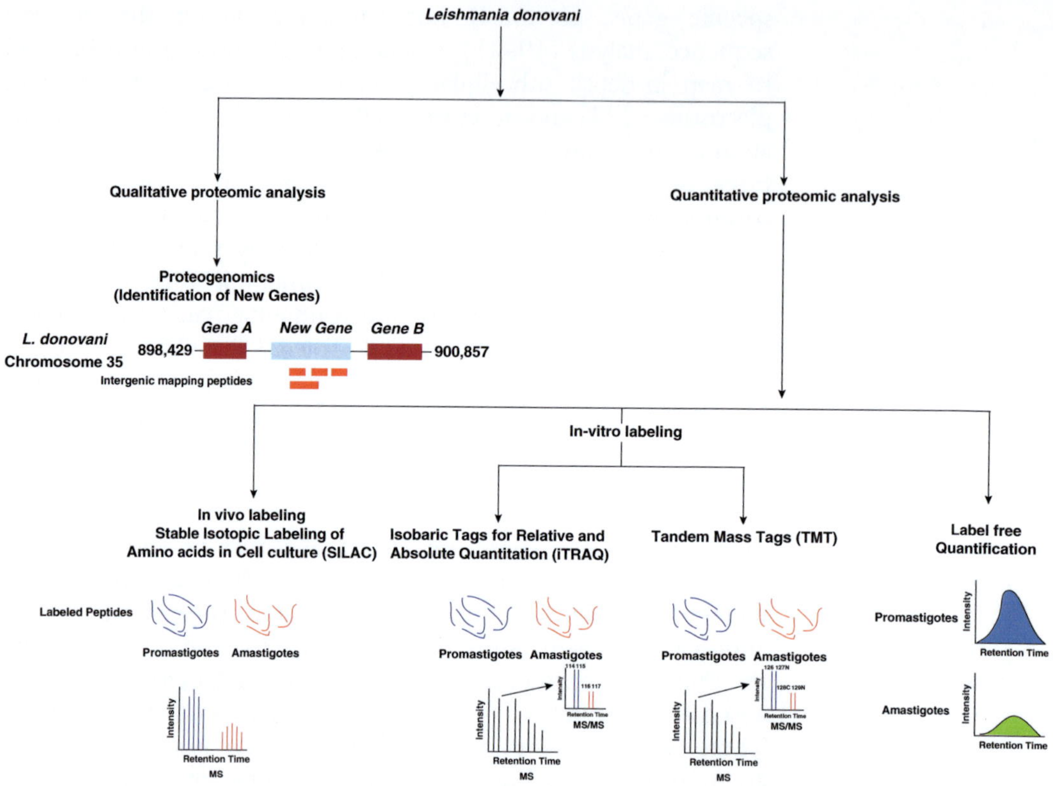

Fig. 1 Detailed workflow for various proteomic analyses (qualitative and quantitative) of *Leishmania donovani* parasites to map the global proteome and phosphoproteome

100 U/ml penicillin. Add 10 mM succinic acid (succinic acid only solubilizes below pH 6) to the M199, adjust to pH 5.5 with HCl and filter sterilize.

2.3 Serum for Amastigote Medium

When purchasing a new batch of serum we recommend that you check *Leishmania* aggregates formation at 5–8 h of differentiation. As indicated below, aggregation is essential for successful differentiation. The factor that induces cell aggregation is sensitive to heat. We recommend purchasing and using non-heat-inactivated serum.

2.4 Cell Lysis and Protein Extraction

1. Lysis buffer: 4% or 2% sodium dodecyl sulfate (SDS) in 50 mM triethyl ammonium bicarbonate buffer (TEABC), protease and phosphatase inhibitor cocktail (Halt Protease and Phosphatase Inhibitor Cocktail, EDTA free, Thermo Fischer) provided as 1 ml solution (100×). Add 10 μl of the cocktail to 1 ml of lysis buffer to get a final concentration of 1×.
2. BCA Protein and peptide estimation kit.

2.5 SDS-PAGE

1. Resolving gel buffer: 1.5 M Tris–HCl, pH 8.8.
2. Stacking gel buffer: 1.0 M Tris–HCl, pH 6.8.

3. 30% acrylamide–bisacrylamide solution: Dissolve 29 g of acrylamide and 1 g of *N*,*N*′-methylenebisacrylamide in 100 ml of water.
4. 10% ammonium persulfate (APS).
5. *N*,*N*,*N*,*N*′-tetramethyl-ethylenediamine (TEMED).
6. Running buffer: 25 mM Tris–HCl, pH 8.3, 0.192 M glycine, 0.1% SDS.
7. Loading buffer (6×): 375 mM Tris–HCl, pH 6.8, 6% SDS, 25% β-mercaptoethanol, 0.1% bromophenol blue (BPB), 45% glycerol.
8. Fixative: methanol–water–glacial acetic acid (5:4:1).

2.6 In-Solution Protein Digestion

1. Reduction solution: 100 mM DTT stock—prepare shortly before use.
2. Alkylation solution: 100 mM (IAA) stock—prepare in the dark, shortly before use.
3. Lysyl Endopeptidase.
4. Lys C solution: 1:100 Lys C enzyme to protein ratio in 50 mM TEABC.
5. Trypsin (modified sequencing grade).
6. Trypsin solution: 1:25 trypsin enzyme to protein ratio in 50 mM TEABC.

2.7 Digested Peptide Cleanup Using C_{18} Sep-Pak Columns

1. Sep-Pak C_{18} Plus Short Cartridge.
2. 100% Acetonitrile (ACN).
3. Solvent A: 0.1% formic acid.
4. Solvent B: 0.1% formic acid, 40% ACN.

2.8 TMT Labeling of Peptides

1. TMT10plex™ Isobaric Label Reagent Set, 1 × 5 mg (Thermo Fisher Scientific).
2. 50 mM TEABC, pH 7.5–8.5, freshly prepared prior to use.
3. 5% (w/v) aqueous hydroxylamine solution.
4. Benchtop centrifuge.
5. Vortex mixer.

2.9 Labeled Peptide Sample Fractionation

1. Solvent A: 10 mM Tetra Ethyl Ammonium Bicarbonate (TEABC) buffer, pH 9.5.
2. Solvent B: 10 mM TEABC buffer, 90% ACN, pH 9.5.
3. Waters XBridge column (Waters Corporation, Milford, MA; 130 Å, 5 μm, 250 × 4.6 mm).
4. HPLC system.

2.10 Phosphopeptide Enrichment

For enrichment of the phosphopeptides either a titanium dioxide or immobilized metal affinity-based batch method will be used.

2.10.1 Titanium Dioxide (TiO_2) Enrichment

1. Titansphere (TiO_2) 100 Å 5 μm.
2. 2,5-Dihydroxybenzoic acid (DHB).
3. 5% Ammonia solution for elution prepared from a 25% ammonia solution.
4. Wash solution 1 (WS1): 80% Acetonitrile in 3% trifluoroacetic acid (TFA).
5. Thermomixer.

2.10.2 Immobilized Metal Affinity Chromatography (IMAC) Enrichment

1. Ni-NTA beads for IMAC (Qiagen).
2. Dibasic sodium phosphate, pH 7.0.
3. 80% Acetonitrile–0.1% TFA.
4. 100 mM EDTA.
5. 10 mM $FeCl_3$.
6. 80% Acetonitrile in 1% trifluoroacetic acid.
7. 500 mM dibasic sodium phosphate, pH 7.0.

2.11 Desalting Using STAGE Tips

1. C_{18} STAGE tips.
2. 100% methanol.
3. 1% formic acid.
4. Solvent A: 0.1% formic acid.
5. Solvent B: 50% acetonitrile–0.1% formic acid.

2.12 LC-MS/MS Analysis

1. A high-resolution mass spectrometer such as LTQ-Orbitrap series (Thermo Electron, Bremen, Germany).
2. A nanoflow HPLC such as Easy-nLCII (Thermo Scientific, Odense, Southern Denmark).
3. Solvent A: 0.1% formic acid.
4. Solvent B: 0.1% formic acid, 95% ACN.

2.13 Mass Spectrometry Data Analysis

1. Latest version of protein data for *L. donovani* downloaded from TriTrypDB.
2. Sequences of common contaminant proteins such as proteases and human keratins.
3. One or multiple search algorithms. Commercially available search algorithms such as SEQUEST or Mascot.

3 Methods

3.1 Principle of TMT Labeling Assay

Tandem Mass Tags (TMT) is an in vitro chemical labeling technique which involves the use of isobaric tags which can label all peptides from a protein digest. TMT reagent is composed of a mass reporter (*m/z*-113-121) for a 10-plex TMT kit, mass normalizer and lastly an amine reactive group (Fig. 2a). There is incorporation of stable isotopes in different combinations within the mass reporter and mass normalizer groups. Upon fragmentation of the TMT-labeled peptide in the mass spectrometer each mass reporter ion from each ten different conditions can be resolved in the MS/MS (MS2) spectrum. The overall mass of the labeled peptides for a particular protein from different conditions will remain the same. Hence, these 10-plex labeled peptides will coelute. The relative intensities of the mass reporter ions denote the relative abundance of the peptide and the mean of all relative abundances of all peptides from each protein represents the relative abundance of the protein in different conditions being in which it is analyzed [31]. The detailed TMT-labeled quantitative proteomic analysis workflow for mapping the proteomic and phosphoproteomic changes during *L. donovani* differentiation is outlined in Fig. 2b.

3.2 Protocol for Axenic Promastigote-to-Amastigote Differentiation

The late log phase promastigote culture of *L. donovani* (cell density 1×10^7 cells/ml) is centrifuged for 10 min at room temperature (RT) and the cell pellet resuspended in prewarmed amastigote medium. The cells are incubated at 37 °C in a 5% CO_2 incubator and the in vitro *L. donovani* differentiation is monitored for up to 120 h. A detailed protocol for undertaking *L. donovani* differentiation is provided in Chapter 3 by Zilberstein.

3.3 Cell Lysis and Protein Extraction

1. *L. donovani* promastigotes (pH 7 and 26 °C) and four different phases (time point 2.5, 24, 48, and 120 h) of amastigote differentiation (pH 5.2 and 37 °C) are analyzed. Wash the cells (1×10^8) from each stage twice in 20 ml ice-cold EARL's salt solution and finally pellet them and keep them frozen (−80 °C) until use.
2. Resuspend the cell pellet in 2% SDS lysis in 50 mM TEABC buffer and heat the cell pellet at 90 °C for 5 min.
3. Sonicate the samples for 3 cycles at 40% amplitude. Keep the tubes on ice for 1 min after each cycle. Centrifuge at 13,200 × *g* for 15 min at 4 °C and transfer the supernatant to a fresh 1.5 ml tube.
4. Estimate the protein amount using a BCA protein estimation kit and load 20 μg of protein on a 10% SDS-PAGE gel to check the integrity of the samples (*see* **Note 1**).

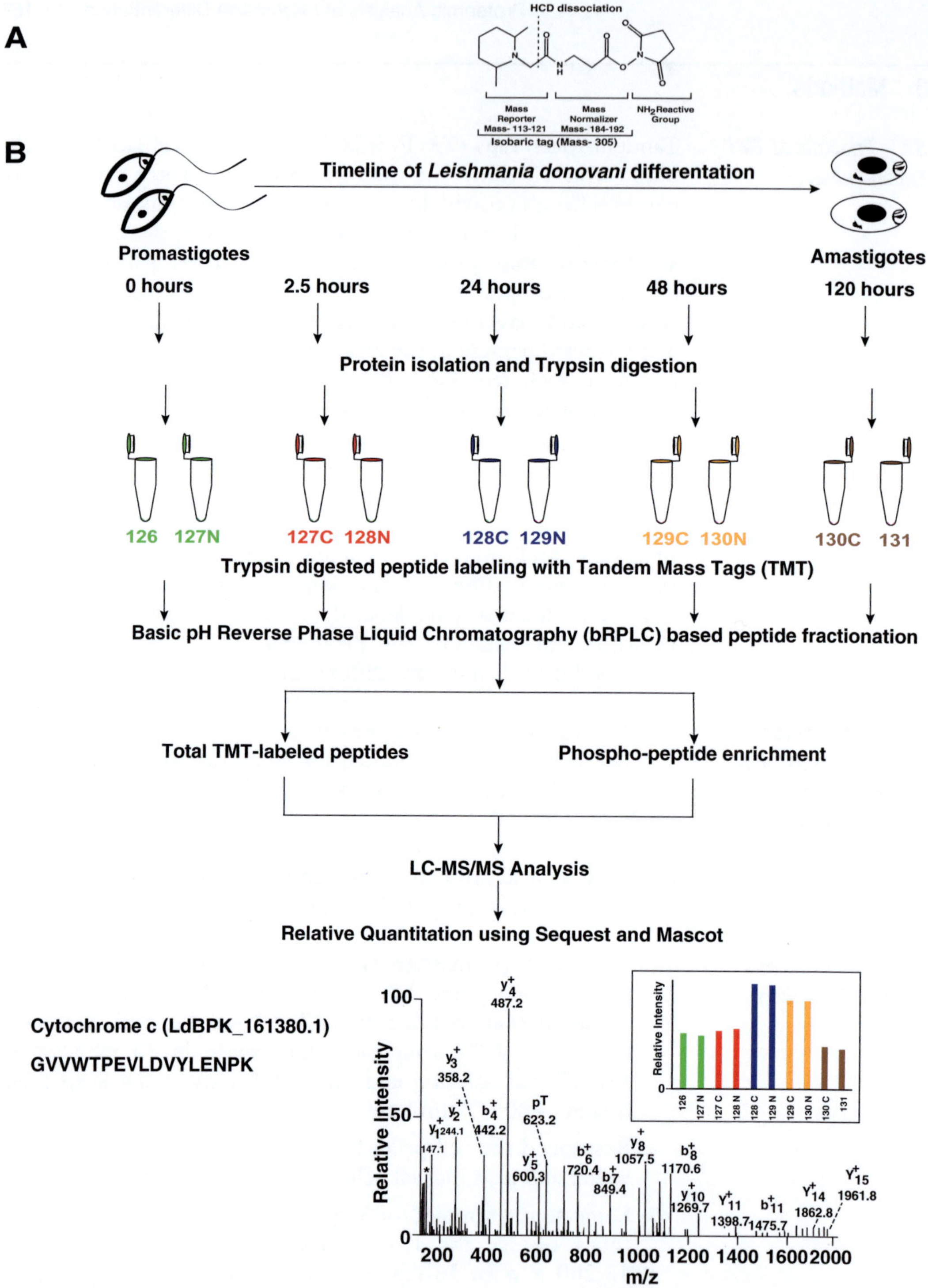

Fig. 2 (**a**) Chemical structure of Tandem Mass Tags (TMT) label used for quantitative proteomic analysis. (**b**) Detailed TMT-labeled quantitative proteomic analysis workflow for mapping the proteomic and phosphoproteomic changes during *Leishmania donovani* stage-specific differentiation

3.4 In-Solution Protein Digestion

1. Take 1 mg of protein from both analyses (**Total proteome and Phosphoproteome**). Add DTT to a final concentration of 5 mM in the samples. Incubate at 60 °C for 20 min.
2. Keep the tubes at room temperature for 10 min and add IAA to a final concentration of 15 mM in the samples. Incubate in dark for 15 min at RT.
3. Add 5 volumes of chilled acetone and incubate the tubes at −20 °C overnight.
4. Centrifuge at 13,200 × *g* at 4 °C for 15 min. Wash the pellet with chilled acetone once and centrifuge again at 13,200 × *g* at 4 °C for 15 min (*see* **Note 2**).
5. Dissolve the pellet in 6 M urea (*see* **Note 3**).
6. Incubate the samples in LysC solution for 4 h at 37 °C.
7. Dilute the samples to <2 M urea with 50 mM TEABC and incubate with Trypsin solution overnight at 37 °C.
8. Load 20 μg of sample on a 10% SDS-PAGE gel to check for digestion efficiency (*see* **Note 4**).
9. If the protein is digested, then acidify the peptide digest with 1% formic acid (pH of the digest should be <3).
10. Clean the samples using Sep-Pak C_{18} columns.

3.5 Digested Peptide Cleanup Using C_{18} Sep-Pak Columns

1. The Sep-Pak C_{18} plus Short Cartridge is connected from the small end to a 10 ml syringe.
2. Pass 6 ml of 100% acetonitrile (ACN) to activate the column.
3. Wash the column twice with 4 ml of solvent A (0.1% formic acid) to equilibrate it.
4. Inject the acidified trypsin digested protein mixture and allow peptide binding to the column for 4 min.
5. Wash the column with 15 ml of solvent A using successively 2, 6, and 7 ml.
6. To elute the peptides wash the column twice with 5 ml of solvent B (0.1% formic acid, 30% ACN) in a 15 ml tube.
7. The eluted peptide solution is dried using a vacuum concentrator.

3.6 TMT Labeling of Peptides

1. Resuspend the entire mixture of digested peptides in 100 μl 50 mM TEABC. Make sure the pH of the solution is in the range of 6.5–8.5. Estimate the peptide amount using a BCA peptide estimation kit. Take 100 μg of peptide digest for TMT labeling (*see* **Note 5**).
2. Bring the TMT reaction kit to room temperature. Dissolve each TMT reagent in 40 μl of anhydrous acetonitrile. Vortex, spin the tubes and keep for 5 min at RT.

3. Add 40 μl TMT reagent to the peptide digests and vortex gently. Incubate the reaction at RT for 1 h (*see* **Note 6**).
4. Take an aliquot of each sample and add 5% hydroxylamine to each of the aliquoted samples to quench the reaction. Pool all samples and proceed for the label check (*see* **Note 7**).
5. Normalize the samples based on the summed label intensities of all PSMs. The samples with the lowest sum should be the baseline for normalization.
6. Quench the reaction with 5% hydroxylamine and incubate for 15 min at RT.
7. Pool all samples and dry the pooled sample using a vacuum concentrator.

3.7 Labeled Peptide Sample Fractionation Using Basic pH Reverse Phase Liquid Chromatography (bRPLC)

1. The dried samples (**step 7**, Subheading 3.6) are reconstituted in 1 ml of 10 mM Tetra Ethyl Ammonium Bicarbonate (TEABC) buffer, pH 9.5.
2. Load the reconstituted TMT-labeled sample on the 30 mm long XBridge C_{18} column.
3. Resolve the TMT-labeled peptide mixture using solvent B (10 mM TEABC buffer, 90% ACN, pH 9.5) gradient (0–100%) for 50 min at a flow rate of 1 ml/min.
4. Collect the fractions in a deep 96-well plate in an LC-autosampler.
5. Pool the fractions into a total of 10–15 fractions or more depending on the mass spectrometer time availability. This is frequently done by pooling equidistant fractions of the bRPLC fractionated sample obtained from the liquid chromatography system (**step 4**).
6. From these 10–15 fractions, 90% of the samples should be taken out for the phosphoproteomic analysis (**step 8** and Subheading 3.8) and the remaining 10% will be used further for the global proteome analysis (**step 7**).
7. Dry the pooled fractions global proteome in a vacuum concentrator and store at −80 °C until mass spectrometry analysis.
8. The pooled TMT-labeled phosphoproteome samples should be lyophilized using a lyophilizer.

3.8 Phosphopeptide Enrichment

Phosphopeptide enrichment can be undertaken by either of the two methods:

3.8.1 Titanium Dioxide (TiO_2) Enrichment

1. Reconstitute the fractions with 100 μl of 5% DHB solution. Ensure the peptides are completely dissolved (*see* **Note 8**).

2. Take an appropriate amount of TiO_2 beads at the ratio 1:4 peptide to TiO_2 beads. Keep tubes in heating block at 60 °C for 15–20 min (*see* **Note 9**).
3. Suspend TiO_2 beads in 100 μl of 5% DHB solution and incubate for 15 min on the rotator at RT. Incubation of TiO_2 with DHB solution results in the material turning brownish.
4. Add an appropriate volume of beads to peptides at a 1:4 ratio and incubate the peptide-DHB-TiO_2 mix on a thermomixer set at 1100 rpm for 15–30 min at RT).
5. Centrifuge the tubes at 1500 × *g* for 1 min and transfer the supernatant to another microfuge tube.
6. Wash the beads with 500 μl WS1 and centrifuge the tubes at 1500 × *g* for 1 min. Discard supernatant. Repeat this step again.
7. Suspend TiO_2 beads in 100 μl WS1 and transfer the entire content to stage-tips packed with two plugs of C_{18} material.
8. Wash the peptide-TiO_2 beads with 100 μl of WS1.
9. In separate tubes (collection tubes), add 40 μl of 4% TFA and place it on ice. Elute phosphopeptides from TiO_2 beads using 5% ammonia solution into collection tubes containing 4% TFA. Repeat elution twice.
10. Dry the samples using a vacuum concentrator.

3.8.2 Immobilized Metal Affinity Chromatography (IMAC) Enrichment

1. Preparation of IMAC beads—Iron-chelated IMAC beads are prepared from Ni-NTA superflow agarose beads that are stripped of nickel with 100 mM EDTA. After stripping wash the beads with 80% Acetonitrile–0.1% TFA. These beads will then be incubated in an aqueous solution of 10 mM $FeCl_3$. Centrifuge for seconds in a tabletop centrifuge at 13,200 × *g* and RT, and discard the $FeCl_3$. Repeat this process twice. After incubation with $FeCl_3$ wash the beads again with 80% Acetonitrile–0.1% TFA. Each step should be repeated twice and the beads are then ready for the phosphopeptide enrichment.
2. Reconstitute each fraction in 80% Acetonitrile–0.1% TFA solution at a concentration of 0.5 μg/μl.
3. Then, enrich the peptide mixture for phosphopeptides with 10 μl freshly prepared Fe-IMAC beads and incubate for 30 min.
4. Pack C_{18} stage-tips and equilibrate with 2 × 100 μl washes of methanol, 2 × 50 μl washes of 50% acetonitrile–0.1% formic acid, and 2 × 100 μl washes of 1% formic acid.
5. Load enriched IMAC beads on packed C_{18} stage-tips and wash twice with 50 μl of 80% acetonitrile–0.1% TFA and 100 μl of 1% formic acid.

6. Elute the phosphorylated peptides from the IMAC beads by washing three times with 70 μl of 500 mM dibasic sodium phosphate, pH 7.0, followed by two washes with 100 μl of 1% formic acid. Finally, all the peptides are eluted from the stage tips with 60 μl of 50% acetonitrile–0.1% formic acid.
7. Concentrate each fraction using a vacuum concentrator.

3.9 C_{18} Stage-Tips Cleanup

1. The C_{18} stage-tips need to be connected to a 5 ml syringe.
2. The C_{18} material in the stage-tips is activated by passing 30 μl of 100% ACN.
3. Samples need to be reconstituted in 30 μl of 0.1% formic acid.
4. Load the sample onto the C_{18} stage-tips and collect the flow through. Repeat this process twice.
5. Wash the column thrice with 30 μl of 0.1% formic acid.
6. Elute the peptide twice with 30 μl of 40% ACN, 0.1% formic acid.
7. Dry the flow through using a vacuum concentrator and store the samples at −80 °C until mass spectrometry analysis (*see* Subheading 3.10).

3.10 LC-MS/MS Analysis

1. The LC-MS/MS method used for analysis of both the TMT-labeled total proteome and phosphoproteome samples of *L. donovani* differentiation will be the same.
2. The dried samples need to be reconstituted in 25 μl of solvent A (0.1% formic acid) and placed in a 96-well plate.
3. Each sample needs to be loaded onto an enrichment column at a flow rate of 3 μl/min. The enrichment column (75 μm × 2 cm) is packed in-house with magic C_{18} AQ (Michrom Bioresources, Auburn, CA, USA) 5 μm particle and 100 Å pore size.
4. Peptide samples are resolved on the analytical column using a linear gradient 7–35% solvent B for 90 min or more. The analytical column has dimensions 75 μm × 25 cm, 5 μm particle and 100 Å pore size packed using nitrogen pressure cell at 2500 psi and is fitted on a flex ion source that is operated at 2.0 kV voltage.
5. The MS data acquisition is in a data dependent manner with full scans in the range of *m/z* 350–2000. Both MS and MS/MS have to be acquired and measured using an Orbitrap mass analyzer. Full MS scans are measured at a resolution of 120,000 at *m/z* 400.
6. Twenty most intense precursor ions are selected for MS/MS and fragmented using a higher-energy collisional dissociation (HCD) method and detected at a mass resolution of 45,000 at *m/z* 400. Automatic gain control for full MS is set to one million ions and for MS/MS is set to 0.05 million ions with a maximum ion injection time of 100 and 200 ms, respectively.

7. Dynamic exclusion is set to 30 s and singly charged ions are rejected. Internal calibration has to be carried out using lock mass option (m/z 445.1200025) from ambient air.

3.11 Mass Spectrometry Data Analysis

For database dependent searches of the mass spectrometry data parasite-specific databases are used.

1. The latest version of the *L. donovani* strain BPKA protein database can be downloaded from TriTrypDB (http://tritrypdb.org/tritrypdb/).
2. To download the protein database as a .fasta file format, click on the downloads tab > click on data files > Current_Release (release-41version)>LdonovaniBPK282A1>fasta>data>TriTrypDB-41_LdonovaniBPK282A1_AnnotatedProteins.fasta (entries $n = 8023$).
3. Open the fasta file in WordPad or Notepad++ and append the contaminants protein list (bovine albumin, porcine trypsin, and other common experimental contaminating proteins). Rename the file as LdonovaniBPK282A1_contaminants.
4. Index the database in the respective search algorithms and in most cases the search algorithms are limited by the mass spectrometer instruments used for the analysis. In our case, most of the data are acquired on the Thermo Orbitrap platform.
5. The Raw MS/MS data (.raw format for Thermo Orbitrap mass spectrometers) obtained from the LC-MS/MS analysis should be searched using the Proteome Discoverer (v 2.1; Thermo Fisher Scientific) suite for protein identification and quantitation.
6. The LC-MS/MS raw data are searched using SEQUEST HT and Mascot (version 2.2.0) search algorithms against LdonovaniBPK282A1_contaminants.
7. The following search parameters are frequently used for database-dependent searches of TMT-labeled peptide sample data.
   (a) Trypsin as a proteolytic enzyme (with up to two missed cleavages).
   (b) Peptide mass error tolerance of 10 ppm.
   (c) Fragment mass error tolerance of 0.05 Da.
   (d) Carbamidomethylation of cysteine (+57.02146 Da).
   (e) TMT tags (+229.162932 Da) on lysine residue and peptide N-termini as fixed modification.
   (f) Oxidation of methionine (+15.99492 Da).
   (g) Phosphorylation (+79.96633 Da) of serine, threonine, and tyrosine residues as variable modifications.

8. The probability of phosphorylation for each Ser/Thr/Tyr site on each peptide is calculated by the PhosphoRS algorithm29. The relative ratio for each phosphopeptide is calculated by dividing the intensity of each phosphorylated peptide over the intensity of the corresponding peptide.

An FDR threshold of ≤1% at peptide and protein level is frequently applied to obtain the list of differentially expressed known proteins identified from the various stages of *L. donovani* differentiated cells.

4 Notes

1. BCA estimation results can be different from the protein amount estimated based on the gel. Normalize all samples based on the gel profile. Any outlier samples should not be included for further downstream steps.
2. Acetone pellet can be stored at −80 °C for 2–3 months.
3. Samples in urea buffer should not be subjected to temperatures >37 °C. Heating the urea buffer will break the urea into isocyanate ions and subsequently leads to carbamylation modification on proteins.
4. If bands are present in the postdigest gel, incubate the sample again for trypsin digestion for 6 h and analyze the samples again by undertaking an SDS-PAGE again.
5. For efficient resuspension of dried peptide digest, sonicate the tubes in a water bath sonicator for 2–5 min. Adjust the volume of the 100 μg peptide digest to 100 μl and make sure the pH of the solution in around 8.
6. Remaining label should be dried using a speed-vac and stored at −80 °C.
7. Labeling efficiency should be >98% at lysine or N-terminus. If the intensities of any of the labels are very low, then do LC-MS/MS analysis for each sample separately to check the labeling efficiency. If the labeling efficiency of any sample is <95%, the sample should be relabeled with fresh TMT reagent.
8. The tubes can be kept on thermomixer set at 1150 rpm for 20 min at 20 °C to ensure complete dissolution.
9. Drying the beads ensures dehydration, otherwise DHB may not bind completely to the beads.

Acknowledgments

This chapter is dedicated to Professor Akhilesh Pandey of Johns Hopkins University (JHU) School of Medicine who was the co-innovator of Stable isotopic labeling of amino acids in cell culture (SILAC) along with Professor Matthias Mann. Dr. Pandey was a research scientist when he joined the group of Prof. Matthias Mann in the University of Southern Denmark. Prof. Pandey was my mentor and he introduced me to proteomics in general and quantitative proteomics including SILAC. While working with him and Dr. Patole, we were able to identify various new genes in *Leishmania* species (*L. donovani* and *L. major*) using the proteogenomics approach. Additionally, we would like to dedicate this chapter to Prof. Dan Zilberstein who is a pioneer in the area in the field of *Leishmania* axenic differentiation. Prof. Zilberstein's research group has established the axenic *L. donovani* differentiation system for in vitro differentiation.

Funding statement: Dr. Harsh Pawar is funded by an Israel Planning and Budgeting Commission (P.B.C.) fellowship.

References

1. Akopyants NS, Matlib RS, Bukanova EN et al (2004) Expression profiling using random genomic DNA microarrays identifies differentially expressed genes associated with three major developmental stages of the protozoan parasite Leishmania major. Mol Biochem Parasitol 136(1):71–86
2. Saxena A, Lahav T, Holland N et al (2007) Analysis of the Leishmania donovani transcriptome reveals an ordered progression of transient and permanent changes in gene expression during differentiation. Mol Biochem Parasitol 152(1):53–65
3. Dillon LA, Okrah K, Hughitt VK et al (2015) Transcriptomic profiling of gene expression and RNA processing during Leishmania major differentiation. Nucleic Acids Res 43 (14):6799–6813
4. Zilberstein (2008) Physiological and biochemical aspects of Leishmania development. In: Myler PJ, Fasel N (eds) Leishmania after the genome. Caister Academic Press, UK, pp 107–122
5. Sunter J, Gull K (2017) Shape, form, function and Leishmania pathogenicity: from textbook descriptions to biological understanding. Open Biol 7(9):170165
6. Naderer T, McConville MJ (2008) The Leishmania-macrophage interaction: a metabolic perspective. Cell Microbiol 10 (2):301–308
7. McConville MJ, de Souza D, Saunders E et al (2007) Living in a phagolysosome; metabolism of Leishmania amastigotes. Trends Parasitol 23 (8):368–375
8. McConville MJ, Saunders EC, Kloehn J et al (2015) Leishmania carbon metabolism in the macrophage phagolysosome—feast or famine? F1000Res 4(F1000 Faculty Rev):938
9. Saunders EC, Naderer T, Chambers J et al (2018) Leishmania mexicana can utilize amino acids as major carbon sources in macrophages but not in animal models. Mol Microbiol 108(2):143–158
10. Tsigankov P, Gherardini PF, Helmer-Citterich M et al (2012) What has proteomics taught us about Leishmania development? Parasitology 139(9):1146–1157
11. Barak E, Amin-Spector S, Gerliak E et al (2005) Differentiation of Leishmania donovani in host-free system: analysis of signal perception and response. Mol Biochem Parasitol 141 (1):99–108
12. Zilberstein D, Blumenfeld N, Liveanu V et al (1991) Growth at acidic pH induces an amastigote stage-specific protein in Leishmania promastigotes. Mol Biochem Parasitol 45 (1):175–178
13. Doyle PS, Engel JC, Pimenta PF et al (1991) Leishmania donovani: long-term culture of axenic amastigotes at 37 degrees C. Exp Parasitol 73(3):326–334

14. Saar Y, Ransford A, Waldman E et al (1998) Characterization of developmentally-regulated activities in axenic amastigotes of Leishmania donovani. Mol Biochem Parasitol 95(1):9–20
15. El Fakhry Y, Ouellette M, Papadopoulou B (2002) A proteomic approach to identify developmentally regulated proteins in Leishmania infantum. Proteomics 2(8):1007–1017
16. Walker J, Vasquez JJ, Gomez MA et al (2006) Identification of developmentally-regulated proteins in Leishmania panamensis by proteome profiling of promastigotes and axenic amastigotes. Mol Biochem Parasitol 147 (1):64–73
17. Pawar H, Renuse S, Khobragade SN et al (2014) Neglected tropical diseases and omics science: proteogenomics analysis of the promastigote stage of Leishmania major parasite. OMICS 18(8):499–512
18. Pawar H, Sahasrabuddhe NA, Renuse S et al (2012) A proteogenomic approach to map the proteome of an unsequenced pathogen—Leishmania donovani. Proteomics 12 (6):832–844
19. Pawar H, Kulkarni A, Dixit T et al (2014) A bioinformatics approach to reanalyze the genome annotation of kinetoplastid protozoan parasite Leishmania donovani. Genomics 104 (6 Pt B):554–561
20. Pawar H, Pai K, Patole MS (2017) A novel protein coding potential of long intergenic non-coding RNAs (lincRNAs) in the kinetoplastid protozoan parasite Leishmania major. Acta Trop 167:21–25
21. Nirujogi RS, Pawar H, Renuse S et al (2014) Moving from unsequenced to sequenced genome: reanalysis of the proteome of Leishmania donovani. J Proteome 97:48–61
22. Jamdhade MD, Pawar H, Chavan S et al (2015) Comprehensive proteomics analysis of glycosomes from Leishmania donovani. OMICS 19(3):157–170
23. Jardim A, Hardie DB, Boitz J et al (2018) Proteomic profiling of Leishmania donovani promastigote subcellular organelles. J Proteome Res 17(3):1194–1215
24. Ong SE, Mann M (2006) A practical recipe for stable isotope labeling by amino acids in cell culture (SILAC). Nat Protoc 1(6):2650–2660
25. Harsha HC, Molina H, Pandey A (2008) Quantitative proteomics using stable isotope labeling with amino acids in cell culture. Nat Protoc 3(3):505–516
26. Dephoure N, Gygi SP (2012) Hyperplexing: a method for higher-order multiplexed quantitative proteomics provides a map of the dynamic response to rapamycin in yeast. Sci Signal 5 (217):rs2
27. Everley RA, Kunz RC, McAllister FE et al (2013) Increasing throughput in targeted proteomics assays: 54-plex quantitation in a single mass spectrometry run. Anal Chem 85 (11):5340–5346
28. Tsigankov P, Gherardini PF, Helmer-Citterich M et al (2013) Phosphoproteomic analysis of differentiating Leishmania parasites reveals a unique stage-specific phosphorylation motif. J Proteome Res 12(7):3405–3412
29. Tsigankov P, Gherardini PF, Helmer-Citterich M et al (2014) Regulation dynamics of Leishmania differentiation: deconvoluting signals and identifying phosphorylation trends. Mol Cell Proteomics 13(7):1787–1799
30. Lahav T, Sivam D, Volpin H et al (2011) Multiple levels of gene regulation mediate differentiation of the intracellular pathogen Leishmania. FASEB J 25(2):515–525
31. Thompson A, Schafer J, Kuhn K et al (2003) Tandem mass tags: a novel quantification strategy for comparative analysis of complex protein mixtures by MS/MS. Anal Chem 75 (8):1895–1904

Chapter 13

CRISPR/Cas9 Technology Applied to the Study of Proteins Involved in Calcium Signaling in *Trypanosoma cruzi*

Noelia Lander, Miguel A. Chiurillo, and Roberto Docampo

Abstract

Chagas disease is a vector-borne tropical disease affecting millions of people worldwide, for which there is no vaccine or satisfactory treatment available. It is caused by the protozoan parasite *Trypanosoma cruzi* and considered endemic from North to South America. This parasite has unique metabolic and structural characteristics that make it an attractive organism for basic research. The genetic manipulation of *T. cruzi* has been historically challenging, as compared to other pathogenic protozoans. However, the use of the prokaryotic CRISPR/Cas9 system for genome editing has significantly improved the ability to generate genetically modified *T. cruzi* cell lines, becoming a powerful tool for the functional study of proteins in different stages of this parasite's life cycle, including infective trypomastigotes and intracellular amastigotes. Using the CRISPR/Cas9 method that we adapted to *T. cruzi*, it has been possible to perform knockout, complementation and in situ tagging of *T. cruzi* genes. In our system we cotransfect *T. cruzi* epimastigotes with an expression vector containing the Cas9 sequence and a single guide RNA, together with a donor DNA template to promote DNA break repair by homologous recombination. As a result, we have obtained homogeneous populations of mutant epimastigotes using a single resistance marker to modify both alleles of the gene. Mitochondrial Ca^{2+} transport in trypanosomes is critical for shaping the dynamics of cytosolic Ca^{2+} increases, for the bioenergetics of the cells, and for viability and infectivity. In this chapter we describe the most effective methods to achieve genome editing in *T. cruzi* using as example the generation of mutant cell lines to study proteins involved in calcium homeostasis. Specifically, we describe the methods we have used for the study of three proteins involved in the calcium signaling cascade of *T. cruzi*: the inositol 1,4,5-trisphosphate receptor ($TcIP_3R$), the mitochondrial calcium uniporter (TcMCU) and the calcium-sensitive pyruvate dehydrogenase phosphatase (TcPDP), using CRISPR/Cas9 technology as an approach to establish their role in the regulation of energy metabolism.

Key words Calcium signaling, CRISPR/Cas9, Endogenous gene tagging, Gene complementation, Gene knockout, Genome editing, Inositol 1,4,5-trisphosphate receptor, Mitochondrial calcium uniporter, Pyruvate dehydrogenase phosphatase, *Trypanosoma cruzi*

Noelia Lander and Miguel A. Chiurillo contributed equally to this work.

Paul A. M. Michels et al. (eds.), *Trypanosomatids: Methods and Protocols*, Methods in Molecular Biology, vol. 2116,
https://doi.org/10.1007/978-1-0716-0294-2_13,

1 Introduction

CRISPR (clustered regularly interspaced short palindromic repeats)/Cas9 (CRISPR-associated gene 9) is a prokaryotic immune system used by many bacteria and most archaea for self-defense against foreign DNA [1, 2]. This efficient system has been repurposed for genome editing in a broad range of organisms, becoming a transformative tool in biology [3–12]. The genetic manipulation of pathogenic protozoans has significantly increased since the emergence of the CRISPR/Cas9 technology [13]. *Trypanosoma cruzi* is the etiologic agent of Chagas disease, a vector-borne tropical disease affecting millions of people worldwide, for which there is no vaccine or satisfactory treatment available. The disease is considered endemic from parts of North America to South America, although over time it has spread to nonendemic countries in Europe, North America, and the Pacific [14]. The genetic manipulation of *T. cruzi* has been historically challenging, as compared to other pathogenic protozoans [15]. However, the use of CRISPR/Cas9 has considerably improved the ability to perform genetic interventions in *T. cruzi*, becoming a powerful tool for studying structural, homeostatic, and metabolic features of this parasite [8, 10, 16–20]. We have adapted the CRISPR/Cas9 system to *T. cruzi* using a methodology that involves the cotransfection of epimastigotes with a vector for expression of Cas9 and a specific single guide RNA (sgRNA), together with a resistance cassette (donor DNA) that allows double strand break repair by homologous recombination [8]. Our method has been successfully used for the generation of stable *T. cruzi* cell lines, where both alleles of the targeted gene have been modified in a time frame of 4–5 weeks, eliminating the need of cell sorting or the selection of clonal populations [8, 16, 21]. Using this strategy we have performed knockout, complementation and in situ tagging of *T. cruzi* genes [8, 16, 17, 20].

Calcium ion (Ca^{2+}) is an important intracellular signal in trypanosomatids that regulates essential cellular processes like host cell invasion [22], differentiation [23], osmoregulation [24], flagellar function [25], life/death decisions [26], and cell bioenergetics [17, 26]. In this chapter we describe the most effective methods to achieve genome editing in *T. cruzi*, using as example the generation of mutant cell lines to study proteins involved in calcium homeostasis and signaling: the inositol 1,4,5-trisphosphate receptor (TcIP_3R) [16], the mitochondrial calcium uniporter (TcMCU) [17] and the calcium-sensitive pyruvate dehydrogenase phosphatase (TcPDP) [20], using CRISPR/Cas9 technology as an approach to establish their role in the regulation of energy metabolism. In addition, we describe the methodology to evaluate the capacity of these mutant cell lines to take up mitochondrial calcium by monitoring the fluorescence of Calcium Green-5N probe in digitonin-permeabilized epimastigotes. Trypanosomes possess a single mitochondrion spread throughout the cell body and its isolation from the rest of the subcellular structures is difficult and time-consuming. Digitonin can be safely used to selectively permeabilize the plasma membrane of *T. cruzi* without affecting the functional integrity of mitochondria [27, 28]. The use of digitonin to permeabilize *T. cruzi* epimastigotes enables to study mitochondrial Ca^{2+} transport in situ [17, 20]. In this assay a decrease in fluorescence correlates with a decrease of extramitochondrial Ca^{2+}, which is concomitant with mitochondrial Ca^{2+} uptake. The method is very useful to evaluate the phenotype of mutant cell lines where genes involved in mitochondrial calcium homeostasis have been ablated.

This chapter has been divided in four sections: endogenous gene tagging, gene knockout, gene complementation, and mitochondrial calcium transport assay for phenotype analysis of calcium-related mutant cell lines. These methods are based on standard procedures published by our group using CRISPR/Cas9 technology.

2 Materials

2.1 Cell Culture

1. *T. cruzi* epimastigotes (Y strain).
2. Liver infusion tryptose (LIT) medium: 68 mM NaCl, 5.3 mM KCl, 56 mM Na_2HPO_4, 0.2% glucose, 0.5% liver infusion, 0.5% trypticase, 0.002% hemin, pH 7.3.
3. Fetal bovine serum (FBS), heat inactivated (storage temperature: −20 °C).
4. Penicillin (10,000 U/ml)/Streptomycin (10 mg/ml) stock solution (storage temperature: −20 °C).
5. Biological safety cabinet (Class II).
6. Culture flasks (T25 and T75).
7. Refrigerated incubator (temperature set at 28 °C).
8. Neubauer counting chamber.

2.2 Amplification and Cloning of sgRNA

1. pUC_sgRNA plasmid (Addgene catalog # 68710) [8].
2. Cas9/pTREX-n plasmid (Addgene catalog # 68708) [8].
3. DNA oligonucleotides (desalted purity).
4. High fidelity *Taq* DNA polymerase.
5. 10 mM deoxynucleotide (dNTP) solution mix
6. *Bam*HI restriction enzyme.
7. Heat labile alkaline phosphatase.

8. Agarose.
9. TAE buffer: 40 mM Tris–acetate, 1 mM EDTA, pH 8.3.
10. DNA molecular weight marker.
11. 10 mg/ml ethidium bromide solution
12. DNA extraction kit from agarose gels.
13. T4 DNA ligase and ligase buffer.
14. *Escherichia coli* DH5α chemically competent cells (storage temperature: −80 °C).
15. LB broth.
16. LB broth with agar.
17. Ampicillin sodium salt.
18. SOC medium.
19. Plasmid DNA extraction kits for miniprep and midiprep.
20. Horizontal electrophoresis chamber.
21. Thermocycler.
22. Gel documentation system.
23. Microvolume spectrophotometer.
24. Tabletop microcentrifuge.
25. Incubator with agitation (temperature set at 37 °C).
26. PCR reaction mix: 1× *Taq* buffer, 1.5 mM $MgCl_2$, 0.2 mM dNTPs, 0.4 μM of each primer, DNA template (purified plasmid or transformant colony), *Taq* DNA polymerase (1 U), made up to a total volume of 20 μl.
27. Sequencing facility.

2.3 Amplification and Purification of Donor DNA

1. Template DNA: plasmid pMOTag23M [29], pMOHX1-Tag4H [16] (for C-terminal endogenous tagging) or plasmid containing Blasticidin-S-deaminase (*Bsd*) gene (for gene knockout).
2. DNA ultramer oligonucleotides (HPLC purity).
3. Agarose.
4. DNA molecular weight marker.
5. 10 mg/ml ethidium bromide solution
6. *Taq* DNA polymerase.
7. Dimethyl sulfoxide (DMSO).
8. Phenol–chloroform–isoamyl alcohol (25:24:1).
9. Ethanol.
10. Equipment for PCR and DNA electrophoresis (**items 20–24**, Subheading 2.2).

2.4 Cell Transfections

1. *T. cruzi* Y strain epimastigotes.
2. Materials for cell culture (Subheading 2.1).
3. Phosphate buffer saline (PBS): 137 mM NaCl, 2.7 mM KCl, 10 mM Na_2HPO_4, 2 mM KH_2PO_4, pH 7.4.
4. Electroporation buffer (Cytomix): 120 mM KCl, 0.15 mM $CaCl_2$, 10 mM K_2HPO_4, 25 mM HEPES, 2 mM EDTA, 5 mM $MgCl_2$, pH 7.6.
5. Electroporation cuvettes (0.4 cm gap).
6. Antibiotics for selection of resistant parasites: G418 disulfate, blasticidin, puromycin dihydrochloride, and hygromycin B.

2.5 Verification of Genome Editing

1. Genomic DNA (gDNA) from control and mutant *T. cruzi* epimastigotes.
2. DNA oligonucleotides (desalted purity).
3. Materials for PCR and DNA electrophoresis (**items 3–7**, Subheading 2.3, and **items 20–24**, Subheading 2.2).
4. Biotin Random Prime Labeling Kit.
5. Chemiluminescent Hybridization and Detection Kit.
6. Nylon membranes, positively charged.
7. Anti-HA monoclonal antibody.
8. Anti-c-Myc monoclonal antibody.

2.6 Gene KO Complementation

1. pTREX-h vector [17].
2. Materials for high fidelity PCR (**items 3–5**, Subheading 2.2).
3. Restriction enzymes.
4. Materials for gene cloning, plasmid purification, and DNA electrophoresis (**items 8–25**, Subheading 2.2).
5. Sequencing facility.

2.7 Mitochondrial Calcium Uptake

1. Three-milliliter disposable fluorometer cuvette equipped with a magnetic stir bar.
2. Calcium Green-5N, hexapotassium salt, cell impermeant. Stock solution: 0.2 mM in water.
3. Carbonyl cyanide 4-(trifluoromethoxy) phenylhydrazone (FCCP). Stock solution: 2 mM in ethanol.
4. Digitonin. Stock solution: 50 mM in DMSO.
5. Ruthenium red. Stock solution: 2 mM in water. Prepared fresh.
6. $CaCl_2$.
7. Sodium succinate.
8. EGTA.

9. Buffer A with glucose (BAG): 116 mM NaCl, 5.4 mM KCl, 0.8 mM $MgSO_4$, 5.5 mM D-glucose and 50 mM HEPES, pH 7.0.
10. Mitochondrial reaction buffer: 125 mM sucrose, 65 mM KCl, 10 mM HEPES-KOH buffer, pH 7.2, 1 mM $MgCl_2$, 2.5 mM potassium phosphate, kept at 28 °C in water bath.
11. A spectrofluorometer equipped with magnetic stirring and a temperature-controlled water bath.

3 Methods

3.1 Cell Culture

1. Culture *T. cruzi* epimastigotes (Y strain) in LIT medium supplemented with 10% FBS (heat inactivated), 100 U/ml penicillin and 100 μg/ml streptomycin at 28 °C [30].
2. Determine the density of *T. cruzi* epimastigotes in culture using a Neubauer counting chamber. *T. cruzi* cultures should be manipulated in a biological safety cabinet (Class II).

3.2 Endogenous Gene Tagging

3.2.1 Selection of Protospacers

1. Go to TriTrypDB (http://tritrypdb.org/tritrypdb/) [31] and download the full sequence of the gene of interest (GOI) plus 200 nucleotides downstream the stop codon of its open reading frame (ORF) (*see* **Note 1**).
2. Select the protospacer region at the 3′ end of the gene, within 50 nt downstream the stop codon. The protospacer is a 20-nt sequence that hybridizes by base-pairing to the sgRNA. It is located upstream a protospacer-adjacent motif (PAM) that determines the Cas9 cut site. Possible protospacers can be found by searching in the gene's coding strand for the sequence 5′-N_{20}-NGG-3′, where N_{20} is the protospacer and NGG is the PAM sequence. Alternatively, search for protospacers in the noncoding DNA strand with the sequence for 5′-CCN-N_{20}–3′. In this case, the protospacer will be the reverse complementary sequence of N_{20} (*see* **Note 2**).
3. Confirm that the chosen protospacers do not generate off-targets of Cas9 in the *T. cruzi* genome. For this purpose use online prediction tools like EuPaGDT (Eukaryotic Pathogen CRISPR guide RNA Design Tool, http://grna.ctegd.uga.edu/) [32].

3.2.2 Amplification and Cloning of sgRNA

1. Design a specific forward primer for each sgRNA to be amplified. Copy and paste the 20-nt protospacer sequence (N_{20}) into the following primer backbone: 5′-GATCGGATCC-N_{20}-GTTTTAGAGCTAGAAATAGC-3′.

2. Use the following common reverse primer to amplify any designed sgRNA: 5′-CAGTGGATCCAAAAAAGCACCGACTCGGTG-3′. Both forward and reverse primers must have a BamHI restriction site (*underlined*).
3. Amplify the sgRNA (PCR volume = 100 μl) using a high fidelity *Taq* DNA polymerase, the specific forward primer, the common reverse primer and plasmid pUC_sgRNA as template. The expected PCR product size is 122 bp.
4. Load 10 μl of the PCR product in a 2% agarose gel prepared in TAE buffer containing 0.5 μg/ml ethidium bromide.
5. Perform horizontal gel electrophoresis at 100 V for 45 min in TAE buffer.
6. Visualize the sgRNA band (122 bp) using a gel documentation system.
7. Purify the remaining DNA volume (90 μl) using a PCR cleanup kit.
8. Prepare restriction reactions to separately digest at least 1 μg of sgRNA (purified PCR product) and 3 μg of plasmid Cas9/pTREX-n with BamHI, and incubate overnight at 37 °C.
9. Dephosphorylate the digested vector with a heat-labile alkaline phosphatase incubating at 37 °C for 30 min.
10. Inactivate the phosphatase by incubation of the reaction at 70 °C for 5 min.
11. Resolve the restriction products by horizontal DNA electrophoresis in a preparative 1.5% agarose gel containing 0.5 μg/ml ethidium bromide in TAE buffer. The expected sizes of the digested fragments are 102 bp (sgRNA) and 11,173 bp (linearized Cas9/pTREX-n).
12. Purify the digested fragments using a kit for DNA extraction from agarose gels.
13. Quantify the DNA fragments using a microvolume spectrophotometer.
14. Perform a ligation reaction by mixing the digested and purified sgRNA (insert) and Cas9/pTREX-n (vector) in a 20:1 molar ratio (insert to vector). Add 3 U of T4 DNA ligase, 5 μl of 2× rapid ligation buffer and ultrapure H_2O to complete a final volume of 10 μl. Incubate the reaction for 15 min at room temperature and then overnight at 4 °C.
15. Transform chemically competent *E. coli* DH5α cells by standard heat-shock transformation protocol with 5 μl of the ligation product.

16. Recover the transformed cells in 500 μl SOC medium for 1 h at 37 °C with shaking (200 rpm).
17. Spread transformed *E. coli* DH5α cells on LB-agar plates supplemented with 100 μg/ml ampicillin. Incubate overnight at 37 °C.
18. Perform PCR from a single colony or using purified plasmid DNA obtained by miniprep as template, to evaluate the insertion and orientation of the sgRNA in Cas9/pTREX-n vector. For this PCR use the specific forward primer designed to amplify sgRNA, and reverse primer HX1: 5′-TAATTTCGCTTTCGTGCGTG-3′. PCR conditions: initial denaturation, 95 °C for 2 min, then 30 amplification cycles (95 °C for 20 s, 60 °C for 20 s, 72 °C for 20 s), and final elongation, 72 °C for 5 min. PCR product expected size: 190 bp (for positive clones with sgRNA inserted in the right orientation).
19. Sequence sgRNA positive clones (sgRNA/Cas9/pTREX-n) using HX1 reverse primer.
20. Isolate ≥75 μg of plasmid DNA from a positive clone by plasmid midiprep. This amount of DNA will be enough to perform at least three transfections. Plasmid DNA should be at a concentration ≥1.25 μg/μl.

3.2.3 Amplification and Purification of Donor DNA

1. Select two homology regions of 100 bp (HR1 and HR2). HR1 will be located upstream the stop codon of the GOI and HR2 will be downstream the Cas9 cut site on the protospacer (3 nt upstream the PAM sequence).
2. Design 120-bp oligonucleotides (ultramers) to amplify the DNA donor for gene tagging as follows: Forward ultramer, 5′-HR1-GGTACCGGGCCCCCCCTCGAG-3′; Reverse ultramer: 5′-HR2 (reverse complementary sequence)-TGGCGGCCGCTCTAGAACTAGTGGAT- 3′. These forward and reverse ultramers have common 3′ end nucleotides to amplify the donor DNA using either pMOTag23M or pMOHX1Tag4H vectors as PCR templates [29].
3. Amplify the DNA donor (a DNA cassette containing HR1, a tag sequence, a gene for antibiotic resistance, and HR2) using pMOHX1Tag4H vector (3×HA tag and hygromycin resistance gene) or pMOTag23M vector (3×c-Myc tag and puromycin resistance gene) as template. PCR conditions using *Taq* DNA polymerase: initial denaturation, 95 °C for 2 min, then 40 amplification cycles (95 °C for 20 s, 63 °C for 20 s, 72 °C for 1 min and 40 s), and a final elongation, 72 °C for 10 min. Perform enough PCRs to obtain ≥75 μg of DNA donor, for at least three transfections.

4. Load 10 μl of PCR product in a 1% agarose gel prepared in TAE buffer and containing 0.5 μg/ml ethidium bromide, then resolve the DNA donor by horizontal gel electrophoresis. PCR product size: 1.5 kb or 1.6 kb, using pMOTag23M or pMOHX1Tag4H as template, respectively.
5. Purify DNA donor by extraction with phenol–chloroform–isoamyl alcohol (25:24:1) and standard ethanol–sodium acetate precipitation. Resuspend DNA in ultrapure H_2O at a final concentration ≥1.25 μg/μl.

3.2.4 Cell Transfections

1. Grow *T. cruzi* epimastigotes to a cell density of 1–2 × 10^7 cells/ml.
2. Centrifuge cells at 1000 × *g* for 7 min.
3. Wash cells once in sterile PBS pH 7.4 at room temperature. Centrifuge at 1000 × *g* for 7 min.
4. Resuspend cells in ice-cold electroporation buffer at a final density of 1 × 10^8 cells/ml.
5. For each transfection, add 400 μl of cell suspension to ice-cold 0.4 cm electroporation cuvettes and gently mix with 25 μg sgRNA/Cas9/pTREX-n plasmid and 25 μg DNA donor. Each DNA should be in a maximum volume of 20 μl. Perform transfections in triplicate.
6. Perform a transfection with Cas9/pTREX-n vector containing a scrambled sgRNA that will not produce any Cas9 cleavage. This scrambled cell line should be used as control when analyzing the phenotype of knockout parasites.
7. Add 10 μl of ultrapure water to one cuvette of cells to use as negative control during the selection process.
8. Keep cuvettes with DNA/cells mixture on ice for 10 min.
9. Electroporate at 1.5 kV and 25 μF applying three pulses with a Bio-Rad Gene Pulser Xcell™ system. Leave cuvettes on ice for ~1 min after each pulse.
10. Leave cells in cuvettes recovering for 15 min at room temperature after electroporation.
11. Transfer cells to T25 culture flasks containing 5 ml LIT medium supplemented with 20% heat-inactivated FBS at room temperature. Then place flasks at 28 °C in an incubator with controlled temperature and refrigeration.
12. Add antibiotics for selection 24 h after transfection. Transfected *T. cruzi* Y strain epimastigotes should be maintained in medium containing 250 μg/ml G418 and 5 μg/ml puromycin (3×c-Myc tagged) or 350 μg/ml hygromycin (3×HA tagged) (*see* **Note 3**).

13. Replace the culture medium with fresh LIT medium supplemented with 20% FBS and antibiotics once a week during the selection of resistant cells (3–4 weeks).
14. Double-resistant parasites can be diluted and maintained in LIT medium supplemented with 10% FBS, after reaching a cell density of 1–2 × 10^7 cells/ml.

3.2.5 Verification of Endogenous Gene Tagging

1. After selection of double resistant parasites, perform genomic DNA (gDNA) extraction from transfectants using standard protocols or commercial kits.
2. Analyze gDNA by PCR to verify the insertion of donor DNA cassette at the 3′ end of the target gene.
3. Design specific forward and reverse primers annealing upstream of the HR1 and downstream of the HR2, respectively. Usually the forward primer anneals on the coding region of the GOI and the reverse primer on the 3′ untranslated region (3′UTR) of the target gene. Oligonucleotides annealing at the 3′end of antibiotic resistance genes present in the donor DNA cassette also can be used as reverse primers: primer RvPuro: 5′-TCAGGCACCGGGCTTGCGGG-3′ for 3×c-Myc tagging and primer RvHygro: 5′-CTATTCCTTTGCCCTCGGAC-3′ for 3×HA tagging.
4. Perform PCR using as template gDNA from wild type (wt) and transfectant cells, and H_2O as negative control. PCR conditions will vary depending on PCR product size and the annealing temperature of the specific primers.
5. Load 10 μl of each PCR product in a 1% agarose gel in TAE buffer containing 0.5 μg/ml ethidium bromide. Resolve the PCR products by horizontal DNA gel electrophoresis to confirm the amplification.
6. Calculate PCR fragment size difference between the wild type locus and the tagged gene. If using a reverse primer annealing downstream HR1, the length of tagged gene would be ~1240 bp longer than the wild type locus (for 3×c-Myc tagging) or ~1350 bp longer than the wild type locus (for 3×HA tagging).
7. Confirm expression of tagged proteins by western blot and immunofluorescence analysis (IFA) using antibodies anti-HA epitope tag or antibodies anti-c-Myc tag (*see* **Note 4**). Figure 1 shows examples of IFAs performed in two cell lines that were endogenously tagged: The IP_3R-3×HA that shows colocalization with vacuolar proton pyrophosphatase (VP1), a marker of acidocalcisomes (Fig. 1a), and TcPDP-3×c-Myc that localizes to mitochondria as shown by colocalization with Mitotracker (MT) in the merged image (Fig. 1b).

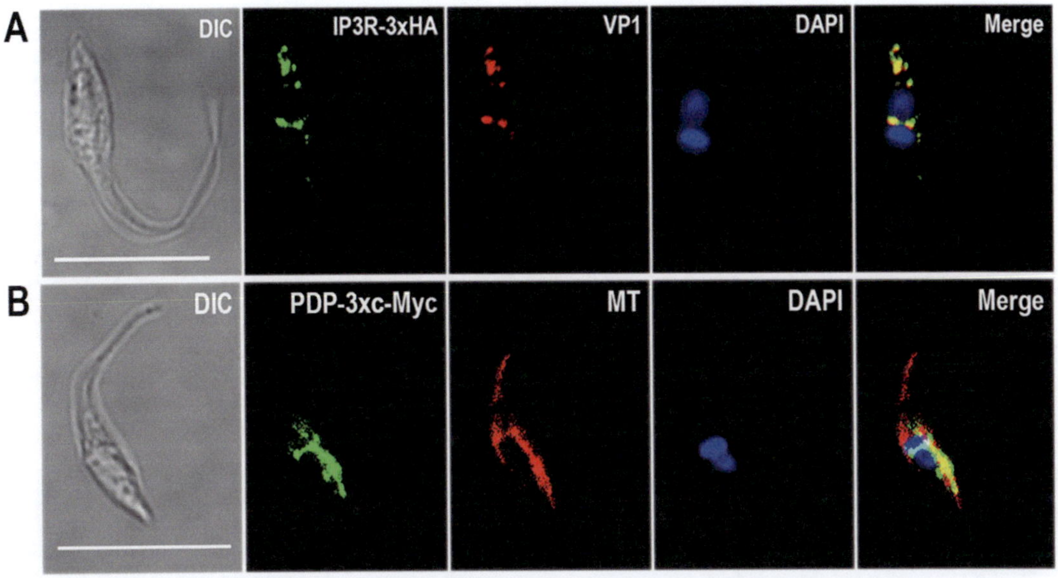

Fig. 1 Immunofluorescence microscopy of mutant cell lines generated by CRISPR/Cas9 for C-terminal tagging of endogenous proteins. (**a**) TcIP_3R endogenous tagging was verified by IFA using antibodies anti-HA epitope tag. Merged image shows colocalization (*yellow*) of TcIP_3R-3×HA (*green*) and VP1 (*red*), a marker of acidocalcisomes. (Reproduced from Lander et al. (2016) (ref. 21) with permission from the *Journal of Biological Chemistry*.) (**b**) TcPDP endogenous tagging was verified by IFA using antibodies anti-c-Myc. Merged image shows colocalization (*yellow*) of TcPDP-3xc-Myc (*green*) and Mitotracker (MT, *red*), a probe that labels mitochondria. DAPI staining (*blue*) and differential interference contrast (*DIC*) images are also shown. Scale bars: 10 μm. (Reproduced from Lander et al. (2018) (ref. 20) with permission from the *Journal of Biological Chemistry*)

3.3 Gene Knockout

3.3.1 Selection of Protospacers for Gene KO

1. Go to TriTrypDB (http://tritrypdb.org/tritrypdb/) [31] and download the full sequence of the GOI plus 200 nucleotides upstream and downstream the start and stop codons, respectively (*see* **Note 1**).
2. Select the protospacer region within the open reading frame (ORF) of the GOI, but always between the homology regions (HR1 and HR2) present in the donor DNA (Fig. 2). Follow protospacer definitions as described above (**step 2**, Subheading 3.2.1).
3. Analyze protospacers to rule out off-targeting as in **step 3**, Subheading 3.2.1.

3.3.2 Amplification and Cloning of sgRNA for Gene KO

1. Follow **steps 1–20**, Subheading 3.2.2.

3.3.3 Amplification and Purification of Donor DNA for Gene KO

1. Select two homology regions of 100 bp (HR1 and HR2). HR1 will be located right upstream the start codon and HR2 will be located right downstream the stop codon of the target gene (*see* **Note 5**) (Fig. 2).

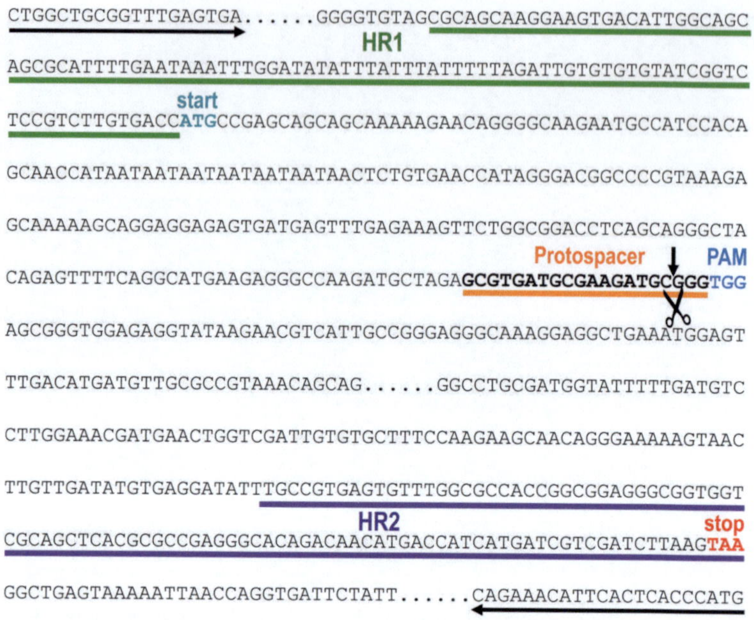

Fig. 2 Molecular design for CRISPR/Cas9-mediated gene knockout of *TcPDP* (gene ID: TcCLB. 506739.200) by homology-directed repair. The scheme shows the genomic DNA sequence of *TcPDP*, including the start codon (start, ATG, dark cyan), the stop codon (stop, TAA, red sequence), the chosen protospacer (bold sequence underlined in orange), the protospacer adjacent motif (PAM, light blue sequence) and the homology regions 1 (HR1) and 2 (HR2) underlined in green and purple, respectively, that were included in the DNA donor cassette to induce DNA repair by homologous recombination. Scissors indicate the Cas9 cut site. HR1 locates right upstream the start codon, while HR2 includes the last 100 nt of the *TcPDP* open reading frame. Arrows indicate forward and reverse primers used to verify the replacement of *TcPDP* by the *Blasticidin-S-deaminase* gene present in the donor DNA. These primers anneal upstream and downstream HR1 and HR2, respectively

2. Design 120-bp ultramers to amplify a DNA cassette to promote double strand break repair by homologous recombination and gene ablation. The forward ultramer will contain the first 20 nucleotides of Blasticidin-S-deaminase gene (*Bsd*) and the reverse ultramer will have the last 20 nucleotides of *Bsd*. Determine the reverse complementary sequence of HR2 (HR2rc). Forward ultramer will be as follows: 5′-HR1- A TGGCCAAGCCTTTGTCTCA-3′. Reverse ultramer will be as follows: 5′-HR2rc-TTAGCCCTCCCACACATAAC- 3′.
3. Amplify the DNA donor containing the ORF of *Bsd* flanked by 100-bp homology arms using a plasmid containing *Bsd* (e.g., pTREX-b) as template. PCR conditions using *Taq* DNA polymerase: initial denaturation, 95 °C for 2 min; then 40 amplification cycles (95 °C for 20 s, 62 °C for 20 s, 72 °C for 45 s),

and a final elongation, 72 °C for 5 min. Perform enough PCRs to obtain ≥75 μg of DNA donor, for at least three transfections.

4. Load 10 μl of PCR product in a 1% agarose gel prepared in TAE buffer and containing 0.5 μg/ml ethidium bromide, then resolve the DNA donor by horizontal gel electrophoresis. PCR product size: 599 bp.
5. Purify donor DNA as in **step 5**, Subheading 3.2.3.

3.3.4 Cell Transfections

1. Follow **steps 1–13** from Subheading 3.2.4.

3.3.5 Verification of Gene KO

1. After selection of double resistant parasites, perform genomic DNA (gDNA) extraction from transfectants using standard protocols or commercial kits.
2. Analyze gDNA by PCR to verify the replacement or disruption of the GOI by the donor DNA cassette.
3. Design specific forward and reverse primers annealing upstream of the HR1 and downstream of the HR2, respectively. Usually these primers anneal on the 5′UTR and the 3′UTR of the target gene, respectively (Fig. 2).
4. Perform PCR using as template gDNA from wild type (wt) and transfectant cells, and H_2O as negative control. PCR conditions will vary depending on PCR product size and the annealing temperature of the specific primers.
5. Load 10 μl of each PCR product in a 1% agarose gel in TAE buffer containing 0.5 μg/ml ethidium bromide. Resolve the PCR products by horizontal DNA gel electrophoresis to confirm the amplification.
6. Calculate PCR fragment size difference between the wild type locus and knockout gene considering the length of GOI replaced by the *Bsd* gene (399 bp).
7. Perform Southern blot analysis to further confirm replacement or disruption of GOI. First, analyze the in silico restriction pattern of a genomic DNA region encompassing 1000–5000 bp upstream and downstream the target gene. The sequence of this region should be retrieved from TriTrypDB. Then select appropriate restriction sites and predict fragment sizes.
8. Digest overnight 25–30 μg of gDNA from wild type and transfectant cell lines using selected restriction enzyme(s).
9. Resolve restriction fragments on a 0.8% agarose gel in TAE buffer containing 0.5 μg/ml ethidium bromide.
10. Transfer DNA fragments to a nylon membrane according to manufacturer's instructions and hybridize with a 200–400 bp biotin-labeled probe spanning the gene locus replaced by the *Bsd* marker.

11. Incubate the membrane with HRP-conjugated streptavidin.
12. Detect the labeling signal using a chemiluminescent detection kit for Southern blot and a digital documentation system or by exposing the membrane to an X-ray film (*see* **Note 6**).

3.4 Gene Complementation of Knockout Mutants Obtained by CRISPR/Cas9

1. To restore the wild type phenotype in knockout cell lines that have been generated by CRISPR/Cas9, reinsert the ablated gene by cloning its full sequence in an expression vector for *T. cruzi*.
2. The ORF of the gene that is going to be reinserted should be modified to eliminate the PAM motif, an NGG sequence downstream the protospacer that is recognized by the assembled sgRNA/Cas9 ribonucleoprotein. Design an overlap extension PCR to eliminate the PAM sequence of the protospacer used to generate the knockout cell line (*see* **Note 7**).
3. Design four primers: FwATG, RvSTOP, FwPAM-mut, and RvPAM-mut. FwPAM-mut and RvPAM-mut primers contain the mutated PAM sequence and the overlapping region.
4. FwATG and RvSTOP primers should have restriction sites for cloning the overlap PCR product into the expression vector (*see* **Note 8**).
5. Perform two PCR reactions, one of them using FwATG and Rv-PAM-mut primers, and another one using Fw-PAM-mut and RvSTOP primers. Use a high fidelity DNA polymerase and *T. cruzi* wild type gDNA as template, in 50-μl reactions. PCR conditions will vary depending on primer sequences and PCR product sizes.
6. Load 10 μl of each PCR product in an agarose gel prepared in TAE buffer containing 0.5 μg/ml ethidium bromide, to visualize the DNA amplicons in a UV transilluminator.
7. Purify the remaining 40-μl of PCR product with a cleanup kit.
8. Quantify the DNA fragments by microvolume spectrophotometry.
9. Perform an overlap extension PCR using FwATG and RvSTOP primers and the two PCR products purified in **step 7** as templates. This PCR should be prepared with a high-fidelity DNA polymerase, in a 50-μl volume, using conditions determined by PCR product size and primer sequences.
10. Load 10 μl of PCR product in an agarose gel prepared in TAE buffer with 0.5 μg/ml ethidium bromide, to visualize the DNA amplicon in a UV transilluminator.
11. Purify the remaining 40-μl of PCR product with a cleanup kit.
12. Quantify the DNA fragment by microvolume spectrophotometry.

13. Digest ≥2 μg of purified PCR product and 3 μg of plasmid pTREX-h or pTREX-p [17] with appropriate restriction enzyme(s). These vectors confer resistance to hygromycin and puromycin, respectively.
14. Perform a ligation reaction to insert the GOI with mutated PAM (GOI-$^{\text{PAM-mut}}$) into pTREX-h vector using an insert to vector molar ratio of 3:1. Add 3 U of T4 DNA ligase, 5 μl of 2× rapid ligation buffer, and ultrapure H_2O to complete a final volume of 10 μl. Incubate the reaction for 15 min at room temperature and then overnight at 4 °C.
15. Transform chemically competent *E. coli* DH5α by standard heat-shock transformation protocol using 5 μl of the ligation product, as previously described (**steps 16** and **17**, Subheading 3.2.2).
16. Pick 4–10 colonies and grow cells in 5 ml LB broth supplemented with 100 μg/ml ampicillin. Incubate overnight at 37 °C.
17. Isolate recombinant plasmids from resistant clones using a plasmid miniprep DNA extraction kit and confirm the presence of the insert by restriction analysis and sequencing.
18. Purify ≥75 μg DNA from a positive clone by plasmid midiprep and concentrate it to reach ≥1.25 μg/μl DNA. This amount of DNA will be enough to perform at least three transfections.
19. Transfect *T. cruzi* Y strain epimastigotes with 25 μg GOI-$^{\text{PAM-mut}}$/pTREX-h or pTREX-p plasmid, as described in Subheading 3.2.4.
20. Select *T. cruzi* complemented cell lines in LIT medium containing 20% heat inactivated FBS, 250 μg/ml G418, 10 μg/ml blasticidin, and 150 μg/ml hygromycin or 5 μg/ml puromycin.
21. Replace the culture medium once a week during the selection period (3–4 weeks), using fresh LIT medium supplemented with 20% FBS and antibiotics.
22. FBS concentration in the culture medium can be reduced to 10% when triple-resistant parasites reach a cell density of 1–2 × 10^7 cells/ml.
23. Check expression of the reconstituted protein by western blot and immunofluorescence analysis (IFA) using either specific antibodies or commercial antibodies labeling an epitope tag included in this protein.
24. Analyze phenotype restoration in the reconstituted cell line, as compared with control and knockout parasites.

3.5 Mitochondrial Calcium Uptake for Phenotype Analysis of CRISPR/Cas9 Mutant Cell Lines Involved in Calcium Homeostasis

1. Grow cell cultures of *T. cruzi* epimastigotes (wild type and knockout cell line) to a cell density of 1–2 × 10^7 cells/ml.
2. Centrifuge cells at 1000 × *g* for 7 min.
3. Wash cells twice in BAG pH 7.0 sterile at room temperature. Centrifuge at 1000 × *g* for 7 min.
4. Resuspend cells in BAG to a density of 1 × 10^9 cells/ml and keep them on ice.
5. For Calcium Green-5N indicator use the following settings in the spectrofluorometer: high sensitivity; acquisition rate, 2 Hz; excitation wavelength, 506 nm; emission wavelength, 532 nm; and both slits set to 2.5 nm. All experiments must be performed at 28 °C with continuous stirring.
6. Add 50 μl of *T. cruzi* epimastigotes (5 × 10^7 cells) to a disposable cuvette with a magnetic stir bar containing 1.95 ml of mitochondrial reaction buffer plus 5 mM succinate (substrate for the respiratory complex), 50 μM EGTA and 0.5 μM Calcium Green-5N (schematic representation in Fig. 3A, panel a).
7. Insert the cuvette into the spectrofluorometer and incubate for 2 min with continuous stirring, then start recording fluorescence levels over time.
8. After recording a short baseline reading (~20 s), add 10 μl of $CaCl_2$ to reach the desired final free Ca^{2+} concentration (Fig. 3A, panel b; and B) (*see* **Note 9**).
9. After stabilization of the trace (~50 s) add digitonin to a final concentration of 50 μM for cell permeabilization (Fig. 3A, panel c; and B). A fluorescence decrease after permeabilization indicates mitochondrial Ca^{2+} uptake (Fig. 3A, panel c, and B).
10. Add FCCP to a final concentration of 4 μM when Ca^{2+} transport reaches the steady-state (lowest stable value) of Calcium Green-5N fluorescence (~500–600 s after permeabilization with digitonin in wild-type epimastigotes) (Fig. 3B). The increase of fluorescence after FCCP addition indicates mitochondrial calcium release promoted by the dissipation of the mitochondrial membrane potential.
11. Finish the trace when fluorescence reaches a value similar to that displayed before permeabilizing with digitonin.
12. Perform a control trace inhibiting MCU-mediated mitochondrial Ca^{2+} transport, by adding ruthenium red to a final concentration of 5 μM into a cuvette with reaction medium, supplements and *T. cruzi* epimastigotes, as in **step 6**. Then repeat **steps 7–11** for this negative control (*see* **Note 10**).

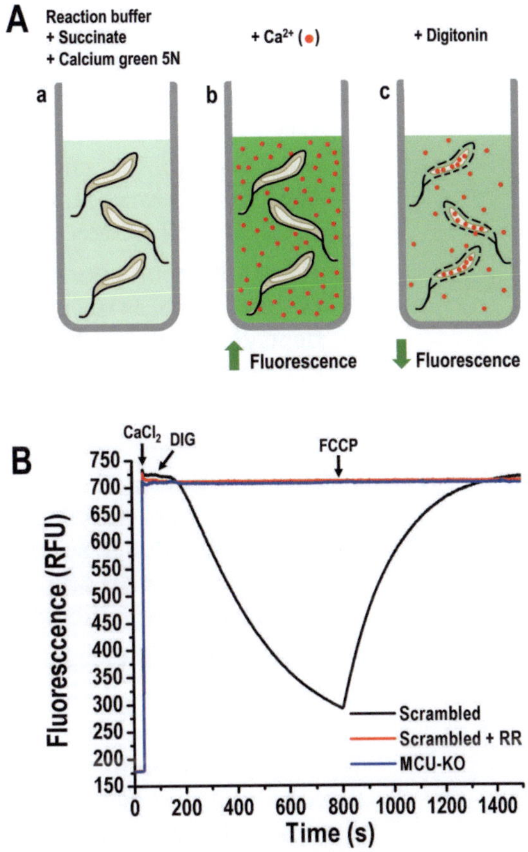

Fig. 3 Mitochondrial calcium uptake of digitonin-permeabilized *T. cruzi* epimastigotes. (**A**) Schematic representation of the fluorometric assay. (Panel **a**) Intact cells are resuspended in reaction buffer containing mitochondrial substrate (succinate) and a fluorescent probe (Calcium Green-5N), that exhibits an increase in fluorescence emission intensity upon binding Ca^{2+}, with little shift in wavelength. (Panel **b**) Fluorescence increases upon addition of Ca^{2+}. Panel (**c**) Digitonin selectively permeabilizes the plasma membrane of the cells, preserving mitochondrial integrity. Then Ca^{2+} is taken up by mitochondria and fluorescence decreases. (**B**) Representative traces of mitochondrial Ca^{2+} uptake by digitonin-permeabilized *T. cruzi* epimastigotes. The traces correspond to control cells (*Scrambled*) in the absence or presence of 5 μM ruthenium red (*RR*), and *MCU-KO* epimastigotes. After recording a short baseline, $CaCl_2$ was added to the cuvette to reach a free Ca^{2+} concentration [Ca^{2+}] of 20 μM in mitochondrial reaction buffer, containing 5 mM succinate and 50 μM EGTA. Mitochondrial Ca^{2+} uptake was started after addition of 50 μM digitonin. The decrease of fluorescence indicates a decrease of extramitochondrial [Ca^{2+}], concomitant with mitochondrial Ca^{2+} uptake. Addition of the uncoupler carbonyl cyanide p-trifluoromethoxylhydrazone (FCCP) completely dissipates the mitochondrial membrane potential, producing mitochondrial calcium release that is observed as an increase in the fluorescence of the probe. Fluorescence is expressed in relative fluorescence units (RFU)

4 Notes

1. *T. cruzi* has a high genetic diversity. For this reason it is necessary to use the most similar genome sequence from TriTrypDB according to the current classification of *T. cruzi* strains [33]. For *T. cruzi* Y strain, we use the Esmeraldo-like haplotype of *T. cruzi* CL Brener curated reference strain.
2. We recommend choosing at least two protospacers for each targeted gene, as the endonuclease efficiency of Cas9 can vary depending on the sgRNA sequence. In addition, the protospacer regions always have to be located between the homology regions present in the Donor DNA (HR1 and HR2).
3. The optimal antibiotic concentration for selection of transfectant parasites should be determined for each specific *T. cruzi* strain, before performing cell transfections. Antibiotic sensitivity can differ due to several factors such as *T. cruzi* strain, time that the cell line has been maintained in the laboratory and even the brand of the antibiotic.
4. Detection of the tagged protein by western blot or IFA depends on its endogenous expression level in *T. cruzi* epimastigotes.
5. The 5′ and 3′ untranslated regions (UTRs) of GOI should be conserved after genome editing because they include sequence elements that are required for the appropriate mRNA processing. If the UTR sequences of the gene are not available in the genome sequence, is incomplete or if the designed strategy involves the disruption or partial elimination of GOI, the sequences of HR1 and HR2 should be selected within the open reading frame of the gene (as in the HR2 selected for TcPDP knockout strategy, Fig. 2).
6. The labeling pattern generated by Southern blot analysis depends on the design of the probe. If the probe corresponds to the sequence of the ablated gene, the signal will be detected only in the control cell line, and absent in the knockout mutant.
7. By eliminating the PAM sequence the constitutively expressed Cas9 and sgRNA will not target the inserted gene. Remove the PAM sequence (NGG) by replacing one of the guanine residues to generate a synonymous mutation or at least a conservative substitution.
8. If there are no specific antibodies against the protein of interest, cells should be transfected with a tagged version of the gene.
9. The amount of $CaCl_2$ required to reach the desired concentration of free Ca^{2+} in the presence of 50 μM EGTA is calculated using the Maxchelator Calculator program, v1.2 (available at https://somapp.ucdmc.ucdavis.edu/pharmacology/bers/maxchelator/CaEGTA-NIST.htm). Free Ca^{2+} concentrations ranging from 5 to

50 μM are usually good to evaluate mitochondrial Ca^{2+} uptake in digitonin-permeabilized epimastigotes using Calcium Green-5N indicator. To fluorometrically determine the concentration of free Ca^{2+} contained in the mitochondrial reaction buffer (expressed in μM) in the presence of Calcium Green-5N probe, use the equation: $[Ca^{2+}] = K_d \times (F - F_{min})/(F_{max} - F)$, where F is any given fluorescence value, F_{min} is the lowest fluorescence reading after the addition of 0.5 mM EGTA, F_{max} is the maximal fluorescence obtained after two consecutive additions of 1 mM $CaCl_2$, and K_d is for Calcium Green-5N, according to manufacturers.

10. The relative rate of mitochondrial calcium uptake can be represented as the absolute value of the slope of the linear regression fit in the linear range of the fluorescent signal (usually between 300 and 350 s). The relative rates of calcium uptake have to be normalized for the control cell lines and/or conditions.

Acknowledgments

We thank Prof. Anibal E. Vercesi (University of Campinas, Brazil) for his encouragement and advice. This work was funded by the U.S. National Institutes of Health (grants AI107663 and AI140421).

References

1. Horvath P, Barrangou R (2010) CRISPR/Cas, the immune system of bacteria and archaea. Science 327(5962):167–170. https://doi.org/10.1126/science.1179555
2. Rath D, Amlinger L, Rath A, Lundgren M (2015) The CRISPR-Cas immune system: biology, mechanisms and applications. Biochimie 117:119–128. https://doi.org/10.1016/j.biochi.2015.03.025
3. Cong L, Ran FA, Cox D, Lin S, Barretto R, Habib N, Hsu PD, Wu X, Jiang W, Marraffini LA, Zhang F (2013) Multiplex genome engineering using CRISPR/Cas systems. Science 339(6121):819–823. https://doi.org/10.1126/science.1231143
4. DiCarlo JE, Norville JE, Mali P, Rios X, Aach J, Church GM (2013) Genome engineering in Saccharomyces cerevisiae using CRISPR-Cas systems. Nucleic Acids Res 41(7):4336–4343. https://doi.org/10.1093/nar/gkt135
5. Jiang W, Zhou H, Bi H, Fromm M, Yang B, Weeks DP (2013) Demonstration of CRISPR/Cas9/sgRNA-mediated targeted gene modification in Arabidopsis, tobacco, sorghum and rice. Nucleic Acids Res 41(20):e188. https://doi.org/10.1093/nar/gkt780
6. Gratz SJ, Cummings AM, Nguyen JN, Hamm DC, Donohue LK, Harrison MM, Wildonger J, O'Connor-Giles KM (2013) Genome engineering of Drosophila with the CRISPR RNA-guided Cas9 nuclease. Genetics 194(4):1029–1035. https://doi.org/10.1534/genetics.113.152710
7. Ghorbal M, Gorman M, Macpherson CR, Martins RM, Scherf A, Lopez-Rubio JJ (2014) Genome editing in the human malaria parasite Plasmodium falciparum using the CRISPR-Cas9 system. Nat Biotechnol 32(8):819–821. https://doi.org/10.1038/nbt.2925
8. Lander N, Li ZH, Niyogi S, Docampo R (2015) CRISPR/Cas9-induced disruption of paraflagellar rod protein 1 and 2 genes in Trypanosoma cruzi reveals their role in flagellar attachment. MBio 6(4):e01012–e01015. https://doi.org/10.1128/mBio.01012-15
9. Sidik SM, Hackett CG, Tran F, Westwood NJ, Lourido S (2014) Efficient genome engineering of Toxoplasma gondii using CRISPR/Cas9. PLoS One 9(6):e100450. https://doi.org/10.1371/journal.pone.0100450

10. Peng D, Kurup SP, Yao PY, Minning TA, Tarleton RL (2015) CRISPR-Cas9-mediated single-gene and gene family disruption in Trypanosoma cruzi. MBio 6(1):e02097–e02014. https://doi.org/10.1128/mBio.02097-14
11. Jinek M, Chylinski K, Fonfara I, Hauer M, Doudna JA, Charpentier E (2012) A programmable dual-RNA-guided DNA endonuclease in adaptive bacterial immunity. Science 337 (6096):816–821. https://doi.org/10.1126/science.1225829
12. Sollelis L, Ghorbal M, MacPherson CR, Martins RM, Kuk N, Crobu L, Bastien P, Scherf A, Lopez-Rubio JJ, Sterkers Y (2015) First efficient CRISPR-Cas9-mediated genome editing in Leishmania parasites. Cell Microbiol 17 (10):1405–1412. https://doi.org/10.1111/cmi.12456
13. Lander N, Chiurillo MA, Docampo R (2016) Genome editing by CRISPR/Cas9: a game change in the genetic manipulation of protists. J Eukaryot Microbiol 63(5):679–690. https://doi.org/10.1111/jeu.12338
14. Forsyth CJ, Hernandez S, Olmedo W, Abuhamidah A, Traina MI, Sanchez DR, Soverow J, Meymandi SK (2016) Safety profile of nifurtimox for treatment of Chagas disease in the United States. Clin Infect Dis 63 (8):1056–1062. https://doi.org/10.1093/cid/ciw477
15. Docampo R (2011) Molecular parasitology in the 21st century. Essays Biochem 51:1–13. https://doi.org/10.1042/bse0510001
16. Lander N, Chiurillo MA, Storey M, Vercesi AE, Docampo R (2016) CRISPR/Cas9-mediated endogenous C-terminal tagging of Trypanosoma cruzi genes reveals the acidocalcisome localization of the inositol 1,4,5-trisphosphate receptor. J Biol Chem 291(49):25505–25515. https://doi.org/10.1074/jbc.M116.749655
17. Chiurillo MA, Lander N, Bertolini MS, Storey M, Vercesi AE, Docampo R (2017) Different roles of mitochondrial calcium uniporter complex subunits in growth and infectivity of Trypanosoma cruzi. MBio 8(3): e00574–e00517. https://doi.org/10.1128/mBio.00574-17
18. Soares Medeiros LC, South L, Peng D, Bustamante JM, Wang W, Bunkofske M, Perumal N, Sanchez-Valdez F, Tarleton RL (2017) Rapid, selection-free, high-efficiency genome editing in protozoan parasites using CRISPR-Cas9 ribonucleoproteins. MBio 8(6): e01788–e01717. https://doi.org/10.1128/mBio.01788-17
19. Costa FC, Francisco AF, Jayawardhana S, Calderano SG, Lewis MD, Olmo F, Beneke T, Gluenz E, Sunter J, Dean S, Kelly JM, Taylor MC (2018) Expanding the toolbox for Trypanosoma cruzi: a parasite line incorporating a bioluminescence-fluorescence dual reporter and streamlined CRISPR/Cas9 functionality for rapid in vivo localisation and phenotyping. PLoS Negl Trop Dis 12(4):e0006388. https://doi.org/10.1371/journal.pntd.0006388
20. Lander N, Chiurillo MA, Bertolini MS, Storey M, Vercesi AE, Docampo R (2018) Calcium-sensitive pyruvate dehydrogenase phosphatase is required for energy metabolism, growth, differentiation, and infectivity of Trypanosoma cruzi. J Biol Chem 293 (45):17402–17417. https://doi.org/10.1074/jbc.RA118.004498
21. Lander N, Chiurillo MA, Vercesi AE, Docampo R (2017) Endogenous C-terminal tagging by CRISPR/Cas9 in Trypanosoma cruzi. Bio Protoc 7(10). https://doi.org/10.21769/BioProtoc.2299
22. Moreno SN, Silva J, Vercesi AE, Docampo R (1994) Cytosolic-free calcium elevation in Trypanosoma cruzi is required for cell invasion. J Exp Med 180(4):1535–1540
23. Lammel EM, Barbieri MA, Wilkowsky SE, Bertini F, Isola EL (1996) Trypanosoma cruzi: involvement of intracellular calcium in multiplication and differentiation. Exp Parasitol 83(2):240–249. https://doi.org/10.1006/expr.1996.0070
24. Rohloff P, Rodrigues CO, Docampo R (2003) Regulatory volume decrease in Trypanosoma cruzi involves amino acid efflux and changes in intracellular calcium. Mol Biochem Parasitol 126(2):219–230
25. Engman DM, Krause KH, Blumin JH, Kim KS, Kirchhoff LV, Donelson JE (1989) A novel flagellar Ca^{2+}-binding protein in trypanosomes. J Biol Chem 264(31):18627–18631
26. Huang G, Vercesi AE, Docampo R (2013) Essential regulation of cell bioenergetics in Trypanosoma brucei by the mitochondrial calcium uniporter. Nat Commun 4:2865. https://doi.org/10.1038/ncomms3865
27. Docampo R, Vercesi AE (1989) Ca^{2+} transport by coupled Trypanosoma cruzi mitochondria in situ. J Biol Chem 264(1):108–111
28. Vercesi AE, Bernardes CF, Hoffmann ME, Gadelha FR, Docampo R (1991) Digitonin permeabilization does not affect mitochondrial function and allows the determination of the mitochondrial membrane potential of Trypanosoma cruzi in situ. J Biol Chem 266 (22):14431–14434
29. Oberholzer M, Morand S, Kunz S, Seebeck T (2006) A vector series for rapid PCR-mediated C-terminal in situ tagging of Trypanosoma

brucei genes. Mol Biochem Parasitol 145 (1):117–120. https://doi.org/10.1016/j.molbiopara.2005.09.002

30. Bone GJ, Steinert M (1956) Isotopes incorporated in the nucleic acids of Trypanosoma mega. Nature 178:2. https://doi.org/10.1038/178308a0
31. Aslett M, Aurrecoechea C, Berriman M, Brestelli J, Brunk BP, Carrington M, Depledge DP, Fischer S, Gajria B, Gao X, Gardner MJ, Gingle A, Grant G, Harb OS, Heiges M, Hertz-Fowler C, Houston R, Innamorato F, Iodice J, Kissinger JC, Kraemer E, Li W, Logan FJ, Miller JA, Mitra S, Myler PJ, Nayak V, Pennington C, Phan I, Pinney DF, Ramasamy G, Rogers MB, Roos DS, Ross C, Sivam D, Smith DF, Srinivasamoorthy G, Stoeckert CJ Jr, Subramanian S, Thibodeau R, Tivey A, Treatman C, Velarde G, Wang H (2010) TriTrypDB: a functional genomic resource for the Trypanosomatidae. Nucleic Acids Res 38(Database issue): D457–D462. https://doi.org/10.1093/nar/gkp851
32. Peng D, Tarleton R (2015) EuPaGDT: a web tool tailored to design CRISPR guide RNAs for eukaryotic pathogens. Microb Genom 1 (4):e000033. https://doi.org/10.1099/mgen.0.000033
33. Zingales B, Andrade SG, Briones MR, Campbell DA, Chiari E, Fernandes O, Guhl F, Lages-Silva E, Macedo AM, Machado CR, Miles MA, Romanha AJ, Sturm NR, Tibayrenc M, Schijman AG, Second Satellite M (2009) A new consensus for Trypanosoma cruzi intraspecific nomenclature: second revision meeting recommends TcI to TcVI. Mem Inst Oswaldo Cruz 104(7):1051–1054

Chapter 14

Application of CRISPR/Cas9-Mediated Genome Editing in *Leishmania*

Wen-Wei Zhang, Patrick Lypaczewski, and Greg Matlashewski

Abstract

CRISPR-Cas9 is an RNA guided endonuclease derived from the bacterium *Streptococcus pyogenes*. Due to its simplicity, versatility, and high efficiency, it has been widely used for genome editing in a variety of organisms including the protozoan parasite *Leishmania*, the causative agent of human leishmaniasis. Compared to the traditional homologous recombination gene targeting method, CRISPR-Cas9 has been shown to be a more efficient method to delete or disrupt *Leishmania* genes, generate point mutations, and add tags to endogenous genes. Notably, the stable CRISPR expression systems were shown to delete multicopy family *Leishmania* genes and genes present in multiploid chromosomes, identify essential *Leishmania* genes, and create specific chromosome translocations. In this chapter, we describe detailed procedures on using the stable CRISPR expression system for genome editing in *Leishmania*. These procedures include CRISPR targeting site selection, gRNA design, cloning single and double gRNA coding sequences into the *Leishmania* CRISPR vector pLdCN, oligonucleotide donor and drug resistance selection donor design, *Leishmania* cell transfection, screening, and isolation of CRISPR-edited mutants. As the principles of gene editing are generally similar, many of these procedures could also apply to the transient *Leishmania* CRISPR systems described by other labs.

Key words CRISPR-Cas9, Genome editing, *Leishmania*, Gene deletion, Gene disruption, Point mutation, Gene tagging

1 Introduction

The commonly used *Streptococcus pyogenes* CRISPR (clustered regularly interspaced short palindromic repeats)-Cas9 is an RNA-guided endonuclease that has been shown to facilitate site-specific DNA cleavage in various organisms [1–6]. For gene editing purposes, the CRISPR-Cas9 system requires at least two components; the Cas9 nuclease and a guide RNA (gRNA) (Fig. 1). The gRNA consists of a 20 nucleotide (nt) guide sequence (protospacer) followed by an 82 nt chimeric sequence derived from the bacterial CRISPR RNA and transactivating RNA [1, 2]. The gRNA and Cas9 nuclease form an RNA–protein complex. The gRNA 20-nt guide sequence, which is complementary to the

Paul A. M. Michels et al. (eds.), *Trypanosomatids: Methods and Protocols*, Methods in Molecular Biology, vol. 2116,
https://doi.org/10.1007/978-1-0716-0294-2_14,

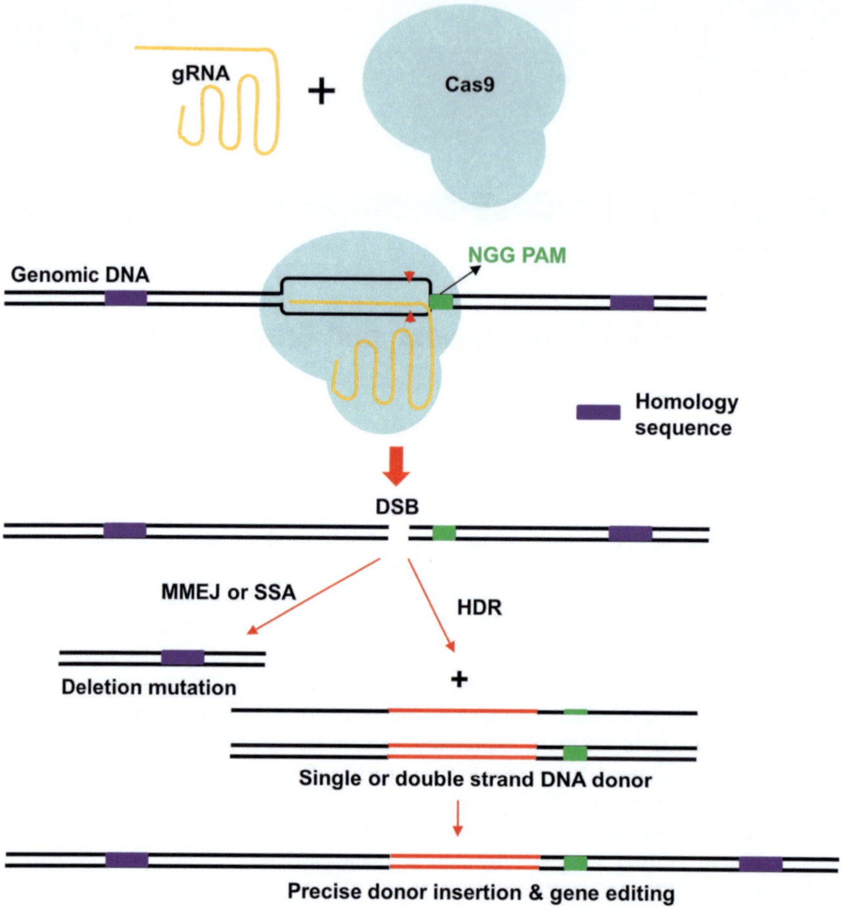

Fig. 1 Scheme of CRISPR-Cas9-mediated genome editing in *Leishmania*. The CRISPR-Cas9 genome editing system consists of at least two components: the gRNA and the Cas9 nuclease. The gRNA forms a ribonucleoprotein complex with Cas9 and guides Cas9 to the specific genomic target site, once the gRNA binds to the complementary target sequence, Cas9 becomes active and generates a double-stranded break (DSB) in the target DNA 3 bp upstream of the NGG PAM site. The DSB is typically repaired in *Leishmania* by microhomology-mediated end joining (MMEJ) or single strand annealing (SSA) with 5–500 bp homology sequences, which can lead to deletions ranging from 10 bp to more than 7000 bp. However, in the presence of donor DNA (repair template), single- or double-stranded DNA with only 25 nt (bp) homology arms flanking the cleavage site, desired mutations such as stop codons, frame shift, point mutations, tags and selection markers can be precisely inserted by homology directed repair (HDR), SSA or MMEJ into the *Leishmania* genome

target DNA sequence, directs the Cas9 nuclease to the specific DNA target site. Once the gRNA binds to the complementary target DNA sequence, the Cas9 nuclease becomes active and cleaves the target DNA three base pair (bp) upstream of the triple nucleotides NGG, known as the protospacer-adjacent motif (PAM), to generate a double-stranded break (DSB) (Fig. 1) [7]. DSBs are lethal to the cell and must be repaired by the cellular machinery either through mutation prone DSB repair pathways such as microhomology-mediated end-joining (MMEJ), single strand annealing (SSA) or through homology directed repair (HDR) [8, 9]. Unlike mammalian cells, *Leishmania* does not have the nonhomologous end-joining (NHEJ) pathway. Instead, *Leishmania* mainly uses MMEJ or SSA to repair DSBs. Repair through the MMEJ or SSA pathway in *Leishmania* often leads to deletion of the targeted gene [10–13]. HDR can be used to introduce a specific DNA sequence with desired mutations or tags [10, 11, 14, 15]. The Cas9 nuclease can be programed to target new sites simply by changing the 20 nt guide sequence of the gRNA. Given its simplicity, efficiency, and versatility, CRISPR-Cas9 has now been widely used for genome engineering in a variety of organisms including human protozoan parasites.

Leishmania protozoans are the causative agents of human leishmaniasis, the second most deadly parasitic disease after malaria. Despite decades of research efforts, there is still no effective vaccine available and the existing antileishmanial drugs are less than ideal with side effects [16]. Due to the lack of an RNA interference pathway in most of the *Leishmania* species [17], gene targeting in *Leishmania* traditionally relied on gene replacement by homologous recombination which requires a minimum of 180 bp flanking sequences and two antibiotic selection markers as *Leishmania* is diploid [18–21]. For genes present in multiploid chromosomes or present in multiple copies, several rounds of targeting are required which is time consuming and often not possible. Although whole genome sequences have been completed for various *Leishmania* species, the biological functions of most genes are unknown [22–26]. CRISPR technology has recently been adapted for use in *Leishmania* and has greatly improved gene editing efficiency [10–13, 27–33]. Compared to the traditional gene targeting method, CRISPR is simpler and more efficient; it has been used to generate gene deletion and disruption mutants, single point mutations, and to tag endogenous genes with or without using a selection marker. Importantly, it has been successfully used to delete multicopy family genes, which was often impossible with the traditional method, and to reveal essentiality of several *Leishmania* genes [10–13, 30].

Thus far, at least five CRISPR systems have been reported for use in *Leishmania* which include two stable expression systems and three transient systems [10–12, 27–31, 34]. In the two stable CRISPR expression systems, the Cas9 nuclease and gRNA are constitutively expressed in the parasites using expression vectors and gRNA transcribed from either the U6 promoter or the ribosomal RNA promoter [10, 11, 27, 30]. Because of the continuous expression of Cas9 and gRNA in the cell, this stable expression system using the ribosomal RNA promoter has been used to delete multicopy family *Leishmania* genes, determine gene essentiality and perform basic gene editing [10, 11]. In the transient expression system relying on the T7 RNA polymerase, the Cas9 and T7 RNA polymerase genes are integrated into the parasite genome and constitutively expressed [28, 34]. Gene editing is then achieved by transiently cotransfecting the Cas9 and T7 RNA polymerase expressing promastigotes with gRNA templates and donor DNA containing antibiotic selection markers or fluorescent protein tags [28, 34]. The second transient system recently reported involves directly transfecting the Cas9 expressing *Leishmania* cells with in vitro synthesized gRNA as well as an antibiotic selection marker donor [31]. The third transient system used a purified recombinant Cas9 protein from *Staphylococcus aureus* (SaCas9) complexed with in vitro-synthesized gRNA to form the ribonucleoprotein complex (RNP) [29]. Gene editing was achieved by transfecting the parasites with the RNP [29]. Compared with the Cas9 and gRNA constitutive expression systems [10, 11, 27, 29], the major advantages of these transient systems [28, 29, 31, 34] are that, once the Cas9 and T7 RNA polymerase expressing *Leishmania* cell line has been established or the SaCas9 recombinant protein purified from bacteria [29], the transient systems are more convenient and faster, as they bypass the DNA cloning procedures, and several gRNA species could be delivered simultaneously. The transient systems may also have lower probability to cause off-target mutations. However, the disadvantages of these transient systems are that it is necessary to develop *Leishmania* lines constitutively expressing T7 polymerase and Cas9 [29, 34] or the need to obtain purified recombinant Cas9 [29]. In the case of SaCas9, the longer PAM (NNGRRT) sequence requirement could also limit the sites available for SaCas9 targeting [12, 29, 35]. Further, how these transient systems will perform on multicopy and essential *Leishmania* genes remains to be determined.

In this chapter, we describe the detailed procedure for carrying out gene editing using the stable plasmid based CRISPR Cas9 expression system [10–12]. This is a versatile system and can be used to delete or disrupt single and multicopy genes, carry out selection with or without antibiotic resistance genes, edit gene codons and establish gene essentiality [10–12]. Depending on the experimental requirements and the investigator preference, one of the other transient or stable CRISPR expression systems can also be considered [27–31, 34]. As the principles of gene editing are similar, many of the procedures described within this chapter also apply to the transient systems.

2 Materials

2.1 Molecular Cloning

1. The pLdCN, pLdCN2, pSPBle, and pSPneogRNA241510 +MT plasmids have been deposited in Addgene (https://www.addgene.org/) with ID no. 84290, 125186, 63561, and 84292, respectively. The pLdCN plasmid is used to coexpress Cas9 and gRNA in *Leishmania*. The pLdCN2 plasmid is

used to coexpress Cas9 and two gRNAs in *Leishmania*. The pSPBle plasmid is used as a template to make donor DNA containing the bleomycin-resistant gene for selection of edited clones. The pSPneogRNA241510+MT plasmid can also be used to make dual gRNAs expressing pLdCN plasmids as detailed below.

2. Guide sequences and other primer oligonucleotides need to be ordered from a local supplier; including primers for PCR, donors, and other locus-specific primers for homologous template construction and gene disruption identification.
3. Common molecular biology reagents: such as *Bbs* I, and other restriction enzymes, T4 DNA ligase, T7 DNA ligase, and T4 Polynucleotide Kinase.
4. TE buffer: 10 mM Tris, 1 mM EDTA, pH 8.0.
5. PCR reagents: high-fidelity DNA polymerases such as the Platinum SuperFi DNA Polymerase, Q5 DNA Polymerase, Taq DNA Polymerase, dNTPs, and other common PCR reagents.
6. Competent bacterial cells such as *Escherichia coli* DH5α.
7. Plasmid purification kit such as the BIO BASIC Plasmid miniprep kit or GeneJET Plasmid Miniprep.
8. Reagents for agarose gel electrophoresis.
9. PCR purification kit and Gel/DNA extraction kit such as GeneJET PCR Purification Kit, Gel Extraction Kit.

2.2 Leishmania Strains and Culture Medium

The common *Leishmania* lab strains such as *L. donovani* 1S/Cl2D, *L. major* Friedlin V9, and *L. mexicana* (MNYC/BZ/62/M379). The culture medium is M199 medium (pH 7.4) supplemented with 10% heat-inactivated fetal bovine serum, 40 mM HEPES (pH 7.4), 0.1 mM adenine, 5 mg/L hemin, 1 mg/L biotin, 1 mg/L biopterin, 50 U/ml penicillin, and 50 μg/ml streptomycin. *Leishmania* promastigotes are routinely cultured at 27 °C and passaged to fresh medium at a 20- to 40-fold dilution once a week.

2.3 Parasite Transfection

1. Depending on the species and strain, *Leishmania* promastigotes from the middle log phase to early stationary phase are usually used for transfection.
2. Tb-BSF buffer [36]: 90 mM Na_2HPO_4, 5 mM KCl, 0.15 mM $CaCl_2$, 50 mM HEPES, pH 7.3.
3. Drug(s) for selection such as G418, phleomycin, hygromycin, and puromycin.
4. Tissue culture supplies such as 25 cm^2 cell culture flasks (T25), 96-well plates, 24-well plates.
5. Electroporation system such as the Nucleofector™ 2b Device from LONZA (*see* **Note 1**).

6. 2 mm gap electroporation cuvettes (Thermo Fisher Scientific).
7. Autoclaved glass Pasteur pipette and transfer bulb.

3 Methods

As outlined in Fig. 2a and b (*see* Drug R donor), the most rapid and direct way to disrupt a gene is to use a single gRNA expressing pLdCN plasmid (follow Subheadings 3.1–3.3) combined with the introduction of a donor DNA fragment containing an antibiotic resistance gene (follow Subheading 3.9). To completely remove a gene from the *Leishmania* genome as shown in Fig. 3, it is necessary to coexpress two gRNAs targeting the 5′ and 3′ end of the same gene (Subheading 3.4). Generally, it is not necessary to completely remove a gene to disrupt its function; this can more easily be achieved by disrupting the gene with a donor DNA fragment containing a selectable marker as outlined in Subheadings 3.1–3.3 and 3.9.

3.1 Selection of CRISPR Targeting Site(s)

To start a CRISPR experiment, the first thing to consider is where the gRNA will target, and the number of gRNAs to be used. For example, a single gRNA targeted to the 5′ half of a gene or sequence encoding functional protein domains is more likely to cause deletion or disruption mutants with more impact on the gene function. Two gRNAs targeted to the 5′ and 3′ flanking sequences of the gene will usually be required to delete the full coding sequence of a gene. To generate a point mutation, the gRNA/Cas9 cleavage site needs to be as close as possible to the desired mutation site. A gRNA designed to target a conserved sequence can be used in different *Leishmania* species. Once the targeting region has been identified, its sequence can then be loaded into design tools to search gRNAs with relatively high activity score as described below.

3.2 gRNA Design

Because most current gRNA design tools were developed from the data of higher eukaryotic cells, they may not accurately predict gRNA activity in *Leishmania* [10, 12]. Nevertheless, to design a gRNA with no off-target site(s) that is likely to be active in *Leishmania*, we recommend using the Eukaryotic Pathogen CRISPR guide RNA Design Tool (EuPaGDT) (http://grna.ctegd.uga.edu/) which ranks a gRNA based on its activity score, off-target sites in the genome and microhomology sequences flanking the double-strand break (DSB) site [37]. CRISPRater (https://crispr.cos.uni-heidelberg.de/) developed from human and mouse data could also be helpful as it can predict gRNA activity with only the guide sequence information [38]. For convenience, one may also directly use the gRNA sequences designed for targeting the

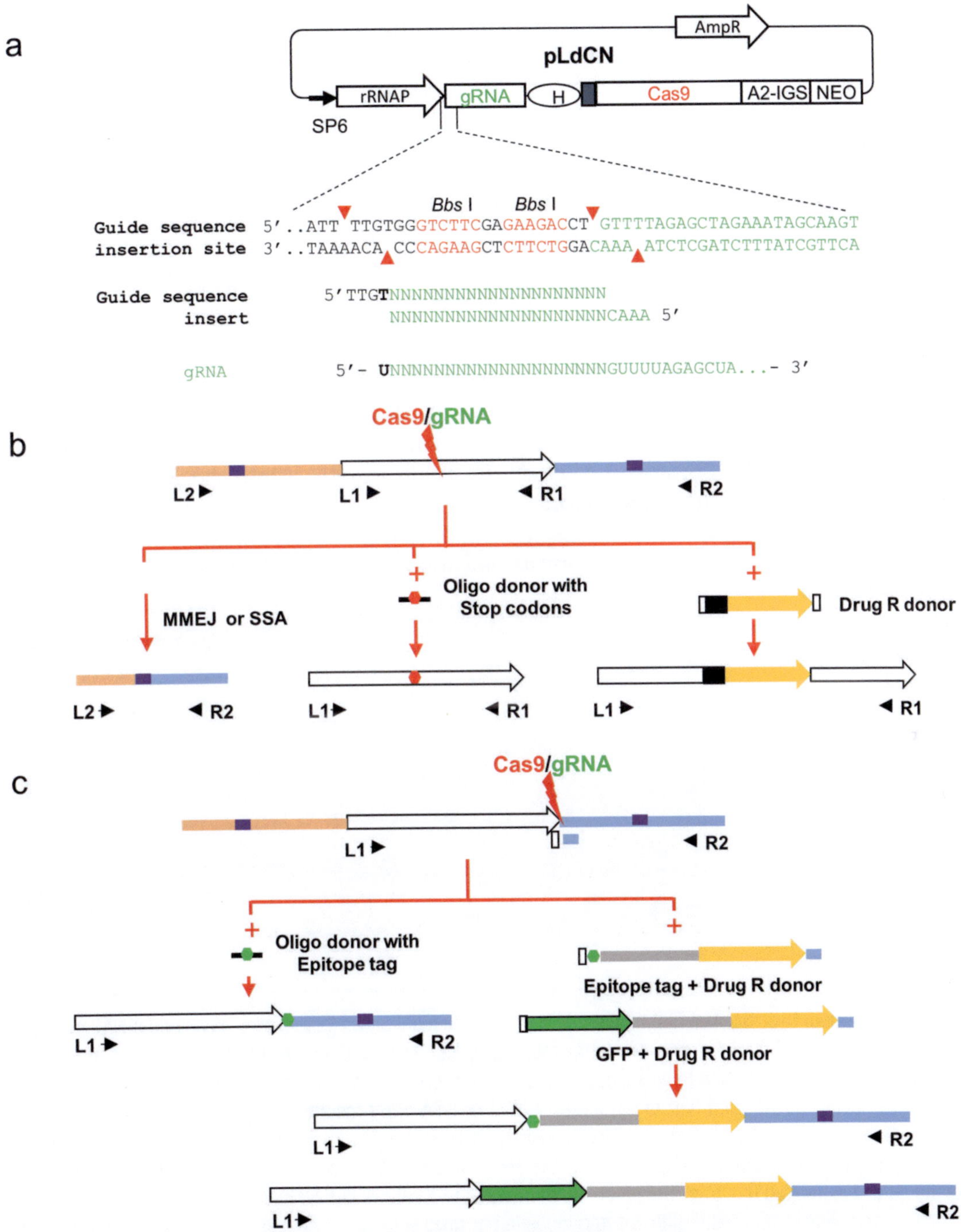

Fig. 2 Gene editing by expressing a single gRNA in *Leishmania*. (**a**) Scheme of the *Leishmania* CRISPR expression vector pLdCN and its guide sequence insertion site. A single gRNA and the *Streptococcus pyogenes* Cas9 nuclease can be stably expressed in pLdCN under the control of *L. donovani* ribosome RNA promoter. rRNAP, *L. donovani* ribosomal RNA promoter; H, Hepatitis delta virus (HDV) ribozyme. The small filled black box in front of Cas9 represents the 92 bp pyrimidine track. *A2-IGS* A2 intergenic sequence, *NEO* neomycin resistance gene, *AmpR* ampicillin resistance gene. The SP6 promoter, which can be used as the sequencing primer to verify the guide sequence insert, is also indicated. The vector size is 9217 bp and the drawing is not

immediate 5′ and 3′ flanking sequences for each of *Leishmania* genes from (http://leishgedit.net/) [28, 34].

3.3 Clone a gRNA Coding Sequence into the Leishmania CRISPR Vector pLdCN

For most gene editing procedures, expression of a single gRNA together with Cas9 is sufficient to enable the introduction of a donor DNA fragment into the target cut site to edit or disrupt a gene or gene family. As illustrated in Fig. 2a, single gRNA guide coding sequences (20 nt) can be ordered as complementary oligos with 5′-TTGT and 5′-AAAC overhangs. For example, for a gRNA targeting site in the genome 'GAAAGCTGATAAAGAAGCGG**AGG**' (PAM sequence NGG shown in bold), order the following two oligos: 5′TTGTGAAAGCTGATAAAGAAGCGG, and 5' AAACCCGCTTCTTTATCAGCTTTC. Note that the NGG PAM sequence (AGG) is part of the genome sequence but not included in the gRNA sequence (green). Use one of the following two protocols to clone the guide sequences into the *Bbs* I sites of the pLdCN vector:

3.3.1 The Traditional Two-Step Digestion and Ligation Cloning Protocol

1. Phosphorylate and anneal each pair of oligos:

3.75 μl	Oligo 1 (100 μM)
3.75 μl	Oligo 2 (100 μM)
1 μl	10× T4 DNA ligase buffer (NEB) (*see* **Note 2**)
1 μl	ddH_2O
0.5 μl	T4 Polynucleotide Kinase (NEB)
10 μl	*Total*
Anneal the oligos in a thermocycler using the following parameters:	
37 °C	30 min

(continued)

Fig. 2 (continued) to scale. The first nucleotide **U** of gRNA is highlighted (black) as *L. donovani* rRNAP initiates transcription at the **T** residue site. (**b**) Gene mutants generated by a single gRNA targeting to its coding sequence. The simplest way to inactivate a *Leishmania* gene is to design a gRNA targeting its coding sequence (ideally in the front half of the gene). MMEJ or SSA often results in large deletions. Single-strand oligonucleotides with stop codons or donors with drug resistant marker genes with 25 nt (bp) homology flanking arms can be used to disrupt the gene following Cas9 double-stranded break to facilitate the isolation of the gene-inactivated mutants. The presence of mutants in a culture can be identified by PCR with a specific primer to the oligo donor, restriction enzyme digestion or drug selection. The oligo donor can also be used to introduce frame shift, point mutations, epitope tags and other modifications. The 92 bp pyrimidine track (the filled black box) is required for trans-splicing of the drug resistance gene. (**c**) Tagging *Leishmania* genes. With CRISPR technology, a gene can be tagged in almost any position of its coding sequence. As an example, this illustration shows how a *Leishmania* gene can be tagged at its 3′ terminus with an oligo donor containing an epitope tag, or GFP together with the drug resistance gene donor. Fluorescence-activated cell sorting may be used to isolate the GFP tagged cells without using the drug resistance gene donor. The primers which can be used to detect these gene editing events are also indicated

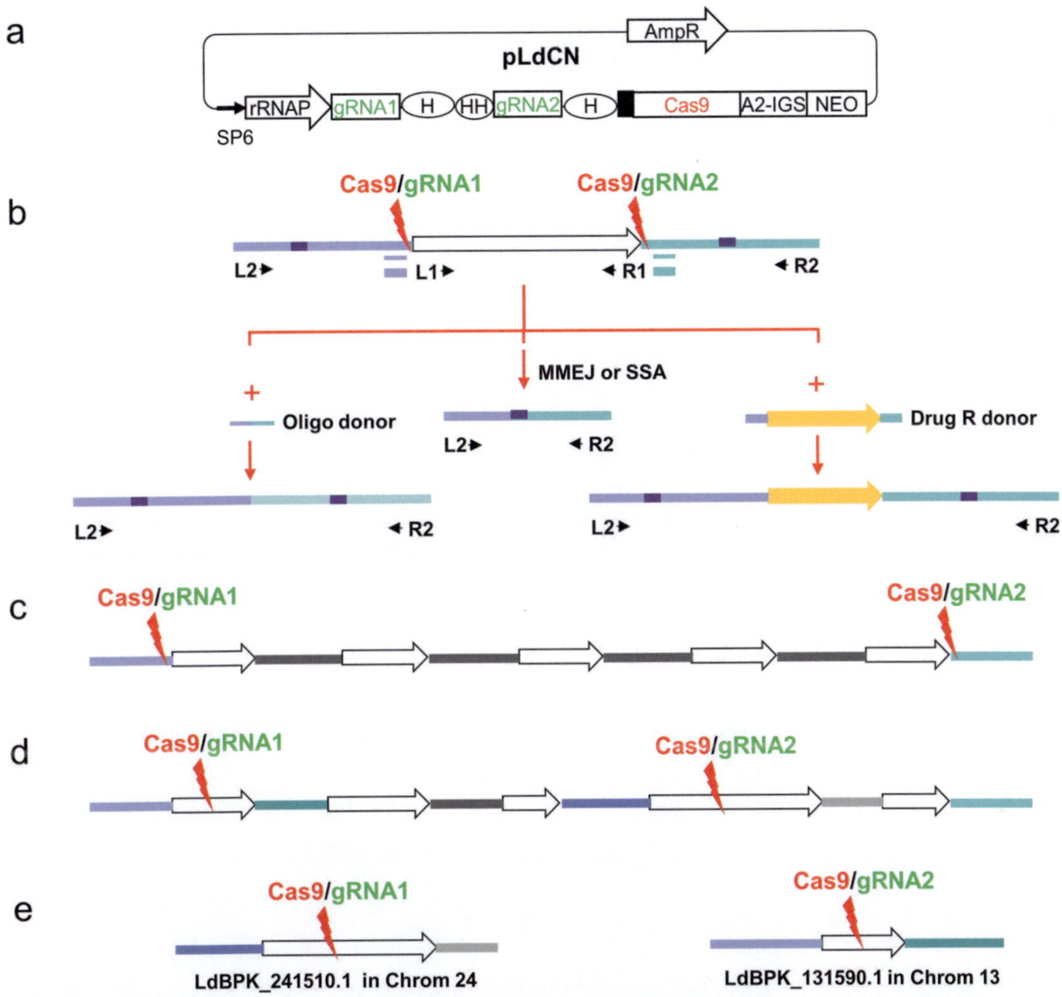

Fig. 3 Gene editing by coexpressing two gRNAs at the same time in *Leishmania* (**a**) Scheme of the *Leishmania* CRISPR vector pLdCN simultaneously expressing two gRNAs and Cas9. *HH* Hammerhead ribozyme. *See* Fig. 2 legend for other abbreviations. (**b**) Complete gene deletion by two gRNAs targeting respectively the 5′ and 3′ flanking sequences of the gene. Compared with single gRNA, the use of double gRNAs significantly increases the gene targeting efficiency (two to tenfold increase) and can be used to delete the whole coding sequence with or without the drug resistance gene donor. The primers which can be used to detect these gene editing events are also indicated. (**c**) Double gRNAs can be used to delete multiple copy family genes. (**d**) Double gRNAs can be used to target two different genes in a single *Leishmania* chromosome. (**e**) Double gRNAs can be used to target genes present in two different chromosomes such as the LdBPK_241510.1 gene in chromosome 24 and the miltefosine transporter (MT) gene (LdBPK_131590.1) in chromosome 13. Cotargeting *MT* and selection for miltefosine resistance cells have been shown to significantly facilitate the isolation of the CRISPR cotargeted gene mutants (*see* **Note 13**). Two different chromosomes targeted simultaneously by two gRNAs can also be used to generate the specific chromosome translocation mutants

Then add 90 μl TE to total volume 100 μl (3.75 μM)	
95 °C	5 min and then ramp down to 25 °C at 5 °C/min

2. Set up the pLdCN plasmid digestion reaction:

X μl	pLdCN (2 μg) (Addgene #84290)
3 μl	10× FastDigest Buffer
3 μl	FastDigest *Bbs* I
Y μl	ddH_2O
30 μl	*Total*
Incubate the digestion reaction at 37 °C for 1 h	

3. Purify the *Bbs* I-digested pLdCN vector directly using a PCR product purification kit following manufacturer's instructions (Thermo Fisher Scientific) and elute the digested pLdCN vector with 30 μl elution buffer.
4. Set up the following ligation reaction:

5.9 μl	*Bbs* I-digested pLdCN (0.39 μg)
3 μl	Phosphorylated and annealed Oligo duplex from **step 1** (3.75 μM)
1 μl	10× T4 DNA ligase buffer
0.1 μl	T4 DNA ligase (Thermo Fisher Scientific)
10 μl	*Total*
Incubate the ligation reaction at room temperature for 1–2 h	

5. Transform competent *E. coli* cells with 5 μl of the ligation reaction, plate and grow overnight at 37 °C.
6. Pick and grow four colonies, prepare plasmid DNA using a minipreparation kit and sequence the plasmids using the SP6 promoter primer and conditions for DNA with secondary structure to verify the clones. Purified pLdCN plasmids can be used to transfect *Leishmania* as detailed below in Subheading 3.5.

3.3.2 The Single-Step Digestion–Ligation Cloning Protocol

The single-step digestion–ligation cloning protocol adapted from Feng Zhang's lab (http://www.genome-engineering.org/crispr/wp-content/uploads/2014/05/CRISPR Reagent-Description-Rev20140509.pdf) is simpler to set up and may increase cloning efficiency. Due to the simultaneous digestion–ligation step, the guide oligos cannot contain any *Bbs* I enzyme recognition sites (i.e., the nucleotide sequence "GAAGAC" or 'GTCTTC').

1. Phosphorylate and anneal each pair of oligos:

1 µl	Oligo 1 (100 µM)
1 µl	Oligo 2 (100 µM)
1 µl	10× T4 DNA Ligase buffer (NEB)
6.5 µl	ddH_2O
0.5 µl	T4 Polynucleotide Kinase (NEB)
10 µl	*Total*
Anneal in a thermocycler using the following parameters:	
37 °C	30 min
95 °C	5 min and then ramp down to 25 °C at 5 °C/min Dilute the annealed oligo 1:250 (250-fold) in TE buffer.

2. Set up the following digestion–ligation reaction: This reaction combines *Bbs* I digestion of the pLdCN plasmid and ligation of the oligonucleotide into the *Bbs* I cut site.

X µl	pLdCN (100 ng) (Addgene #84290)
2 µl	Phosphorylated and annealed Guide duplex from **step 1** (1:250 dilution)
2 µl	10× FastDigest buffer
1 µl	10 mM DTT
1 µl	10 mM ATP
1 µl	FastDigest *Bbs* I (Thermo Fisher Scientific)
0.5 µl	T7 DNA ligase
Y µl	ddH_2O
20 µl	*Total*
Incubate the ligation reaction in a thermocycler:	
37 °C	5 min
23 °C	5 min Cycle the previous two steps for six cycles (total run time 1 h)
4 °C	Hold until ready to proceed

3. Transform competent *E. coli* cells with 5 µl of the ligation reaction from **step 2**, plate and grow overnight at 37 °C.
4. Pick and grow four colonies, prepare plasmid DNA using a minipreparation kit and sequence the plasmids using the SP6

promoter primer and conditions for DNA with secondary structure to verify the clones. Purified pLdCN plasmids can be used to transfect *Leishmania* as detailed below in Subheading 3.5.

3.4 Clone Two gRNA Guide Coding Sequences into Leishmania CRISPR Vector pLdCN

To delete a complete gene sequence, delete multicopy family genes, cotarget two different genes or generate specific chromosomal translocations, and to improve the gene targeting efficiency, two (or more) gRNAs can be simultaneously expressed in pLdCN vector (Fig. 3a) (*see* **Note 3**). One of the following two protocols (3.4.1 or 3.4.2) can be used to express two gRNA sequences from a single vector. The pLdCN2 (Addgene 125186) vector was recently engineered to simplify the cloning of two guide RNA sequences in a single vector (protocol 3.4.2).

3.4.1 The Cloning Protocol Using PCR Generated DNA Cassette

To express two gRNAs in the pLdCN vector, first use PCR to generate a DNA cassette that contains the two gRNA sequences separated by self-splicing ribozyme sequences as shown in Fig. 3a. To insert two gRNA coding sequences into the pLdCN vector with PCR and a single cloning step, an example for targeting the A2 *Leishmania* gene [11] is shown below:

1. The two A2 gene gRNA targeting sites are as follows: a, CCACAAGCGGACGCACGCTGCGG; b, ACCTTGGCTGCTGTTGCCAGGCGG.
2. Design and order the following two primers which contain respectively the A2 gRNA a and b guide coding sequence (in Green), a *Bbs* I site (in Red) and the pSPneogRNA241510+MT plasmid sequence (in Black):

   A2 a 5' ATCGAAGACCTTTGTCCACAAGCGGACGCACGCTG GTTTTAGAGCTAGAAATAGCAAG

   A2 b 5' ATCGAAGACCCAAACCCTGGCAACAGCAGCCAAGGT CACCATGACGAGCTTACTC

3. Use the pSPneogRNA241510+MT plasmid (Addgene #84292) as template, carry out a PCR reaction to obtain the following 276 bp PCR product which contains the coding sequences of gRNAa, HDV (in Blue) and Hammerhead (in Purple) ribozymes, and gRNAb guide (*see* also Fig. 3a). This PCR product is then cloned into the pLdCN vector after *Bbs* I digestion as cloning the oligo duplex described above in Subheading 3.3.

```
ATCGAAGACCTTTGTCCACAAGCGGACGCACGCTGGTTTTAGAGCTA
TAGCTTCTGGAAACAGGTGTTCGCCTGCGTGCGACCAAAATCTCGAT

GAAATAGCAAGTTAAAATAAGGCTAGTCCGTTATCAACTTGAAAAAG
CTTTATCGTTCAATTTTATTCCGATCAGGCAATAGTTGAACTTTTTC

TGGCACCGAGTCGGTGCTTTTTTGGCCGGCATGGTCCCAGCCTCCTC
ACCGTGGCTCAGCCACGAAAAAACCGGCCGTACCAGGGTCGGAGGAG

GCTGGCGCCGGCTGGGCAACATGCTTCGGCATGGCGAATGGGACGGA
CGACCGCGGCCGACCCGTTGTACGAAGCCGTACCGCTTACCCTGCCT

TCTCACCATCTGATGAGTCCGTGAGGACGAAACGAGTAAGCTCGTCA
AGAGTGGTAGACTACTCAGGCACTCCTGCTTTGCTCATTCGAGCAGT

TGGTGACCTTGGCTGCTGTTGCCAGGGTTTGGGTCTTCGAT
ACCACTGGAACCGACGACAACGGTCCCAAACCCAGAAGCTA
```

3.4.2 The Single-Step Digestion–Ligation Cloning Protocol for Two gRNA

To further simplify the cloning of two guide RNA sequences into a single vector, we generated the pLdCN2 plasmid containing *Bbs* I sites generating four unique ends that ensures the proper insertion and orientation of two pairs of oligonucleotides with the vector and the interspaced ribozyme sequences (required for gRNA processing) as shown in Fig. 4. For versatility and economy, the primer pair used for insertion at site 1 is cross-compatible with the single gRNA expression vector pLdCN. The primer pair used for insertion at site 2 is unique to pLdCN2 and requires the inclusion of a GT:CA pair at the 3′ end of the guide sequence (highlighted in green bold in Fig. 4.) as the *Bbs* I site in site two cuts into the gRNA scaffold on the vector. Make sure the guide oligos do not contain any *Bbs* I enzyme recognition sites (i.e., the nucleotide sequence 'GAAGAC' or 'GTCTTC').

1. Phosphorylate and anneal each pair of oligos in the same reaction:

1 μl	Oligo 1a (100 μM)
1 μl	Oligo 1b (100 μM)
1 μl	Oligo 2a (100 μM)
1 μl	Oligo 2b (100 μM)
1 μl	10× T4 DNA Ligase buffer (NEB)
4.5 μl	ddH_2O
0.5 μl	T4 Polynucleotide Kinase (NEB)
10 μl	*Total*
Anneal in a thermocycler using the following parameters:	

(continued)

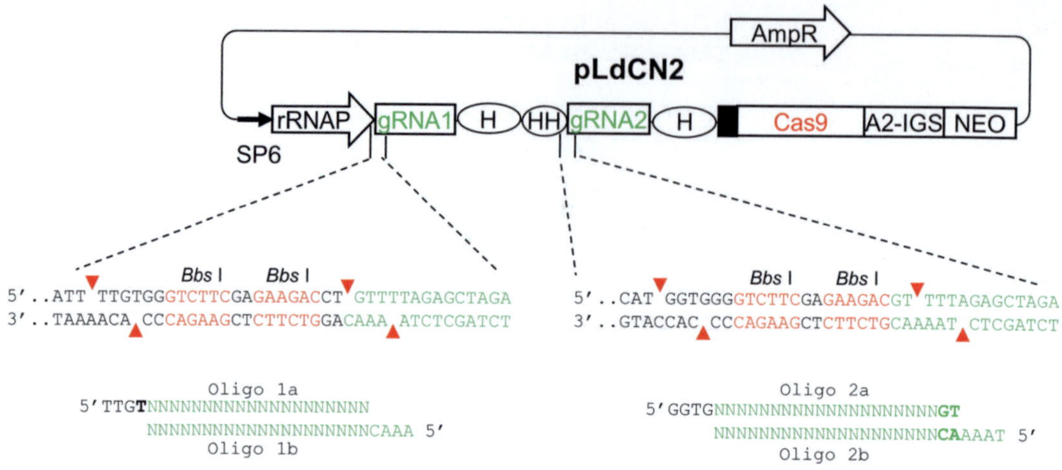

Fig. 4 Representation of the pLdCN2 vector used to express two gRNAs using primer pairs as inserts in a single-tube digestion–ligation reaction into a Cas9-expressing plasmid. rRNAP, *L. donovani* ribosomal RNA promoter; gRNA1, scaffold of the first gRNA; *H* Hepatitis delta virus (HDV) ribozyme, *HH* Hammerhead ribozyme, *gRNA2* scaffold of the second gRNA. Refer to Fig. 2 legend for other abbreviations. The guide sequence insertion sites 1 and 2 are enlarged to show the *Bbs* I recognition sites (in red) and cleavage sites (red arrows) with resulting overhangs. Guide sequences (N_{20}) can be inserted into pLdCN2 by using partially complementary primers resulting in overhangs matching insert site 1 or 2 (TTGT/CAAA; GGTG/AAAT, respectively). Overhangs used for insert site 1 are cross compatible with the single insert site pLdCN plasmid. Overhangs used for site 2 are unique to pLdCN2. Insert site 2 further requires a GT:CA 2 bp sequence be appended to the N_{20} guide sequence for proper insertion (in bold). These 2 base pairs are not part of the recognition sequence and will not affect the targeting of gRNA2

37 °C	30 min
95 °C	5 min and then ramp down to 25 °C at 5 °C/min
Dilute the annealed oligos 1:250 (250-fold) in TE buffer.	

2. Set up the following digestion–ligation combination reaction: This reaction combines both plasmid digestion with *Bbs* I and ligation of the two oligonucleotides into site 1 and site 2 of the *Bbs*I-digested plasmid.

X µl	pLdCN2 (100 ng) (Addgene #125186)
2 µl	Phosphorylated and annealed Guide duplexes from **step 1** (1:250 dilution)
2 µl	10× FastDigest buffer
1 µl	10 mM DTT
1 µl	10 mM ATP
1 µl	FastDigest *Bbs* I
0.5 µl	T7 DNA ligase

(continued)

Y µl	ddH_2O
20 µl	*Total*
Incubate the digestion–ligation reaction in a thermocycler:	
37 °C	5 min
23 °C	5 min Cycle the previous two steps for six cycles (total run time 1 h)
4 °C	Hold until ready to proceed

3. Transform competent *E. coli* cells with 5 µl of the ligation reaction from **step 2**, plate and grow overnight at 37 °C.
4. Pick and grow four colonies, prepare plasmid DNA using a minipreparation kit and sequence the plasmids using the SP6 promoter primer and conditions for DNA with secondary structure to verify the clones. The purified pLdCN2 plasmids can be used to transfect *Leishmania* as detailed below in Subheading 3.5.

As with the pLdCN vector expressing a single gRNA (Subheading 3.3), an oligonucleotide donor or an antibiotic selection gene containing donor can be designed for integration into the double gRNA targeting sites to improve editing efficiency.

3.5 Transfection of Leishmania with pLdCN Plasmid or Donor DNA

1. 2×10^7 *Leishmania* promastigotes (middle log phase to early stationary phase) are harvested by centrifugation at 4000 rpm ($1500 \times g$) in a benchtop centrifuge for 5 min.
2. Wash once with 200 µl Tb-BSF buffer.
3. Resuspend the parasites in 100 µl Tb-BSF buffer.
4. Add 2–5 µg of the pLdCN or pLdCN2 plasmid from Subheading 3.3 or 3.4 in less than 20 µl volume into the above *Leishmania* promastigotes suspension and mix well.
5. Transfer the above parasites and DNA mix solution into a 2-mm gap electroporation cuvette.
6. Place the cuvette into the Nucleofector™ 2b Device and perform the transfection using program U-33.
7. Transfer the electroporated parasites into a 25 cm^2 flask containing 5 ml culture medium using an autoclaved glass Pasteur pipette or a sterile transfer bulb.
8. Add G418 to the culture at 50 µg/ml the following day, to select for the pLdCN(2) plasmid-transfected cells.
9. Monitor drug selection of the transfection culture daily. If needed, change the culture with fresh medium once every 5 days, and increase the G418 concentration to 100 µg/ml.

10. Once the pLdCN(2) transfected cell culture is established, these cells can be subsequently transfected with the donor DNA (*see* Subheading 3.8 below for use of donor DNA); 4–8 μl of 100 μM oligonucleotide donor DNA or 2–4 μg of purified PCR product donor DNA is used for each transfection (*see* **Note 4**).
11. Cells can be repeatedly transfected with an oligonucleotide donor DNA at 2–3 day intervals, up to a total of four transfections to improve gene editing efficiency [11].
12. The drug selection for integration of the donor DNA (if the donor contains an antibiotic resistance gene) should start 1–2 days after the transfection with a drug resistance gene containing donor to allow time for the donor DNA integration into the genome and expression of the resistance gene. If the bleomycin resistance gene donor is used, add 50 μg/ml phleomycin initially and then increase to 100 μg/ml once the cultures start to look healthy.
13. The transfected *Leishmania* cultures can sometimes be incubated at 33 °C or 37 °C for 2–3 days to improve gene editing efficiency [10].

3.6 Isolate the CRISPR Edited Mutants

To isolate the CRISPR edited mutants, transfected *Leishmania* promastigotes can be cloned by limiting dilution in 96-well plates containing G418 (*see* **Note 5**). The clones are then expanded in a 24-well plate for genomic DNA extraction [39], PCR, and other analyses. Depending on the editing efficiency, several cloning methods can be used to isolate the edited mutants.

1. For experiments with high editing efficiency (editing frequency > 10%) or if the edited mutants can be selected with an antibiotic selection marker using a donor DNA, the transfected cells or the drug resistant cells can be cloned either by directly inoculating 1–3 promastigotes in 100 μl per well in a 96-well plate or by serial twofold dilution until the single cell per well is reached (limiting dilution) (*see* **Note 6**).
2. For experiments with low editing efficiency (editing frequency < 10%) and when the edited mutants cannot be selected with a drug, for example for gene editing with an oligonucleotide donor, the transfectants can be cloned in following way. Inoculate 5–20 promastigotes in 150 μl per well in two to three 96-well plates. Once the cells in these plates have grown up, pool a portion of the cells from 8–12 wells (take 100 μl cells from each of these wells), extract the genomic DNA, and perform PCR analysis to identify the presence of the mutant. If the desired gene editing can be detected in these pooled wells, continue cloning cells from the individual wells until the desired edited mutant is detected by PCR and has been single cell cloned.

3. It is possible that after a first round of cloning, promastigotes with only a single gene allele mutated (deleted or disrupted) are isolated. In this case, the single allele edited mutants should be further cultured and recloned until mutants with all alleles edited have been isolated.
4. Since alteration of the gene sequence (deletion, disruption or point mutation) could result in phenotype changes, pay attention to clones with different phenotypes such as reduced growth rate, changes in size or motility, drug resistance and others. Because the mutant promastigotes often grow slower than the wild-type promastigotes, it is important to clone these CRISPR transfectants early to avoid overgrowth by the wild-type promastigotes.

3.7 Generate Gene Deletion Mutants Without Using a Donor

Generally, it is always better to use a donor DNA to repair the Cas9 cut site to improve the gene targeting efficiency and specifity, since the double strand breaks in *Leishmania* are mainly repaired by MMEJ or SSA which often cause large deletions [10–13]. However, it is possible to directly isolate the CRISPR deletion mutants without using a donor, for example in targeting of the miltefosine transporter gene [10, 12], the A2 gene family [11] and the arginine transporter (AAP3) gene [13]. If a donor is not used, it is important to obtain pure clones and to use several PCR primer pairs with various distances flanking the Cas9 cleavage site to identify the deletion junctions (*see* Fig. 2b) (*see* **Note 7**). If a gene targeted is flanked by direct repeated sequences, the gene will most likely be deleted by the SSA mechanism, therefor primers flanking these direct repeat sequences can be conveniently used to detect the gene deletion mutants resulting from SSA [12].

Due to the low efficacy of double-strand DNA break repair in *Leishmania*, the double allelic mutation frequency using CRISPR without using a donor ranges from <1% to 10% depending on the gRNA used and the length of time post transfection [10]. However, the use of multiple gRNAs, extended culture (months posttransfection) and development of new CRISPR methods could improve the targeting efficiency to ease isolation of the donor-free gene deletion mutants [10, 11].

3.8 Generate Gene Edited Mutants by Using an Oligonucleotide Donor

As discussed above, double strand DNA break repair with MMEJ or SSA can lead to large unpredictable deletions which are often difficult to detect and verify [10, 41]. A single strand sense oligonucleotide with only 25 nt homology arms flanking the Cas9 cleavage site can be used as a source of DNA to repair the double strand break to introduce stop codons, frame shift, single point mutations, restriction sites, small epitope tags and others (Figs. 2b, c and 3) (*see* **Note 8**). An example using an oligonucleotide donor with stop codons to disrupt the *L. donovani* miltefosine transporter gene [10] is shown below.

```
gRNA   5'- UGUCCAGGCGCAGUGGAUGCGUUUUA...- 3'
LdMT 1110 TGAAGTGTGCAAAGTGGTCCAGGCGCAGTGGATGCGGGTGGACTGCCTCATGATGGAGTACATG 1173

5' TGCAAAGTGGTCCAGGCGCAGTGGATGAGTAGGTAGTGCGGGTGGACTGCCTCATGATGGA 3'
```
Oligonucleotide donor with stop codons

↓

```
TGAAGTGTGCAAAGTGGTCCAGGCGCAGTGGATGAGTAGGTAGTGCGGGTGGACTGCCTCATGATGGAGTACATG
```

Sequential transfection of pLdCN plasmid containing promastigotes with an oligonucleotide donor at 2- to 3-day intervals (as soon as enough G418 resistant cells have recovered) up to a total of four transfections can significantly improve the gene editing efficiency [11]. After the last oligonucleotide donor transfection, the *Leishmania* promastiogtes should be immediately cloned in 96 well plates to avoid overgrowth by the unedited cells. A PCR primer specific to the edited site and/or the inclusion of a restriction site within the oligonucleotide donor can greatly help to identify the gene edited mutants. To avoid the edited site being recut by the gRNA/Cas9 complex, some nucleotides in the seed region of the protospacer and the PAM site should also be mutated or deleted [11]. The oligonucleotide donor can also be used to generate a precise deletion between two gRNA targeting sites (Fig. 3b) or targeted chromosomal translocation between two chromosome targeting sites [10, 11].

3.9 Generate Gene Disrupted Mutants by Using an Antibiotic Resistance Selection Marker Donor

To facilitate the isolation of gene disrupted mutants, donor DNA containing a selection marker such as an antibiotic resistance gene flanked by 25 bp homology arms can be introduced into the Cas9 cleavage site(s) of the open reading frame (ORF) sequence (Figs. 2 and 3) (*see* **Note 9**). An example using the bleomycin resistance gene as a donor generated by PCR for disrupting the *L. donovani* LdBPK_241510.1 gene [10] is shown below.

```
                         3'-...AUUUUGACCGACGUCUUGCUGUGGU-5' gRNALd241510
     LdBPK_241510
5592 GGATCCTGCGCCTACTGTGCCGAGGTGCCTTGGCTGCAGAACGACACCATCCGCGCCAACATCGTG 6057
     CCTAGGACGCGGATGACACGGCTCCACGGAACCGACGTCTTGCTGTGGTAGGCGCGGTTGTAGCAC

CGCCTACTGTGCCGAGGTGCCTTGGATCTTCAT-Ble-AGGACTGACTGCAGAACGACACCATCCGCGCCA
GCGGATGACACGGCTCCACGGAACCTAGAAGTA-Ble-TCCTGACTGACGTCTTGCTGTGGTAGGCGCGGT
```
Ble donor PCR product 584 bp

↓

```
ATCCTGCGCCTACTGTGCCGAGGTGCCTTGGATCTTCAT-Ble-AGGACTGACTGCAGAACGACACCATCCGCGCCAACATCG
TAGGACGCGGATGACACGGCTCCACGGAACCTAGAAGTA-Ble-TCCTGACTGACGTCTTGCTGTGGTAGGCGCGGTTGTAGC
```
Insertion of 534 bp *Ble* expression cassette

To generate a donor DNA with a bleomycin resistance gene, it is necessary to start with the pSPBle plasmid that contains the bleomycin resistance gene (Addgene #63561). Design the following two specific donor primers which consist of 20 nt of pSPBle plasmid sequence (in Red) and 25 nt of sequence flanking the Cas9 cleavage site (in Black and Green) (example shown for the LdBPK_241510.1 gene below). The pSPBle plasmid is used as the PCR template to make the 584 bp bleomycin resistance gene donor PCR product (The 92 bp pyrimidine track upstream of the bleomycin resistance gene needed for trans-splicing is underlined).

```
241510BleF
 5' CGCCTACTGTGCCGAGGTGCCTTGGATCTTCATCGGATCGGGTAC
241510BleR
 5' TGGCGCGGATGGTGTCGTTCTGCAGTCAGTCCTGCTCCTCGGCCA
```

```
CGCCTACTGTGCCGAGGTGCCTTGGATCTTCATCGGATCGGGTACCGA
GCTCTCTCTTCTCCTTCCCCTCTCTCTCCTCTCTCCTCTCTCCAGAGC
TCTCTCTTCTCCTTCCCCTCTCTCTCCTCTCTCCTCTCTCCAGAGCTC
GAATTCATCGATGATATCAGATCCCCAACTAGATATCACCATGGCCAA
GTTGACCAGTGCCGTTCCGGTGCTCACCGCGCGCGACGTCGCCGGAGC
GGTCGAGTTCTGGACCGACCGGCTCGGGTTCTCCCGGGACTTCGTGGA
GGACGACTTCGCCGGTGTGGTCCGGGACGACGTGACCCTGTTCATCAG
CGCGGTCCAGGACCAGGTGGTGCCGGACAACACCCTGGCCTGGGTGTG
GGTGCGCGGCCTGGACGAGCTGTACGCCGAGTGGTCGGAGGTCGTGTC
CACGAACTTCCGGGACGCCTCCGGGCCGGCCATGACCGAGATCGGCGA
GCAGCCGTGGGGGCGGGAGTTCGCCCTGCGCGACCCGGCCGGCAACTG
CGTGCACTTCGTGGCCGAGGAGCAGGACTGACTGCAGAACGACACCAT
CCGCGCCA
```

Following PCR, run the product on an agarose gel to verify the size (584 bp) and purify the PCR product from the agarose gel. Transfect the PCR product containing the bleomycin resistance gene donor into the pLdCN plasmid containing promastigotes as described in Subheading 3.5 (*see* **Note 10**).

Likewise, a fluorescent protein coding sequence alone or together with a selection marker can be used to tag the gene of interest (Fig. 2) [10, 28]. As reported by Beneke et al., the use of two selection marker donors can further enhance the gene targeting efficiency [28, 34]. Small epitope tags together with a selection marker can also facilitate isolation of the gene-tagged mutants (Fig. 2).

3.10 Delete Multicopy Family Genes

Compared with the traditional gene targeting methods, one of the major advantages of CRISPR technology is that the gRNA and Cas9 complex stably expressed will continuously scan the genome and generate targeted double-strand breaks until all target sites have been deleted or mutated. The stable CRISPR expression system has been successfully used to delete the multicopy A2 family genes which have more than 11 copies distributed in four clusters on chromosome 22 of *L. donovani* 1SCL2D parasites [11]. To delete multicopy family genes, it is possible to use either a single gRNA targeted to the gene internally (Fig. 2) or two gRNAs, one targeted to the 5′ flanking sequence of the gene cluster and the other to the 3′ flanking sequence (Fig. 3c). A prolonged culture time and the use of an oligonucleotide donor or drug selection marker donor will increase the efficiency of targeting multicopy genes.

3.11 Target Essential Leishmania Genes

Because some *Leishmania* chromosomes are multiploid ranging from 3 to 5 chromosomes and *Leishmania* is well known to be capable of randomly amplifying its genes by using the direct or inverted repeat sequences to form circular or linear amplicons [12, 23, 24, 40, 41], it is often difficult and time consuming (more than two rounds of gene targeting are required) to determine whether a gene is essential for the viability of *Leishmania* with the traditional homologous recombination gene targeting method. CRISPR technology has greatly reduced the effort and time required to reveal the essentiality of *Leishmania* genes [10–12]. To determine whether a gene is essential for *Leishmania*, a single or double gRNAs together with an antibiotic selection marker donor should be used for maximal gene targeting efficiency. Once one allele of the essential gene has been disrupted or deleted, as evidenced by PCR analysis, there will be a reduced rate of proliferation compared with targeting nonessential genes. It will be possible to directly observe some of these CRISPR targeted cells dying in culture, especially after cloning into the 96-well plate since the gRNA and Cas9 will continuously scan the genome to search for the last essential gene target site to disrupt resulting in cell death. Depending on the targeting efficiency, 10–50% of these cells could be seen dying after cloning in the 96-well plate. These essential gene knockout promastigotes usually can still grow and divide slowly for about 1–2 weeks forming clumps in the wells before final cell death (lysis) [10–12]. This could be due to the time required to dilute and degrade the remaining mRNA and protein after all copies of the essential gene have been knocked out. PCR analysis will show the wild-type gene band persists in surviving single knockout *Leishmania* cells (*see* **Note 11**).

To facilitate the direct observation of dying cells following CRISPR gene targeting of essential genes, add cells into 96-well plates.

1. Inoculate 1–3 promastigotes in 100 μl per well in a 96-well plate.
2. Carefully examine each of the wells under a microscope in the following days and mark the wells with live parasites.

3. Monitor the promastigote growth daily, mark the wells with poorly growing promastigotes, focus on these wells thereafter until all the promastigotes in these wells are dead.
4. Expand the cultures of surviving promastigote wells in a 24-well plate, extract genomic DNA and perform PCR to confirm that the wild-type gene band persists in the surviving clones.
5. If required, additional selection markers or an oligonucleotide donor with silent mutations can be used to further confirm the essentiality of the gene.

3.12 Gene Tagging

As described above, oligonucleotide and PCR products can be used to introduce an epitope tag or a fluorescent protein into the Cas9 cleavage site to tag the gene of interest (Fig. 2c). The ability to tag a gene in its genomic locus will help to accurately measure the native gene expression at the protein level and should be especially useful for genes which are difficult to clone due to their large size or presence of repeated sequences such as the A2 family genes. With the help of cell sorting, cells with GFP or other fluorescent proteins tagged into an endogenous gene could be selected without using an antibiotic selection marker.

3.13 Gene Complementation

Like in mammalian cells, with carefully designed gene-specific gRNAs, CRISPR-Cas9 induced off-target mutations should be low in *Leishmania*. Nevertheless, to exclude the possibility of an observed phenotype change resulting from off-site targeting and other unexpected genetic changes such as deletion of neighboring genes during the CRISPR process [12], as occurs with traditional gene targeting, it is necessary to add back the wild-type gene to complement the knockout mutant to determine if it is possible to restore the wild-type phenotype. Gene complementation can be achieved by episomal expression of the wild-type gene [12, 25, 41, 42], or by reusing CRISPR technology to insert the wild-type gene back into the locus (*see* **Note 12**). Since the selection marker donor (if used) has been inserted into the genome, and the pLdCN CRISPR vector can remain in the parasites for weeks, even in the absence of G418 after gene editing, it is important to consider whether the addback wild-type gene can be similarly targeted by the remaining CRISPR vector, and whether an episomal expression vector with a new selection marker is needed to express the addback gene [10].

3.14 Generate Targeted Chromosome Translocations

One may consider using CRISPR to generate specific chromosome translocations to study polycistronic transcription control, gene amplification, chromosome replication, stability, and others. Two gRNAs each targeting specific sites from two different chromosomes are cloned into the pLdCN2 vector and expressed simultaneously in the cell (Fig. 3e), an antibiotic selection marker donor should help to isolate the cells with targeted chromosome translocation [11].

4 Notes

1. The electroporation method using Bio-Rad Gene Pulser Electroporation System with Cytomix buffer can also be used for labs not yet equipped with LONZA Nucleofector™ System [10].
2. T4 Polynucleotide Kinase is used for 5′ phosphorylation of the oligos for subsequent ligation into the pLdCN(2) vector and requires in the reaction the presence of ATP which is provided by the DNA ligase buffer (1 mM ATP at 1× final concentration). However, the T4 Polynucleotide Kinase buffer itself usually does not contain ATP as T4 Polynucleotide Kinase is mostly used for end radiolabeling of DNA or RNA probes where the [γ-^{32}P]ATP is additionally added for the 5′ End-Labeling reaction.
3. If required, with the PCR cassette approach, more than two gRNAs in tandem array can be cloned into the pLdCN vector. Alternatively, other CRISPR vectors such as pLdCH (Addgene #84291) can be used to clone additional gRNAs.
4. The amount of oligonucleotide donor used has not been systematically tested; one may try different quantities to find the most efficient dose.
5. G418 drug pressure should be maintained in the culture medium to retain the pLdCN plasmid in these *Leishmania* cells until the desired gene editing mutant has been obtained.
6. Since it is difficult to evenly distribute 1 promastigote per well in a 96-well plate, adding 2–3 promastigotes per well will reduce the number of empty wells (with no promastigotes).
7. Sometimes, due to the presence of wild-type dead promastigotes, the faint wild-type band could be present in PCR products in some of the knockout clones; this can be verified by recloning these promastigotes.
8. Likely because the antisense oligonucleotide could hybridize to the corresponding mRNA to reduce its availability as the repair template, we have successfully generated the single amino acid replacement mutant of the RAD51 protein with the sense oligonucleotide donor but not with the antisense oligo donor [11].

9. For a first-time user of CRISPR gene editing and the experimental goal being simply to knockout (inactivate) a single gene, we recommend to first express a single gRNA in pLdCN (Subheadings 3.1–3.3) and selection with an antibiotic resistance gene donor (Subheading 3.9) because this will be the simplest and most direct way to obtain the disrupted gene mutant. For researchers who already have the first-hand CRISPR experience and are familiar with basic molecular biology and parasitology techniques, they can take more challenging and advanced approaches such as gene targeting without using a donor or using an oligonucleotide donor to tag a gene or edit a gene (Subheading 3.8) or express two-gRNAs from pLdCN2 (Subheading 3.4).
10. Besides the bleomycin resistance gene, other drug resistance genes such as the puromycin and hygromycin resistance genes could also be used as the selection marker donor. As reported by Beneke et al. [28], the raw PCR product donor without purification can be directly used for transfection. As the single-strand DNA donor could be more efficient than the double-strand DNA donor, the PCR product donor can be heat-denatured and sterilized immediately before transfection.
11. Since DSB repair is not efficient in *Leishmania* and nonrepaired DSB is lethal to the cell, some of these promastigote deaths could also be triggered by DSBs which are not promptly repaired [12]. Cell deaths observed in targeting nonessential genes are most likely caused by nonrepaired DSB. Contrary to cell deaths resulting from knockout of essential genes, cells with nonrepaired DSB usually cannot replicate before death.
12. To re-CRISPR the cell, the pLdCN vector can be removed from the cells by culturing in G418-free medium for about 2 months. Alternatively, other CRISPR vectors such as pLdCH (Addgene#84291) with the hygromycin resistance marker can be used for subsequent CRISPR targeting. In addition, we recently developed a novel *Staphylococcus aureus* Cas9 (SaCas9) expression vector pLdSaCN (Addgene#123261) which uses NNGRRT PAM sequences, has similar or improved gene editing efficiency compared with the *Streptococcus pyogenes* Cas9 expression vector pLdCN. The same guide sequence cloning strategy is used for pLdSaCN vector [12].
13. Cotargeting the miltefosine transporter (MT) gene can significantly facilitate isolation of the gene edited mutants. However, mutation of the *MT* gene could also reduce the parasite infectivity and virulence.

Acknowledgments

This work was supported by the Canadian Institute of Health Research grant MOP125996 to G.M. and a doctoral training award from the Fonds de recherche du Québec—Santé (FRQS) to P.L.

References

1. Jinek M, Chylinski K, Fonfara I, Hauer M, Doudna JA, Charpentier E (2012) A programmable dual-RNA-guided DNA endonuclease in adaptive bacterial immunity. Science 337:816–821
2. Cong L, Ran FA, Cox D, Lin S, Barretto R, Habib N, Hsu PD, Wu X, Jiang W, Marraffini LA, Zhang F (2013) Multiplex genome engineering using CRISPR/Cas systems. Science 339:819–823
3. Mali P, Esvelt KM, Church GM (2013) Cas9 as a versatile tool for engineering biology. Nat Methods 10(10):957–963
4. Doudna JA, Charpentier E (2014) Genome editing. The new frontier of genome engineering with CRISPR-Cas9. Science 346 (6213):1258096
5. Hsu PD, Lander ES, Zhang F (2014) Development and applications of CRISPR-Cas9 for genome engineering. Cell 157(6):1262–1278
6. Knott GJ, Doudna JA (2018) CRISPR-Cas guides the future of genetic engineering. Science 361(6405):866–869
7. Nishimasu H, Ran FA, Hsu PD, Konermann S, Shehata SI, Dohmae N, Ishitani R, Zhang F, Nureki O (2014) Crystal structure of Cas9 in complex with guide RNA and target DNA. Cell 156(5):935–949
8. Her J, Bunting SF (2018) How cells ensure correct repair of DNA double-strand breaks. J Biol Chem 293(27):10502–10511
9. Sallmyr A, Tomkinson AE (2018) Repair of DNA double-strand breaks by mammalian alternative end-joining pathways. J Biol Chem 293(27):10536–10546
10. Zhang WW, Matlashewski G (2015) CRISPR-Cas9-mediated genome editing in Leishmania donovani. MBio 6(4):e00861
11. Zhang WW, Lypaczewski P, Matlashewski G (2017) Optimized CRISPR-Cas9 genome editing for Leishmania and its use to target a multigene family, induce chromosomal translocation and study DNA break repair mechanisms. mSphere 2(1):e00340–e00316. https://doi.org/10.1128/mSphere.00340-16
12. Zhang WW, Matlashewski G (2019) Single-Strand Annealing Plays a Major Role in Double-Strand DNA Break Repair following CRISPR-Cas9 Cleavage in Leishmania. mSphere 4:e00408–19. https://doi.org/10.1128/mSphere.00408-19
13. Goldman-Pinkovich A, Kannan S, Nitzan-Koren R, Puri M, Bar-Avraham Y, McDonald JA, Sur A, Zhang WW, Matlashewski G, Madhubala R, Michaeli S, Myler PJ, Zilberstein Dan (2019) The hunger games: sensing host arginine is essential for Leishmania parasite virulence. bioRxiv 751610. https://doi.org/10.1101/751610
14. Böttcher R, Hollmann M, Merk K, Nitschko V, Obermaier C, Philippou-Massier J, Wieland I, Gaul U, Förstemann K (2014) Efficient chromosomal gene modification with CRISPR/cas9 and PCR-based homologous recombination donors in cultured Drosophila cells. Nucleic Acids Res 42(11):e89. https://doi.org/10.1093/nar/gku289
15. Paix A, Wang Y, Smith HE, Lee CY, Calidas D, Lu T, Smith J, Schmidt H, Krause MW, Seydoux G (2014) Scalable and versatile genome editing using linear DNAs with microhomology to Cas9 sites in Caenorhabditis elegans. Genetics 198(4):1347–1356
16. Burza S, Croft SL, Boelaert M (2018) Leishmaniasis. Lancet 392(10151):951–970. https://doi.org/10.1016/S0140-6736(18)31204-2
17. Lye LF, Owens K, Shi H, Murta SM, Vieira AC, Turco SJ, Tschudi C, Ullu E, Beverley SM (2010) Retention and loss of RNA interference pathways in trypanosomatid protozoans. PLoS Pathog 6(10):e1001161
18. Cruz A, Beverley SM (1990) Gene replacement in parasitic protozoa. Nature 348 (6297):171–173

19. Tobin JF, Laban A, Wirth DF (1991) Homologous recombination in Leishmania enriettii. Proc Natl Acad Sci U S A 88(3):864–868
20. Cruz A, Coburn CM, Beverley SM (1991) Double targeted gene replacement for creating null mutants. Proc Natl Acad Sci U S A 88 (16):7170–7174
21. Papadopoulou B, Dumas C (1997) Parameters controlling the rate of gene targeting frequency in the protozoan parasite Leishmania. Nucleic Acids Res 25(21):4278–4286
22. Peacock CS, Seeger K, Harris D, Murphy L, Ruiz JC, Quail MA et al (2007) Comparative genomic analysis of three Leishmania species that cause diverse human disease. Nat Genet 39(7):839–847
23. Downing T, Imamura H, Decuypere S, Clark TG, Coombs GH, Cotton JA et al (2011) Whole genome sequencing of multiple *Leishmania donovani* clinical isolates provides insight into population structure and mechanisms of resistance. Genome Res 21 (12):2143–2156
24. Rogers MB, Hilley JD, Dickens NJ, Wilkes J, Bates PA, Depledge DP et al (2011) Chromosome and gene copy number variations allow major structural change between species and strains of *Leishmania*. Genome Res 21 (12):2129–2142
25. Zhang WW, Ramasamy G, McCall LI, Haydock A, Ranasinghe S, Abeygunasekara P, Sirimanna G, Wickremasinghe R, Myler P, Matlashewski G (2014) Genetic analysis of Leishmania donovani tropism using a naturally attenuated cutaneous strain. PLoS Pathog 10 (7):e1004244
26. Lypaczewski P, Hoshizaki J, Zhang WW, McCall LI, Torcivia-Rodriguez J, Simonyan V, Kaur A, Dewar K, Matlashewski G (2018) A complete Leishmania donovani reference genome identifies novel genetic variations associated with virulence. Sci Rep 8 (1):16549
27. Sollelis L, Ghorbal M, MacPherson CR, Martins RM, Kuk N, Crobu L, Bastien P, Scherf A, Lopez-Rubio JJ, Sterkers Y (2015) First efficient CRISPR-Cas9-mediated genome editing in Leishmania parasites. Cell Microbiol 17 (10):1405–1412
28. Beneke T, Madden R, Makin L, Valli J, Sunter J, Gluenz E (2017) A CRISPR Cas9 high-throughput genome editing toolkit for kinetoplastids. R Soc Open Sci 4:170095. https://doi.org/10.1098/rsos.170095
29. Soares Medeiros LC, South L, Peng D, Bustamante JM, Wang W, Bunkofske M, Perumal N, Sanchez-Valdez F, Tarleton RL (2017) Rapid, selection-free, high-efficiency genome editing in protozoan parasites using CRISPR-Cas9 ribonucleoproteins. MBio 8:e01788–e01717
30. Ishemgulova A, Hlaváčová J, Majerová K, Butenko A, Lukeš J, Votýpka J, Volf P, Yurchenko V (2018) CRISPR/Cas9 in Leishmania mexicana: a case study of LmxBTN1. PLoS One 13(2):e0192723
31. Fernandez-Prada C, Sharma M, Plourde M, Bresson E, Roy G, Leprohon P, Ouellette M (2018) High-throughput Cos-Seq screen with intracellular Leishmania infantum for the discovery of novel drug-resistance mechanisms. Int J Parasitol Drugs Drug Resist 8 (2):165–173. https://doi.org/10.1016/j.ijpddr.2018.03.004
32. Beneke T, Demay F, Hookway E, Ashman N, Jeffery H, Smith J, Valli J, Becvar T, Myskova J, Lestinova T, Shafiq S, Sadlova J, Volf P, Wheeler RJ, Gluenz E, Hill KL (2019) Genetic dissection of a Leishmania flagellar proteome demonstrates requirement for directional motility in sand fly infections. PLOS Pathogens 15(6):e1007828
33. Giri, S, Shaha, C (2019) Leishmania donovani parasite requires Atg8 protein for infectivity and survival under stress. Cell Death Dis 10:808. https://doi.org/10.1038/s41419-019-2038-7
34. Beneke T, Gluenz E (2019) LeishGEdit: A Method for Rapid Gene Knockout and Tagging Using CRISPR-Cas9. Methods Mol Biol 1971:189–210. https://doi.org/10.1007/978-1-4939-9210-2_9
35. Ran FA, Cong L, Yan WX, Scott DA, Gootenberg JS, Kriz AJ, Zetsche B, Shalem O, Wu X, Makarova KS, Koonin EV, Sharp PA, Zhang F (2015) In vivo genome editing using Staphylococcus aureus Cas9. Nature 520 (7546):186–191
36. Schumann Burkard G, Jutzi P, Roditi I (2011) Genome-wide RNAi screens in bloodstream form trypanosomes identifydrug transporters. Mol Biochem Parasitol 175(1):91–94
37. Peng D, Tarleton R (2015) EuPaGDT: a web tool tailored to design CRISPR guide RNAs for eukaryotic pathogens. Microb Genom 1 (4):e000033
38. Labuhn M, Adams FF, Ng M, Knoess S, Schambach A, Charpentier EM, Schwarzer A, Mateo JL, Klusmann JH, Heckl D (2018) Refined sgRNA efficacy prediction improves large- and small-scale CRISPR–Cas9 applications. Nucleic Acids Res 46(3):1375–1385
39. Medina-Acosta E, Cross GA (1993) Rapid isolation of DNA from trypanosomatid protozoa using a simple 'mini-prep' procedure. Mol Biochem Parasitol 59(2):327–329

40. Grondin K, Roy G, Ouellette M (1996) Formation of extrachromosomal circular amplicons with direct or inverted duplications in drug-resistant Leishmania tarentolae. Mol Cell Biol 16(7):3587–3595
41. Ubeda JM, Raymond F, Mukherjee A, Plourde M, Gingras H, Roy G, Lapointe A, Leprohon P, Papadopoulou B, Corbeil J, Ouellette M (2014) Genome-wide stochastic adaptive DNA amplification at direct and inverted DNA repeats in the parasite Leishmania. PLoS Biol 12(5):e1001868
42. Zhang WW, Matlashewski G (2015) Screening Leishmania donovani complex-specific genes required for visceral disease. Methods Mol Biol 1201:339–361

Chapter 15

Next-Generation Analysis of Trypanosomatid Genome Stability and Instability

Emma M. Briggs, Catarina A. Marques, Joao Reis-Cunha, Jennifer Black, Samantha Campbell, Jeziel Damasceno, Daniella Bartholomeu, Kathryn Crouch, and Richard McCulloch

Abstract

Understanding the rate and patterns of genome variation is becoming ever more amenable to whole-genome analysis through advances in DNA sequencing, which may, at least in some circumstances, have supplanted more localized analyses by cellular and genetic approaches. Whole-genome analyses can utilize both short- and long-read sequence technologies. Here we describe how sequence generated by these approaches has been used in trypanosomatids to examine DNA replication dynamics, the accumulation of modified histone H2A due to genome damage, and evaluation of genome variation, focusing on ploidy change.

Key words Next-generation sequencing, DNA replication, MFA-seq, ChIP-seq, DNA damage, Single nucleotide polymorphisms, Copy number variation, Ploidy

1 Introduction

The genome is the crucible of life for cellular organisms. Accurate copying and transmission of DNA content from parent to offspring is needed for the propagation of cellular life. However, the genetic content cannot remain unchanged, since alterations in sequence are needed for adaptation to changing or hostile environments, and are the basis for selection by evolution. Normally these content changes accumulate slowly and often occur in a limited way, such as through single base changes or small insertions and deletions, subtly altering the protein and RNA products that are encoded. Other changes are more dramatic, either because they happen at high rates or because they occur through larger scale changes in the genome. These dramatic changes are not frequently found as examples of evolution but instead are normally genetically programmed reactions that reflect specific aspects of organism biology and

Paul A. M. Michels et al. (eds.), *Trypanosomatids: Methods and Protocols*, Methods in Molecular Biology, vol. 2116,
https://doi.org/10.1007/978-1-0716-0294-2_15,

development. Prominent examples of such adaptive change are immunoglobulin gene rearrangements during B- and T-cell development [1, 2], mating type switching during yeast life cycles [3], and genome reconstruction in a range of ciliates [4–6]. In all cases, understanding of the timing, rate and mechanism of such dramatic change relative to the slower accrual of evolution-directing mutations is greatly aided by mapping the nature and location of the changes. Such questions are hugely easier to address, and more comprehensively evaluated, using next generation sequencing approaches that study such biology on a genome-wide scale.

Trypanosomatids—parasites within the wider order Kinetoplastae—provide a rich source of adaptive change, including frequent changes in the content and location of genes encoding the critical variant surface glycoprotein coat that underlies immune evasion by antigenic variation in *Trypanosoma brucei* [7], and the remarkable levels of genome-wide mosaic aneuploidy and gene amplification that are seen during *Leishmania* growth and dissemination [8, 9]. All such processes are amenable to analysis through next generation sequencing. Here, we provide details of three broad approaches that have been applied to date to understand the reactions that underlie stable transmission and directed variation in trypanosomatid genome content. First, we explain how the initiation and progression of DNA replication has been mapped by Marker Frequency Analysis (MFA-seq) [10, 11]; elsewhere, we have discussed how this approach compares with other strategies to map replication initiation, either using next generation sequencing or not [12]. Second, we explain how sites of DNA damage may be mapped in trypanosomatids [13], exploiting chromatin immunoprecipitation of histone γH2A, a phosphorylated variant of core histone H2A, on residue Thr130, which is generated in response to a range of DNA insults [14, 15]. Third, whole-genome sequencing, to date using Illumina methodology, can be exploited to map patterns of single nucleotide polymorphism (SNP) accumulation during growth [16], to determine patterns of chromosome and gene copy number variation (CNV) [17–19], and to predict structural changes, such as translocations [16, 20]; here, as an example, we describe the evaluation of chromosome CNV (CCNV) in *Leishmania major*, using freely available files and datasets. We have described each of the three approaches such that they can be followed individually, rather than relying on cross-checking on materials and protocols between the approaches.

2 Materials

2.1 MFA-seq Analysis of Replication Dynamics

2.1.1 Cell Preparation and Staining with Propidium Iodide

1. 1× PBS supplemented with 5 mM of EDTA.
2. 100% methanol (at 4 °C) or 1% formaldehyde (methanol-free) diluted in 1× PBS (*see* **Note 1**).
3. Propidium iodide (Sigma Aldrich).
4. RNase A (Sigma Aldrich).
5. Triton X-100 (Promega).
6. BD Falcon™ 12 × 75 mm (5 ml) tube with a 35 μm nylon mesh cell strainer cap (BD Biosciences, Cat. No. 352235) or other type of tube compatible with the FACS system being used.

2.1.2 Cell Sorting, DNA Extraction, and NGS

1. Fluorescence-activated cell sorting (FACS) system (e.g., BD FACSAria™ Cell Sorter).
2. Lysis Buffer: 1 M NaCl, 10 mM EDTA, 50 mM Tris–HCl pH 8.0, 0.5% SDS, 0.4 mg/ml Proteinase K, and 0.8 μg/ml of glycogen [21].

2.1.3 Genomic DNA Extraction and Sequencing

1. DNeasy Blood and Tissue DNA extraction kit (Qiagen).
2. Nextera® XT DNA Sample Preparation kit (Illumina) or Tru-Seq® DNA Sample Preparation kit (Illumina).
3. Illumina MiSeq 250 bp paired-end sequencing system or Illumina HiSeq 100 bp paired-end sequencing system.

2.1.4 Marker Frequency Analysis

All analysis can be run on a computer running UNIX or Linux with version 2.7 or higher of Python. The following **software** needs to be installed before MFA-seq analysis can be run.

1. FastQC (http://www.bioinformatics.babraham.ac.uk/projects/fastqc/).
2. fastq-mcf (https://github.com/ExpressionAnalysis/ea-utils/blob/wiki/FastqMcf.md).
3. Bowtie2 (http://bowtie-bio.sourceforge.net/bowtie2/index.shtml).
4. Samtools (http://www.htslib.org).
5. Bedtools (https://bedtools.readthedocs.io/en/latest/).
6. pysam package (https://pypi.org/project/pysam/) (version 0.8.3 recommended).
7. mfaseq.py (https://github.com/CampbellSam/MFAseq).
8. ggplot2 (https://ggplot2.tidyverse.org) and R package (https://www.r-project.org), or Prism (GraphPad software Inc.).

The following files must be obtained prior to the analysis:

1. adapters.fa—.fa file containing the adapter sequences used in the library preparation and sequencing processes.
2. refgenome.fa—fasta file containing the reference genome to which the sequencing data are going to be aligned to. This can be obtained from TriTrypDB.org (Downloads → Data Files → Current_Release).

2.2 ChIP-seq Analysis of γH2A Distribution

2.2.1 Chromatin Immunoprecipitation

1. ChIP-IT Express Enzymatic Kit (Active Motif®).
2. Anti-γH2A antibody.
3. Formaldehyde (methanol-free).
4. Serum-free media, as appropriate for trypanosomatids.
5. Dounce homogenizer.
6. Magnetic rack.

2.2.2 Library Preparation

1. TrueSeq ChIP Library Preparation kit (Illumina).

2.2.3 qPCR

1. SYBR™ Select Master Mix (ThermoFisher).

2.2.4 Data Analysis

All analyses can be carried out on a computer running UNIX or Linux with the following software installed:

1. FastQC (http://www.bioinformatics.babraham.ac.uk/projects/fastqc/).
2. TrimGalore (https://www.bioinformatics.babraham.ac.uk/projects/trim_galore/).
3. Bowtie2 (http://bowtie-bio.sourceforge.net/bowtie2/index.shtml).
4. Samtools (http://www.htslib.org).
5. DeepTools (https://deeptools.readthedocs.io/en/develop/).

2.3 Next Generation Analysis of Instability

2.3.1 Hardware

1. A computer running UNIX, Linux or is suitable for all the procedures detailed here (*see* **Note 23**).

2.3.2 Datasets

1. To perform chromosomal copy number variation (CCNV) evaluations, a chromosome-level assembly of the desired reference genome, as well as whole-genome sequencing reads preferentially in FASTQ format with at least 20× of coverage is needed. Lower genome coverages could be used; however, they can compromise the ploidy analysis. The advantage of using FASTQ instead of fasta reads is the base quality information, which can be used to more accurately identify SNPs and genomic alterations. Although not required in all ploidy

estimation methodologies, the use of a General Feature Format (GFF) file containing the genome coordinates of all annotated genes could be important to perform CCNV in complex genomes or to polish the ploidy estimation.

Genomic reads generated by Illumina (https://www.illumina.com/documents/products/illumina_sequencing_introduction.pdf) are suggested due to their high depth and base quality; however, this analysis can also be performed with reads from other technologies as 454 [22] and Ion torrent (https://www.thermofisher.com/br/en/home/brands/ion-torrent.html) [23]. The use of long-reads such as generated by the PacBio Sequel/RSII (https://www.pacb.com/smrt-science/smrt-sequencing/) and Oxford Nanopore (https://nanoporetech.com/) to perform ploidy estimations is possible, but this analysis would need a different toolset from the one described in this chapter.

2. Chromosome-level assembly of the *Leishmania major* Friedlin reference genome (version 41), available at TriTrypDB (http://tritrypdb.org/tritrypdb/). Version 41 was used for the analysis described here, but new versions can also be used:

   http://tritrypdb.org/common/downloads/Release_41/LmajorFriedlin/fasta/data/TriTrypDB-41_LmajorFriedlin_Genome.fasta.

3. General Feature Format (GFF) file containing the genome coordinates of all annotated genomic features (*see* **Note 1**), also available at TriTrypDB: http://tritrypdb.org/common/downloads/Release_41/LmajorFriedlin/gff/data/TriTrypDB-41_LmajorFriedlin.gff.

4. Files with whole genome short sequencing reads (100 bases) from a *Leishmania major* isolate. The file we will use here is in a FASTQ format and can be downloaded from the Sequence Read Archive (SRA) of the National Center for Biotechnology Information (NCBI): https://www.ncbi.nlm.nih.gov/sra/?term=SRR6369659 (*see* **Notes 24–28**).

2.3.3 Software (See Note 29)

1. *SRAtoolkit*. Package used to easily download and process reads from the NCBI SRA database.

   Download link: https://www.ncbi.nlm.nih.gov/sra/docs/toolkitsoft/.

   Documentation link: https://www.ncbi.nlm.nih.gov/books/NBK242621/.

2. *FASTQC*. Program used to evaluate the quality of FASTQ reads.

   Download link: https://www.bioinformatics.babraham.ac.uk/projects/download.html#fastqc.

Documentation link: https://www.bioinformatics.babraham.ac.uk/projects/fastqc/.

3. *Trimmomatic*. Program used to evaluate and remove low quality reads and adapter sequences. Download link: http://www.usadellab.org/cms/?page=trimmomatic.
   Documentation link: http://www.usadellab.org/cms/uploads/supplementary/Trimmomatic/TrimmomaticManual_V0.32.pdf.
4. *BWA*. Software used to map reads in a low-divergent genome.
   Download link: https://sourceforge.net/projects/bio-bwa/.
   Documentation link: http://bio-bwa.sourceforge.net/bwa.shtml.
5. *SAMtools*. SAMtools is a group of tools that allow the user to manipulate files in SAM or BAM formats.
   Download link: http://www.htslib.org/download/.
   Documentation link: http://www.htslib.org/doc/samtools.html.
6. *BCFtools*. A set of tools that manipulate Variant Call Format (VCF) files.
   Download link: https://samtools.github.io/bcftools/.
   Documentation link: https://samtools.github.io/bcftools/bcftools.html.
7. *BEDtools*. A group of tools to evaluate and compare genome alignment and annotation features.
   Download link: https://bedtools.readthedocs.io/en/latest/content/installation.html.
   Documentation link: https://bedtools.readthedocs.io/en/latest/content/bedtools-suite.html.
8. *GATK*. A group of tools with a focus on variant discovery and genotyping.
   Download link: https://software.broadinstitute.org/gatk/download/.
   Documentation link: https://software.broadinstitute.org/gatk/documentation/.
9. *R*. R is a free software environment for statistical computing and graphics.
   Download link: https://cran.r-project.org/mirrors.html.
   Documentation link: https://www.r-project.org/.
10. *R library "ggplot"*.
    Documentation link: https://www.rdocumentation.org/packages/ggplot2/versions/3.1.0/topics/ggplot.
11. *Picard Tools*. Command line tools for manipulating high-throughput sequencing data.
    Download link: https://broadinstitute.github.io/picard/.

Documentation link: https://broadinstitute.github.io/picard/command-line-overview.html.

12. *vcflib*. A C++ library for parsing and manipulation VCF files. Download and documentation link: https://github.com/vcflib/vcflib.

3 Methods

3.1 Mapping Replication Initiation by MFA-seq

All steps are done at room temperature, unless stated otherwise. All volumes are for the processing of 1×10^8 cells (*see* **Note 2**). The fixing protocols are different for *T. brucei* procyclic form cells and bloodstream form cells (*see* **Note 1**).

3.1.1 Cell Preparation and Staining with Propidium Iodide—T. brucei Procyclic Cell Forms and L. major/L. mexicana Promastigote Cells

1. From a log-phase culture (1×10^7 cells/ml *T. brucei* procyclic form cells; 5×10^6 cells/ml *L. major* or *L. mexicana* promastigote form cells), collect 1×10^8 cells by centrifuging for 10 min at $1000 \times g$.
2. Wash the pellet in 10 ml of 1× PBS supplemented with 5 mM EDTA (*see* **Note 3**), and centrifuge again for 10 min at $1000 \times g$.
3. Resuspend the cells in 1.2 ml of 1× PBS supplemented with 5 mM EDTA, and add 2.8 ml of ice-cold 100% methanol, in a drop-wise fashion while vortexing gently; the final fixing solution will be of 70% methanol, and the concentration of 2.5×10^7 cells/ml (*see* **Note 4**).
4. Wrap the tube in aluminum foil, and store at 4 °C (from overnight to up to 3 weeks) until the sorting.
5. Centrifuge the cells for 10 min at $1000 \times g$, at 4 °C.
6. Wash the pellet in 1 ml of 1× PBS supplemented with 5 mM EDTA, and centrifuge again for 10 min at $1000 \times g$, at 4 °C.
7. Resuspend the pellet in 4 ml of 1× PBS supplemented with 5 mM EDTA, 10 μg/ml of propidium iodide, and 10 μg/ml of RNase A.
8. Incubate for 45 min at 37 °C, protected from light.
9. Transfer the cells to a 5 ml BD Falcon™ tube through the 35 μm nylon mesh cell strainer cap.
10. Keep the cells on ice and protected from light.

3.1.2 Cell Preparation and Staining with Propidium Iodide—T. brucei Bloodstream Form Cells

1. From a log-phase culture (1×10^6 cells/ml *T. brucei* bloodstream form cells), collect 1×10^8 cells by centrifuging for 10 min at $1000 \times g$.
2. Wash the pellet in 10 ml of 1× PBS supplemented with 5 mM EDTA (*see* **Note 3**), and centrifuge again for 10 min at $1000 \times g$.

3. Resuspend the pellet first in 500 μl of 1× PBS, and then add 9.5 ml of 1% formaldehyde in 1× PBS.
4. Incubate the cells for 10 min at room temperature.
5. Centrifuge the cells for 10 min at 1000 × *g*.
6. Wash the pellet in 10 ml of 1× PBS, and then centrifuge for 10 min at 1000 × *g*.
7. Resuspend the cells in 4 ml of 1× PBS, so to have a final concentration of 2.5×10^7 cells/ml (*see* **Note 4**).
8. Wrap the tube in aluminum foil, and store at 4 °C (from overnight to up to 3 weeks) until the sorting.
9. Centrifuge the cells for 10 min at 1000 × *g*.
10. Resuspend the pellet, first in 1 ml of 0.01% Triton X-100 diluted in 1× PBS, and then add the remaining 9 ml of 0.01% Triton X-100 diluted in 1× PBS; incubate for 30 min at room temperature.
11. Centrifuge the cells for 10 min at 700 × *g* (*see* **Note 5**).
12. Wash the cells in 10 ml of 1× PBS, and then centrifuge for 10 min at 1000 × *g*.
13. Resuspend the pellet first in 4 ml of 1× PBS with 10 μg/ml of propidium iodide, and 100 μg/ml of RNase A.
14. Incubate for 1 h at 37 °C, protected from light.
15. Transfer the cells to the 5 ml BD Falcon™ tube through the 35 μm nylon mesh cell strainer cap.
16. Keep the cells on ice and protected from light.

3.1.3 Cell Sorting into G1, S, and G2/M Phase Subpopulations

1. Immediately before introducing the sample into the sorting machine, gently vortex and refilter the sample through the cell strainer cap.
2. Run the samples through the FACS machine—the settings (*see* **Note 6**) will vary between systems and different FACS facilities will have different protocols of use in place—contact them first before running the experiment. Propidium iodide is excited by the 488 nm or 561 nm lasers and detected by the 695/40 nm or 610/20 nm detectors (respectively).
3. On the FACS machine software, create the following plots: side scatter area (SSC-A) vs forward scatter area (FSC-A), and PE area (PE-A) vs PE width (PE-W).
4. Initially, run ~ 50,000 events to get an idea of the quality of the sample and to set the gates for the sorting. First, the SSC vs FSC scatter plot will inform on the shape of the cells, while the PE-A vs PE-W scatter will allow you to draw a gate to include only singlet events (excluding agglomerates of cells). From this gate, generate a histogram of cell count vs PE-A. This will allow

you to see the "typical" cell cycle profile. On this graph, set the gates to sort cells in G1, S (can be divided into early S and late S populations), and G2/M phase populations.

5. Sort the samples into the different populations (*see* **Note 7**) into collection tubes (*see* **Note 8**) containing 200 μl of lysis buffer; the collection chamber was kept at 4 °C (*see* **Note 9**). If various collection tubes are needed, keep them on ice until the next step.
6. After the sorting, homogenize the sorted cells and lysis solution, and incubate for 2 h at 55 °C (*see* **Note 10**).
7. The lysate can be stored at −20 °C, for later gDNA extraction (*see* **Note 11**), or used straight for gDNA extraction.

3.1.4 gDNA Extraction from the G1, S and G2/M Phase Subpopulations

With the exception of the lysis one, all steps are as described in the instructions of the Qiagen DNeasy Blood and Tissue kit.

1. Thaw frozen lysates at 37 °C and, in the case of multiple sorting sessions, pool per cell cycle stage; take note of the total volume per sample.
2. To each sample, add 100% ethanol, in a volume that corresponds to one-third of the sample's volume, and vortex thoroughly.
3. Transfer 800 μl onto a DNeasy Mini spin column (Qiagen).
4. Centrifuge for 1 min at 6000 × *g* and discard the flow-through.
5. Repeat **steps 3** and **4** until all the lysate has been passed through the column.
6. Wash the column with 500 μl of buffer AW1 (Qiagen).
7. Centrifuge for 1 min at 6000 × *g* and discard the flow-through.
8. Add 500 μl of buffer AW2 (Qiagen) to the column.
9. Centrifuge for 3 min at 20,000 × *g* and discard the flow-through.
10. Transfer the column to a 1.5 ml Eppendorf and add 50 μl of Buffer AE (Qiagen).
11. Centrifuge for 1 min at 6000 × *g*.
12. Store the gDNA at −20 °C, until needed for library prep.

3.1.5 Sequencing Library Preparation

Library preparation and sequencing were performed at facilities such as the Glasgow Polyomics at the University of Glasgow, or Eurofins Genomics (Germany). Seek advice on which kit and sequencing system to use, as these evolve rapidly and more efficient ones might be available at the time of your experiment. In our work we have used the following:

1. DNA libraries were prepared with the Nextera® XT DNA Sample Preparation kit (Illumina) or the TruSeq® DNA Sample Preparation kit (Illumina), according to the manufacturer instructions.
2. The samples were multiplexed and sequenced using either the Illumina MiSeq paired-end 250 bp sequencing system or the Illumina HiSeq paired-end sequencing system, according to the manufacturer instructions.

3.1.6 Marker Frequency Analysis

1. Assess the quality of the sequenced data (.fastq files) using the FastQC software package, a quality control tool. Type "FastQC" on the command line/terminal; if installed, it opens a graphical interface in which the files are uploaded and analyzed. The results are shown in a graph showing quality score versus position in read. Decide on a threshold—in our studies we have used a threshold score of 20.
2. Back in the command line/terminal, use the fastq-mcf tool to simultaneously trim the sequencing reads according to the defined threshold (in this case, 20), and remove the sequences of the adaptors used for the library preparation and sequencing processes.

```
# Type fastq-mcf -h to open the help information on
this tool; it will provide information on the
commands used.
fastq-mcf -h

# -q allows to define the quality threshold; -w
window size for the quality trimming; adapters.fa
refers to the file that has the adapter sequences; -o
output file; only the files for the bloodstream
form early S (BSF_ES_L001_R1.fastq and
BSF_ES_L001_R2.fastq) are shown as an example; there
are two files per sample as the sequencing was
paired-end. This will generate files containing the
trimmed sequences (e.g.
BSF_ES_L001_R1_TRIMMED.fastq).
 fastq-mcf -q 20 -w 5 adapters.fa
$BSF_ES_L001_R1.fastq BSF_ES_L001_R2.fastq -o
BSF_ES_L001_R1_TRIMMED.fastq -o
BSF_ES_L001_R2_TRIMMED.fastq
```

3. Align the trimmed files onto the reference genome using bowtie2 and prepare the output for downstream analysis by using samtools to convert the output to binary format and sort it by coordinate. For convenience, this can be achieved by piping the output of bowtie2 directly to samtools, thus preventing the generation of a large intermediate file.

```
# First need to index the reference genome.
bowtie2-build refgenome.fa indexed_refgenome

# Align the trimmed sequences to the indexed
reference genome. Use the --very-sensitive-local
option - this does not attempt to map 100% of the
read, it will try to map as much of it as it can,
while tolerating the not complete mapping of its
ends; -p leads bowtie2 to run a defined number of
parallel search threads, with each of these running
on a different processor or core - this will depend
on the computer or server/cluster service being used
(in this example is 4); -x will tell bowtie2 where
to find the indexed reference genome; -1 and -2 are
used in the case of paired-end reads, these inform
bowtie2 where to find the forward (-1) and reverse
(-2) reads; bowtie2 will generate the .sam file
containing the actual alignment, as well as a .log
file, which is a report of the alignment, including
statistics and information on the overall alignment
rate. Pipe the output directly to samtools to
convert the output to binary BAM format and sort it.
bowtie2 -p 4 --very-sensitive-local -x
indexed_refgenome -1 BSF_ES_L001_R1_TRIMMED.fastq -2
BSF_ES_L001_R2_TRIMMED.fastq 2> BSF_ES.log |
samtools view -bS - | samtools sort - -o BSF_ES.bam
```

4. Index the BAM file using samtools. The index is required for many downstream analysis steps.

```
# Create an index for each alignment file using
SAMtools index
samtools index input.bam
```

5. Apply custom MFAseq Python script to perform marker frequency analysis. The script used to perform the MFAseq analysis is available at https://github.com/CampbellSam/MFAseq. Python version 2.7 or higher is required to run this script and the pysam package (version 0.8.3 recommended) is also a dependency that must be installed prior to running the analysis. Running the mfaseq.py script on the command line with no input will provide usage instructions that are also available in the script header. Two alignment files are the only required input but the window size and output file can also be specified as input parameters if necessary. This script will produce output in wiggle format (.wig) that can then be viewed as a custom track on EuPathDB using the GenomeBrowser tool or plotted for visualization using ggplot in R or Python. Details to alter the appearance of the EuPathDB track are also included within

the script and will normally be printed as standard out when the output file is generated. The .wig data can also be imported to excel and plotted in Excel or Prism (GraphPad). Bigwig output can be visualized on other genome viewers, such as IGV.

```
# The Python script will calculate a read depth
ratio between the two sets of alignments for a
specified window size along each chromosome and
output these values as a list in .wig format. The
default window size is 2500bp and the ratio is
calculated as first alignment file/second alignment
file.
mfaseq.py --file1 alignmentFile1.srt.bam --file2
alignmentFile2.srt.bam --window [window size in
bases] --wig [output file name - defaults to
standard out]
```

3.2 Localization of DNA Damage by γH2A ChIP-seq

For the ChIP procedure described in Subheadings 3.2.1–3.2.5, all buffers and reagents are supplied in the ChIP-IT Express Enzymatic Kit (Active Motif®), with the exceptions of appropriate serum-free medium, formaldehyde, and an anti-γH2A antibody.

3.2.1 Chromatin Extraction and Enzymatic Shearing

1. Harvest 1 × 10^8 parasites via centrifugation at 1200 × *g* for 10 min, at 4 °C. Remove media from cell pellet.
2. Resuspend parasites in 10 ml Fixation Solution consisting of 10% formaldehyde in appropriate medium (serum-free). Incubate with agitation at room temperature for 5 min (*see* **Note 12**).
3. Add 1 ml of 10× Glycine to halt fixation.
4. Centrifuge at 1200 × *g* for 10 min, at 4 °C, to pellet parasites. Pour off supernatant.
5. Resuspend in 10 ml 1× Glycine and incubate with agitation for 5 min at room temperature. Centrifuge as before to pellet parasites.
6. Resuspend parasites in 10 ml ice-cold 1× PBS and pellet again via centrifugation at 1200 × *g* for 10 min, at 4 °C. Remove all PBS by pouring and pipetting. At this stage the pellet may be stored at −80 °C.
7. Resuspend cells in 1 ml ice-cold Lysis Buffer supplemented with 5 μl protease inhibitor cocktail (PIC) and 5 μl phenylmethylsulfonyl fluoride (PMSF). Pipette and vortex gently to resuspend. Transfer to a 1.5 ml Eppendorf and incubate the on ice for 30 min. During this time prepare the Enzymatic Shearing Cocktail Solution by adding 1 μl of the Enzyme Shearing Cocktail to 99 μl 50% glycerol.

8. Transfer samples in the Lysis Buffer to a Dounce homogenizer and Dounce with ten strokes on ice. Ensure cells have lysed by checking 10 μl in a hemocytometer under a phase contrast microscope. Continue to Dounce until cells have lysed and nuclei are released (*see* **Note 13**).
9. Transfer lysed cells to a 1.5 ml Eppendorf. Centrifuge at 2400 × *g* for 10 min, at 4 °C, to isolate the nuclei. Carefully remove and discard the supernatant.
10. Resuspend the nuclei in 350 μl Digestion Buffer (supplemented with 1.75 μl 100 mM PMSF and 1.75 μl PIC). Incubate at 37 °C for 5 min.
11. Add 17 μl of prepared Enzymatic Shearing Cocktail solution to each sample and incubate at 37 °C for 5 min (*see* **Note 14**).
12. To stop the shearing reaction, add 7 μl ice-cold 0.5 M EDTA. Incubate on ice for 10 min.
13. Centrifuge the sheared chromatin at 18,000 × *g* for 10 min, at 4 °C.
14. Transfer the supernatant, containing sheared chromatin, into 1.5 ml Eppendorf tubes as 50 μl aliquots. Chromatin can be used immediately for downstream steps or stored at −80 °C.

3.2.2 DNA Clean Up, Quantification and Shearing Check

1. If frozen, thaw one 50 μl aliquot on ice. Add 150 μl dH_2O to the sample, then 10 μl 5 M NaCl.
2. Incubate at 65 °C for 4–16 h to reverse the cross-links.
3. Add 1 μl RNase A and incubate at 37 °C for 15 min.
4. Add 10 μl Proteinase K and incubate at 42 °C for 1.5 h.
5. (a) Quantify the sample (*see* **Note 15**). Multiple the resulting concentration by 4.42 to account for dilution of the sample in the above steps and calculate the DNA content of prepared chromatin. Concentrations >15 ng/μl are expected.

   (b) Assess shearing efficiency. Add 4 μl of 6× loading dye to 16 μl of sample and load 5 and 10 μl to wells of a 1% TAE agarose gel. Run at 100 V for 1 h to observe fragment sizes. If optimal, shearing should result in 200–1500 bp bands.

3.2.3 Chromatin-Immunoprecipitation (ChIP)

For immunoprecipitation of γH2A we used 11 μl of antibody (produced in house).

1. If frozen, thaw chromatin on ice. Transfer 10 μl of chromatin to a 1.5 ml Eppendorf and store at −20 °C. This will serve as the Input sample and will be used in downstream steps.

2. Set up ChIP reaction(s) as per the table below (*see* **Note 16**). **It is important to add the antibody last.**

Reagent	Volume
Protein G magnetic beads	25 μl
ChIP buffer 1	20 μl
Sheared chromatin[a]	61–150 μl
Protease inhibitor cocktail	2 μl
dH_2O	Up to final volume 200 μl
Antibody (1–3 μg)	*X* μl
Total volume	*200 μl*

[a]As little as 1 μg of chromatin can be used successfully depending upon the target (*see* **Note 17**)

3. Incubate on an end-to-end rotator at 4 °C overnight.
4. Spin tubes briefly to collect liquid from inside the cap.
5. Place tubes on a magnetic rack and allow beads to gather to the side of the tubes.
6. Carefully remove the supernatant and discard.
7. Remove tubes from the magnetic rack and add 800 μl of ChIP Buffer 1. Fully resuspend the beads by pipetting up and down to wash (*see* **Note 18**).
8. Replace tubes on the magnetic rack. Wash as before with 800 μl ChIP Buffer 2.
9. Perform a second wash with 800 μl ChIP Buffer 2. After this final wash step, remove as much supernatant as possible. Use a 200 μl pipette if necessary.
10. To elute, resuspend the washed beads in 50 μl Elution Buffer AM2.
11. Incubate for 15 min on an end-to-end rotator, at room temperature.
12. Briefly spin tubes to collect liquid from inside the cap.
13. Add 50 μl Reverse Cross-linking Buffer to the beads and mix by pipetting up and down.
14. Place tubes on the magnetic rack and allow the beads to pellet. Transfer the supernatant, which contains the eluted chromatin, into a fresh 1.5 ml Eppendorf. This is the Elute sample.
15. Retrieve the Input sample of chromatin and thaw on ice. Add 88 μl of ChIP Buffer 2 and 2 μl 5 M NaCl to the Input chromatin only.

16. Incubate both the ChIP Elute and Input samples at 65 °C for 2.5 h (*see* **Note 19**). The samples can be stored at −20 °C at this point if necessary.
17. Return the tubes to room temperature and spin briefly to remove any liquid from the cap. Add 1 μl Proteinase K and mix well.
18. Incubate at 37 °C for 1 h. During this step place the Proteinase K Stop Solution at room temperature for at least 30 min.
19. Return the samples to room temperature and add 2 μl Proteinase K Stop Solution. Briefly spin tubes. DNA can now be used immediately for downstream analysis or stored at −20 °C.

3.2.4 ChIP-qPCR

DNA acquired from ChIP reactions can be used in qPCR analysis to compare the presence of a specific DNA sequence in Eluted samples relative to Input, and hence infer if binding of the target (i.e., γH2A) takes place at that sequence. Primer efficiency must be ascertained before use.

1. Dilute Input DNA 1:10 in dH_2O (*see* **Note 20**). qPCR needs to be performed with both Input and Eluted samples for each primer pair.
2. For each reaction combine 1 μl DNA (diluted Input or Elute), 400 nM each primer, 1× SYBR Select Master Mix, and H_2O to a final volume of 20 μl. We recommend performing each reaction in triplicate, as well as performing an H_2O negative control for each primer pair.
3. Perform qPCR with the following conditions: 50 °C for 2 min and 95 °C for 2 min, followed by 40 cycles of 95 °C for 15 s, 59 °C for 15 s, and 72 °C for 1 min. Take fluorescence intensity measurements during the extension step (72 °C for 1 min) of each cycle.
4. Calculate the average C_T for each condition from the three replicate values.
5. Calculate the percentage of Input sequence in the Elute sample using the table below.

	Raw average Input C_T (10%)	**Adjust Input to 100%**	**Raw average Elute C_T**	**Percentage input**
Calculation	Average of three C_T values	Ct input—3.322[a]	Average of three C_T values	$100 \times 2^{(\text{adjusted input} - \text{Elute})}$
Example	28.5	25.178	30.6	2.33%

[a]The number of cycles to subtract is calculated from the dilution factor used (i.e., for a 1:10 dilution, log2 of 10 is 3.322)

3.2.5 ChIP-seq

For library preparation we recommend the TrueSeq ChIP Library Preparation kit from Illumina. The following steps then must be followed for both the Input and Elute sequencing files.

1. Assess read quality using FASTQC. This is done in the same manner as for MFA-seq (*see* Subheading 3.1.6).
2. Trim reads to remove Illumina adaptor sequences and based with quality scores <20.

```
# This can be done using Trim Galore, which will by
default remove Illumina adapter sequences and bases
with a Phred score < 20. Trim_galore also has a
database of adaptors used in commercial library prep
kits and will trim these if they are found. Custom
adaptors can be supplied at the command line.
 # For single-end reads
 trim_galore <file>

 #For paired-end reads
 trim_galore -paired <reads1File> <reads2File>
```

3. Map to the reference genome using Bowtie2 in "very-sensitive" mode and prepare BAM files for downstream analysis. This can be performed in the same manner as for MFA-seq (*see* Subheading 3.1.6) and will first require a reference genome. If single end reads are used, the command can be altered as follows:

```
 bowtie2 -p 4 --very-sensitive-local -x
indexed_refgenome -U <readsFile> 2> BSF_ES.log |
samtools view -bS - | samtools sort - -o
<output.bam>
```

4. In order to avoid mapping artefacts, remove reads with a MapQ value <0 using SAMtools (*see* **Note 21**).

```
 # This is done with the SAMTools view function
 Samtools view -h -q 1 <input.bam> > <output.bam>

 # Create an index for each alignment file using
SAMtools index
 samtools index input.bam
```

5. To obtain the resulting ChIP signal across the genome, the read-depth of Elute samples is calculated relative to the corresponding Input sample. SES normalisation is recommended [24]. This can be done using the bamCompare tool from Deeptools (*see* **Note 22**).

```
 #Use bamCompare to calculate signal enrichment
normalized to Input
bamCompare -b1 <Elute.bam> -b2 <Input.bam> --
scaleFactorsMethod SES -o output.bw
```

6. For further analysis, the resulting normalized signal enrichment file (in bigwig format) can be directly used with Deeptools computeMatrix, plotHeatmap, and plotProfile tools. This can be used to plot ChIP signal across specific regions of interest (e.g., coding regions), which can be supplied as a bed format file of coordinates. Bigwig output can also be visualized on genome viewers, such as IGV.

3.3 Next Generation Sequencing to Examine Genome Variation

3.3.1 Download Data Sets

In the command line (*see* **Note 30**), use wget and fastqdump to download the appropriated data files (*see* **Note 31**):

```
#For the genome reference file:
>wget <link-to-genome-file>
Example command:
>wget
http://tritrypdb.org/common/downloads/release41
/LmajorFriedlin/fasta/data/TriTrypDB-
41_LmajorFriedlin_Genome.fasta.

#For the GFF file:
>wget <link-to-GFF-file>
Example command:
> wget
http://tritrypdb.org/common/downloads/release-
41/LmajorFriedlin/gff/data/TriTrypDB-
41_LmajorFriedlin.gff.

# Download the whole genome sequencing reads:
> fastq-dump.2.8.1 --split-files <Read.file.ID>
Example command:
> fastq-dump.2.8.1 --split-files SRR6369659
```

3.3.2 Run FastQC to Evaluate the Read Library Quality

FastQC evaluates the quality of the read libraries and generate several report files. Among them, the *.html file contains the summary of the results (Fig. 1a, b). It is desirable that the mean read quality is higher than phred 30, meaning one expected error in 1000 bases (*see* **Note 32**).

```
# For the file containing one group of the read pair
> fastqc <read.libray1> <read.libray2>
Example command:
> fastqc SRR6369659_1-paired.fastq
SRR6369659_2-paired.fastq
```

3.3.3 Run Trimmomatic

Trimmomatic will exclude low quality reads, remove positions with low quality at the extremities of the quality reads and adaptors sequences.

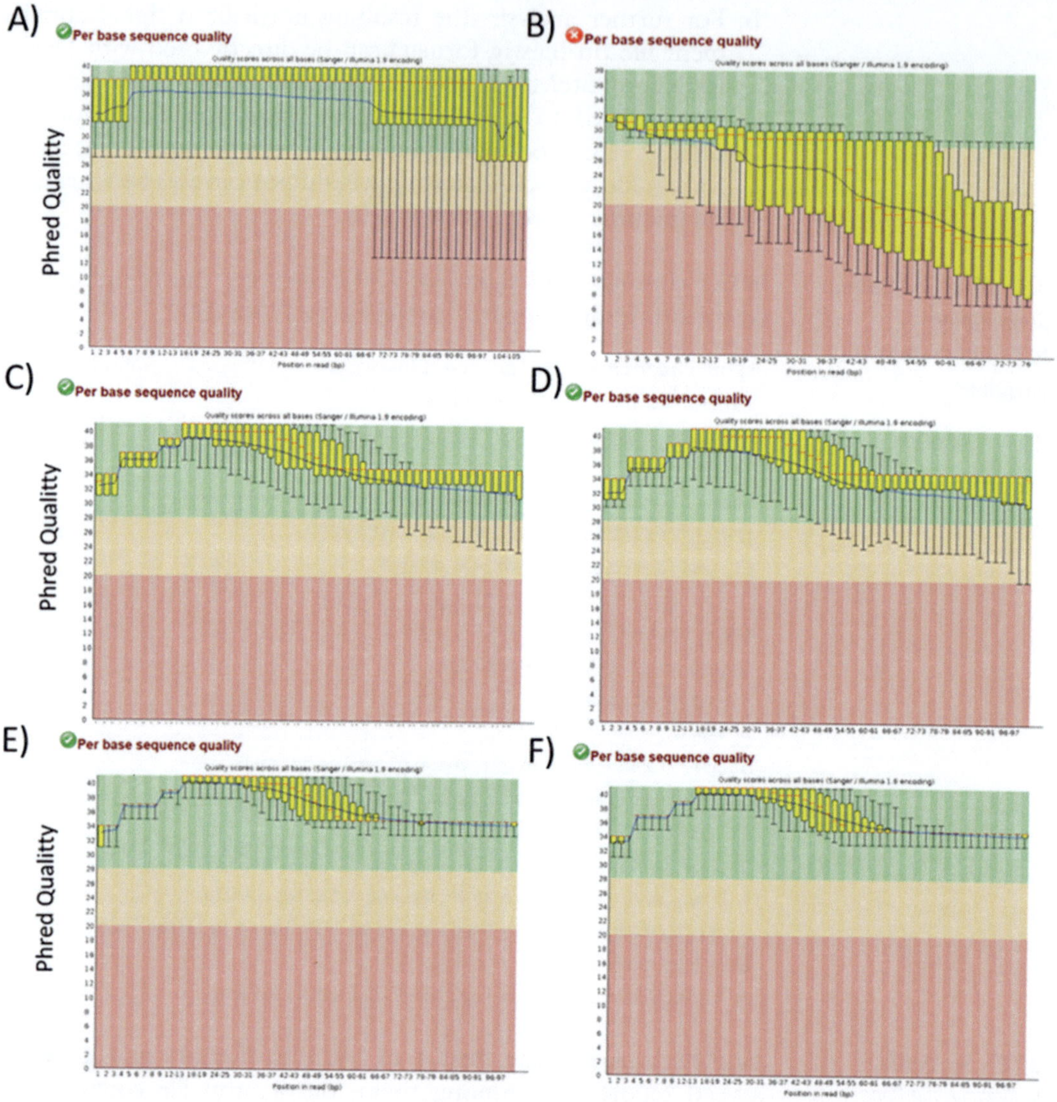

Fig. 1 FastQC read libraries base quality. In this image the *X* axis denotes the phred base quality and the *Y* axis represents the read position. (**a**) Read library with a mean quality higher than 30. (**b**) Read library with a mean quality lower than 30. Read libraries (**c**) SRR6369659_1.fastq and (**d**) SRR6369659_2.fastq before the trimming step. Read libraries (**e**) SRR6369659_1.fastq and (**f**) SRR6369659_2.fastq after the trimming step

```
#Trimmomatic runs as follow:
> java -jar trimmomatic-0.33.jar PE -phred33 <Read-
file-1.fastq> <Read-file-2.fastq>
<Paired_output_1.fastq> <Unpaired_output_1.fastq>
<Paired_output_2.fastq> <Unpaired_output_2.fastq>
ILLUMINACLIP:<Adapters fasta file>:<seed
mismatches>:<palindrome clip threshold>:<simple clip
threshold> LEADING:<quality> TRAILING:<quality>
SLIDINGWINDOW:<window size>:<required quality>
```

```
MINLEN:<size>
Example command:
> java -jar Trimmomatic-0.33/trimmomatic-
0.33.jar PE -phred33 SRR6369659_1.fastq
SRR6369659_2.fastq SRR6369659_1-paired.fastq
SRR6369659_1-UNpaired.fastq SRR6369659_2
-paired.fastq SRR6369659_2-UNpaired.fastq
ILLUMINACLIP:all_adapters:2:30:10 LEADING:25
TRAILING:25 SLIDINGWINDOW:5:30 MINLEN:50
```

Trimmomatic can be run using single-end or paired-end read libraries. The above example represents the command line by using paired-end reads, which requires two input files, `Read-file-1.fastq` and input file 2 is `Read-file-2.fastq`. Trimmomatic will generate four output files. The output files `Paired_output_1.fastq` and `Paired_output_2.fastq` contain the reads that have a corresponding high quality read pair with each other. On the other hand, the output files `Unpaired_output_1.fastq` and `Unpaired_output_2.fastq` contain the reads that did not have a high quality pair with each other.

At the end of the process, Trimmomatic will generate a summary of the process, as in the example below:

```
Input Read Pairs: 21125144 Both Surviving: 15021842
(71.11%) Forward Only Surviving: 1980418 (9.37%)
Reverse Only Surviving: 1406608 (6.66%) Dropped:
2716276 (12.86%)
```

This means that from the `21125144` reads present in the input files, `15021842 (71.11%)` were of high quality in both pair-end read files, `1980418 (9.37%)` were of high quality only in the first read library, `1406608 (6.66%)` were of high quality only in the second read library and `2716276 (12.86%)` presented low quality in both libraries, and were excluded. A comparison of the quality of read libraries before and after the trimming step can be seen in Fig. 1.

3.3.4 Mapping the Reads to the Reference Genome

BWA-MEM maps the filtered reads to the reference genome, generating an alignment file in Sequence Alignment/Map (SAM) format.

```
#Index the Reference genome
> bwa index <Reference-genome.fasta>
Example command:
> bwa index TriTrypDB-
41_LmajorFriedlin_Genome.fasta

#Align reads to the reference genome using BWA-mem:
> bwa mem -M <reference.genome.fasta>
```

```
<Paired_output_1.fastq> <Paired_output_2.fastq> >
Mapped-file.sam
Example command:
> bwa mem -M TriTrypDB-
41_LmajorFriedlin_Genome.fasta SRR6369659_1-
paired.fastq SRR6369659_2-paired.fastq >
SRR6369659-Mapped-file.sam
```

If necessary, the user could use all the "paired" and "unpaired" reads in this mapping analysis to improve the depth of coverage. To that end, it is possible to combine all reads in a single file, with the command:

```
> cat <Paired_output_1.fastq>
<Unpaired_output_1.fastq> <Paired_output_2.fastq>
<Unpaired_output_2.fastq> >
<allreads_file_name.fastq>

> bwa mem -M <reference.genome.fasta>
<allreads_file_name.fastq> > <All-reads-Mapped-
file.sam>
```

The samtools flagstat command generates a report (Mapped-file-info) with information on the number and proportion of mapped reads and number and proportion of properly paired mapped reads.

```
#Check alignment results using SAMtools flagstat:
> samtools flagstat <Mapped-file.sam> > <Mapped-
file-info>
Example command:
> samtools flagstat SRR6369659-Mapped-file.sam
> SRR6369659-Mapped-file-info
```

The flagstat results in the "SRR6369659-Mapped-file-info" can be seen below:

```
30055150 + 0 in total (QC-passed reads + QC-failed
reads)
11466 + 0 secondary
0 + 0 supplementary
0 + 0 duplicates
25150804 + 0 mapped (83.68% : N/A)
30043684 + 0 paired in sequencing
15021842 + 0 read1
15021842 + 0 read2
25081734 + 0 properly paired (83.48%: N/A)
25133580 + 0 with itself and mate mapped
5758 + 0 singletons (0.02%: N/A)
29784 + 0 with mate mapped to a different chr
22208 + 0 with mate mapped to a different chr
(mapQ>=5)
```

In summary, flagstat result showed that from the 30055150 reads in the input files, 25150804(83.68%) mapped in the reference genome TriTrypDB-41_LmajorFriedlin_Genome.fasta, where 25081734(83.48%) of the reads were properly paired (*see* **Note 33**).

3.3.5 Filter Alignment File by Mapping Quality and Convert .sam File to .bam

```
# Use SAMtools to filter the alignment file and
convert to the binary bam file.
> samtools view -bh <Mapped-file.sam> -q <30> -o
<Mapped-file-q30.bam>
Example command:
> samtools view -bh SRR6369659-Mapped-file.sam
-q30 -o SRR6369659-Mapped-file-q30.bam
```

Samtools view flag "-b" converts the SAM to a BAM compact file, while the flag "-q 30" filter the alignment file to only report reads that presented a mapping quality higher than Phred 30. Finally, the flag "-h" generates a header for the BAM file.

3.3.6 Sort .bam File

Samtools sort sorts alignments based on leftmost coordinates. This sorting is required by the majority of the downstream programs that work with alignment files.

```
# Sort the bam alignment file
> samtools sort <Mapped-file-q30.bam> -o <Mapped-
file-q30-sorted.bam>
Example command:
> samtools sort SRR6369659-Mapped-file-q30.bam
-o SRR6369659-Mapped-file-q30-sorted.bam
```

Generate the read depth coverage of each position in each chromosome

```
#Estimate the read depth of coverage in each genomic
position
> bedtools genomecov -ibam <Mapped-file-q30-
sorted.bam> -g <reference.genome.fasta> -d >
<Genome-coverage.bed>
Example command:
> bedtools genomecov -ibam SRR6369659-Mapped-
file-q30-sorted.bam -g TriTrypDB-
41_LmajorFriedlin_Genome.fasta -d > SRR6369659-
coverage.bed
```

The flag "-d" BEDTools will generate a file reporting the depth of coverage in each position of each chromosome. This file can be used to estimate the mean genome coverage as well as the mean coverage for each chromosome.

3.3.7 Estimate the Mean Genome Coverage

```
#Count the number of nucleotides in the reference
genome
> wc -l <Genome-coverage.bed> | awk '{print $1}' >
<Genome-positions>
Example command:
> wc -l SRR6369659-coverage.bed | awk '{print
$1}' > SRR6369659-Genome-positions
```

This command will count and save, in the "`Genome-positions`" file, the number of lines in the file "`Genome-coverage.bed`", which is equivalent to the number of nucleotides in the evaluated genome. In the example, the "`SRR6369659-Genome-positions`" contains the number "`32855095`".

```
#Estimate the sum of the read depth coverage (RDC)
of all genomic positions:
cat <Genome-coverage.bed> | awk '{print totalsize+=
$3}' | tail -n1 > <Genome-RDC>
Example command:
awk '{print totalsize += $3}' SRR6369659-
coverage.bed | tail -n1 > SRR6369659-Genome-RDC
```

This command will sum the RDC of each position in the genome. In the example, the "`SRR6369659-Genome-positions`" contains the number "`2144501882`". This value can vary if different mapper programs or versions are used.

The genome mean RDC can be obtained by dividing "`Genome-RDC`" by the "`Genome-positions`". In the example, by dividing 2144501882 by 32855095, the mean genome coverage of ~ 65×.

3.3.8 Estimate the Chromosomal Somy by RDC

```
#Generate a list with all chromosome names:
> cat <Genome-coverage.bed> | awk '{print $1}' |
sort -u > <Chromosome-IDs>
Example command:
> cat SRR6369659-coverage.bed | awk '{print
$1}' | sort -u > SRR6369659-Chromosome-IDs

# Generate a table containing the normalized
chromosome copy number based on the ratio between
the mean genome RDC and the mean genome RDC.
> for i in $(cat <Chromosome-IDs>); do awk -v i="$i"
'$1 == i {print $0}' <Genome-coverage.bed> | awk -v
i="$i" ' {sum += $3} {NR} END {print
i","(sum/NR)/<genome_RDC>}' >> <CCNV-Table.csv>;
done
Example command:
> for i in $(cat SRR6369659-Chromosome-IDs); do
awk -v i="$i" '$1 == i {print $0}' SRR6369659-
```

```
coverage.bed | awk -v i="$i" ' {sum += $3} {NR}
END {print i","(sum/NR)/65}' >>
SRR6369659_CCNV_Table.csv; done
```

In this command line, the "genome_RDC" corresponds to the mean genome coverage, estimated in the 3.3.6 step, which is "65" in the example command.

The output CCNV-Table.csv file contains two columns separated by a coma (","), where the first column contains the chromosome ID and the second one contains the chromosomal copy number estimation. In this CCNV estimation, values of "0.5," "1," and "2" denotes that the chromosome has, respectively, "0.5", "1," or "2" copies per haploid genome. This means that, if the studied genome is mainly diploid, a value of "1" in this estimation represent two chromosomal copies (one per haploid genome), whereas a value of "1.5" represent three copies and a value of "2" represent four copies. An example of the table generated can be seen in Fig. 2.

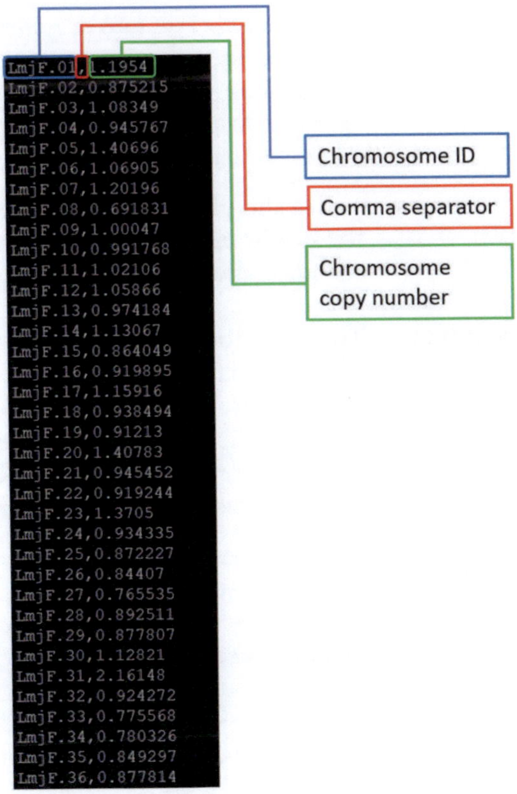

Fig. 2 Chromosome copy number estimation table

3.3.9 Generate a CCNV Plot

The CCNV plot will be generated in "R".

```
#Install R library "ggplot2"
>install.packages("ggplot2")
#Load the R library "ggplot2"
>library(ggplot2)
#Open the file CCNV-Table.csv
>Table <- read.table(file = "<CCNV-Table.csv>", sep
= ",")
#Generate the plot using ggplot
> ggplot(Table, aes(x=V1, y=V2)) + geom_bar(stat =
"identity") + labs(x = "Chromosomes", y = "Copies
per haploid genome") +
theme(axis.text.x=element_text(angle=90)) +
ggsave("<CCNV_plot1.png>", width = 10, height = 7
plot= last_plot(), dpi = 300)
Example command:
>library(ggplot2)
>Table <- read.table(file =
"SRR6369659_CCNV_Table.csv", sep = ",")
>ggplot(Table, aes(x=V1, y=V2)) + geom_bar(stat
= "identity") + labs(x = "Chromosomes", y =
"Copies per haploid genome") +
theme(axis.text.x=element_text(angle=90)) +
ggsave("SRR6369659_CCNV-CCNV_plot1.png", width
= 10, height = 7 plot= last_plot(), dpi = 300)
```

In this plot, each bar corresponds to one chromosome, where the height of the bar corresponds to the number of copies of that chromosome for each haploid genome (Fig. 3).

3.3.10 Restrict the Somy Estimation to Coding Sequences (CDSs) Regions

The chromosomal somy estimation could be restricted to CDSs. This optional step removes the biased impact of non-CDS repetitive regions, as well as the bias from "N" blocks in the reference genome, improving the somy estimation. Hence, this step is highly recommended in repetitive, "N" rich genome drafts. The CCNV estimation using only CDSs-filtered regions can be seen in Fig. 3b.

```
#Filter only the CDS regions from the GFF file and
sort the annotation file
>awk '$3=="CDS"{print $0}' <File.gff> | sort -k1,1 -
k4,4n > <File-CDS.gff>
Example command:
>awk '$3=="CDS"{print $0}' TriTrypDB
-41_LmajorFriedlin.gff | sort -k1,1 -k4,4n >
TriTrypDB-41_LmajorFriedlin-CDS.gff

#Merge redundant CDS regions using bedtools merge
> bedtools merge -i <File-CDS.gff> > <File-CDS-
```

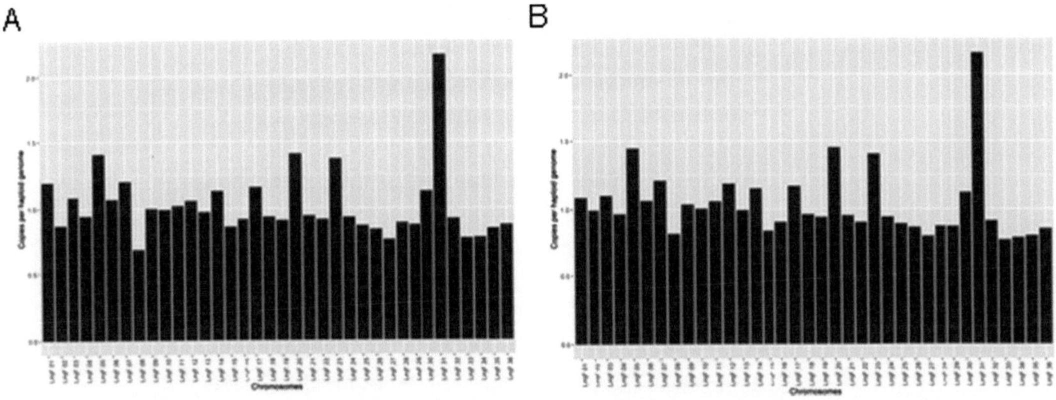

Fig. 3 Chromosome copy number estimation by RDC. In this image, each chromosome is represented by a black bar, where the height of the bar represents the chromosomal copy number per haploid genome. (**a**) Chromosome copy number estimation using the whole chromosomal sequence. (**b**) Chromosome copy number estimation using only coding sequences

```
merged.gff>
Example Command:
>bedtools merge -i TriTrypDB-41_LmajorFriedlin-
CDS.gff > TriTrypDB-41_LmajorFriedlin-CDS-merged.gff

#Generate a Genome-coverage.bed compatible with
bedtools intersect:
> awk '{print $1"\t"$2"\t"$2"\t"$3}' <Genome-
coverage.bed> > <Genome-coverage.bed-form>
Example command:
> awk '{print $1"\t"$2"\t"$2"\t"$3}'
SRR6369659-coverage.bed > SRR6369659-
coverage.bed-form

#Filter the Genome-coverage.bed-form file using the
CDS coordinates with
the program bedtools intersect
> bedtools intersect -a <Genome-coverage.bed-for> -b
<File-CDS-merged.gff> | awk '{print $1"\t"$2"\t"$4}'
> <GFF-filtered-CDS.bed>
Example command:
> bedtools intersect -a SRR6369659-
coverage.bed-form -b TriTrypDB-
41_LmajorFriedlin-CDS-merged.gff | awk '{print
$1"\t"$2"\t"$4}' > SRR6369659-GFF-filtered-
CDS.bed

# Count the number of nucleotides in CDSs in the
filtered reference genome:
> wc -l <GFF-filtered-CDS.bed> | awk '{print $1}' >
```

```
<CDS-Genome-positions>
Example command:
> wc -l SRR6369659-GFF-filtered-CDS.bed | awk
'{print $1}' > SRR6369659-CDS-Genome-positions

#Estimate the sum of the RDC of all CDSs genomic
positions:
cat <GFF-filtered-CDS.bed> | awk '{print totalsize+=
$3}' | tail -n1 > <CDS-Genome-RDC>
Example command:
awk '{print totalsize += $3}' SRR6369659-GFF-
filtered-CDS.bed | tail -n1 > SRR6369659-CDS-
Genome-RDC

#Estimate the genome coverage based on CDS regions:
Divide the value in "CDS-Genome-RDC" for the value
in "SRR6369659-CDS-Genome-positions"
Example command:
Divide the value in SRR6369659-CDS-Genome-RDC
(1131730860) for the value in SRR6369659-CDS-
Genome-positions (16255649), obtaining ~69.62,
which represent the genome coverage based on
CDSs regions

#Generate a list with all chromosome names:
> cat <GFF-filtered-CDS.bed> | awk '{print $1}' |
sort -u > <Chromosome-IDs>
Example command:
> cat SRR6369659-GFF-filtered-CDS.bed | awk
'{print $1}' | sort -u > SRR6369659-GFF-
filtered-Chromosome-IDs

# Generate a table containing the normalized
chromosome copy number based on the ration between
the mean genome RDC and the mean genome RDC.
> for i in $(cat <Chromosome-IDs>); do awk -v i="$i"
'$1 == i {print $0}' <GFF-filtered-CDS.bed> | awk -v
i="$i" ' {sum += $3} {NR} END {print
i","(sum/NR)/<genome_RDC>}' >> <CCNV-Table.csv>;
done
Example command:
> for i in $(cat SRR6369659-GFF-filtered-
Chromosome-IDs); do awk -v i="$i" '$1 == i
{print $0}' SRR6369659-GFF-filtered-CDS.bed |
awk -v i="$i" ' {sum += $3} {NR} END {print
i","(sum/NR)/69}' >> SRR6369659_CCNV_Table-
CDS.csv; done
```

```
#Generate the plot in R using ggplot (Fig. 3b)
> library(ggplot2)
> Table <- read.table(file = "<CCNV-Table-CDS.csv>",
sep = ",")
> ggplot(Table, aes(x=V1, y=V2)) + geom_bar(stat =
"identity") + labs(x = "Chromosomes", y = "Copies
per haploid genome") +
theme(axis.text.x=element_text(angle=90)) +
ggsave("<CCNV_plot-CDS.png>", width = 10, height =
7, plot= last_plot(), dpi = 300)
Example command:
> library(ggplot2)
> Table <- read.table(file =
"SRR6369659_CCNV_Table-CDS.csv", sep = ",")
> ggplot(Table, aes(x=V1, y=V2)) +
geom_bar(stat = "identity") + labs(x =
"Chromosomes", y = "Copies per haploid genome")
+ theme(axis.text.x=element_text(angle=90)) +
ggsave("SRR6369659-CCNV_plot-CDS.png", width =
10, height = 7, plot= last_plot(), dpi = 300)
```

3.3.11 Chromosomal Somy Estimations Based on Allele Frequency Analysis

The chromosomal somy estimations based on allele frequency analysis can be performed using any SNP caller program. In this example we will use GATK. This estimation is based on the proportion of reads that correspond to each allele in heterozygous positions. Initially, generate an index and sequence dictionary required to run GATK and mark PCR duplicated reads.

```
#Format files to run GATK:
Index fasta reference genome with BWA:
>bwa index <reference.genome.fasta>
Index fasta reference using samtools:
Example command:
>bwa index TriTrypDB-
41_LmajorFriedlin_Genome.fasta

>samtools faidx <reference.genome.fasta>
Create a sequence dictionary using Picard
Example command:
>samtools faidx TriTrypDB-
41_LmajorFriedlin_Genome.fasta

>java -jar CreateSequenceDictionary.jar R=
<reference.genome.fasta> O= <reference.genome.dict>
Assigns all the reads in a file to a single new
read-group
>java -jar picard-tools-
1.119/AddOrReplaceReadGroups.jar
```

```
SORT_ORDER=coordinate I=<file.bam> O=$<file-RG.bam>
RGID=<ID> RGSM=<ID> RGPU=unit11 RGLB=Lib1
RGPL=ILLUMINA
Example command:
java -jar picard-tools-
1.119/AddOrReplaceReadGroups.jar
SORT_ORDER=coordinate I=SRR6369659-Mapped-file-
q30-sorted.bam o=SRR6369659-Mapped-file-q30-
sorted-RG.bam RGID=ID RGSM=ID RGPU=unit11
RGLB=Lib1 RGPL=ILLUMINA

Mark duplicated reads originated by PCR:
>java -jar picard-tools-1.119/MarkDuplicates.jar
I=<file-RG.bam> O=<file-RG.DD.bam> M=<file-
MarkDuplicates.metrics.tmp.txt>
Example command:
java -jar picard-tools-1.119/MarkDuplicates.jar
I=SRR6369659-Mapped-file-q30-sorted-RG.bam
O=SRR6369659-Mapped-file-q30-sorted-RG-DD.bam
M=MarkDuplicates.metrics.tmp.txt
```

Next, generate the SNP call file in VCF format using GATK.

```
#Index the bam file with the de-duplicated reads:
>samtools index <file-RG.DD.bam>
Example command:
samtools index SRR6369659-Mapped-file-q30-
sorted-RG-DD.bam

#Re-align reads
>java -jar GenomeAnalysisTK.jar -T
RealignerTargetCreator -R <reference.genome.fasta> -
I <file-RG.DD.bam> -o <file-intervals.tmp.list>
Example command:
java -jar GenomeAnalysisTK.jar -T
RealignerTargetCreator -R TriTrypDB-
41_LmajorFriedlin_Genome.fasta -I SRR6369659-
Mapped-file-q30-sorted-RG-DD.bam -o SRR6369659-
intervals.tmp.list

>java -jar GenomeAnalysisTK.jar -T IndelRealigner -R
<reference.genome.fasta> -I <file-RG.DD.bam> -
targetIntervals <file-intervals.tmp.list> -o <file-
realign.tmp.bam>
Example command:
java -jar GenomeAnalysisTK.jar -T
IndelRealigner -R TriTrypDB-
41_LmajorFriedlin_Genome.fasta -I SRR6369659-
```

```
Mapped-file-q30-sorted-RG-DD.bam -
targetIntervals SRR6369659-intervals.tmp.list -
o SRR6369659-Mapped-file-q30-sorted-RG-DD-
SNPs.bam

#Call SNPS:
java -jar GenomeAnalysisTK.jar -T HaplotypeCaller -R
<reference.genome.fasta> -I <file-realign.tmp.bam> -
ploidy 2 -stand_call_conf 30 -stand_emit_conf 10 -o
<file-SNPs-indels.vcf>
Example command:
java -jar GenomeAnalysisTK.jar -T
HaplotypeCaller -R TriTrypDB-
41_LmajorFriedlin_Genome.fasta -I SRR6369659-
Mapped-file-q30-sorted-RG-DD-SNPs.bam -ploidy 2
-stand_call_conf 30 -stand_emit_conf 10 -o
SRR6369659-SNPs-Indels.vcf

#Filter vcf file (optional):
>vcflib/bin/vcffilter -f "DP > 9" -f "QUAL >10"
<file-SNPs-indels.vcf> > <file-SNPs-filter.tmp.vcf>
Example command:
/media/data/joao/VCFlib.dir/vcflib/bin/vcffilte
r -f "DP > 9" -f "QUAL >10" SRR6369659-SNPs-
Indels.vcf > SRR6369659-SNPs-Indels-filt.vcf

#Recover only SNP calls
>java -jar GenomeAnalysisTK.jar -T SelectVariants -R
<reference.genome.fasta> -V <file-SNPs-
filter.tmp.vcf> -selectType SNP -o <file-only-
SNPs.vcf>
Example command:
java -jar
/home/bioinfo/bin/GenomeAnalysisTK.jar -T
SelectVariants -R ../../TriTrypDB-
41_LmajorFriedlin_Genome.fasta -V SRR6369659-
SNPs-Indels-filt.vcf -selectType SNP -o
SRR6369659-SNPs-filt.vcf
```

After obtaining the VCF file containing all the SNP positions, filter only the heterozygous positions and generate the allele frequency ratio for the whole genome as well as for each chromosome (Figs. 4 and 5):

```
#Convert the VCF output to a table
>java -jar GenomeAnalysisTK.jar -R
<reference.genome.fasta> -T VariantsToTable -V
<file-only-SNPs.vcf> -F CHROM -F POS -F REF -F ALT -
```

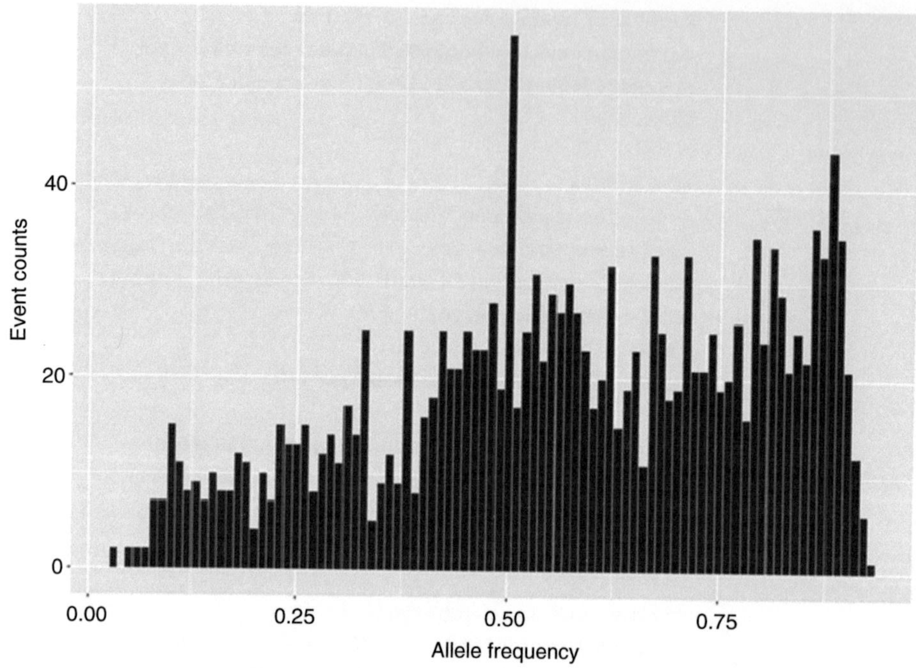

Fig. 4 Genome ploidy estimation based on allele frequency ratios. In this image, the *X* axis denotes the allele frequency ratio of heterozygous positions, while the *Y* axis represents the number of heterozygous positions that present a given allele frequency ratio. The higher peak in 0.5 shows that the majority of the heterozygous positions present a similar RDC in both allele variants, supporting an overall diploid genome

```
GF GT -GF AD -o <file-only-SNPs.table>
Example command:
java -jar GenomeAnalysisTK.jar -R TriTrypDB-
41_LmajorFriedlin_Genome.fasta -T
VariantsToTable -V SRR6369659-SNPs-filt.vcf -F
CHROM -F POS -F REF -F ALT -GF GT -GF AD -o
SRR6369659-SNPs-filt.table

#Remove the header from the table file:
>tail -n +2 <file-only-SNPs.table> > <file-only-
SNPs.NH.table>
Example command:
tail -n +2 SRR6369659-SNPs-filt.table >
SRR6369659-SNPs-filt-NH.table

#Generate the overall genome ploidy based on allele
frequency ratio across the genome with two decimal
values. Obs: The number of decimal values can be
changed to 1 or 3 by respectively replacing the
"%0.2f\n" for "%0.1f\n" or "%0.3f\n",
>awk '{print $6}' <file-only-SNPs.NH.table> | sed
s'/,/\t/' | awk '{if ($1>=5 && $2>=5) print $0}' |
```

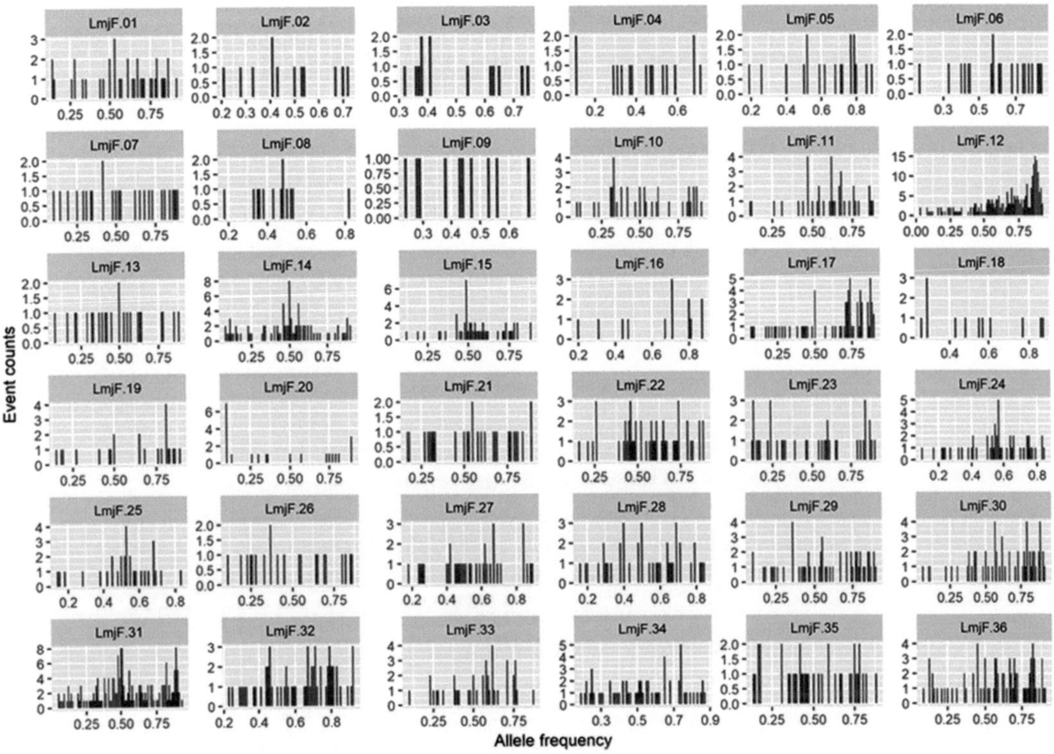

Fig. 5 Chromosomal somy estimation based on allele frequency ratios. In this image, each box corresponds to a chromosome. In each box, the *X* axis denotes the allele frequency ratio of heterozygous positions, while the *Y* axis represents the number of heterozygous positions that present a given allele frequency ratio. As the number of heterozygous SNPs in *Leishmania* is low, the chromosome somy estimation based on allele frequency is compromised

```
awk '$3 = $1+$2{printf "%0.2f\n",$1/$3}' | sort |
uniq -c | awk '{print $2"\t"$1}' > <whole-genome-
allele-frequency>
Example command:
awk '{print $6}' SRR6369659-SNPs-filt-NH.table
| sed s'/,/\t/' | awk '{if ($1>=5 && $2>=5)
print $0}' | awk '$3 = $1+$2{printf
"%0.2f\n",$1/$3}' | sort | uniq -c | awk
'{print $2"\t"$1}' > SRR6369659-whole-genome-
allele-frequency

#Plot the whole genome allele frequency using "R"
(Fig. 4).
library(ggplot2)
Table <- read.table(file = "whole-genome-allele-
frequency", sep = "\t")
ggplot(Table, aes(x=V1, y=V2)) + geom_bar(stat =
"identity") + labs(x = "Allele frequency", y =
```

```
"Event counts") + ggsave("Genome-Allele-
frequency.png", width = 10, height = 7,
plot= last_plot(), dpi = 300)
Example command:
library(ggplot2)
Table <- read.table(file = "SRR6369659-whole-
genome-allele-frequency", sep = "\t")
ggplot(Table, aes(x=V1, y=V2)) + geom_bar(stat
= "identity") + labs(x = "Allele frequency", y
= "Event counts") + ggsave("SRR6369659-whole-
genome-allele-frequency.png", width = 10,
height = 7, plot= last_plot(), dpi = 300)

#Generate a chromosomal somy estimation based on the
allele frequency of each chromosome (Fig. 5).
cat <file-only-SNPs.NH.table> | sed s'/,/\t/' | awk
'$8=$6+$7{if ($6>=5 && $7>=5) printf
$1","" %0.2f\n",$6/$8}' | sort | uniq -c | sed
s'/,/\t/' | awk '{print $1"\t"$3"\t"$2}' > <Alelle-
Frequency-chromosomes>
Example command:
cat SRR6369659-SNPs-filt-NH.table | sed
s'/,/\t/' | awk '$8=$6+$7{if ($6>=5 && $7>=5)
printf $1","" %0.2f\n",$6/$8}' | sort | uniq -c
| sed s'/,/\t/' | awk '{print $1"\t"$3"\t"$2}'
> Alelle-Frequency-chromosomes

#Plot the chromosomal somy estimation based on the
allele frequency of each chromosome using "R"
library(ggplot2)
Table <- read.table(file = "<Alelle-Frequency-
chromosomes>", sep = "\t")
ggplot(Table, aes(x=V2, y=V1)) + facet_wrap(.~V3,
scales = "free") + geom_bar(stat = "identity") +
labs(x = "Allele frequency", y = "Event counts") +
ggsave("chromosome-allele-frequency.png", width =
10, height = 7, plot= last_plot(), dpi = 300)

Example command:
library(ggplot2)
Table <- read.table(file = "Alelle-Frequency-
chromosomes", sep = "\t")
ggplot(Table, aes(x=V2, y=V1)) +
facet_wrap(.~V3, scales = "free") +
geom_bar(stat = "identity") + labs(x = "Allele
frequency", y = "Event counts") +
ggsave("SRR6369659-chromosome-allele-
frequency.png", width = 10, height = 7, plot=
last_plot(), dpi = 300)
```

As the low number of heterozygous SNPs compromises the chromosomal somy estimation by allele frequency in *Leishmania*, we have also performed this analysis in a highly heterozygous *T. cruzi* clone, obtained from the Y strain (Fig. 6). *T. cruzi* Y clone 2 genomic read library can be obtained from NCBI SRA (ID: SRX3453758), while the *T. cruzi* CL Brener Esmeraldo-like haplotype reference genome can be obtained from TriTypDB (https://tritrypdb.org/common/downloads/release-42/TcruziCLBrenerEsmeraldo-like/fasta/data/TriTrypDB-42_TcruziCLBrenerEsmeraldo-like_Genome.fasta). The commands used to generate the following plot are the same as the one used to generate the *Leishmania* estimations.

4 Notes

MFA-seq Analysis of Replication Dynamics

1. As a fixing agent, methanol is used for *T. brucei* procyclic cells and *Leishmania* promastigote cells. Insufficient *T. brucei* bloodstream form cells could be retrieved after fixing with methanol; instead, fixation with 1% formaldehyde (methanol-free) allows the retrieval of a sufficient number of cells.
2. The number of cells needed is variable depending upon how many cells are needed for downstream applications; for this protocol we recommend preparing 3×10^8 cells for each sorting session. If other numbers of cells are to be used, adjust the volumes used in the protocol accordingly.
3. Washing in 1× PBS in the presence of EDTA prevents cell aggregation.
4. A final concentration of 2.5×10^7 cells/ml is ideal for the following steps in the protocol; if denser, the cells start to form aggregates.
5. After formaldehyde fixation the cells seem to become more fragile, so the speed used in the centrifugation was reduced from $1000 \times g$ to $700 \times g$.
6. Settings such as flow and event threshold rates will vary depending on the machine; this will impact the hours that will be needed to obtain the desirable number of cells (e.g., a machine that sorts a max. of 3000 events per second vs one that does it at 10,000 events per second).
7. The number of cells needed depends on the application. The minimum number of cells we have used is 1×10^6 cells in each of the S phase subpopulations (early and late).
8. The type of tubes will depend on the machine used.

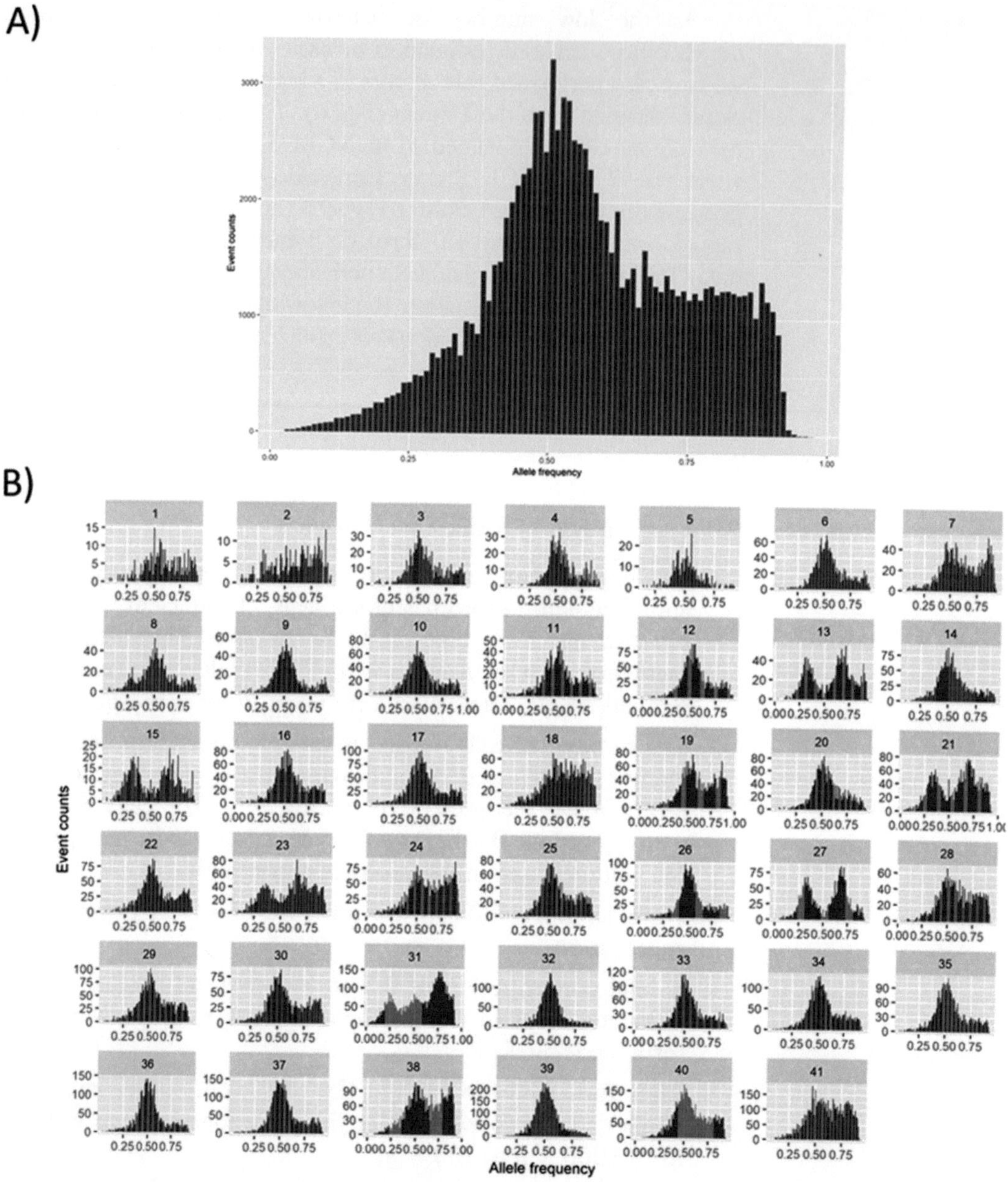

Fig. 6 *T. cruzi* Y clone 2 ploidy and somy estimation based on allele frequency ratios. In this image, the *X* axis denotes the allele frequency ratio of heterozygous positions, while the *Y* axis represents the number of heterozygous positions that present a given allele frequency ratio. (**a**) Whole-genome ploidy. The peak in 0.5 shows that the majority of the heterozygous positions present a similar RDC in both allele variants, supporting an overall diploid genome. (**b**) Chromosomal somy estimation, where each box corresponds to a chromosome. The majority of the chromosomes present a peak in 0.50, suggesting disomy. However, chromosomes 13, 15, 21, 23, and 27 presented peaks in ~0.33 and ~0.66 suggesting trisomy, while the chromosome 31 presented peaks in 0.25, 0.50, and 0.75 suggesting tetrasomy

9. The SDS in the lysis buffer will precipitate at 4 °C, giving it a 'blurry' look; this is ok during collection and remember to mix it thoroughly after sorting and before lysis.
10. The temperature and incubation period allow for the reversal of the formaldehyde crosslinking.
11. If several sorting sessions are needed to obtain the desired number of cells, store the lysate at −20 °C and extract gDNA from the samples of the different sorting sessions at the same time (e.g., if three sessions were run to obtain enough cells in S phase, pool the extracts from the three sessions and extract the gDNA using a single column).

Localization of DNA Damage by γH2A ChIP-seq

12. Do not exceed fixation time as cells will be difficult to lyse.
13. It may be helpful to observe cells before lysis for comparison. If cells are successfully lysed numerous nuclei should appear as black dots and cell bodies will appear "ghostly". It is important that the Dounce homogenizer is tight fitting for optimal lysis.
14. Shearing has been optimized for *T. brucei* chromatin. Incubation for 5 min results in fragments between 200 and 1500 bp in length. Shearing time may require optimization for other genomes.
15. Quantification has been carried out using a Qubit. If using a spectrometer for quantification, the DNA must be cleaned up by phenol–chloroform prior to quantification. Column purification is not recommended as protein may clog the column.
16. When performing multiple samples to compare, that is, treatment vs control, use the same quantity of chromatin (ng) per IP reaction.
17. Depending on the target, more chromatin may need to be added to the ChIP reaction in order to achieve a high enough concentration of DNA in the eluted sample for downstream analysis. If vastly more chromatin is required, the number of cells used for chromatin extraction can be increased. However, the volumes of Fixation Solution, Glycine, 1× PBS, Lysis Buffer (as well as the supplements PIC and PMSF), Digestion Buffer (plus PIC and PMSF), Enzymatic Shearing Cocktail and 0.5 M EDTA must all be scaled accordingly. For example, double all reagents when the protocol is started with 2×10^8 parasites.
18. When washing the samples, it is important to prevent the beads from drying; therefore, perform wash steps one tube at a time.
19. When large amounts of chromatin have been used, and so the samples contain higher concentrations of proteins, this step can be extended.

20. If little DNA is available for analysis, input DNA can be diluted further and eluted DNA can also be diluted. However, these must be corrected for accurately when calculating Input percentage.
21. This is especially important when analyzing regions of highly similar sequences such as *T. brucei* VSG genes.
22. When targeting γH2A, it is likely that some nonspecific binding to the unphosphorylated H2A histone occurs. Therefore, it may be useful to compare ChIP signal enrichment between control and treatment samples (e.g., wild-type and mutant). This can also be done via Deeptools using the bigwigCompare tool.

Next Generation Sequencing to Examine Genome Variation

23. The examples shown here were executed on an Ubuntu 10.10 server with a 2.8-GHz CPU. For 32 million reads, at least 4 GB of RAM is required. More RAM may need to if more deeply sequenced samples are used.
24. Although not required for all ploidy estimation methodologies, the use of a GFF file can increase accuracy when performing CCNV analysis in complex genomes. This optional step removes the biased impact of non-CDS repetitive regions, as well as the bias from "N" blocks in the reference genome, improving the somy estimation.
25. The Illumina platform usually yields reads with the deepest and highest base quality. However, reads from other platforms, such as 454 and Ion torrent, can also be used.
26. Long-reads, such as generated by the PacBio Sequel/RSII and Oxford Nanopore platforms, are also suitable for ploidy estimations. The .bam file can be generated using BlasR (https://github.com/PacificBiosciences/blasr), and the following steps described in this chapter can be used.
27. It is preferable to use FASTQ format, rather than fasta format, because it encodes not only the sequence information itself, but also the base quality information. This is essential for accurate detection of SNPs and other types of structural alterations.
28. Coverage of at least 20× is desirable. Using lower genome coverages can compromise sensitivity and accuracy of any structural variation analysis.
29. All software used here are compatible with the Linux operational systems, such as Fedora and Ubuntu. Some of them are also compatible with macOS; however, all of the examples were performed on Linux.

30. A guide on how to work with bash in command line can be seen in: https://www.cs.wcupa.edu/rkline/linux/bash-basics.html. A beginner guide can be seen here: https://www.lifewire.com/guide-to-bash-part-1-hello-world-2202041 and here https://www.bash.academy/.
31. In our example, we are using a paired-end read library from the *L. major* genome. Thus, when downloading it using fastq-dump, the use of "--split-files" flag is mandatory. By doing so, reads from each pair will be split into two different files. When using single-end read libraries, the aforementioned flag is not needed.
32. It is not advisable to use read libraries with a mean read quality lower than 20. Such libraries will reduce the SNP call precision and compromise the accuracy of downstream analysis.
33. We suggest that read libraries in which more than 50% of the read were dropped should not be used in CCNV analysis. As the proportion of excluded reads is not necessarily similar to all chromosomes, this could lead to detection of false variation in chromosome copy number.

Acknowledgement

This work was supported by the BBSRC [BB/K006495/1, BB/M028909/1, BB/N016165/1], the European Commission [RECREPEMLE], and the Wellcome Trust [206815, 083485, 089172]. The Wellcome Centre for Integrative Parasitology is supported by core funding from the Wellcome Trust [104111].

References

1. Roth DB (2014) V(D)J recombination: mechanism, errors, and fidelity. Microbiol Spectr 2. https://doi.org/10.1128/microbiolspec.MDNA3-0041-2014
2. Hwang JK, Alt FW, Yeap LS (2015) Related mechanisms of antibody somatic hypermutation and class switch recombination. Microbiol Spectr 3:MDNA3-0037-2014
3. Lee CS, Haber JE (2015) Mating-type gene switching in Saccharomyces cerevisiae. Microbiol Spectr 3:MDNA3-0013-2014
4. Yao MC, Chao JL, Cheng CY (2014) Programmed genome rearrangements in tetrahymena. Microbiol Spectr 2. https://doi.org/10.1128/microbiolspec.MDNA3-0012-2014
5. Yerlici VT, Landweber LF (2014) Programmed genome rearrangements in the ciliate oxytricha. Microbiol Spectr 2. https://doi.org/10.1128/microbiolspec.MDNA3-0025-2014
6. Betermier M, Duharcourt S (2014) Programmed rearrangement in ciliates: paramecium. Microbiol Spectr 2. https://doi.org/10.1128/microbiolspec.MDNA3-0035-2014
7. McCulloch R, Morrison LJ, Hall JP (2015) DNA recombination strategies during antigenic variation in the African trypanosome. Microbiol Spectr 3:MDNA3-0016-2014
8. Dumetz F, Imamura H, Sanders M, Seblova V, Myskova J, Pescher P, Vanaerschot M, Meehan CJ, Cuypers B, De Muylder G et al (2017) Modulation of aneuploidy in Leishmania donovani during adaptation to different in vitro and in vivo environments and its impact on gene expression. MBio 8:e00599-17
9. Lachaud L, Bourgeois N, Kuk N, Morelle C, Crobu L, Merlin G, Bastien P, Pages M, Sterkers Y (2014) Constitutive mosaic aneuploidy

is a unique genetic feature widespread in the Leishmania genus. Microbes Infect 16:61–66

10. Tiengwe C, Marcello L, Farr H, Dickens N, Kelly S, Swiderski M, Vaughan D, Gull K, Barry JD, Bell SD et al (2012) Genome-wide analysis reveals extensive functional interaction between DNA replication initiation and transcription in the genome of *Trypanosoma brucei*. Cell Rep 2:185–197
11. Marques CA, Dickens NJ, Paape D, Campbell SJ, McCulloch R (2015) Genome-wide mapping reveals single-origin chromosome replication in Leishmania, a eukaryotic microbe. Genome Biol 16:230
12. Marques CA, McCulloch R (2018) Conservation and variation in strategies for DNA replication of kinetoplastid nuclear genomes. Curr Genomics 19:98–109
13. Briggs E, Crouch K, Lemgruber L, Lapsley C, McCulloch R (2018) Ribonuclease H1-targeted R-loops in surface antigen gene expression sites can direct trypanosome immune evasion. PLoS Genet 14:e1007729
14. Glover L, Horn D (2012) Trypanosomal histone gammaH2A and the DNA damage response. Mol Biochem Parasitol 183:78–83
15. Stortz JA, Serafim TD, Alsford S, Wilkes J, Fernandez-Cortes F, Hamilton G, Briggs E, Lemgruber L, Horn D, Mottram JC et al (2017) Genome-wide and protein kinase-focused RNAi screens reveal conserved and novel damage response pathways in Trypanosoma brucei. PLoS Pathog 13:e1006477
16. Damasceno JD, Obonaga R, Silva GLA, Reis-Cunha JL, Duncan SM, Bartholomeu DC, Mottram JC, McCulloch R, Tosi LRO (2018) Conditional genome engineering reveals canonical and divergent roles for the Hus1 component of the 9-1-1 complex in the maintenance of the plastic genome of Leishmania. Nucleic Acids Res 46:11835–11846
17. Reis-Cunha JL, Rodrigues-Luiz GF, Valdivia HO, Baptista RP, Mendes TAO, de Morais GL, Guedes R, Macedo AM, Bern C, Gilman RH et al (2015) Chromosomal copy number variation reveals differential levels of genomic plasticity in distinct Trypanosoma cruzi strains. BMC Genomics 16:499
18. Almeida LV, Coqueiro-Dos-Santos A, Rodriguez-Luiz GF, McCulloch R, Bartholomeu DC, Reis-Cunha JL (2018) Chromosomal copy number variation analysis by next generation sequencing confirms ploidy stability in Trypanosoma brucei subspecies. Microb Genom 4. https://doi.org/10.1099/mgen.0.000223
19. Rogers MB, Hilley JD, Dickens NJ, Wilkes J, Bates PA, Depledge DP, Harris D, Her Y, Herzyk P, Imamura H et al (2011) Chromosome and gene copy number variation allow major structural change between species and strains of Leishmania. Genome Res 21:2129–2142
20. Laffitte MC, Leprohon P, Hainse M, Legare D, Masson JY, Ouellette M (2016) Chromosomal translocations in the parasite Leishmania by a MRE11/RAD50-independent microhomology-mediated end joining mechanism. PLoS Genet 12:e1006117
21. Azuara V (2006) Profiling of DNA replication timing in unsynchronized cell populations. Nat Protoc 1:2171–2177
22. Margulies M, Egholm M, Altman WE, Attiya S, Bader JS, Bemben LA, Berka J, Braverman MS, Chen YJ, Chen Z et al (2005) Genome sequencing in microfabricated high-density picolitre reactors. Nature 437:376–380
23. Quail MA, Smith M, Coupland P, Otto TD, Harris SR, Connor TR, Bertoni A, Swerdlow HP, Gu Y (2012) A tale of three next generation sequencing platforms: comparison of Ion Torrent, Pacific Biosciences and Illumina MiSeq sequencers. BMC Genomics 13:341
24. Diaz A, Park K, Lim DA, Song JS (2012) Normalization, bias correction, and peak calling for ChIP-seq. Stat Appl Genet Mol Biol 11:9

Part III

Molecular Biology and Genetics

Chapter 16

Transcription Factor Analysis in Trypanosomatids

Arthur Günzl, Ankita Srivastava, and Ujwala Gosavi

Abstract

Known transcription factors of trypanosomatid organisms are extremely divergent in amino acid sequence to their counterparts in other eukaryotes. Sequence similarity is so limited that factors have been primarily identified by functional and structural studies. In addition, trypanosomatids may have evolved factors that are specific to this group of organisms. Under these circumstances, an in vitro transcription system is invaluable as it allows for unambiguous determination of a factor's transcriptional role. Here we describe procedures for the preparation of transcriptionally active extracts, detail in vitro transcription reactions, and specify the particular strategy necessary to detect template-derived RNA in this system. As examples of how to use this system, we describe factor depletion from extract and antibody-mediated interference with a factor's transcriptional function. Furthermore, we detail a promoter pull-down assay that makes use of the extracts and facilitates analysis of a factor's interaction with promoter DNA.

Key words In vitro transcription, Extract preparation, Primer extension, Radiolabeling of DNA, Promoter pull-down assay

1 Introduction

Annotation of the completed TriTryp genomes revealed only few transcription factors such as the TATA box binding protein TBP (originally named TRF4), the helicase subunits of transcription factor (TF)IIH, and the TFIIB-related factor 1 [1, 2]. This scarcity of factors correlated with unusual modes of transcription. In trypanosomatids, unrelated protein coding genes are organized in directional gene arrays that are transcribed polycistronically, tRNA genes are associated with small RNA genes driving their expression, and spliced leader (SL) RNA genes are the only noncoding RNA genes transcribed by RNA polymerase (pol) II in monocistronic fashion [3, 4]. However, trypanosomatids have many more transcription factors as originally believed. For example, it now appears that trypanosomatids possess orthologs of each and every general transcription factor that assemble a transcription preinitiation complex at and recruit RNA pol II to the SL RNA gene promoter, comprising the factors SNAPc, TFIIA, TFIIB, TFIIH/E, a TFIIF-

Paul A. M. Michels et al. (eds.), *Trypanosomatids: Methods and Protocols*, Methods in Molecular Biology, vol. 2116,
https://doi.org/10.1007/978-1-0716-0294-2_16,

like factor, and a mediator complex [5–14]. The amino acid sequences of these factors are extremely divergent from their counterparts in other eukaryotes. This is best illustrated by the trypanosome mediator complex MED-T of which nine subunits were identified [13]. While the factor structurally resembled the head domain of yeast mediator and had the functional properties of a mediator complex, none of the trypanosome subunits exhibited recognizable sequence homology to any of the known mediator subunits of other organisms. Similarly, the class I transcription factor A or CITFA, an initiation factor for RNA pol I-mediated transcription, consists of the dynein light chain LC8 and seven proteins that are conserved only among trypanosomatids [15, 16].

Trypanosomatids likely harbor additional transcription factors which are either too divergent to be identified bioinformatically or are specific to these evolutionary early-branched organisms. For example, the structures of trypanosomatid tRNA and 5S rRNA genes are similar to their counterparts in other eukaryotes, yet TFIIIA and the multisubunit TFIIIC, which are important factors for RNA pol III-mediated transcription of these genes, have not been identified in trypanosomatids so far. Furthermore, the recent identification of promoter elements for the transcription of protein coding gene arrays in *Trypanosoma brucei* [17] and cell cycle-regulated, gene-specific promoters in *Leishmania donovani* [18] suggest the presence of yet to be identified DNA-binding proteins that facilitate transcription from these promoters. Finally, *T. brucei* harbors a multifunctional RNA pol I that transcribes the large rRNA gene unit (*RRNA*) as in other organisms as well as the genes of its major cell surface proteins VSG and procyclin [19]. The *RRNA,* VSG, and procylin gene promoters differ structurally, and the latter two are developmentally regulated, indicating that additional factors to CITFA are required to productively initiate transcription from these promoters [20].

There are several approaches to analyze a putative transcription factor in vivo. Chromatin immunoprecipitation (ChIP) assays can reveal whether a protein occupies promoters, and gene silencing or conditional gene knockout experiments combined with RNA analysis may uncover effects of factor depletion on RNA abundances. For transcription factor analysis, it is most telling when nascent or newly synthesized RNA is investigated. In this respect, it should be noted that metabolic labeling of RNA with 4-thiouridine has been successfully applied in *T. brucei* [21]. In addition, a permeabilized cell system has been established in *T. brucei* in which radiolabeled ribonucleotides or bromo-UTP are efficiently incorporated into newly synthesized RNA [22, 23]. However, caveats of these methods are that they either do not provide functional transcription data (ChIP) or cannot rule out that observed effects on RNA abundance are secondary in nature. This is particularly problematic when the factor under investigation does not exhibit any sequence similarity to known factors from model organisms and does not harbor a recognizable DNA-binding domain. An in vitro transcription system, however, provides the means to explicitly determine the transcriptional function of a factor. The key step in establishing such a system is the generation of transcriptionally active, cell-free extracts. This has been pioneered in *T. brucei* with a nuclear extract that supported accurately initiated transcription by RNA pol III [24] and of SL RNA genes by RNA pol II [25]. A slightly modified extract established a comparable system in another trypanosomatid, *Leptomonas seymouri* [26]. Furthermore, a *T. brucei* "whole-cell extract" (WCE), in which nuclear proteins were extracted into the soluble cytoplasmic fraction, proved to be active in SL RNA gene and RNA pol I-mediated transcription [27, 28]. While these extracts were established on a large scale in procyclic trypanosomes, the WCE could also be achieved on a small scale and was successfully applied to bloodstream form trypanosomes [29] and therefore may be the method of choice for trypanosomatid species that cannot be easily grown to large numbers. A transcription system for protein coding gene arrays, however, has not been established yet.

A key problem in preparing trypanosome extracts is that the cells are difficult to break due to their robust microtubule-based cytoskeleton and their spindle-like cell shape. The harsh treatments necessary to achieve quantitative cell breakage lead to genomic DNA contamination of extracts that is difficult to eliminate. While the use of a labeled ribonucleotide and a specific DNA template generates a detectable RNA of defined size in cell-free systems of other organisms, the addition of a labeled ribonucleotide to trypanosome extracts results in RNA smears even in the absence of template DNA [24]. The strategy to circumvent this general labeling activity and specifically detect template-derived RNA is based on the insertion of a ~20 bp-long, unrelated oligonucleotide tag sequence ~50–120 bp downstream of the transcription initiation site (TIS) in template DNA. The resulting transcripts can then be specifically detected by primer extension assays (Fig. 1). Moreover, since the reverse transcriptase extends a primer to the 5′ end of an RNA, the size of the extension product reveals whether transcription initiation on the template was accurate. For *T. brucei*, tagged templates were generated and successfully transcribed for the SL RNA gene (SLins19) and the RNA pol I-transcribed rRNA (Rib-trm), VSG (VSG-trm), metacyclic (m)VSG (1.61-trm, 1.63 trm), and procyclin genes (GPEET-trm, originally termed PARP-trm) [25, 27, 30].

Once the in vitro system for a particular promoter/gene is established, it offers various ways to probe or confirm the function of a putative transcription factor. For example, the conditional gene silencing system in *T. brucei* [31] enables the comparison of transcriptional activities in extracts from uninduced cells and from cells

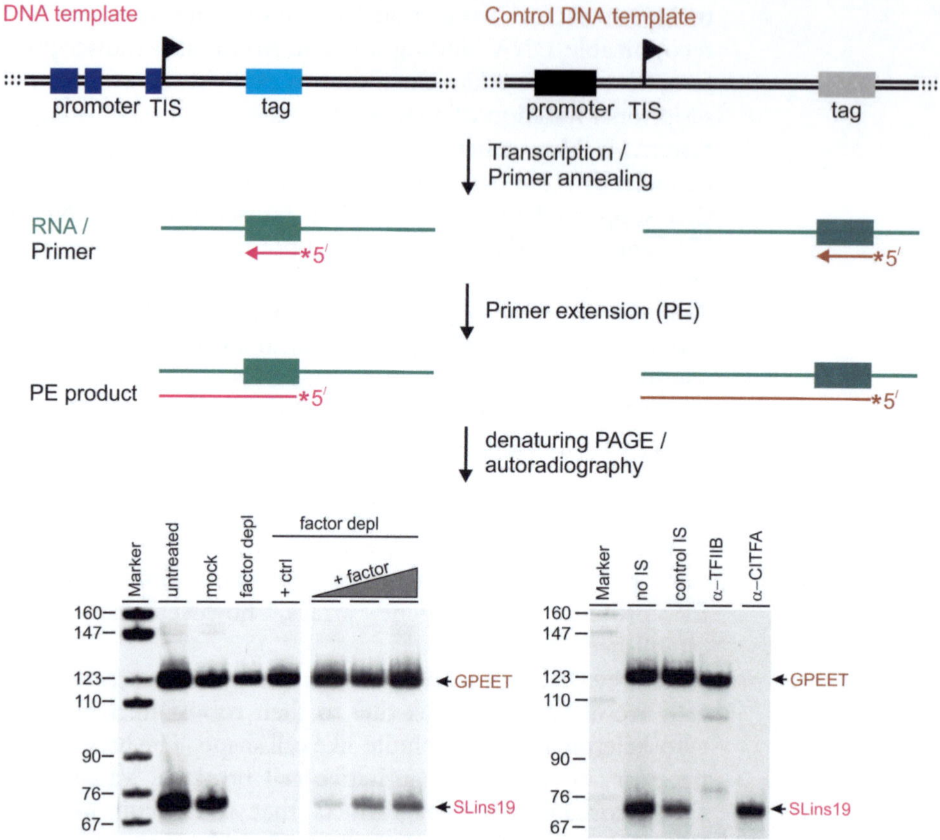

Fig. 1 In vitro transcription assay. Template DNAs harbor a promoter region with essential sequence elements (dark blue and black rectangles), the transcription initiation site (TIS, indicated by a flag), and unrelated tag sequences downstream of the TIS. The tags are placed at different distances from the flag to generate differently sized transcription signals. After the transcription reaction, total RNA is prepared and radiolabeled, tag-complementary oligonucleotides are annealed to template-derived transcripts. Reverse transcription extends these primers until the enzyme reaches the 5′ ends of the RNAs. Finally, radiolabeled extension products are separated on denaturing 50% urea/6% PAA gels and visualized by autoradiography. The bottom panels show cotranscription of the SLins19 and GPEET-trm templates. SLins19 contains the RNA pol II-recruiting promoter of the SL RNA gene, and GPEET-trm the RNA pol I-specific GPEET procyclin promoter template. On the left, an essential basal factor for RNA pol II transcription was depleted from extract (factor depl) which specifically abolished SLins19 transcription. Mock treatment of extract with control beads did not have this specific effect. Adding back purified factor (+ factor) partially restored SLins19 transcription in a dose-dependent manner whereas a similarly derived control factor (+ ctrl) did not restore transcription. As shown on the right, treatment of extract with anti-TFIIB immune serum (α-TFIIB) or with anti-CITFA serum (α-CITFA) abolished SLins19 and GPEET-trm transcription, respectively, whereas a nonspecific immune serum (control IS) had no effect on GPEET transcription and marginally affected SLins19 transcription

in which a factor has been depleted [12, 32]. If gene silencing is not an option, removal of a factor from extract by immunoprecipitation is an alternative and can abolish transcription of a specific template in vitro (Fig. 1, bottom left) [9, 12–14, 32]. Finally, preincubation of extract with an antibody against the endogenous factor often

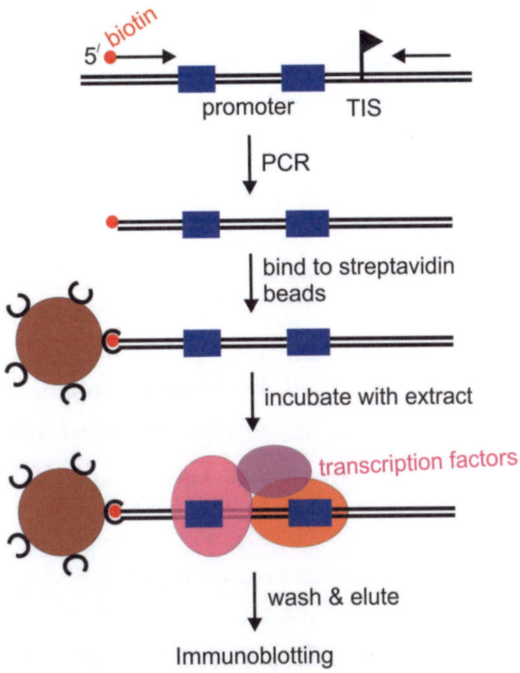

Fig. 2 Schematic outline of the promoter pull-down assay. A promoter region is amplified by PCR with one oligonucleotide carrying a biotin group at its 5′ end. The biotinylated promoter DNA is coupled to streptavidin beads and incubated with extract under transcription conditions. After washing the beads, DNA-bound proteins are eluted in SDS buffer and analyzed by standard immunoblotting. Blue rectangles and the flag denote promoter sequence elements and the transcription initiation site (TIS), respectively

interferes with its function, affecting transcription (Fig. 1, bottom right) [9, 12, 14, 32].

Another use of extracts is the promoter pull-down assay, which can reveal the interaction between a transcription factor and its cognate promoter (Fig. 2). The assay does not require cross-linking of proteins and is less stringent than an electric mobility gel shift assay (EMSA). For example, EMSA could not be established with factors that bind to the SL RNA gene promoter whereas the promoter pull-down assay readily revealed binding of a SNAPc subunit to this promoter [33]. While meaningful EMSAs often require a purified fraction of the transcription factor, promoter pull-downs typically work well with crude extracts. However, the latter assay requires detection of the factor by immunoblotting. Hence, it is only feasible if an antibody against the factor is available or extract is prepared from cells that express a tagged version of the factor that can be detected through the tag. Once established, the pull-down assay can be used to probe the DNA–protein interaction of a factor by mutating promoter elements.

2 Materials

All buffers should be prepared with RNase-free water and analytical grade reagents.

2.1 Extract Preparation

1. 5 L round, flat-bottomed glass flask, stirrer, and stirring magnet.
2. 15 ml "tight" glass Dounce homogenizer (Wheaton, Millville, NJ, USA) for large-scale preparations (*see* **Note 1**).
3. 800 μm Low Binding Silica Beads (OPS Diagnostics, Lebanon, NJ, USA) for small-scale preparations.
4. 15- and 50-ml Falcon tubes.
5. Amicon Ultra-4 centrifugal filtering unit (Millipore Sigma, St. Louis, MO, USA) with a molecular weight cutoff of 10 kDa.
6. A Dewar with liquid nitrogen for shock-freezing of extract aliquots (alternatively, a dry-ice bath can be used).
7. Tryp wash: 100 mM NaCl, 3 mM $MgCl_2$, 20 mM Tris–HCl pH 7.5.
8. Transcription buffer (incomplete): 150 mM sucrose, 20 mM L-glutamic acid, 10 mM HEPES–KOH pH 7.7, 3 mM $MgCl_2$. Complete the buffer just before use by making it 1 mM dithiothreitol (DTT), 10 μg/ml leupeptin, and 10 μg/ml aprotinin (complete transcription buffer aliquots can be stored at −20 °C and should be kept on ice after thawing) (*see* **Note 2**).
9. EDTA-free complete protease inhibitor cocktail (Millipore Sigma): Dissolve one tablet in 1 ml incomplete transcription buffer, aliquot, and store at −20 °C.
10. HS (high-salt) buffer (store aliquots at −20 °C): 150 mM sucrose, 1.5 M KCl, 20 mM Hepes–KOH pH 7.7, 3 mM $MgCl_2$.
11. 1 M dithiothreitol (DTT) dissolved in water and stored at −20 °C in 1 ml aliquots.
12. 3 M KCl.

2.2 *In Vitro* Transcription Analysis

2.2.1 *In Vitro* Transcription Reaction and RNA Preparation

1. Template DNA (1 μg/μl) in the form of a plasmid (*see* **Note 3**) and a standard nontemplate plasmid DNA such as pUC19 (1 μg/μl).
2. Transcription buffer (*see* above).
3. 10× salts: 0.2 M L-glutamic acid, 0.2 M Hepes–KOH pH 7.7, 30 mM $MgCl_2$, 72 mM DTT, 3.5 mM EDTA, 8.9 mM EGTA, 100 μg/ml leupeptin, 100 μg/ml aprotinin. Prepare a 1-ml aliquot and store at −20 °C.

4. 25% polyethylene glycol (PEG; w/v). Prepare 1-ml aliquots and store at −20 °C.
5. 0.5 M creatine phosphate. Store in 0.1 ml aliquots at −20 °C.
6. 12 mg/ml creatine kinase. Prepare freshly every time with incomplete Transcription buffer. Creatine kinase activity is highly unstable and will not survive a freeze–thaw cycle.
7. 10 mM NTP mix (10 mM of ATP, CTP, GTP, UTP; 100 mM stocks of each nucleotide are available from Millipore Sigma [Roche]).
8. TRIzol™ LS Reagent (ThermoFisher Scientific, Grand Island, NY, USA).
9. 20 mg/ml Glycogen, RNase-free (Millipore Sigma [Roche]).
10. DNase I (10 U/μl), RNase-free (Millipore Sigma [Roche]); includes 10× DNase I buffer.
11. Buffered phenol–chloroform–isoamyl alcohol (25/24/1, v/v/v) and chloroform.
12. 100% ethanol, 70% ethanol, 3 M sodium acetate (NaOAc) pH 7.0.

2.2.2 Factor Depletion from Extract

1. IgG Sepharose® 6 Fast Flow (Millipore Sigma).
2. Transcription buffer (*see* above).

2.2.3 Antibody-Mediated Transcription Inhibition

1. Immune serum or purified antibody against the endogenous transcription factor to be analyzed.
2. Preimmune serum and/or nonspecific immune serum/antibody of same origin.

2.2.4 Radiolabeling of Oligonucleotides and DNA Marker

1. Oligonucleotide to be labeled (100 ng/μl).
2. T4 Polynucleotide Kinase (PNK) (New England Biolabs, Ipswich, MA, USA); includes 10× PNK buffer.
3. [γ-^{32}P]ATP, 6000 Ci/mmol (PerkinElmer, Waltham, MA, USA).
4. Marker pBR322, *Msp*I-digested (1 μg/μl, New England Biolabs).
5. DNA Polymerase I, Large (Klenow) Fragment (New England Biolabs), includes 10× Klenow buffer.
6. [α-^{32}P]dCTP, 3000 Ci/mmol (PerkinElmer).
7. 5 mM dGAT mix (5 mM of dGTP, dATP, dTTP) (100 mM stocks of each nucleotide are available from Millipore Sigma [Roche].
8. Micro Bio-Spin 6 columns (Bio-Rad, Hercules, CA, USA).
9. Čerenkov counter.

2.2.5 Primer Extension Reaction and Denaturing Polyacrylamide Gel Electrophoresis (PAGE)

1. SuperScript Reverse Transcriptase (ThermoFisher Scientific), includes 5× first strand buffer and 0.1 M DTT aliquots.
2. 10 mM dNTP mix.
3. 5′-^{32}P-endlabeled oligonucleotide(s) (*see* Subheading 3.2.4).
4. Radiolabeled DNA marker (*see* Subheading 3.2.4).
5. 10×/1× Tris–Borate–EDTA (TBE) buffer: For 1 L of 10× TBE buffer dissolve 108 g of Tris base and 55 g of boric acid in 900 ml of water. Add 40 ml of 0.5 M EDTA, pH 8.0. Make up volume to 1 L, autoclave and store at room temperature.
6. Urea loading buffer: 50% (w/v) urea in 1× TBE buffer, 0.1% (w/v) xylene cyanol, 0.1% (w/v) bromophenol blue.
7. System for vertical gel electrophoresis which includes glass plates (~18 cm × 20 cm), 0.4 mm thick spacers and comb, electrophoresis chamber, and a high voltage power supply.
8. 50% urea/1× TBE solution: dissolve 500 g urea in 100 ml 10× TBE buffer and water to a volume of 1 L, filter solution and store at room temperature in a dark glass bottle.
9. 50% urea/20% PAA/1× TBE solution: dissolve 500 g urea in 500 ml of 40% polyacrylamide (PAA) solution (29:1, Fisher Scientific, Fair Lawn, NJ, USA), 100 ml 10× TBE buffer and water to a volume of 1 L, filter solution and store at room temperature in a dark glass bottle.
10. 10% ammonium persulfate (APS, w/v), prepare a 1-ml aliquot and store at 4 °C up to 1 week.
11. Tetramethylethylenediamine (TEMED).
12. Heating block.
13. Whatman paper.
14. Vacuum gel dryer.
15. X-ray film (Research Products International, Mt. Prospect, IL, USA), intensifying screens, film cassettes and film developer.

2.3 Promoter Pull Down Assay

1. Oligonucleotides for promoter DNA amplification, one of which should be synthesized with a 5′–terminal biotin group.
2. QIAquick Gel Extraction Kit (Qiagen, Germantown, MD, USA).
3. Paramagnetic Streptavidin Dynabeads M-280 (ThermoFisher).
4. 2x B&W buffer: 10 mM Tris–HCl, pH 7.5, 1 mM EDTA, 2 M NaCl.
5. A magnetic stand to collect paramagnetic beads, for example the Magna GrIP™ Rack (Millipore Sigma).

6. TK_{20} buffer: 150 mM sucrose, 20 mM Hepes–KOH pH 7.7, 20 mM potassium L-glutamate, 20 mM KCl, 3 mM $MgCl_2$, 2.5% (w/v) polyethylene glycol, 0.2 mM EDTA, 0.5 mM EGTA, 4 mM DTT, 10 μg/ml leupeptin, 10 μg/ml aprotinin.
7. Bovine serum albumin.
8. Polyvinylpyrrolidone (PVP10, Millipore Sigma).
9. TN_{40} buffer: 150 mM sucrose, 20 mM Tris–HCl pH 8.0, 40 mM NaCl, 3 mM $MgCl_2$, 0.5 mM DTT, 10 μg/ml leupeptin, 10 μg/ml aprotinin.

3 Methods

3.1 Extract Preparation

Several techniques have been used to break trypanosome cells including Stansted Cell Disruptor and French Press. However, only two procedures reliably produced transcriptionally active extracts, namely repeated cycles of vortexing cells in the presence of glass beads followed by shock-freezing and thawing the sample (small scale), and the use of a glass Dounce homogenizer (large scale). For extract preparations, all solutions should be ice-cold and Eppendorf and Falcon tubes precooled on ice before use.

3.1.1 Small-Scale WCE Preparation

1. Before harvesting cells, place a vortexer and the liquid nitrogen Dewar in a cold room. Wash an Amicon Ultra-4 centrifugal filtering unit twice by passing 2 ml of water through the filter device at 4000 × *g*. This washing step is important because the filter unit contains trace amounts of glycerol that needs to be removed.
2. Grow 2–3 × 10^9 trypanosomes to mid-log phase and pellet cells at 2700 × *g* and 2 °C for 10 min. Discard the supernatant. Resuspend cells in 10 ml of Tryp wash, transfer cells to a 15-ml Falcon tube, and spin as before. Repeat the washing step once with Tryp wash and once with incomplete Transcription buffer, increasing the centrifugation speed to 3300 × *g* in the last step to counter the viscosity of the sucrose-containing Transcription buffer. Record packed cell volume (PCV; should be around 0.25 ml).
3. Resuspend cells in one PCV of complete Transcription buffer, transfer cells to a precooled 1.5-ml microcentrifuge tube, and incubate cells on ice for 20 min. The Transcription buffer is slightly hypotonic, causing the cells to swell moderately. During incubation, equilibrate the glass beads in incomplete Transcription buffer, cut the top of a blue 1-ml tip and transfer 0.2 ml of beads to the cell suspension. Just prior to breaking the cells, mix 20 μl of protease inhibitor cocktail into the suspension.

4. Cells are broken in the cold room by five cycles of vortexing, shock-freezing and thawing the suspension. Vortex the cell suspension at full power for 1 min, let it sit on ice for 1 min and then repeat the vortexing step. Shock-freeze the suspension in liquid nitrogen and thaw it in your hands for the next cycle.
5. For the protein extraction procedure, have a precooled 1.5-ml tube containing 60 μl of ice-cold HS buffer ready. Take off the broken cell suspension from the glass beads all at once (best by pushing a yellow tip on top of a blue tip) and rapidly mix the suspension with the HS buffer aliquot. The rapid mixing with high salt buffer will minimize nuclear lysis. Incubate the broken cell suspension for 20 min on ice and intermittently (~three times) flick/invert the tube during this period.
6. To separate the extract from nuclei and insoluble cell debris, spin the tube in a cooling microcentrifuge at 25,000 × *g* and 2 °C for 10 min. Transfer the extract (~500 μl) to a new precooled tube using a 200 μl-pipette.
7. Reduce the salt concentration of the extract by adding an equal volume of complete Transcription buffer, and concentrate the extract in the prewashed Amicon Ultra-4 filter unit at 4000 × *g* and 2 °C to a volume of 150–200 μl.
8. Prepare 50-μl aliquots in precooled 1.5 ml-tubes, shock-freeze the extract, and store at −80 °C.

3.1.2 Large-Scale WCE Preparation

1. Grow 4 L of procyclic trypanosomes (*see* **Note 4**) to mid-log phase (1×10^7 cells/ml) in a 5 L round flat-bottom glass flask using a stirrer and a stirring magnet. Harvest cells in 500-ml centrifugation bottles at 3000 × *g* and 2 °C for 10 min. Resuspend cell pellets in 5 ml of Tryps wash each. Transfer and combine the cell suspensions in a 50-ml Falcon tube. Pellet cells again at 3000 × *g* and 2 °C for 7 min and discard the supernatant without disturbing the cell pellet.
2. Wash cells twice with 40 ml of Tryps wash and spin as above. Determine the packed cell volume (PCV), which should be 5–7 ml.
3. Resuspend and wash cells once in 30 ml of ice-cold incomplete transcription buffer. Centrifuge at 3300 × *g* and 2 °C for 10 min. The increase in centrifugation speed is necessary to counter the viscosity of the sucrose-containing transcription buffer. Remove the supernatant and resuspend cells in one PCV of incomplete transcription buffer so that the total volume is ~10–14 ml. Incubate the cells on ice for 20 min.
4. During this incubation, prepare the glass Dounce homogenizer by washing it once with 100% ethanol, three times with water, and once with incomplete Transcription buffer. Place the

homogenizer in an ice bucket so that it touches the bottom. In this way, it cannot break through the ice during douncing. Transfer cells to the homogenizer.

5. Prior to douncing, add DTT to a final concentration of 1 mM and leupeptin and aprotinin to final concentrations of 10 μg/ml. Dilute a 2 μl sample of the cell suspension in 38 μl of Tryps wash for microscopic analysis.
6. Vigorously dounce the solution until about 70–80% of the trypanosomes are broken. Dependent on the tightness of the homogenizer, this may take 3–10 min. To assess cell breakage, take 2 μl samples, dilute and compare them to the unbroken cell sample under the microscope at 400× magnification.
7. Prepare 1-ml aliquots of broken cell suspension, shock-freeze them in liquid nitrogen and store them at −80 °C. Shock-freezing is an important step since it appears to disrupt cells that have not been broken by douncing.
8. Transcription extract can be prepared from one aliquot at a time. Thaw a 1-ml aliquot of broken cell suspension in your hands and place on ice. Add 100 μl of HS buffer to a new tube, then transfer and rapidly mix the broken cell suspension with HS buffer to minimize nuclear lysis. Incubate the extract on ice for 20 min and flick/invert the tubes during this period three times.
9. Separation of extract from nuclei and cell debris, dilution and concentration of extract, and preparation and storage of transcription extract aliquots should be carried out as detailed in Subheading 3.1.1, **steps 6–8**. Note that the soluble extract before dilution is ~600 μl in this procedure and the final volume of the extract after concentration should be between 200 and 250 μl.

3.1.3 Nuclear Extract Preparation (Large Scale)

The preparation of 1-ml aliquots of broken cell suspension is identical to the previous protocol (Subheading 3.1.2, **steps 1**–7). For nuclear extract preparation a single 1-ml aliquot of broken cell suspension is treated as follows:

8. Spin the suspension at 16,000 × *g* and 2 °C for 10 min. Discard the supernatant and wash pellet with 900 μl of complete Transcription buffer by gently resuspending the pellet, inverting and flicking the tube. Do not use the pipette for this purpose because nuclei may get damaged.
9. Repeat the spin, discard the supernatant, and resuspend the pellet in 520 μl of complete transcription buffer. For extraction, mix in, drop-by-drop, 80 μl of 3 M KCl (final KCl concentration of 400 mM). Incubate the extract on ice for 20 min and flick/invert the tubes during this period three times.

10. Except for the fact that this extract needs to be diluted with 2.5 volumes of complete Transcription buffer instead of an equal volume, separation of extract from nuclei and cell debris, dilution and concentration of extract, and preparation and storage of extract aliquots should be carried out as detailed in Subheading 3.1.1, **steps 6–8**. Note that the nuclear extract has a lower protein concentration and should be more concentrated than WCE (e.g., from ~600 μl before dilution to a final volume of 150 to maximal 200 μl).

3.2 In Vitro Transcription Analysis

The method consists of the in vitro transcription reaction, the subsequent RNA analysis by primer extension, and separation and detection of the radiolabeled extension products by denaturing PAGE and autoradiography, respectively. Accordingly, we provide protocols for radiolabeling of oligonucleotides and the DNA size marker pBR322-*Msp*I. In addition, we describe how to deplete an extract of a factor and use immune sera to inactivate a factor in extract.

3.2.1 In Vitro Transcription Reaction and RNA Preparation

1. Thaw or prepare all reagents and place on ice. Set a water bath at 28 °C.
2. Set up the following 38-μl reaction (*see* **Note 5**): 1.6 μl of template plasmid DNA (do not use more than 1 μg of a single template in a reaction; if there is only one template per reaction, then add nontemplate DNA to a final total DNA amount of 1.6 μg [*see* **Note 6**]), 2.24 μl of 10× salts, 4 μl of PEG, 1.6 μl of creatine phosphate, 1.6 μl of creatine kinase, 10.96 μl of water, 8 μl of complete Transcription buffer, and 8 μl of extract. Incubate the reaction for 10 min on ice.
3. Add 2 μl of NTP mix to the reaction and incubate transcription reaction for 1 h at 28 °C.
4. Stop the reaction and prepare total RNA from the reaction as follows: add 60 μl of water, 300 μl of TRIzol reagent, and 60 μl of chloroform to the reaction, vortex the sample for 1 min and incubate on ice for 10 min. Separate the lower red organic phase from the upper colorless aqueous phase by centrifugation in a microcentrifuge at top speed and room temperature for 5 min. Transfer the aqueous phase (200 μl) to a new microcentrifuge tube and mix well with 1 μl of glycogen (glycogen serves as a carrier for efficient RNA precipitation) and 600 μl of ethanol. Precipitate RNA by spinning the sample in a microcentrifuge at top speed and room temperature for 10 min. Discard the supernatant, briefly spin again and remove trace amounts of liquid. Wash the pellet twice with 70% ethanol and air-dry pellet for 5–10 min.

5. To remove all template DNA from the RNA preparation, it is important to treat the sample with DNase as follows: Dissolve RNA pellet in 90 μl of water at 65 °C for 10 min, vortex sample, and place the tube back on ice. Mix the sample with 10 μl of 10× DNase I buffer and 1 μl of DNase I. Incubate sample at 37 °C for 1 h. Stop the reaction and extract RNA with 100 μl of buffered phenol–chloroform–isoamyl alcohol and, subsequently, with 100 μl of chloroform. Transfer the aqueous phase to a new tube, precipitate RNA with 30 μl of 3 M NaOAc and 600 μl of 100% ethanol, and wash RNA pellet twice with 70% ethanol. Air-dry the pellet and proceed to the primer extension reaction. Please note, that RNA preparations are best stored in 70% ethanol (second wash) at −20 °C.

3.2.2 Factor Depletion from Extract

A factor can be depleted from extract at different preparation steps by standard immunoprecipitation (IP). We have obtained best results when extract was subjected to IP after extraction and before dilution with transcription buffer to reduce the salt concentration (between **steps 6** and 7 of Subheading 3.1.1). Furthermore, for factor depletion we routinely prepared extracts from cell lines that exclusively expressed a transcription factor fused to a PTP tag. The PTP tag is a composite tag for tandem affinity purification and includes tandem protein A domains [34]. Hence, IgG beads can be used for efficient removal of a PTP-tagged factor from extract. However, any bead-bound antibody that efficiently precipitates a factor can be used instead. To ensure that the IP procedure does not inactivate the transcription reaction nonspecifically, mock depletion with control beads (e.g., protein A or protein G beads) and cotranscription of an unaffected template are valuable controls (Fig. 1). The gold standard though is when adding back the factor to extract—either in recombinant form or from an independent purification (*see* **Note** 7)—activates transcription in a dose-dependent manner (Fig. 1).

1. Wash and equilibrate 50 μl of settled IgG beads (100 μl of 1:1 slurry) twice with 0.8 ml complete Transcription buffer, pelleting the beads at 3000 × *g* and 4 °C for 1 min.
2. Add undiluted extract (~500 μl) to beads and slowly rotate tube at 4 °C for 1 h. Spin sample at 3000 × *g* and 2 °C for 2 min. Transfer supernatant, that is, depleted extract, to a new, precooled tube and continue with extract preparation by diluting the extract with complete Transcription buffer as described in Subheading 3.1.1, **step** 7.

3.2.3 Antibody-Mediated Transcription Inhibition

1. The 40-μl in vitro transcription reaction is carried out as described in Subheading 3.2.1 with the following modification: 6 μl of extract (instead of 8 μl) is mixed with 1 μl of a polyclonal immune serum (*see* **Note 8**) directed against the

factor and 1 μl of complete Transcription buffer, and incubated on ice for 30 min. The extract is then added to the transcription reaction and the procedure carried out as described. As an essential control, a reaction with preimmune or a nonspecific immune serum of the same origin should be carried out in parallel.

3.2.4 Radiolabeling of Oligonucleotides and DNA Marker

Please note that working with radioactive nucleotides standardly requires special training of personnel and institutional approval of a radiation safety protocol, specifying where and how experiments are conducted, radioactivity is monitored and radioactive waste is disposed (*see* **Note 9** for nonradioactive alternatives).

1. For ^{32}P-5′-end labeling of an oligonucleotide to be used in primer extension reactions, set up the following 20 μl reaction: 14.3 μl of water, 2 μl of 10× PNK buffer, 2 μl of oligonucleotide solution (100 ng/μl), 1.2 μl of [γ-^{32}P]ATP, and 0.5 μl of PNK. Incubate at 37 °C for exactly 30 min.
2. Separate unincorporated radionucleotides from oligonucleotides by gel filtration using Micro Bio-Spin 6 columns as follows: Remove tip and cap of the column, place it in a 2 ml microcentrifuge tube (tubes come with the columns), and dry column with a 2 min spin at 1100 × *g* and room temperature. Wash the column with 600 μl of water, repeating the spin. Transfer the PNK reaction to the center of the dried column, place the column in a fresh 1.5 ml microcentrifuge tube and spin at 1100 × *g* and room temperature for 4 min. Discard the column and dilute the oligonucleotide solution with 150 μl of water. Store at −20 °C.
3. Radiolabeling of a DNA size marker will allow for direct comparison of primer extension products with DNA fragments of known size in denaturing PAGE. *Msp*I-digested pBR322 can be labeled with radiolabeled dCTP due to 5′-CG overhangs that can be filled in with Klenow enzyme. Set up a 20-μl labeling reaction as follows: 1.0 μl of digested DNA marker, 1 μl of 5 mM dGAT mix, 2 μl of 10× Klenow buffer, 10 μl of water, 5 μl of [α-^{32}P]dCTP, and 1 μl of Klenow enzyme. Incubate reaction at 37 °C for 30 min and remove unincorporated nucleotides via a Micro Bio-Spin 6 column as described in **step 2**. Store at −20 °C.

3.2.5 Primer Extension Reaction and Denaturing PAGE

1. Resuspend the dried RNA pellet generated from the in vitro transcription reaction (Subheading 3.2.1) in 11.5 μl of water, and add 4 μl of 5× first strand buffer and 1 μl of labeled oligonucleotide (10.5 μl water/2 μl oligonucleotide when two primers are used in parallel). Anneal primers to RNA by heating the sample to 70 °C for 5 min, followed by an incubation on ice for 5 min.

2. Set up reverse transcription reaction by adding 2 μl of 0.1 M DTT, 1 μl of 10 mM dNTP mix, and 0.5 μl of reverse transcriptase to the annealing reaction. Incubate at 42 °C for 45 min.
3. Precipitate labeled DNA by mixing the reaction with 2.5 μl of 3 M NaOAc and 60 μl of 100% ethanol. Spin sample for 7 min at top speed and room temperature in a microcentrifuge, remove all liquid, air-dry the pellet and resuspend DNA in 10 μl of Urea loading buffer.
4. Dilute labeled DNA marker (Subheading 3.2.4, **step 3**) in Urea loading buffer such that a 5 μl sample generates about 20 counts per second in a Čerenkov counter.
5. For denaturing PAGE, assemble two glass plates with spacers and seal the plates with packaging tape except for the top part. For a 6% PAA gel (*see* **Note 10**), mix 7.5 ml of 50% urea/20% PAA/1×TBE solution with 17.5 ml of 50% urea/1× TBE solution, 0.15 ml of 10% APS, and 15 μl of TEMED. Immediately pour the gel, insert the comb and let the gel polymerize for at least 30 min in horizontal position. Clamps may be used to tighten the plates during polymerization.
6. After removing tape and comb, assemble plates into the electrophoresis chamber, add 1× TBE buffer to the chamber, and prerun gel at 700 V for 30 min. Before loading, heat the DNA marker for 5 min and the PE samples for 1 min in a 100 °C heating block, briefly spin the samples, and load 5 μl of each sample into the wells which need to be cleaned just before loading, for example with a Pasteur pipette. Run the gel at 700 V until the fast blue reaches the bottom of the gel. Disassemble glass plates, pick up the gel on Whatman paper and dry it in a vacuum gel dryer. Expose the gel to an X-ray film in a film cassette, best with an intensifying screen at −80 °C. Expect exposure times of 3–16 h. Develop film.

3.3 Promoter Pull-Down Assay

When designing primers to amplify a promoter region, it is important to provide ~20 bp of additional sequence around the known promoter elements to provide a DNA platform for factor binding. Moreover, if the sequence elements of a promoter have been characterized, a most valuable control for this assay is to analyze a comparable DNA in which the promoter element(s) have been mutated. Once the assay is established for a particular transcription factor, a refined mutational analysis of the promoter region can reveal the critical nucleotides for factor binding.

1. Generate biotinylated promoter DNA by PCR in which one of the oligonucleotides carries a biotin group at its 5′ end. Gel-purify the amplification product, using the QIAquick gel extraction kit.

2. For each assay, couple 500 ng of the PCR product to 100 μg of Streptavidin Dynabeads M-280 as follows: Vortex manufacturer's beads vial for 30 s and transfer 10 μl of beads solution (10 μg/μl) to a new microcentrifuge tube. Wash the beads with 0.8 ml of 1× B&W buffer, collecting the beads on a magnet for 2 min. Resuspend beads in 100 μl of 2× B&W buffer and add DNA resuspended in 100 μl of water. Slowly rotate the tube for 15 min at room temperature. Collect the biotinylated DNA-coated beads and wash three times with 0.8 ml of 1× B&W buffer.
3. Block the beads with 0.5 ml of TK_{20} buffer, containing 5 mg/ml bovine serum albumin and 5 mg/ml PVP10, by slowly rotating the tube for 30 min at room temperature. Wash the beads twice with 0.5 ml TK_{20} buffer.
4. Set up an in vitro transcription reaction as described in Subheading 3.2.1, **steps 2** and **3** using the DNA-coated beads as template (*see* **Note 11**). Incubate the reaction for 15 min on ice and for 15 min at 27 °C. Wash the beads three times with 0.5 ml of TK_{20} buffer and once with 0.5 ml of TN_{40} buffer (*see* **Note 12**).
5. Elute proteins in 40 μl of 1× SDS loading buffer at 70 °C for 5 min and analyze sample by standard immunoblotting.

4 Notes

1. We standardly use the 15-ml Dounce homogenizer because it is less likely to break. However, the extracts were originally established with the smaller 7-ml "tight" Dounce homogenizer from Wheaton and this homogenizer is more suitable when the PCV of pelleted cells is in the range of 2–4 ml.
2. In other systems, the "viscous" ingredient of transcription buffers most often is glycerol and not sucrose. However, trypanosomatid extracts typically harbor glycerol kinase activity which, in the presence of even trace amounts of glycerol, can rapidly deplete ATP pools [24].
3. We have always used circular plasmid DNA in transcription reactions because linearization of a plasmid template just downstream of the tag did not result in a transcription signal, that is, primer extension product. However, we learned that trypanosome RNA pols fall off linear templates before reaching the linearization site. Accordingly, transcription signals were achieved when the plasmid was linearized ~40 bp downstream of the tag (A.G., unpublished results). It is therefore likely that PCR-amplified DNA templates will work in these systems.

4. Four liters of procyclic trypanosome culture will produce the maximal amount of broken cell suspension from a 5 L glass flask and allow for the use of the sturdy 15 ml-glass Dounce homogenizer. However, 2–3 L (2–3 × 10^{10} cells) of culture is sufficient when the 7-ml Dounce homogenizer is used (*see* **Note 1**).
5. While the 40-μl reaction described has resulted in robust transcription signals, downscaling the reaction to 25 μl has worked, too [29]. It is recommended when extract is precious. For example, it requires 2 L of *T. brucei* bloodstream form culture to prepare extract on the small scale.
6. The reactions work best if they contain a total of 40 μg/ml plasmid DNA. However, individual templates have different concentration optimums in different extracts. In most cases, the optimum is 7.5 μg/ml; therefore, nontemplate plasmid DNA such as pUC19 needs to be added for optimal activity. The extra DNA likely sequesters nonspecific DNA-binding activities that can interfere with transcription. With the exception of the GPEET-trm template which works best at 40 μg/ml in extracts prepared from procyclics, template concentrations above 25 μg/ml were found to be deleterious.
7. Transcription reconstitution is most convincing when the factor for add back is expressed and purified from a different system (e.g., *Escherichia coli* or wheat germ extract). However, this is only feasible if the factor comprises not more than one or two proteins. In cases of larger protein complexes such as TFIIH (nine subunits) or CITFA (eight subunits) we have used endogenous factor of high purity that was isolated from extract by tandem affinity purification. Although the protein amounts necessary for successful transcription reconstitution may vary among factors, amounts in the range of 10–100 ng were sufficient in our hands.
8. Inactivation of a factor by an antibody is not a given because the antibody needs to bind to and block a functionally important domain. Since a polyclonal antibody/immune serum likely recognizes more than one epitope on a factor, its blocking potential is greater than that of a monoclonal antibody.
9. The generation and detection of radiolabeled primer extension products as described here is very sensitive and requires relatively few procedural steps. On the other hand, radiolabeled nucleotides are expensive and short-lived, and working with radioactive materials is tightly regulated. Thus, nonradioactive labeling methods such as the use of biotin- or fluorescent-labeled primers may be suitable alternatives [35–37].

10. If primer extension products smaller than 70 nt are investigated, an 8% PAA/50% urea gel will offer better resolution.
11. The promoter pull-down assay will most likely be successful under conditions of a functional transcription reaction which ensure that relevant transcription factors interact with the promoter. However, a transcriptionally active extract is not a prerequisite for this assay and promoter–factor interaction may also occur in inactive extracts.
12. The specified buffers provide the lowest stringency conditions we used successfully in this assay. However, once a pull-down has been achieved, increasing the salt concentration of the TK and TN buffers and/or adding a non-ionic detergent will increase the specificity of the assay. For example, CITFA was pulled down using 0.1% Tween 20-containing TK_{40} and TN_{80} buffers, in which the KCl and NaCl concentrations of the specified TK_{20} and TN_{40} buffers were increased to 40 and 80 mM, respectively, whereas a TK_{150} buffer abolished CITFA binding to its cognate promoter.

Acknowledgments

We thank previous collaborators and laboratory members for their help in developing this technology. Specifically, we thank Elisabetta Ullu, Christian Tschudi, Gabrielle Laufer, and Gabriel Schaaf for their help in developing the in vitro transcription systems, and Bernd Schimanski and Jens Brandenburg for establishing the promoter pull-down assay. This work was supported by grants R56 AI130747 and R21 AI142149 to A.G., and grant R01 AI028798 on which A.G. is a coinvestigator. All grants are from the National Institute of Allergy and Infectious Diseases of the US National Institutes of Health.

References

1. Ruan JP, Arhin GK, Ullu E, Tschudi C (2004) Functional characterization of a *Trypanosoma brucei* TATA-binding protein-related factor points to a universal regulator of transcription in trypanosomes. Mol Cell Biol 24:9610–9618
2. Ivens AC, Peacock CS, Worthey EA, Murphy L, Aggarwal G, Berriman M, Sisk E, Rajandream MA, Adlem E, Aert R et al (2005) The genome of the kinetoplastid parasite, *Leishmania major*. Science 309:436–442
3. Nakaar V, Tschudi C, Ullu E (1995) An unusual liaison: small nuclear and cytoplasmic RNA genes team up with tRNA genes in trypanosomatid protozoa. Parasitol Today 11:225–228
4. Gilinger G, Bellofatto V (2001) Trypanosome spliced leader RNA genes contain the first identified RNA polymerase II gene promoter in these organisms. Nucleic Acids Res 29:1556–1564
5. Das A, Bellofatto V (2003) RNA polymerase II-dependent transcription in trypanosomes is associated with a SNAP complex-like transcription factor. Proc Natl Acad Sci U S A 100:80–85
6. Schimanski B, Nguyen TN, Günzl A (2005) Characterization of a multisubunit transcription factor complex essential for spliced-leader RNA gene transcription in *Trypanosoma brucei*. Mol Cell Biol 25:7303–7313

7. Das A, Zhang Q, Palenchar JB, Chatterjee B, Cross GA, Bellofatto V (2005) Trypanosomal TBP functions with the multisubunit transcription factor tSNAP to direct spliced-leader RNA gene expression. Mol Cell Biol 25:7314–7322
8. Palenchar JB, Liu W, Palenchar PM, Bellofatto V (2006) A divergent transcription factor TFIIB in trypanosomes is required for RNA polymerase II-dependent spliced leader RNA transcription and cell viability. Eukaryot Cell 5:293–300
9. Schimanski B, Brandenburg J, Nguyen TN, Caimano MJ, Günzl A (2006) A TFIIB-like protein is indispensable for spliced leader RNA gene transcription in *Trypanosoma brucei*. Nucleic Acids Res 34:1676–1684
10. Lee JH, Nguyen TN, Schimanski B, Günzl A (2007) Spliced leader RNA gene transcription in *Trypanosoma brucei* requires transcription factor TFIIH. Eukaryot Cell 6:641–649
11. Lecordier L, Devaux S, Uzureau P, Dierick JF, Walgraffe D, Poelvoorde P, Pays E, Vanhamme L (2007) Characterization of a TFIIH homologue from *Trypanosoma brucei*. Mol Microbiol 64:1164–1181
12. Lee JH, Jung HS, Günzl A (2009) Transcriptionally active TFIIH of the early-diverged eukaryote *Trypanosoma brucei* harbors two novel core subunits but not a cyclin-activating kinase complex. Nucleic Acids Res 37:3811–3820
13. Lee JH, Cai G, Panigrahi AK, Dunham-Ems S, Nguyen TN, Radolf JD, Asturias FJ, Günzl A (2010) A TFIIH-associated mediator head is a basal factor of small nuclear spliced leader RNA gene transcription in early-diverged trypanosomes. Mol Cell Biol 30:5502–5513
14. Srivastava A, Badjatia N, Lee JH, Hao B, Günzl A (2018) An RNA polymerase II-associated TFIIF-like complex is indispensable for SL RNA gene transcription in *Trypanosoma brucei*. Nucleic Acids Res 46:1695–1709
15. Brandenburg J, Schimanski B, Nogoceke E, Nguyen TN, Padovan JC, Chait BT, Cross GA, Günzl A (2007) Multifunctional class I transcription in *Trypanosoma brucei* depends on a novel protein complex. EMBO J 26:4856–4866
16. Nguyen TN, Nguyen BN, Lee JH, Panigrahi AK, Günzl A (2012) Characterization of a novel class I transcription factor A (CITFA) subunit that is indispensable for transcription by the multifunctional RNA polymerase I of *Trypanosoma brucei*. Eukaryot Cell 11:1573–1581
17. Wedel C, Forstner KU, Derr R, Siegel TN (2017) GT-rich promoters can drive RNA pol II transcription and deposition of H2AZ in African trypanosomes. EMBO J 36:2581–2594
18. Chandra U, Yadav A, Kumar D, Saha S (2017) Cell cycle stage-specific transcriptional activation of cyclins mediated by HAT2-dependent H4K10 acetylation of promoters in *Leishmania donovani*. PLoS Pathog 13:e1006615
19. Günzl A, Bruderer T, Laufer G, Schimanski B, Tu LC, Chung HM, Lee PT, Lee MG (2003) RNA polymerase I transcribes procyclin genes and variant surface glycoprotein gene expression sites in *Trypanosoma brucei*. Eukaryot Cell 2:542–551
20. Günzl A (2012) In: Bindereif A (ed) RNA metabolism in trypanosomes, vol 28. Springer Press, New York, pp 1–27
21. Pena AC, Pimentel MR, Manso H, Vaz-Drago R, Pinto-Neves D, Aresta-Branco F, Rijo-Ferreira F, Guegan F, Pedro Coelho L, Carmo-Fonseca M et al (2014) *Trypanosoma brucei* histone H1 inhibits RNA polymerase I transcription and is important for parasite fitness *in vivo*. Mol Microbiol 93:645–663
22. Ullu E, Tschudi C (1990) Permeable trypanosome cells as a model system for transcription and trans-splicing. Nucleic Acids Res 18:3319–3326
23. Dossin FM, Schenkman S (2005) Actively transcribing RNA polymerase II concentrates on spliced leader genes in the nucleus of *Trypanosoma cruzi*. Eukaryot Cell 4:960–970
24. Günzl A, Tschudi C, Nakaar V, Ullu E (1995) Accurate transcription of the *Trypanosoma brucei* U2 small nuclear RNA gene in a homologous extract. J Biol Chem 270:17287–17291
25. Günzl A, Ullu E, Dörner M, Fragoso SP, Hoffmann KF, Milner JD, Morita Y, Nguu EK, Vanacova S, Wünsch S et al (1997) Transcription of the *Trypanosoma brucei* spliced leader RNA gene is dependent only on the presence of upstream regulatory elements. Mol Biochem Parasitol 85:67–76
26. Huie JL, He P, Bellofatto V (1997) *In vitro* transcription of the *Leptomonas seymouri* SL RNA and U2 snRNA genes using homologous cell extracts. Mol Biochem Parasitol 90:183–192
27. Laufer G, Schaaf G, Bollgönn S, Günzl A (1999) *In vitro* analysis of alpha-amanitin-resistant transcription from the rRNA, procyclic acidic repetitive protein, and variant surface glycoprotein gene promoters in *Trypanosoma brucei*. Mol Cell Biol 19:5466–5473
28. Laufer G, Günzl A (2001) *In-vitro* competition analysis of procyclin gene and variant surface glycoprotein gene expression site

transcription in *Trypanosoma brucei*. Mol Biochem Parasitol 113:55–65

29. Park SH, Nguyen TN, Günzl A (2012) Development of an efficient *in vitro* transcription system for bloodstream form *Trypanosoma brucei* reveals life cycle-independent functionality of class I transcription factor A. Mol Biochem Parasitol 181:29–36
30. Ginger ML, Blundell PA, Lewis AM, Browitt A, Günzl A, Barry JD (2002) *Ex vivo* and *in vitro* identification of a consensus promoter for VSG genes expressed by metacyclic-stage trypanosomes in the tsetse fly. Eukaryot Cell 1:1000–1009
31. Wirtz E, Leal S, Ochatt C, Cross GAM (1999) A tightly regulated inducible expression system for conditional gene knock-outs and dominant-negative genetics in *Trypanosoma brucei*. Mol Biochem Parasitol 99:89–101
32. Nguyen TN, Schimanski B, Günzl A (2007) Active RNA polymerase I of *Trypanosoma brucei* harbors a novel subunit essential for transcription. Mol Cell Biol 27:6254–6263
33. Schimanski B, Laufer G, Gontcharova L, Günzl A (2004) The *Trypanosoma brucei* spliced leader RNA and rRNA gene promoters have interchangeable TbSNAP50-binding elements. Nucleic Acids Res 32:700–709
34. Schimanski B, Nguyen TN, Günzl A (2005) Highly efficient tandem affinity purification of trypanosome protein complexes based on a novel epitope combination. Eukaryot Cell 4:1942–1950
35. Mackey J, Darfler M, Nisson P, Rashtchian A (1993) Use of random primer extension for concurrent amplification and nonradioactive labeling of nucleic acids. Anal Biochem 212:428–435
36. Lloyd AL, Marshall BJ, Mee BJ (2005) Identifying cloned *Helicobacter pylori* promoters by primer extension using a FAM-labelled primer and GeneScan analysis. J Microbiol Methods 60:291–298
37. Wang H, Ayala JC, Benitez JA, Silva AJ (2014) The LuxR-type regulator VpsT negatively controls the transcription of rpoS, encoding the general stress response regulator, in *Vibrio cholerae* biofilms. J Bacteriol 196:1020–1030

Chapter 17

Identifying Trypanosome Protein–RNA Interactions Using RIP-Seq

Elisha Mugo and Esteban D. Erben

Abstract

Trypanosomatids rely primarily on posttranscriptional mechanisms for the control of gene expression, with regulation of RNA processing, localization, degradation, and translation by RNA-binding proteins (RBPs). To determine the mechanisms by which RBPs control gene expression in trypanosomatids, transcriptome-wide identification of mRNA targets and mapping of the RNA-binding site is required. Here we present our most current RIP-Seq (RNA immunoprecipitation followed by high-throughput sequencing) protocol that we generally apply to elucidate RNA/protein interactions in *Trypanosoma brucei*. The technique provides valuable information about the workings of messenger ribonucleoprotein (mRNP) networks and trypanosome gene expression mechanisms.

Key words RNA-binding proteins, RNA Immunoprecipitation (RIP), Protein characterization, mRNA target identification

1 Introduction

In eukaryotic cells, there is not always a correspondence between mRNA transcript levels and the final amount of protein produced. RNA-Binding Proteins (RBPs) contribute to the final amount of protein product produced by regulating all events from transcription of the mRNA to its nucleocytoplasmic export, its subcellular localization in the cytoplasm, its translation, and its mode and rate of degradation. The mRNAs are present as messenger ribonucleoprotein particles (mRNPs), which include not only proteins that bind directly to the mRNA but also additional proteins that are recruited via protein–protein interactions. This set of proteins may change dynamically and all these processes are coordinated to generate a gene expression profile unique under a specific condition. Each mRNA often contains binding-sites for many RBPs and each RBP may associate with more than one mRNA, giving rise to complex regulatory networks. Thus, one of the challenges to assess the impact of RBPs on posttranscriptional gene regulation is

Paul A. M. Michels et al. (eds.), *Trypanosomatids: Methods and Protocols*, Methods in Molecular Biology, vol. 2116, https://doi.org/10.1007/978-1-0716-0294-2_17,

identifying their mRNA targets in a cellular context. A popular approach to characterize ribonucleoprotein complexes associated with specific RBPs at a global level relies on immuno- or affinity-purification procedures followed by identification of the associated RNA. Initial genome-wide attempts to identify associated transcripts employed microarrays (RIP-ChIP: RNA-Binding Protein Immunoprecipitation-Microarray (Chip) Profiling) [1] and once next-generation sequencing was established, RNA sequencing (RIP-Seq: RNA-Binding Protein Immunoprecipitation followed by deep sequencing) [2]. In general, the steps that have to be followed for an RIP experiment are quite similar regardless of the cell line, protein studied or the antibody or affinity purification method employed. The protocol often involves cross-linking of proteins to RNA, followed by immunoprecipitation or affinity purification of the protein–RNA complexes. The recovered RNPs are washed extensively, and then released and dissociated into RNA and protein components. Isolated RNA is then used to make a cDNA library that is subjected to RNA sequencing (RNA-Seq) and/or qPCR for pilot experiments or validation. It is worth to notice that RIP-Seq allows, unlike the CLIP family of techniques (e.g., PAR-CLIP [3] or iCLIP [4]), for the detection of RNA components of RNPs that are not directly bound to the RBP of interest. Thus, the disadvantages of RIP-Seq compared to these techniques include lack of actually RBP binding site identification and nonspecific RNA interaction identification [5].

Yet RIP-Seq has provided several valuable insights into post-transcriptional gene networks in trypanosomes; for example, Clayton and coworkers were able to show that mRNAs bound by the zinc-finger protein ZC3H11, including those encoding refolding chaperones, escape heat-induced translation inhibition [6–8]. Recently the same group also showed that a single RNA-binding protein, RBP10, promotes the bloodstream-form trypanosome differentiation [9]. In both cases, the authors were able to identify not only the target mRNAs those proteins bind but also the binding-sites and the mechanism of action. Thus, while precise locations of the binding site may sometimes be difficult or impossible to determine by this technique, in some cases it has proven feasible. In this chapter, we describe our most current RIP-Seq method and introduce basic computational aspects of RNA motif finding.

2 Materials

We recommend that throughout this method, all standard precautions should be taken to minimize RNAse contamination. RNA samples must be handled with gloves and kept on ice. All buffers and solutions should be either purchased or be prepared with nuclease-free water. Phenol-containing solutions should be handled under a fume cabinet, and phenol waste must be disposed of in accordance with lab safety regulations. We assume that readers are familiar with *Trypanosoma brucei* cell culture and genetic manipulation, thus this is not described here.

2.1 Cell Line

To isolate the RNA targets associated with the protein of interest, the lysate is immunoprecipitated (or affinity purified) with an antibody directed toward the protein of interest. In the example described below, RBP10 is tagged with a tandem affinity purification (TAP) tag at the N-terminus as described at Mugo and Clayton [9]. The tagged protein is immunoprecipitated with IgG Sepharose beads and the mRNPs eluted by TEV cleavage (*see* **Note 1**). While in this protocol we describe the use of Sepharose beads, we have successfully immunoprecipitated mRNP complexes using both Sepharose and magnetic beads.

2.2 Cell Harvesting and In Vivo UV Cross-Linking

1. 1× Phosphate-buffered saline (PBS): Add about 800 ml water to a 1 L beaker. Weigh 8 g NaCl, 0.2 g of KCl, 1.44 g of Na_2HPO_4, 0.24 g of KH_2PO_4. Mix and adjust pH 7.4 with HCl. Make up to 1 L with water. Dispense the solution into aliquots and sterilize by autoclaving (20 min, 121 °C, liquid cycle). Store at room temperature.
2. Petri dishes (145 × 20 mm).
3. FCS-free HMI-9 medium.
4. Liquid nitrogen.
5. Sterile centrifuge tubes.
6. 50 ml Falcon tubes.
7. UV cross-linker (e.g., Stratalinker 2400).

2.3 RNA Immunoprecipitation

1. IP buffer: 20 mM Tris–HCl, pH 7.5, 150 mM NaCl, 0.1% Nonidet P-40 (NP-40). To make 50 ml IP buffer add 1 ml of 1 M Tris–HCl, pH 7.5, 1.875 ml of 4 M NaCl, and 50 μl of NP-40 to 47.075 ml of nuclease-free ddH_2O.
2. Lysis buffer: 10 mM Tris–HCl, pH 7.5, 10 mM NaCl, 2000 U RNasin (Promega), 10 μg/ml leupeptin, 1× complete protease Inhibitor without EDTA (Roche), 0.1% (v/v) NP-40. To make 5 ml lysis buffer add 50 μl of 1 M Tris–HCl, pH 7.5, 12.5 μl of 4 M NaCl, and 5 μl of NP-40 to 4.8575 ml of nuclease free ddH_2O. At the time of use add 50 μl of 40 U/μl RNasin (Promega), 25 μl of 2 mg/ml leupeptin, and one tablet protease inhibitor cocktail (without EDTA).
3. TEV cleavage buffer: 20 mM Tris–HCl, pH 7.5, 150 mM NaCl, 0.1% NP-40, 0.5 mM EDTA, 1 mM DTT, 200 U/ml RNasin (Promega). To make 10 ml TEV cleavage buffer add

12.5 μl of 0.4 M EDTA to 9.9275 ml of IP buffer (as above). At the time of use add 10 μl of 1 M DTT, and 50 μl of 40 U/μl RNasin (Promega).

4. IgG Sepharose beads suspension (e.g., Fastflow-Amersham Biosciences).
5. Polyprep chromatography columns (0.8 × 4 cm).
6. TEV protease.
7. Proteinase K.
8. Trifast FL reagent (Peqlab, Germany) or similar guanidinium thiocyanate–phenol reagent.
9. 4× Laemmli buffer.

3 Methods

3.1 Sample Collection and In Vivo UV Cross-Linking

1. Grow ~2 × 10^9 RBP10$^{TAP/-}$ cells in HMI-9 medium supplemented with proper antibiotics (*see* **Note 2**).
2. Harvest cells by centrifugation at 2300 × *g* for 10 min at 4 °C and resuspend the cell pellet in 50 ml of ice cold FCS-free HMI-9 media. Kept on ice.
3. Split the concentrated cells into two petri culture dishes without their lids on ice and irradiate the cells at a distance of ~10 cm from the UV source. Irradiate with 0.4 J/cm^2 at 254 nm (*see* **Note 3**).
4. Transfer the cross-linked sample to a 50 ml Falcon tube and pellet the cells by centrifugation at 2300 × *g* for 10 min at 4 °C.
5. Discard the supernatant, resuspend the pellet in 10 ml of ice-cold PBS and then spin down the cells again.
6. Carefully remove and discard the supernatant without disturbing the pellet. The cell pellet is either used immediately for immunoprecipitation or snap frozen in liquid nitrogen and stored at −80 °C until use.

3.2 Cell Lysis and RNA Immunoprecipitation

1. Thaw frozen cell pellet on ice; for the next steps proceed in the cold room and work on ice.
2. While waiting for the samples to thaw, begin to wash the IgG Sepharose beads.
3. Transfer 200 μl IgG Sepharose bead suspension to a polyprep chromatography column. Add 8 ml of IP buffer (*see* Subheading 2.3), mix slowly on a rotator in the cold room for 5 min and stand on a column holder to let the beads settle (~5 min) at the bottom. Remove the cap at the bottom of the column to discard the wash solution by gravity flow.

4. Repeat the washing step one more time. While waiting for the beads to settle, begin to lyse the cell pellet.
5. For lysis, resuspend each sample with 4 ml of cold lysis buffer (*see* Subheading 2.3), to then lyse the cells by passing 15–20 times through a 21 G needle.
6. Clear the cell lysate by spinning down at 15,000 × *g* for 10 min at 4 °C.
7. Transfer the supernatant to a new Falcon tube, measure the volume (~3.5 ml are collected) and then adjust NaCl concentration to 150 mM (lysis buffer already contains 10 mM of NaCl; add 35 μl of 4 M NaCl per ml of lysis buffer).
8. Take 20 μl of the lysate from each sample, transfer to an Eppendorf tube and then resuspend in 5 μl of 4× Laemmli buffer. This serves as the input (I) sample for Western blot analysis.
9. Incubate the rest of the cell lysate with the washed IgG Sepharose beads (*see* Subheading 2.3) and mix slowly on a mini-rotator for 2 h at 4 °C.
10. After incubation, leave the beads to settle at the bottom of column for 10 min, then collect the flow through (FT) into a new falcon tube and keep it on ice (a sample aliquot is taken as described in **step 8** above; this forms the FT sample for immunoblotting).
11. Wash the beads three times with 8 ml of IP buffer and one time with 8 ml of TEV cleavage buffer (*see* Subheading 2.3).
12. To elute RNA–RBP complex, add 1 ml TEV cleavage buffer containing 150 U of TEV protease, mix slowly on a mini-rotator for 2–3 h at 4 °C (or shorter times if incubation temperature is higher). *See* **Note 4**.
13. After incubation, collect the TEV eluate by gravity into a new tube and keep it on ice (take ~1.5% of the TEV eluate (E) sample for Western blotting).
14. Transfer the rest of the TEV eluate sample into an Eppendorf tube and then incubate with proteinase K to digest the cross-linked protein. To 100 μl of the TEV eluate sample add 50 μg of proteinase K, 8 mM EDTA, and 0.2% SDS. Incubate at 42 °C for 30 min. Do the same with 500 μl of the flow through sample (scale up proteinase K reaction accordingly) collected in **step 10**. This sample serves as a background control and is used to estimate transcript enrichment by subsequent RNA-seq or qPCR.
15. After proteinase K treatment, RNA is isolated from both eluate and flow through fractions using Trifast FL reagent.

16. To 250 μl of proteinase K treated sample add 750 μl of Trifast FL reagent, and perform RNA extraction following the manufacturer's protocol. Trifast reagent is phenol based and the procedure requires chloroform; therefore, RNA isolation must be carried under a fume hood. During RNA precipitation, add glycogen/glycoblue to help visualize trace amounts of RNA.
17. Dissolve recovered RNA in 10 μl of water and quantify (*see* **Note 5**). Concentration of the bound RNA is usually very low (0.25–1 μg per purification). RNA samples are kept at −80 °C for long-term storage.

3.3 Important Controls

1. Assess the efficiency of the pulldown by Western blot analysis of the collected samples (input, flow-through, and eluate) as shown in Fig. 1a. The flow-through must show more than 50% target protein depletion to follow up with RNA analysis.
2. Check the quality of the purified RNA (input, flow-through, and eluate samples) by Northern blotting (Fig. 1b). To detect ribosomal RNA (rRNA), the formaldehyde gel is stained with ethidium bromide. Alternatively, after blotting onto Nytran membranes stain the blot with methylene blue. Three rRNA

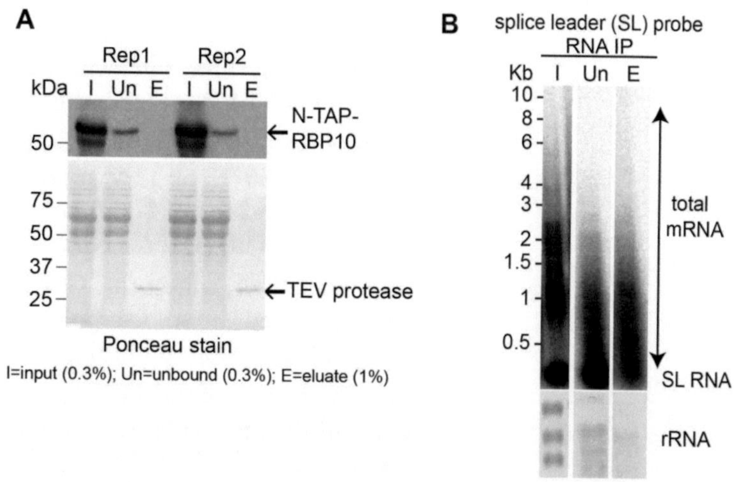

Fig. 1 Purification of mRNAs bound by RBP10. (**a**) Cells expressing TAP-tagged RBP10 were UV-irradiated, protein was affinity-purified with IgG, samples were run on a denaturing SDS-PAGE and protein detected with rabbit anti-PAP antibody. "I" refers to the input (cell lysate), "Un" (unbound) refers to the unbound fraction and "E" (eluate) refers to the bound fraction. Each sample represents approximately the same number of input trypanosomes. Ponceau staining served as loading control. (**b**) The recovered RNA fractions after proteinase K treatment from all three samples were analyzed by Northern blot. Total mRNA was detected by hybridization with a splice leader probe and ribosomal RNAs stained by methylene blue. Only slight degradation on mRNA is detected

bands should be present in the input and flow-through samples; none should be detected in the eluate sample unless the RBP of interest binds rRNAs. The blot is then hybridized with gene specific probes in case RNA targets are known, or with either an abundant and unspecific probe (e.g., tubulin) or with a splice leader probe for a global overview of the transcripts. These controls are relevant to check both RNA integrity and specificity of the assay.

3. To identify common contaminants (sticky transcripts), a pull-down is performed using parental cells (where RBP of interest is untagged) or cells where unrelated protein is tagged.

3.4 Computational Analysis

Although the bioinformatics analysis is fundamental to this protocol, it is not described here. Chapter 6 (Mulindwa et al.) in this volume provides a detailed discussion and further considerations on both sample preparation and bioinformatics analysis. Although DEseq program [10] may not appear applicable to RIP-Seq analysis, it has proven useful to us. As an alternative approach, ASPeak [11] or RIPSeeker [12] may serve as better options as these methods determine local, strand-specific enrichment of RBP binding relative to an empirically measured background.

3.5 Motif Discovery

We normally use the MEME suite software (http://meme-suite.org) to discover the motifs (if any) into the protein-bound RNAs [13]. The MEME program is not only powerful but also extremely easy to run on a web browser. It only considers the RNA sequence and not the structure for which many other alternatives exist [14]. Despite ignoring secondary structure, the method is often successful, presumably because many RBPs generally bind short ungapped RNA sequences. DREME, another MEME suite package, may also be used to discover short motifs relatively faster than MEME with the advantage that can handle much larger datasets. This is a very brief summary of how to use the public MEME web application to discover motifs in your sequence data.

1. Open the MEME web application (http://meme-suite.org/tools/meme) in your web browser.
2. In the section titled "Input the primary sequences" you may upload a FASTA file containing your sequences by selecting "Upload sequences" and setting the name of the file containing your sequence data in the box labeled "Choose File." Alternatively, you can paste the sequence data directly into a text box by selecting "Type in sequences." The sequences you type in must be in FASTA format, including the header lines. The sequences to be analyzed are downloaded from TriTrypDB [15]. In general, the motifs are localized into the 3′UTR so we normally start the analysis by downloading all the 3′UTR sequences >20 nts. For the missing 3′UTR, manual annotation

can be done using the RNA-Seq reads and/or detected poly (A) sites available at TriTrypDB's databases or alternatively, simply using 200 nts downstream of each ORF. As background control, a list containing 3′UTRs from the unbound mRNAs may be used.

3. Set the motif discovery mode. Here the user provide one set of sequences and MEME discovers motifs enriched in this set (Classic mode) or more conveniently, provide two set of sequences, and MEME discovers motifs that are enriched in the first (Elution) set relative to the second (Flow-through) (possible on both "Discriminative" or "Differential Enrichment" modes).
4. Set the site distribution model:

   If you expect each sequence to contain one or zero instances of a particular motif, select the "Zero or one per sequence" model. This is the default, and usually a good starting point. If you expect each sequence to contain any number of instances of a motif, select the "Any number of repetitions" model.
5. Adjust any of the other parameters on the page. The quality and quantity of MEME's output is quite sensitive to its search parameters and using the defaults is usually a good starting point.
6. Click on the "Start Search" button. You will be sent an e-mail with a link to your job's results.

By default, MEME will find three motifs. You should always check the *E*-value of the motifs found by MEME as sometimes the motifs found will not be statistically significant. Generally, biologically relevant motifs have really small E-values. The user must have in mind that not all sequences obtained in the elution (or negative control) are needed to find a motif. It is better to have as input, a clean sequence set and to remove sequences which look unusual or repetitive as this would override any differences in specific motifs. Although identifying bona fide RNA-binding sites can be challenging, the protocol described here is a good starting point and may provide a first hint on the motifs or regions involved. To identify functional interactions from a vast number of targets (and probable sites) identified in RIP-Seq screens it is good idea to integrate diverse layers of complementary information. For instance, knockdown or overexpression of the RBP of interest followed by global transcriptome analyses can not only provide new biological insights but also deliver an integrated view of the posttranscriptional regulatory network [9, 16].

4 Notes

1. The TAP tag consists of two IgG binding domains of *Staphylococcus aureus* protein A (ProtA) and a calmodulin binding peptide (CBP) separated by a TEV protease cleavage site. The TAP tag approach is advantageous because it also allows for the isolation of protein complexes at high purity [17]. Any other tag providing means of removing the intact mRNP complex from the beads by competitive elution may be used (flag, myc, HA, etc.). We prefer to use the N-terminal tag as this maintains expression of the target protein under the control of its natural 3′UTR, hence maintains endogenous levels of mRNA and protein (unless protein degradation is affected). Knocking out the second allele is optional but it ensures the in situ tagged protein is functional (if the gene is essential) and implies that virtually all the target mRNP should be recovered.
2. The amount of the starting material has to be determined experimentally due to the variations of both RBP abundance and target mRNAs. We found 1–3 $\times$ 10^9 cells at mid-log phase (0.8–1 $\times$ 10^6 cells/ml) to be sufficient for most RBPs tested in our group. In general, more material is needed for proteins with destabilizing effect on targets or for components of the degradation machinery.
3. Keep the petri dishes containing cells on a tray half filled with ice to maintain cold conditions during cross-linking. It is important to process the cells quickly; therefore, if you are dealing with a large number of cells, proceed with small sets while leaving the remaining in culture. The use of UV cross-linking is advised, as it was demonstrated that mRNPs complexes might arise from associations generated after cell lysis, potentially misleading the true landscape of the RNA–protein interactions that occurs in vivo [5]. Also, by fixing the protein–RNA interactions by UV, potentially more stringent washes can be performed decreasing the background signal while capturing also weak interactions. On the other hand, the use of UV cross-linking requires additional manipulation of the sample, which increases the processing time and may adversely affect the quality of isolated RNA. We have successfully performed RIP-Seq analysis on both conditions (i.e., we have identified real mRNA targets); however, we have not compared this systematically.
4. The duration of the cleavage reaction is empirically determined. We have observed that 3 h at 16 °C or 1.5 h at room temperature typically digest >90% of the TEV-fusion protein.

5. Since the expected RNA concentration in the eluates is low, it is recommended to quantify the sample with Qubit Fluorometer or similar device. In this range of concentration, NanoDrop generally overestimates the amount.

Acknowledgments

We thank Christine Clayton for her continuous support and all former and current CC lab members who have contributed to improve this and many other techniques.

References

1. Tenenbaum SA, Carson CC, Lager PJ et al (2000) Identifying mRNA subsets in messenger ribonucleoprotein complexes by using cDNA arrays. Proc Natl Acad Sci U S A 97:14085–14090
2. Licatalosi DD, Mele A, Fak JJ et al (2008) HITS-CLIP yields genome-wide insights into brain alternative RNA processing. Nature 456:464–469
3. Hafner M, Landthaler M, Burger L et al (2010) Transcriptome-wide identification of RNA-binding protein and microRNA target sites by PAR-CLIP. Cell 141:129–141
4. Konig J, Zarnack K, Rot G et al (2010) iCLIP reveals the function of hnRNP particles in splicing at individual nucleotide resolution. Nat Struct Mol Biol 17:909–915
5. Mili S, Steitz JA (2004) Evidence for reassociation of RNA-binding proteins after cell lysis: implications for the interpretation of immunoprecipitation analyses. RNA 10:1692–1694
6. Droll D, Minia I, Fadda A et al (2013) Post-transcriptional regulation of the trypanosome heat shock response by a zinc finger protein. PLoS Pathog 9:e1003286
7. Minia I, Clayton C (2016) Regulating a post-transcriptional regulator: protein phosphorylation, degradation and translational blockage in control of the trypanosome stress-response RNA-binding protein ZC3H11. PLoS Pathog 12:e1005514
8. Minia I, Merce C, Terrao M et al (2016) Translation regulation and RNA granule formation after heat shock of procyclic form *Trypanosoma brucei*: many heat-induced mRNAs are also increased during differentiation to mammalian-infective forms. PLoS Negl Trop Dis 10:e0004982
9. Mugo E, Clayton C (2017) Expression of the RNA-binding protein RBP10 promotes the bloodstream-form differentiation state in *Trypanosoma brucei*. PLoS Pathog 13:e1006560
10. Anders S, Huber W (2010) Differential expression analysis for sequence count data. Genome Biol 11:R106
11. Kucukural A, Ozadam H, Singh G et al (2013) ASPeak: an abundance sensitive peak detection algorithm for RIP-Seq. Bioinformatics 29:2485–2486
12. Li Y, Zhao DY, Greenblatt JF et al (2013) RIPSeeker: a statistical package for identifying protein-associated transcripts from RIP-Seq experiments. Nucleic Acids Res 41:e94
13. Bailey TL, Boden M, Buske FA et al (2009) MEME SUITE: tools for motif discovery and searching. Nucleic Acids Res 37:W202–W208
14. Achar A, Saetrom P (2015) RNA motif discovery: a computational overview. Biol Direct 10:61
15. Aslett M, Aurrecoechea C, Berriman M et al (2010) TriTrypDB: a functional genomic resource for the Trypanosomatidae. Nucleic Acids Res 38:D457–D462
16. Najafabadi HS, Lu Z, MacPherson C et al (2013) Global identification of conserved post-transcriptional regulatory programs in trypanosomatids. Nucleic Acids Res 41: D8591–D8600
17. Puig O, Caspary F, Rigaut G et al (2001) The tandem affinity purification (TAP) method: a general procedure of protein complex purification. Methods 24:218–229

Chapter 18

The Tethering Assay: A Simple Method for the Characterization of mRNA-Fate Regulators

Elisha Mugo and Esteban D. Erben

Abstract

In trypanosomatids, posttranscriptional controls are very important in regulation of individual gene expression. These are achieved through combinatorial sets of RNA-binding proteins (RBPs) which recognize RNA regulatory motifs or regions of secondary structure within RNAs. To analyze the potential functional impact of an RBP on their mRNA targets, we have applied a robust technique called tethering assay. In this method, the protein under study is attached to an mRNA reporter through an artificial RNA–protein interaction. Therefore, the functional activity of a protein can be analyzed independently of its intrinsic ability to bind to RNA. By making use of a cell line expressing a chloramphenicol acetyltransferase (CAT) reporter mRNA, we have characterized dozens of novel mRNA-fate regulators in cultured *Trypanosoma brucei*. After induction of the candidate fusion protein, the effect on the reporter expression is determined by a rapid CAT assay. The protocol is simple and typically takes one working day for analysis of a single protein and controls. In this chapter, we provide a description of materials and methods for the tethering method and should allow the assay to be successfully deployed in any laboratory with minimal user training.

Key words Tethering, RNA-binding proteins, mRNA fate, Lambda N-peptide, Translation, RNA stability

1 Introduction

Much, if not all of the control of gene expression of developmentally regulated genes in *Trypanosoma brucei* is conferred via cis-regulatory elements in the untranslated region (UTR) of a given mRNA [1]. These cis-regulatory elements may be recognized by RNA-binding proteins (RBPs) dictating transcript localization, stability and/or translation in a specific spatiotemporal manner. Whereas by bioinformatics analysis, more than 150 RBPs were inferred to exist in the *T. brucei* genome, system-wide identification of RBPs by interactome capture in the bloodstream form increased this number to far more than 200 proteins [2, 3]. To address the role of specific mRNA-fate regulators on mRNA metabolism and function we normally perform a tethering function assay [4– 12]. The method, originally

Paul A. M. Michels et al. (eds.), *Trypanosomatids: Methods and Protocols*, Methods in Molecular Biology, vol. 2116, https://doi.org/10.1007/978-1-0716-0294-2_18,

devised to analyze the role of poly A-binding protein (PABP) on mRNA stability [13], provides a simple means to the study of suspect regulators of mRNA metabolism that have unknown target specificity and/or functional activity [14]. In this technique, the protein under study is brought to the UTR of an mRNA reporter through an artificial RNA-protein interaction. Hence, the functional activity of a protein can be studied independent of its intrinsic ability to bind to RNA. This assay has been applied successfully for numerous proteins in diverse organisms and in *T. brucei* has proven useful in (1) the identification of posttranscriptional mRNA regulators [2, 4, 6–10], (2) mapping of functional domains [5, 12], and (3) for dissecting functional maps of protein complexes [11].

Although there are several alternatives for the tether of the fusion protein, we make use of the bacteriophage lambda-N protein. The N-protein regulates bacterial transcriptional antitermination by binding to a 15-nucleotide RNA hairpin, called boxB, within nascent transcripts. We have chosen the N-protein for its small size (22 amino acids) and its high affinity for the boxB RNA (K_d = 22 nM in vitro) [15]. The choice of reporter mRNA is dictated by the effect to be assayed, and so far, we have successfully used the following as reporters for mRNA-fate regulators: blasticidin resistance gene (Blasticidin S-deaminase, BSD), phosphoglycerate kinase B (PGKB), green fluorescent protein (GFP) and more generally, chloramphenicol acetyltransferase (CAT) [4–12]. The use of CAT as reporter has several advantages: the *CAT* gene is not endogenous to trypanosomatids, the enzyme can be easily assayed, and minute amounts of activity are rapidly detectable. Here we present a detailed protocol to perform a tethering assay to find proteins implicated in posttranscriptional regulation in *Trypanosoma brucei.*

2 Materials

Prepare all solutions using ultrapure water and analytical grade reagents. Disposal of radioactive wastes must be in accordance with radiation protection regulations.

2.1 Reagents

1. 1× Phosphate-buffered saline (PBS): Add about 800 ml water to a 1 L beaker. Weigh 8 g NaCl, 0.2 g of KCl, 1.44 g of Na_2HPO_4, 0.24 g of KH_2PO_4. Mix and adjust pH 7.4 with HCl. Make up to 1 L with water. Dispense the solution into aliquots and sterilize by autoclaving (20 min, 121 °C, liquid cycle). Store at room temperature.

2. CAT assay buffer (100 mM Tris–HCl buffer, pH 7.8). Add about 80 ml water to a 0.2 L beaker. Weigh 1.21 g Tris base. Mix and adjust pH with concentrated 12.1 N HCl (about 559 μl). Make up to 100 ml with water. Autoclave and store at 4 °C.
3. Tetracycline solution: Weigh 50 mg tetracycline, transfer to a 15 ml Falcon tube and add 10 ml ethanol to make a 5 mg/ml solution. Make aliquots and keep solution at −20 °C. Protect from light.
4. Chloramphenicol solution: Weigh 4 mg chloramphenicol, transfer to a 15 ml Falcon tube and add 10 ml ethanol to make a 0.4 mg/ml solution. Make aliquots and keep solution at −20 °C.
5. Protease inhibitors.
6. Butyryl-1-^{14}C-CoA. To make the working solution, dilute stock to 10 μCi/ml in 10 mM sodium acetate (pH 5.0). Make aliquots and store them at −80 °C.
7. Scintillation Cocktail (e.g., Ultima Gold F, PerkinElmer).
8. Scintillation vials.
9. Bradford reagent.
10. BSA 100 μg/ml.

2.2 Equipment

1. Scintillation counter (e.g., LS6000IC, Beckman).
2. Spectrophotometer.

3 Methods

3.1 Construction of a CAT Reporter-Expressing Cell Line

The procedures used in the assembling of cell strains are standard in the field of molecular parasitology and are not described here. The CAT-expressing vectors may be inserted into the tubulin locus or rDNA intergenic region allowing its constitutive transcription by Pol II or Pol I, respectively. These plasmids have five copies (or none for the negative control) of the lambda N-peptide recognition site *boxB* inserted immediately between the CAT reporter sequence and the *actin* 3′UTR [2, 4, 6, 7]. The *actin* 3′UTR was chosen because it is well-characterized and not developmentally regulated. For expression of lambda fusion proteins, the genes of interest are cloned into the pHD1743, so that the resulting plasmid encodes a fusion protein, lambdaN-ORF-myc. The expression of the transgene is driven by the *EP* promoter and is regulated by tetracycline. Alternatively, we have assembled plasmids that incorporate the Gateway cassette, which may facilitate the effort required for cloning [2, 6].

3.2 Important Controls

It is necessary to confirm that (1) the overexpressed tethered protein alone does not have an impact on cell growth, and (2) any observed change on reporter activity should occur only in cis (that is, when the protein is bound to the mRNA). To control for possible effect on cell growth, the impact of the fusion protein overexpression on cell proliferation needs to be evaluated. To control for possible trans-acting effects, the fusion protein is expressed alongside a reporter that lacks the *boxB* binding sites. We generally include also the tethering of a "neutral" protein such as GFP, with little to none effect on reporter expression. This set of controls can ensure that an observed effect is specific to the protein of interest, and occurs only when it is associated with the mRNA [14, 16].

3.3 Assay of Chloramphenicol Acetyltransferase (CAT Assay)

The rapid two-phase CAT assay described here utilizes butyryl Coenzyme A (CoA) as the labeled substrate. In this assay, the ^{14}C-labeled butyryl group of butyryl CoA is transferred to the chloramphenicol molecule by the CAT enzyme. While the butyryl CoA remains in the aqueous phase so it does not give any scintillation, the ^{14}C-labeled butyryl-chloramphenicol turns more hydrophobic and diffuses linearly over time into the organic phase of the cocktail. Direct liquid scintillation counting of the two-phase reaction mix in the vial provides quantitative data reflecting the CAT activity. Thus, the rate of the enzymatic reaction is directly proportional to the concentration of CAT protein in the sample. This assay can be completed in few hours, is linear over a wide range of magnitude and can detect tiny amounts of CAT.

1. For a single CAT assay, harvest about 1×10^7 trypanosomes (~10 ml) from tetracycline induced and uninduced cultures at mid-log phase by centrifugation at 1000 × *g* for 5 min at 4 °C. Be sure to include also trypanosomes that did receive and did not receive a CAT gene as these are your reference and negative control, respectively (*see* Subheading 3.2 and **Note 1**).
2. Discard supernatant from cell pellet and resuspend in 1 ml cold PBS and transfer to an Eppendorf tube.
3. Spin down the cells at 1000 × *g* at 4 °C for 5 min and repeat the wash once more with PBS.
4. Resuspend the cell pellet by pipetting with 200 μl of CAT assay buffer supplemented with protease inhibitors and snap-freeze the cells into liquid nitrogen. Thaw samples on ice (thawing takes a few minutes). Vortex briefly.
5. Repeat freeze–thaw cycle one more time.
6. Centrifuge the cell lysates at 10,000 × *g* for 3 min at 4 °C and transfer the supernatant to a new Eppendorf microfuge tube. At this point, all cell extracts can be frozen, or they can be processed immediately.

7. Determine protein concentration by Bradford assay. For this, prepare a standard curve by pipetting into 1 ml cuvettes, 800 µl of water containing 0, 1, 2, 4, 8, 12, 16, and 20 µg of BSA (from a 100 µg/ml stock). For each cell lysate, add 5 µl sample into 795 µl of water. To each cuvette, add 200 µl of Bradford reagent, mix by pipetting and incubate for 5 min at room temperature. Set the spectrophotometer to 595 nm. Zero the instrument with the blank sample and measure the absorbance of the standards and unknown samples.

3.3.1 Radioactive Kinetic Assay

1. Make up a master mix as follows, in a 5 ml tube:
   2 ml of CAT assay buffer.

   20 µl of 40 mg/ml chloramphenicol stock solution.

   100 µl Butyryl-1-^{14}C-CoA working solution.

   This is enough for nine assays [i.e., three samples induced/uninduced plus negative control (GFP) and blank (cells without CAT)].
2. Distribute 1–2 µg of cell extract into labeled microfuge tubes filled with up to 50 µl CAT buffer at 4 °C (*see* **Note 2**).
3. To each tube add 200 µl master mix and transfer immediately to a prelabeled scintillation vial. From now on everything is radioactive so should be treated appropriately.
4. Gently overlay with 4 ml scintillation cocktail and put on the vial caps without mixing.
5. Load vials into the scintillation counter and start measurement on the ^{14}C channel as soon as possible. Counting will be repeated approximately every 20–30 min to get a time course of the reaction (*see* **Note 3**).
6. Work out the relative CAT activity for each sample.

3.3.2 CAT Activity Quantification

Analysis of the data for the CAT analysis is best done on a spreadsheet like Excel. A specific example on the activation of CAT expression along six time points by the protein Tb927.7.2780 is shown in Fig. 1. We normally include, together with the induced and uninduced samples, cells that carry (reference) and do not carry the CAT enzyme (blank). The slopes are calculated easily and normalized to the reference value (*see* **Notes 4** and **5**).

4 Notes

1. While we routinely induce protein synthesis overnight for ~18–24 h, different time points may be evaluated depending on the assay evaluated. For instance, tethering of the

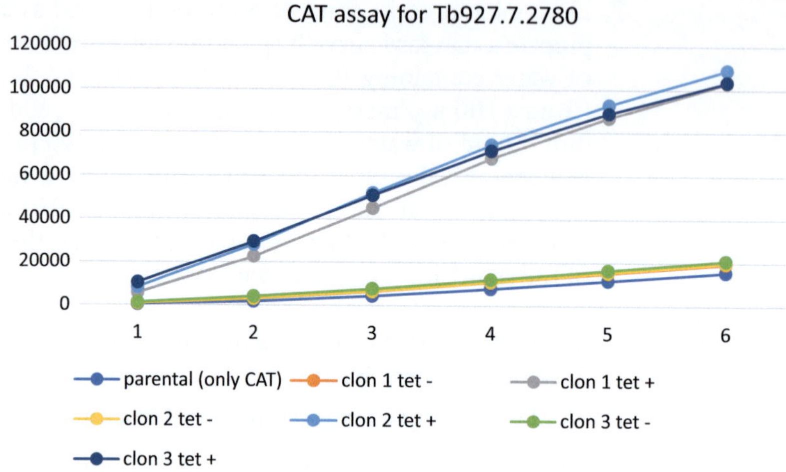

Fig. 1 Data spreadsheet from the CAT assay analysis of reporter cells expressing lambda-tagged Tb927.7.2780. Expression of CAT in cells expressing Tb927.7.2780 protein was assayed after 24 h tetracycline induction and CAT activities were calculated relative to a control with no lambda-N protein as described

cap-binding complex factor 4EIP to a CAT reporter for 24 h, decreases the mRNA reporter level to <10% which may be difficult to detect.

2. The volume used can also vary but do not exceed 50 μl. Note the protein amount required will depend on the expected CAT activity. For instance, use more protein if working with a protein known to be a repressor of gene expression or a component of the degradation machinery.
3. CAT assays are performed in the linear range of the assay.
4. The use of lambda-GFP as reference protein is convenient when the clones are leaky (i.e., when display active transcription even in the absence of tetracycline) which makes relative CAT activity measures difficult to normalize.
5. The activity of the test protein might be context dependent. Therefore, negative results (i.e., absence of an effect after tethering) does not mean necessarily the putative RBP is inactive or nonfunctional.

Acknowledgments

We thank Christine Clayton for her continuous support and all former and current CC lab members who have contributed to improve this and many other techniques.

References

1. Clayton C (2013) The regulation of trypanosome gene expression by RNA-binding proteins. PLoS Pathog 9:e1003680
2. Lueong S, Merce C, Fischer B, Hoheisel JD, Erben ED (2016) Gene expression regulatory networks in *Trypanosoma brucei*: insights into the role of the mRNA-binding proteome. Mol Microbiol 100:457–471
3. Erben ED (2018) High-throughput methods for dissection of trypanosome gene regulatory networks. Curr Genomics 19:78–86
4. Wurst M, Seliger B, Jha BA, Klein C, Queiroz R, Clayton C (2012) Expression of the RNA recognition motif protein RBP10 promotes a bloodstream-form transcript pattern in *Trypanosoma brucei*. Mol Microbiol 83:1048–1063
5. Mugo E, Clayton C (2017) Expression of the RNA-binding protein RBP10 promotes the bloodstream-form differentiation state in *Trypanosoma brucei*. PLoS Pathog 13:e1006560
6. Erben ED, Fadda A, Lueong S, Hoheisel JD, Clayton C (2014) A genome-wide tethering screen reveals novel potential post-transcriptional regulators in *Trypanosoma brucei*. PLoS Pathog 10:e1004178
7. Delhi P, Queiroz R, Inchaustegui D, Carrington M, Clayton C (2011) Is there a classical nonsense-mediated decay pathway in trypanosomes? PLoS One 6:e25112
8. Droll D, Minia I, Fadda A, Singh A, Stewart M, Queiroz R, Clayton C (2013) Post-transcriptional regulation of the trypanosome heat shock response by a zinc finger protein. PLoS Pathog 9:e1003286
9. Chakraborty C, Clayton C (2018) Stress susceptibility in *Trypanosoma brucei* lacking the RNA-binding protein ZC3H30. PLoS Negl Trop Dis 12:e0006835
10. Ouna BA, Stewart M, Helbig C, Clayton C (2012) The *Trypanosoma brucei* CCCH zinc finger proteins ZC3H12 and ZC3H13. Mol Biochem Parasitol 183:184–188
11. Farber V, Erben E, Sharma S, Stoecklin G, Clayton C (2013) Trypanosome CNOT10 is essential for the integrity of the NOT deadenylase complex and for degradation of many mRNAs. Nucleic Acids Res 41:1211–1222
12. Singh A, Minia I, Droll D, Fadda A, Clayton C, Erben E (2014) Trypanosome MKT1 and the RNA-binding protein ZC3H11: interactions and potential roles in post-transcriptional regulatory networks. Nucleic Acids Res 42:4652–4668
13. Coller JM, Gray NK, Wickens MP (1998) mRNA stabilization by poly(A) binding protein is independent of poly(A) and requires translation. Genes Dev 12:3226–3235
14. Coller J, Wickens M (2002) Tethered function assays using 3′ untranslated regions. Methods 26:142–150
15. Austin RJ, Xia T, Ren J, Takahashi TT, Roberts RW (2002) Designed arginine-rich RNA-binding peptides with picomolar affinity. J Am Chem Soc 124:10966–10967
16. Coller J, Wickens M (2007) Tethered function assays: an adaptable approach to study RNA regulatory proteins. Methods Enzymol 429:299–321

Chapter 19

RNA-Binding Proteins and Their Targets in *Trypanosoma brucei*: Single Nucleotide Resolution Using iCLIP and iCLAP

Sameer Dixit, Juan D. Alfonzo, and Julius Lukeš

Abstract

RNA-binding proteins (RBPs) are critical to posttranscriptional gene regulation. Therefore, characterization of the RNA molecules bound by RBPs in vivo represent a key step in elucidating their function. The recently developed iCLIP technique allows single nucleotide resolution of the RNA binding footprints of RBPs. We present the iCLIP technique modified for its application to *Trypanosoma brucei* and most likely other kinetoplastid flagellates. By using the immuno- or affinity purification approach, it was successfully applied to the analysis of several RBPs. Furthermore, we also provide a detailed description of the iCLIP/iCLAP protocol that shall be particularly suitable for the studies of trypanosome RBPs.

Key words RNA-binding proteins (RBPs), iCLIP, iCLAP, Posttranscriptional gene regulation

1 Introduction

Posttranscriptional gene regulation is critical for the maintenance and control of gene expression levels [1]. Interestingly, *Trypanosoma brucei* lacks regulation at the transcriptional level, which means that it has to rely extensively on posttranscriptional mechanisms [2]. Numerous RNA-binding proteins (RBPs) are known to be involved in posttranscriptional gene regulation [3]. To elucidate the role of a given RBP, it is important to characterize its RNA targets in vivo. However, initially developed approaches such as RIP-sequencing lack sufficient resolution and specificity to identify binding sites of the studied RBPs [4]. The relatively recently established in vivo UV cross-linking and immunoprecipitation (CLIP) technique provides high specificity and single nucleotide resolution [5]. Still, a significant drawback of the CLIP protocol is the use of 3′ and 5′ adapters during library preparation. This feature makes the CLIP protocol insufficient in capturing truncated cDNAs at the reverse transcriptase step. Hence, a CLIP variant called individual-nucleotide resolution CLIP (iCLIP) has been developed, which

Paul A. M. Michels et al. (eds.), *Trypanosomatids: Methods and Protocols*, Methods in Molecular Biology, vol. 2116, https://doi.org/10.1007/978-1-0716-0294-2_19,

uses 3′ adapters and incorporates a circularization step that allows an efficient capture of truncated cDNAs [6].

Most of the abovementioned techniques were developed in cells that lacked flagella and consequently were immotile. We have successfully applied the iCLIP technique and its variant that uses a two-step-based affinity purification (iCLAP) to the study of three RBPs that participate in the uridine-insertion/deletion type of RNA editing in the mitochondrion of *T. brucei* [7, 8]. While our protocol for the iCLIP library preparation remains generally the same as the original iCLIP protocol developed previously [9], some modifications have been made. Hence, we provide the iCLIP or iCLAP protocols that can be easily applied to the studies of RBPs in *T. brucei* and other kinetoplastid flagellates.

2 Materials

2.1 iCLIP Buffers

1. iCLIP lysis buffer: 100 mM Tris–HCl (pH 7.5), 100 mM NaCl, 0.1% SDS, 1% NP-40, 1× protease inhibitor (freshly prepared).
2. iCLIP high-salt wash buffer: 100 mM Tris–HCl (pH 7.5), 1 M NaCl, 1 mM EDTA, 1% NP-40, 0.1% SDS.
3. PNK buffer: 20 mM Tris–HCl (pH 7.5), 10 mM $MgCl_2$, 0.2% Tween 20.
4. PK buffer: 100 mM Tris–HCl (pH 7.5), 50 mM NaCl, 10 mM EDTA.

2.2 iCLAP Buffers

1. iCLAP lysis buffer: 50 mM Tris–HCl (pH 7.5), 1.5 mM $MgCl_2$, 10% glycerol, 250 mM NaCl, 0.5% NP-40, 0.1% SDS, 2.5 mM beta-mercaptoethanol (freshly prepared), 1× protease inhibitor (freshly prepared).
2. iCLAP wash buffer: 50 mM Tris–HCl (pH 7.5), 300 mM NaCl, 0.1% NP-40, 2.5 mM beta-mercaptoethanol.
3. TEV cleavage buffer: 50 mM Tris–HCl (pH 7.5), 100 mM NaCl, 0.1% NP-40, 2.5 mM beta-mercaptoethanol.
4. His-binding buffer: 50 mM Tris–HCl (pH 7.5), 100 mM NaCl, 0.1% NP-40, 10 mM imidazole.
5. Urea buffer: 50 mM Tris–HCl (pH 7.5), 100 mM NaCl, 0.1% NP-40, 10 mM imidazole, 7 M urea.
6. PNK buffer: 20 mM Tris–HCl (pH 7.5), 10 mM $MgCl_2$, 0.2% Tween 20.
7. PK buffer: 100 mM Tris–HCl (pH 7.5), 50 mM NaCl, 1 mM EDTA.

2.3 UV-Cross Linking

Stratalinker UV cross-linker 2400, Protease inhibitor cocktail, IgG Sepharose beads, Anti-RNase, RNAse I, Turbo DNase, T4 PNK plus 10× PNK buffer, RNasin, Protein spin columns, T4 RNA Ligase I, γ-^{32}P-ATP, Phosphate buffered saline (PBS), Falcon tubes, Shrimp alkaline phosphatase, Protein G Dynabeads, IgG Sepharose 6 fast flow affinity resin, His-Tag Isolation Dynabeads.

2.4 SDS-PAGE and Nitrocellulose Transfer

4–12% NuPAGE gels, electrophoresis chamber, transfer apparatus (Life Technologies), LDS-4X sample buffer, prestained protein marker, nitrocellulose membrane, sponge pads for XCell II blotting, 20× transfer buffer, 20× MOPS-SDS running buffer, Whatman filter paper GE Healthcare, Film (Fuji).

2.5 RNA Isolation

Proteinase K, 19 G syringe needles, phenol and chloroform, phase lock gel heavy tube (VWR), glycogen, 3 M sodium acetate (pH 5.5).

2.6 Reverse Transcription

PCR tubes, dNTPs, Superscript III (Life Technologies), 5× First-strand buffer (Life Technologies), dithiothreitol, 1 M HEPES, TE buffer.

2.7 cDNA Isolation and PCR Amplification

2× TBE-urea loading buffer (Life Technologies), 6% TBE-urea precast gels (Life Technologies), low molecular weight marker, TBE running buffer, SYBR Green II (Life Technologies), 19 G syringe needle, glass prefilters (Whatman), phase lock gel heavy (VWR), Costar SpinX column (Corning Incorporation), 10× CircLigase buffer, CircLigase II (Cambio), $MnCl_2$, BamHI (Fermentas), Fast digest buffer (Fermentas), Accurprime Supermix I (Life Technologies), SYBR Green I (Life Technologies).

2.8 Trypanosome Culture

Procyclic form of *T. brucei* strain Lister 427 29-13 cell line was cultured using SDM79 with appropriate selection drugs as previously mentioned [7, 8].

3 Methods

3.1 UV Cross-Linking of T. brucei (Fig. 1): Day 0

1. Grow trypanosomes in SDM79 medium with appropriate selection by drugs to a density of 2×10^7 cells/ml.
2. Use the culture from **step 1** as a starting culture to scale up to 1000 ml. If required, add tetracycline to express protein of interest (*see* **Note 1**).
3. Harvest the cells once they reach a density of 2×10^7 cells/ml, by spinning them down at 2600 rpm (~950 rcf) for 10 min.
4. Resuspend the pellet in 20 ml of cold PBS and split it into 2×10 ml in two 15 ml Falcon tubes.

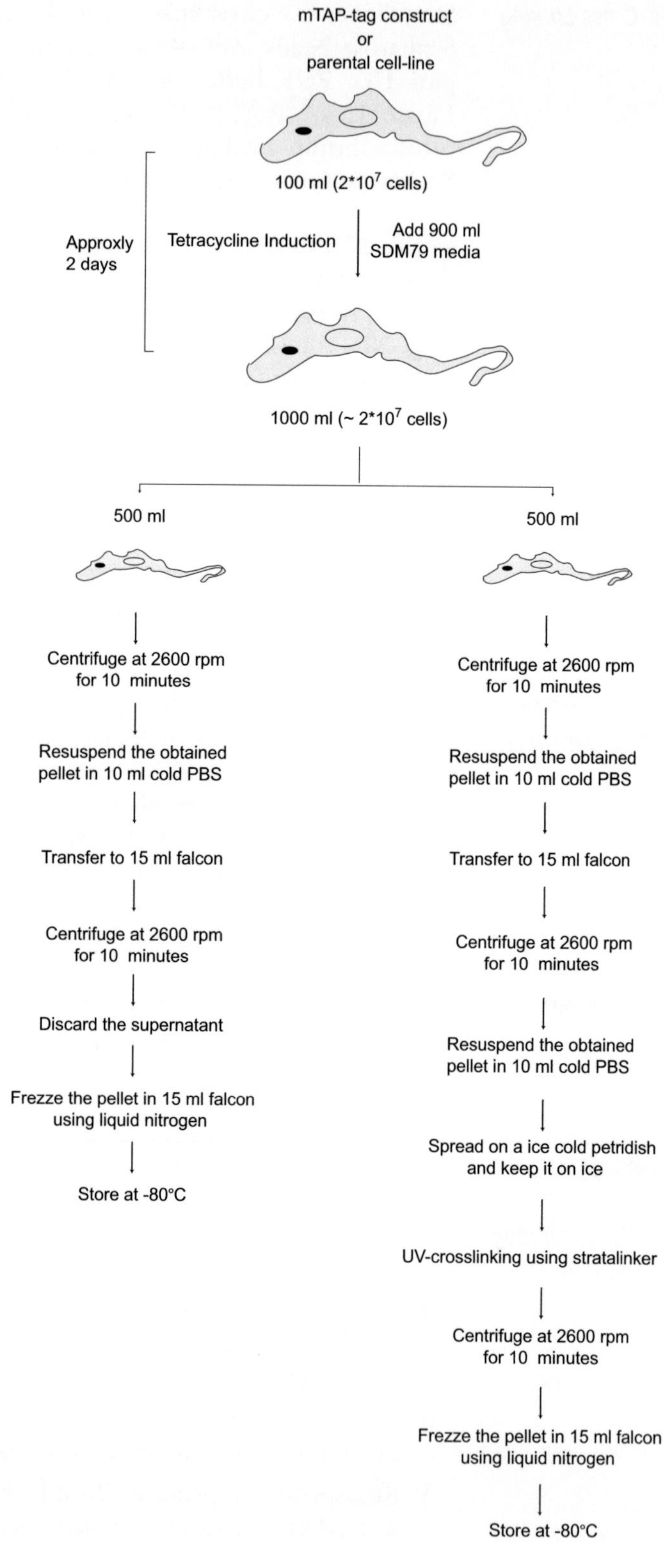

Fig. 1 Schematic depiction of the in vivo UV cross-linking protocol in trypanosomes

5. Spin both Falcon tubes at 2600 rpm (~950 rcf) for 10 min and carefully discard the supernatants.
6. Freeze one pellet in liquid nitrogen and keep it at −80 °C until use in the iCLIP experiment. Label the tube as non-UV-cross-linked pellet that is required as a negative control for the subsequent iCLIP protocol (*see* **Note 2**).
7. Resuspend the second pellet in 10 ml cold PBS and use it for UV cross-linking.
8. Spread the trypanosomes from **step 7** onto a prechilled petri dish (140 mm diameter) and keep them on ice.
9. Take the petri dish along with ice tray from **step 8** and UV irradiate trypanosomes in the Stratalinker.
10. Transfer the UV irradiated cells from the petri dish to a 15 ml Falcon tube and spin them at 2600 rpm for 10 min (*see* **Note 3**).
11. Carefully discard the supernatant and freeze the tube in liquid nitrogen. Label it as UV-cross-linked pellet and keep it at −80 °C until its use in the iCLIP experiment (*see* **Note 4**).

3.2 iCLIP (In Vivo Cross-Linking and Immunoprecipitation): Day 1 (Fig. 2)

3.2.1 Lysate Preparation

1. Thaw the UV- and non-UV-cross-linked pellets on ice (~15 min) and resuspend them in 1.5 ml cold lysis buffer, which is freshly supplemented with protease inhibitor (*see* **Note 5**).
2. Clean the sonicator tip with RNAseZap and then with milliQ water.
3. Sonicate both samples (5–10 pulses each 30 s at 50% amplitude with 20 s pause in-between) (*see* **Note 6**).
4. Transfer the lysate to a fresh 1.5 ml microcentrifuge tube and spin it for 10 min at maximum speed of 16,110 × *g* at 4 °C in a benchtop centrifuge (*see* **Note 7**).
5. Transfer the supernatant into a fresh tube (leave some to prevent carryover). We usually get enough supernatant that is diluted and used to carry out simultaneously several control immunoprecipitation assays (*see* **Note 8**).

3.2.2 Partial RNA Digestion

1. Prepare a dilution of RNAse I at 1:500 (low RNase treatment) and 1:50 (high RNase treatment) in cold lysis buffer under the hood (*see* **Note 8**).
2. Add 10 μl of low RNase I dilution (1:500) and 2 μl of Turbo DNase per 1.5 ml of freshly prepared lysate (from **step 5**, Subheading 3.2.1) (*see* **Note 9**).
3. Incubate the lysate at 37 °C for 3 min while shaking at 800 rpm in a thermomixer.
4. Place the reaction on ice for 3 min (*see* **Note 10**).

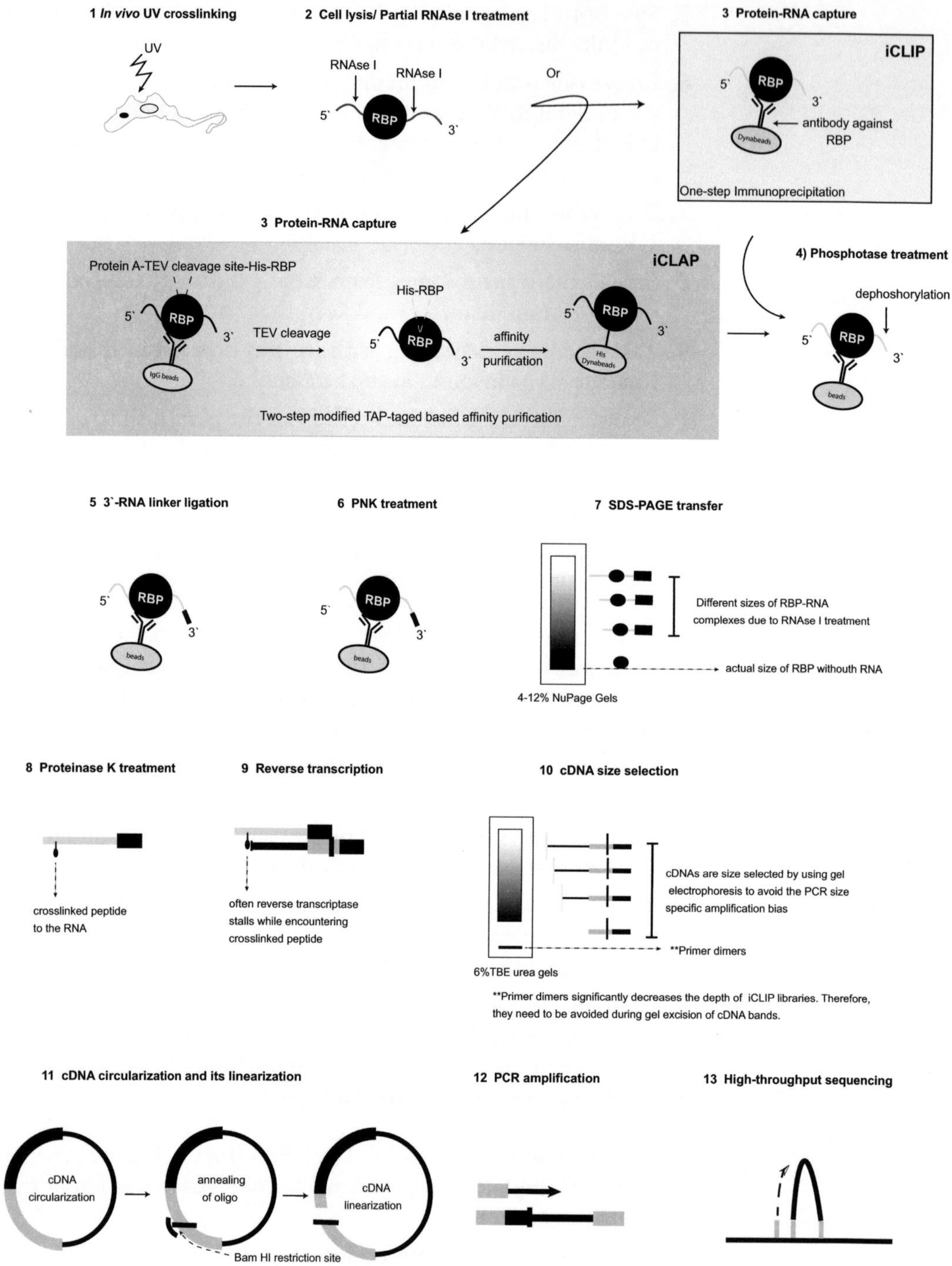

Fig. 2 Preparation of the iCLIP or iCLAP libraries

3.2.3 Bead Preparation

1. Rotate the protein G dynabeads, that come in the form of a suspension, for 5 min on a rotator. Take 100 μl of resuspended protein G dynabeads in the 1.5 ml microcentrifuge tube per immunoprecipitation (IP) assay (*see* **Note 11**).
2. Stack the microcentrifuge tube containing protein G dynabeads into the magnetic rack for 45 s (usually it takes ~45 s for the beads to settle close to the magnetic side of the microcentrifuge tube) and carefully pipette out all the residual buffer.
3. Wash the protein G dynabeads 3× with 500 μl cold lysis buffer (each wash for 5 min at 4 °C).
4. Resuspend protein G dynabeads into 200 μl cold lysis buffer and add an already optimized amount of the antibody (*see* **Note 12**).
5. Let the tube rotate for 45 min at 4 °C.
6. Wash the antibody-coupled protein G dynabeads 3× for 5 min in cold lysis buffer at 4 °C.
7. The protein G dynabeads are now ready for immunoprecipitation. Keep them on ice until you are ready to proceed to the next step.

3.2.4 Immuno-precipitation

1. Add 1.5 ml of lysate (from **step 4** of partial RNA digestion, Subheading 3.2.2) to antibody-coupled protein G dynabeads (from **step** 7 of bead preparation, Subheading 3.2.3).
2. Incubate the dynabeads on a rotator for 1 h at 4 °C.
3. Use the magnetic rack to discard the supernatant from the dynabeads.
4. Wash the dynabeads 2× with 500 μl of high-salt wash buffer for 2 min each at 4 °C.
5. Wash the dynabeads 2× with 500 μl of PNK buffer for 2 min each at 4 °C.
6. Resuspend the dynabeads in 1 ml of PNK buffer.
7. Transfer 100 μl of resuspended dynabeads into a new microcentrifuge tube and leave it at 4 °C overnight. It will be used next day for the 5′ radiolabeling of RNA (*see* Subheading 3.4 and also **Note 13**).
8. For each sample prepare the 3′ RNA dephosphorylation master mix:

   8 μl water.

   1 μl of 10× Shrimp alkaline phosphatase (SAP) buffer.

   1 μl of Shrimp alkaline phosphatase (SAP).

   (*See* **Note 14**).

9. Remove the supernatant from the remaining 900 μl of dynabeads and resuspend the beads in 10 μl of 3′ RNA dephosphorylation master mix.
10. Incubate the reaction at 37 °C for 20 min.
11. Wash the dynabeads on a rotator 2× with 500 μl of high-salt wash buffer for 2 min each at 4 °C (*see* **Note 15**).
12. Wash them on a rotator 2× with 500 μl of PNK buffer for 2 min each at 4 °C.
13. Prepare the 3′ RNA linker ligation mix per sample:

    3.5 μl water.

    0.75 μl 10× RNA ligase buffer.

    2.5 μl PEG 400.

    0.25 μl T4 RNA ligase 1.

    0.1 μl RNase OUT.

    3 μl linker L3.
14. Remove the supernatant from **step 12** and resuspend the beads in 10 μl of the 3′ RNA linker ligation mix.
15. Place the microcentrifuge tube overnight at 16 °C for linker ligation. After this step go directly to Subheading 3.4.

3.3 iCLAP Protocol (In Vivo Cross-Linking and Affinity Purification Protocol)

This is a separate protocol that uses a modified TAP-tag (protein of interest with His_6-TEV protease cleavage site-protein A) to purify a given protein–RNA complex from trypanosomes. It uses a two-step affinity purification, while the downstream cDNA library preparation remains the same as the one used in iCLIP.

3.3.1 Preparation of the Lysate: Day 1 (Fig. 2)

1. Thaw UV- and non-UV-cross-linked pellets on ice (~15 min) and resuspend them in 1.5 ml cold iCLAP lysis buffer, which is freshly supplemented with the protease inhibitor (*see* **Note 5**).
2. Clean the sonicator tip with RNAseZap and then with milliQ water.
3. Sonicate both samples (five pulses each 30 s at 50% amplitude, with 20 s pause in-between) (*see* **Note 6**).
4. Transfer 1.5 ml lysate to a fresh 1.5 ml microcentrifuge tube and spin for 10 min at maximum speed of 16,000 × *g* at 4 °C (*see* **Note 7**).
5. Transfer the supernatant to a fresh 1.5 ml microcentrifuge tube (leave some supernatant to prevent carryover).

3.3.2 Partial RNA Digestion

Same as partial RNA digestion in Subheading 3.2.2.

3.3.3 Preparation of IgG Sepharose Beads

1. Add 300 μl of IgG Sepharose beads into a 1.5 ml microcentrifuge tube and spin it at 200 × *g* for 30 s. Keep the microcentrifuge tube on ice and let the IgG beads settle for ~45–60 s. Once the IgG beads are settled, discard the supernatant (*see* **Note 16**).
2. Add 1 ml of cold iCLAP lysis buffer to the IgG beads and let it spin on a rotator for 5 min at 4 °C. Spin the microcentrifuge tube at 1200 rpm for 30 s, and afterward keep the tube on ice for 45 s. Once beads are fully settled, discard the supernatant.
3. Wash the IgG beads 3× with the iCLAP lysis buffer.
4. Keep the equilibrated IgG beads on ice until the lysate is ready.

3.3.4 IgG Sepharose-Based Affinity Purification

1. Once the lysates are ready, dilute them in the iCLAP lysis buffer by bringing the total volume to 10 ml and use a fresh 15 ml Falcon tube to load both equilibrated IgG beads and diluted lysis buffer.
2. Let them incubate for 2 h at 4 °C on a rotator.
3. Wash IgG beads in wash buffer 3× for 5 min each.
4. Resuspend IgG beads in 1 ml of TEV cleavage buffer and transfer it to a 1.5 ml tube.
5. Wash the IgG beads in 1 ml TEV cleavage buffer 3× for 5 min each.
6. After the last wash, resuspend the IgG beads in 100 μl of TEV cleavage buffer and 20 μl of homemade GST-TEV protease (depending upon the batch but usually ~20 U) (*see* **Note 17**).
7. For TEV protease cleavage, keep the tube in a thermomixer at 18 °C while shaking at 1000 rpm.
8. After 2 h, transfer the beads along with the supernatant to a 1.5 ml protein purification column and spin the column at 250 × *g* for 1 min (*see* **Note 18**).
9. Collect the flow-through into a separate 1.5 ml tube.
10. Add 1.2 ml of His-binding buffer to a flow-through and keep it on ice until His-dynabeads are ready.

3.3.5 Preparation of His-Dynabeads

1. Transfer 100 μl of the His-dynabeads into a fresh 1.5 ml tube and remove the supernatant from the beads using a magnetic rack (*see* **Note 19**).
2. Wash the His-dynabeads on a rotator with 1 ml of His-binding buffer 3× for 2 min at 4 °C.

3.3.6 His Dynabeads-Based Affinity Purification

1. Resuspend the collected flow-through from **step 10** (Subheading 3.3.4) to already equilibrated His-dynabeads from **step 2** (Subheading 3.3.5).
2. Let them incubate on a rotator for 1 h at 4 °C.

3. Wash the His-dynabeads on a rotator with 500 μl of urea wash buffer 2× for 5 min each at 4 °C.
4. Wash the His-dynabeads on a rotator with 1 ml of PNK buffer 2× for 2 min each at 4 °C.
5. Resuspend the His-dynabeads in 1 ml PNK buffer.
6. Transfer 100 μl of resuspended His-dynabeads into a new tube and leave it at 4 °C overnight (will be used the next day for 5′ radiolabeling).
7. Prepare 3′ RNA dephosphorylation master mix per sample:

   8 μl nuclease-free water.

   1 μl of 10× shrimp alkaline phosphatase (SAP) buffer.

   1 μl of shrimp alkaline phosphatase (SAP).
8. Remove the supernatant from the remaining 900 μl of the His-dynabeads and resuspend the beads in 10 μl of 3′ RNA dephosphorylation master mix.
9. Incubate the reaction at 37 °C for 20 min.
10. Wash the His-dynabeads on a rotator with 500 μl of high-salt wash buffer 2× for 2 min each at 4 °C.
11. Remove the supernatant and on a rotator wash the His-dynabeads with 500 μl PNK buffer 2× for 2 min each at 4 °C.
12. Next step is a 3′-linker ligation of the RNA. Prepare a L3 linker ligation mix per sample:

    0.75 μl 10× RNA ligase buffer.

    3.5 μl water.

    2.5 μl PEG 400.

    0.25 μl T4 RNA ligase 1.

    0.1 μl RNase OUT.

    3 μl linker L3.
13. Remove the PNK buffer from the His-dynabeads (**step 11**) and resuspend them in 10 μl of the L3 linker ligation mix.
14. Keep the tube overnight at 16 °C.

3.4 SDS-PAGE and Transfer of Protein–RNA Complexes to Nitrocellulose Membrane: Day 2

From here on, all subsequent steps are the same for both the iCLIP and iCLAP protocols. In case you want to carry out the iCLIP protocol, go directly from Subheading 3.2.4 to this subheading, or in case of the iCLAP protocol, go directly from Subheading 3.3.6 to this subheading.

1. Next day prepare a hot PNK master mix for 5′ radiolabeling of the RNA per sample:

   0.2 μl T4 PNK.

0.4 μl 10× PNK buffer.

0.4 μl γ-^{32}P-ATP.

2 μl nuclease-free water.

2. For iCLIP: remove 100 μl of the protein G dynabeads from **step** 7 (Subheading 3.2.4), discard the supernatant using the magnetic rack and resuspend them in the hot PNK master mix. While, for iCLAP: remove 100 μl of the His-dynabeads from **step 6** (Subheading 3.3.6), discard the supernatant and resuspend them in the hot PNK master mix. In both cases mix the samples well and incubate them at 37 °C for 10 min (keep in mind that the beads are now radioactively hot).
3. Dilute 4× NuPage protein loading dye to 1.5× and prepare a 10-well 4–12% NuPage Bis-Tris gel with 1× MOPS running buffer.
4. For iCLIP: remove 900 μl of the protein G dynabeads from **step 15** (Subheading 3.2.4) and discard the linker ligation mix.

   For iCLAP: remove 900 μl of the His-dynabeads from **step 14** (Subheading 3.3.6) and discard the linker ligation mix.

   Wash the dynabeads once with 500 μl of PNK wash buffer for 2 min at 4 °C. These beads are radioactively cold and contain 3′ RNA linkers.
5. Discard the PNK wash buffer from the above step and resuspend the cold dynabeads into 25 μl of 1.5× NuPage loading dye.
6. After 10 min incubation discard the hot PNK mix from the hot dynabeads.
7. Pool the radioactively cold and hot dynabeads together using 25 μl of 1.5× NuPage loading dye.
8. Heat the dynabeads for 10 min at 70 °C.
9. Collect 25 μl of 1.5× NuPage supernatant from the dynabeads using the magnetic rack.
10. Load the supernatant directly into one well of the 4–12% NuPage Bis-Tris gel. In case of more samples leave one lane free between the samples to decrease the chances of RNA cross contamination.
11. Load the prestained marker for the reference in the last well and run the gel for 45 min at 180 V.
12. After the run is finished, cut the bottom of the gel that contains free ATP and discard it in a solid radioactive waste bin.
13. Transfer the remaining gel onto a nitrocellulose membrane using a Novex wet transfer apparatus and Novex transfer buffer supplemented with 20% methanol. The condition used for transfer is 2 h at 45 V and 4 °C.

14. Once the transfer is finished, rinse the membrane in sterile cold PBS and wrap it with Saran wrap.
15. Transfer the membrane into a cassette and expose the film at −80 °C. Analyze the exposure at three different time points (suggested times are 30 min, 1 h, and overnight).

3.5 RNA Isolation: Day 3

1. Analyze the overnight exposure and place the developed autoradiogram precisely over the nitrocellulose membrane.
2. Use the autoradiogram as a reference to mark the square that needs to be cut out of the nitrocellulose membrane with a marker that corresponds to the protein–RNA complex of your interest (*see* **Note 20**).
3. Take the marked nitrocellulose membrane out of the cassette and use a fresh scalpel to cut the marked area into tiny pieces.
4. Place the tiny nitrocellulose membrane pieces into a fresh 1.5 ml tube and add to it 200 μl of PK buffer.
5. Add 10 μl of proteinase K into the tube and incubate it in a thermomixer at 1000 rpm for 10 min at 37 °C.
6. After 10 min incubation add 200 μl of PK buffer that contains 7 M urea and incubate the tube for another 20 min at 37 °C.
7. Transfer the supernatant carefully without taking the membrane pieces from the microcentrifuge tube to a 2 ml phase lock gel tube.
8. Add 400 μl acidic phenol and chloroform–isoamyl alcohol to the 2 ml phase lock gel tube and incubate the reaction at 30 °C while shaking at 1000 rpm for 5 min (do not vortex).
9. After 5 min spin the phase lock gel tube at maximum speed in a benchtop centrifuge.
10. Carefully transfer the upper aqueous layer to a fresh 1.5 ml tube (leave some to avoid the carryover) and add to it 1 μg of glycogen, 50 μl of 3 M sodium acetate (pH 5.5), and 1 ml of 100% ethanol.
11. Precipitate RNA overnight at −20 °C (alternatively for 1 h at −80 °C).

3.6 Reverse Transcriptase: Day 4

1. Take out the tube with the precipitated RNA and spin it for 30 min at 13,000 rpm and 4 °C.
2. Carefully remove the supernatant without disturbing the pellet, add 500 μl of 70% ethanol and spin the samples for 15 min at 13,000 rpm and 4 °C.
3. Carefully remove the supernatant without disturbing the pellet and let the pellet dry for 5–10 min at room temperature.
4. Once the pellet is dry, resuspend the (usually invisible) pellet in 6 μl of nuclease-free water.

5. Dilute RCLIP primers to 0.1 μM (mix 2.5 μl water and 0.5 μl primer from 2 μM stock) (*see* **Note 21**).
6. Prepare dNTP–primer mix in a PCR tube (include one tube for reverse transcriptase (RT)-control in 6 μl of nuclease-free water):

   0.5 μl RPCLIP primer specific for L3 linker (0.1 pmol/μl; from **step 5**).

   0.5 μl dNTP Mix (10 mM each).

   (*See* **Note 22**).
7. Transfer 6 μl of RNA (from **step 4**) to the already prepared dNTP–primer mix in a PCR tube (from **step 6**).
8. Place the PCR tube in the PCR cycler machine and start the RT thermal program:

   *70 °C for 5 min.

   Hold at **25 °C until the RT mix is added.

   42 °C for 20 min.

   50 °C for 40 min.

   4 °C hold.

   While the samples are being denatured at *70 °C for 5 min, prepare a master mix for the RT reaction (including RT control) per sample:

   2 μl 5× RT buffer.

   0.5 μl DTT (0.1 M).

   0.25 μl Superscript III RT (200 U/μl).

   Once the temperature reaches **25 °C, add 2.75 μl of freshly prepared RT master mix to each PCR tube and mix well.
9. Take the tubes out from the cycler, add 90 μl of TE buffer, transfer it to new 1.5 ml tube, add 0.5 μl glycogen and 15 μl sodium acetate and mix well.
10. Add 300 μl of ethanol, mix well and precipitate the RNA overnight at −20 °C (alternatively for 1 h at −80 °C).

3.7 Size Selection of cDNA: Day 5

1. Take the tube with the overnight precipitated cDNA out and spin it for 30 min at 13,200 rpm and 4 °C.
2. Carefully remove the supernatant without disturbing the pellet, add 500 μl of 70% ethanol and spin the samples for 15 min at 13,200 rpm and 4 °C.
3. Carefully remove the supernatant without disturbing the pellet, let the pellet dry for 10 min at room temperature, and resuspend it in 6 μl of nuclease-free water.
4. To 6 μl of this cDNA add another 6 μl of 2× TBE-urea loading buffer.

5. Heat the samples for 3 min at 70 °C.
6. Place a precasted 6% of TBE-urea gel in a gel running chamber and fill it with 1× TBE running buffer.
7. Load 12 μl of cDNA (from **step 5**) using a long pipette tip. It is important to flush the urea from the wells using a needle just before loading of the cDNA. Always leave one lane free between the samples to avoid possible cross contamination. Also load a DNA size marker.
8. Run the gel at 180 V for exactly 40 min.
9. After the run is finished, cut the last lane with the DNA size marker and incubate it for 15 min in 25 ml TBE buffer with 1 μl of SYBR Green II. Take a scan for a DNA size marker using ChemiDoc and print the result by making sure it is in size exactly to 100% scale.
10. Use the printed DNA size marker result from the above step as a reference to excise the size selected cDNA from the TBE-urea gel.
11. Cut out bands from the gel in 3 sizes of approximately 60–90, 90–120, and 120–200 nucleotides and place them in three different 1.5 ml tubes (*see* **Note 23**).
12. Add 400 μl of TE buffer to each tube and crush the gel into fine pieces using the plunger from a 1 ml syringe.
13. Incubate the gel pieces in the tube at 37 °C for 2 h in a thermomixer while shaking at 200 × *g*.
14. Add 1 cm of glass prefilter to a Costar SpinX column and transfer it into a fresh 1.5 ml tube.
15. Transfer the supernatant from the tube containing gel pieces onto the Costar SpinX column.
16. Spin the Costar tube for 2 min at maximum speed at room temperature.
17. Keep the flow-through (usually ~350 μl) and add 40 μl of sodium acetate, 0.5 μl glycogen, and 1 ml of 100% ethanol.
18. Precipitate the RNA overnight at −20 °C (alternatively for 1 h at −80 °C).

3.8 cDNA Circulation and Linearization: Day 6

1. Take the tube with the overnight precipitated cDNA out and spin it for 30 min at 13,200 rpm and 4 °C.
2. Carefully remove the supernatant without disturbing the pellet, add 500 μl of 70% ethanol and spin the samples for 15 min at 13,200 rpm and 4 °C.
3. Carefully remove the supernatant without disturbing the pellet and let it dry for 10 min at room temperature.

4. While the pellet is left to dry, prepare the cDNA circularization ligation mix:

   6.5 μl nuclease-free water.

   0.8 μl CircLigase buffer II.

   0.4 μl 50 mM $MnCl_2$.

   0.3 μl Circligase II.

5. Resuspend the dry pellet in 8 μl of ligation mix and transfer it to a fresh PCR tube.
6. Incubate the PCR tube for 1 h at 60 °C in PCR thermocycler, which is then set up for 4 °C on hold.
7. During the 4 °C on hold, prepare the oligo annealing mix:

   26 μl nuclease-free water.

   3 μl Fast digest buffer.

   1 μl of 10 mM CutC4 (complimentary DNA for BamHI restriction in next step).

8. Change the thermocycler settings to:

   95 °C for 2 min.

   70 cycles starting with 95 °C for 1 min, and decreasing the temperature by 1 °C in every cycle with the final temperature being 25 °C.

   25 °C on hold.

9. Add 2 μl of BamHI to the PCR tubes and change the thermocycler settings to 37 °C for 40 min (*see* **Note 24**).
10. Following the restriction digestion, add 60 μl of TE buffer and transfer the samples to a fresh 1.5 ml tube, to which add 0.5 μl of glycogen, 15 μl sodium acetate, and 300 μl 100% ethanol and mix everything properly.
11. Precipitate RNA overnight at −20 °C (alternatively for 1 h at −80 °C).

3.9 PCR Amplification: Day 7

1. Take out the tube with the overnight precipitated cDNA and spin it for 30 min at 13,000 rpm and 4 °C.
2. Carefully remove the supernatant without disturbing the pellet, add 500 μl of ice cold 70% ethanol and spin the samples for 15 min at 13,000 rpm and 4 °C.
3. Carefully remove the supernatant and let the pellet dry for about 10 min at room temperature.
4. Resuspend the dry pellet in 11 μl of nuclease-free water.
5. Prepare a PCR master mix in a PCR tube as follows:

   1 μl of cDNA (from **step 4**).

   9 μl of nuclease-free water.

   0.5 μl of P5/P3 Solexa primer mix (10 μM each).

6. Place the PCR tube into the PCR thermocycler with the following settings:

   95 °C for 10 min.

   95 °C for 10 s, 65 °C for 30 s, 68 °C for 30 s (20–25 cycles).

   72 °C 3 min.

   25 °C on hold.

7. Resolve the PCR products on a 1% agarose gel or 6% TBE-urea gel by loading 7 μl of the cDNA and stain it using 3 μl SYBR Green I for 10 min in 30 ml of 1× TBE.
8. Depending on the results, pool the PCR products from different size fractions into a single microcentrifuge tube (*see* **Note 25**).

4 Notes

1. While scaling up to a larger volume, you can skip adding the drugs to reduce the costs.
2. This is an important negative control which shall be done for every new RNA binding protein. This will allow the visualization of the background levels of pulled-down RNA with the target protein in the absence of UV cross-linking.
3. Since the UV treatment might lead to UV-induced activation of the DNA damage repair pathway, spin and freeze the cells in liquid nitrogen after UV cross-linking as quickly as possible. For successful UV cross-linking keep the Petri dish about 5 cm from the UV lamp in the Stratalinker.
4. Use the frozen pellets to carry out the iCLIP or iCLAP experiments within a month.
5. Use freshly made buffers which have been filtered through 0.22-μm filters.
6. Avoid foaming and ensure that during the process, the samples remain cold. Depending on the machine used, the duration of sonication and the amplitude have to be optimized before the initial experiment.
7. It is critical to optimize the lysate concentration used for the immunoprecipitation assay. We use 5 and 10 mg/ml of protein for the iCLIP and iCLAP experiments, respectively.
8. The high RNase treatment of the lysate is required only during the initial set up of the iCLIP assay and serves two purposes (*see* Fig. 3a). Firstly, it is used as a positive control to determine the specificity of the pull down of the protein–RNA complexes. Due to the high RNase treatment, it makes RNA to appear as a sharp band (usually ~5 kDa above the molecular weight of the

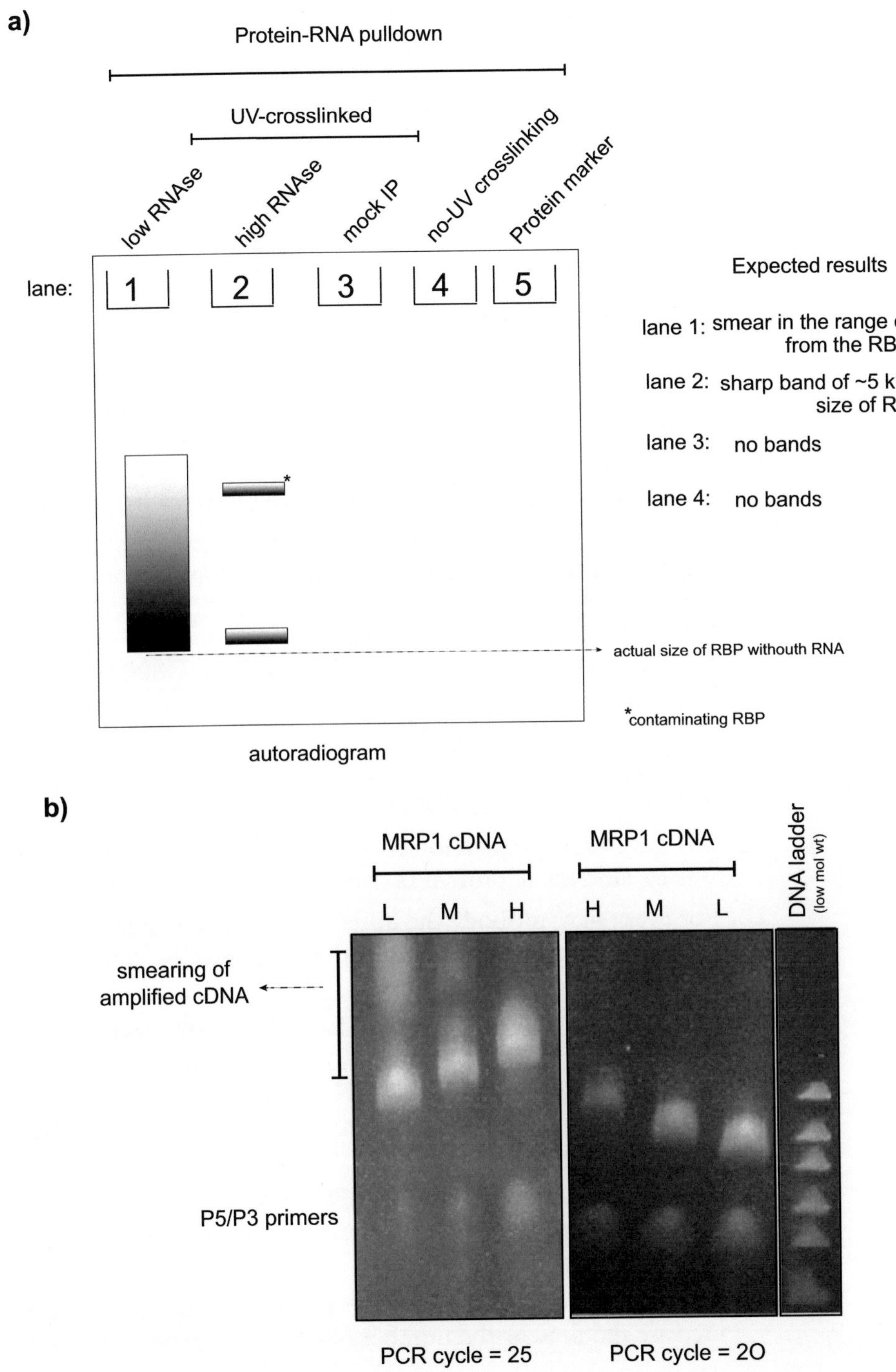

Fig. 3 Key steps in the iCLIP/iCLAP analysis. (**a**) Analysis of copurified RNA–protein complexes. The autoradiogram depicts the expected results and necessary controls. Low RNase I (lane 1) treated RNA–protein complex usually results in a smear and is used for preparation of the cDNA library. The high RNase I (lane 2) treated RNA–protein complex yields a sharp band. Mock immunoprecipitation (lane 3) and non-UV-cross-

protein of interest) in the autoradiogram as compared to a smear in case of low RNase-treated lysate. Therefore, if you obtain more than one radiolabeled RNA band in the autoradiogram, it possibly reflects the presence of another contaminating RBP. This will likely demand optimization of the protocol to obtain higher stringency in the pull-down experiments. Otherwise, if the contaminating RBP(s) have a considerable size difference with the RBP of interest, then you can still excise the target band from the nitrocellulose membrane. At this point you must carry out the other control immunoprecipitation (IP) assays to verify the stringency of IPs, which include non-UV-cross-linked and mock IPs with high RNase treatment. In both cases, this should not yield a radiolabeled RNA band. If all the controls work properly, proceed with the iCLIP library preparation protocol. Lastly, the use of RNase I is recommended given it has no base preference for its activity.

9. After all control IPs have been performed, you shall perform the iCLIP protocol for final library preparation. It requires low RNase treatment of the lysates and optimization for every new batch of RNase I. It is suggested that you test several low RNAse treatment conditions (1:250, 1:500, 1:800) (*see* ref. 9). In our hands, a 1:500 RNase dose was used to make both the iCLIP and iCLAP libraries.
10. For better reproducibility of the iCLIP libraries, be consistent with the timing of the RNase treatment.
11. For the initial optimization of IPs (including control IPs) use a smaller amount of protein G dynabeads (~50 μl) per IP assay.
12. For every new antibody the initial experiment requires testing the optimal antibody concentration that will be coupled to dynabeads.
13. At this point separate the dynabeads into 100 and 900 μl fractions. The 100 μl fraction will be used for 5′ RNA radiolabeling while the lack of a 3′ RNA linker will prevent reverse transcription. The 900 μl fraction will be used for 3′ RNA linker attachment.
14. Before the 3′-linker is ligated to RNA, it must be dephosphorylated, since the T4 RNA ligase cannot add ends to the cyclic 2–3′ phosphate groups.
15. To increase the specificity of the immunoprecipitation you can increase the time or the number of high salt washes.

Fig. 3 (continued) linked RNA–protein pull-down in the presence of high RNase I treatment (lane 4) serve as additional negative controls. (**b**) Optimization of the MRP1 iCLIP libraries. The first panel shows the final MRP1 iCLIP library PCR carried out using 25 cycles that resulted in a smear. Decreasing the number of PCR cycles to 20 resulted in sharper bands

16. Protein spin columns can be used for easy washing and resuspension of the IgG beads.
17. It is important to use homemade GST-TEV protease since most commercially available TEV proteases contain a His tag. This will create a problem in the second step of His-tag purification of the protein complex.
18. The time for TEV protease cleavage might vary depending upon the batch of TEV protease or the RBP of interest and therefore requires initial optimization.
19. One can also use nickel- or copper-based Sepharose beads. However, it is easier to work with dynabeads, since some downstream steps require resuspension of beads in smaller volumes. For example, 3′ RNA dephosphorylation and linker ligation uses 10 μl of total master mix.
20. The cross-linked RNA adds additional weight to the RBP. Therefore, if there is no other contaminating RBP in the vicinity (as already determined from the high RNase treated pull-down experiment), cut out the nitrocellulose membrane ~20–60 kDa above the expected molecular weight of the actual RBP.
21. In the original iCLIP protocol, the authors tested all the available RTCLIP primers. In their examination RTCLIP primers 1, 2, 6, 9, 10, and 13–16 were more efficient. As every RTCLIP primer contains a unique barcode, it allows the pooling of various iCLIP libraries to a single lane by using different RTCLIP primers. Every time prepare a fresh dilution of RCLIP primers (0.1 μM). Names and sequences of all primers used in the iCLIP/iCLAP protocol are provided in Fig. 4.
22. Remember to include the negative control for the reverse transcriptase reaction.
23. Use a fresh scalpel for samples with different RTCLIP primer barcodes. Cut the higher band first and then move downward to avoid cross contamination of primer dimers (runs around ~51 nt). It is crucial to avoid primer dimers in the library preparation, as they considerably decrease its depth.
24. Circularization and linearization make the identification of UV-cross-linked peptide position easy to decipher by bioinformatics, since the first nucleotide after the removal of the adapter from iCLIP sequence becomes the UV-cross-linked site.
25. The aim is to pool different size fractions in a ratio that will allow similar sequencing depths for each fraction (*see* Fig. 3b).

Primer's name	Sequence Information
RT1	/5Phos/NNAACCNNNAGATCGGA AGAGCGTCGTGgatcCTGAACCGC
RT2	5Phos/NNACAANNNA GATCGGAAGAGCGTCGTGgatcCT GAACCGC
RT3	/5Phos/NNATTGNNNAGATCGGA AGAGCGTCGTGgatcCTGAACCGC
RT4	/5Phos/NNAGGTNNNAGATCG GAAGAGCGTCGTGgatcCTGAA CCGC
RT6	/5Phos/NNCCGGNNNAGATC GGAAGAGCGTCGTGgatcCTGAA CCGC
RT7	/5Phos/NNCTAANNNAGATCGGA AGAGCGTCGTGgatcCTGAACCGC
RT8	/5Phos/NNCATTNNNAGATCGGA AGAGCGTCGTGgatcCTGAACCGC
RT9	/5Phos/NNGCCANNNAGATCGG AAGAGCGTCGTGgatcCTGAACCGC
RT11	/5Phos/NNGGTTNNNAGATCGGAAGAGCGTCGTGgatcCTGAACCGC
RT12	/5Phos/NNGTGGNNNAGA TCGGAAGAGCGTCGTGgatcCT GAACCGC
RT13	/5Phos/NNTCCGNNNAGATCGGAA GAGCGTCGTGgatcCTGAACCGC
RT14	/5Phos/NNTGCCNNNAG ATCGGAAGAGCGTCGTGgatc CTGAACCGC
RT15	/5Phos/NNTATTNNNAGATCGGAA GAGCGTCGTGgatcCTGAACCGC
RT16	/5Phos/NNTTAANNNAGATCGGAAG AGCGTCGTGgatc CTGAACCGC
Cut oligo	GTTCAGGATCCACGACGCTCTTCaaaa
L3 linker	rAppAGATCGGAAGAGCGGTTCAG/ddC/
P5	AATGATACGGCGACCACCGAGA TCTAC ACTCTTTCCCTACACGA CGCTCTTCCGATCT
P3	CAAGCAGAAGACGGCATACGA GATCGGTCTCGGCATTCCTGCTGAACCGCTCTTCCGATCT

Fig. 4 Primers required for preparation of the library

Acknowledgments

Support from the Czech Grant Agency (18-15962S), ERC CZ (LL1601) and the ERD Funds, project OPVVV (16_019/0000759) (all to J.L.) is acknowledged.

References

1. Zhao BS, Roundtree IA, He C (2017) Post-transcriptional gene regulation by mRNA modifications. Nat Rev Mol Cell Biol 18:31–42
2. Clayton C (2013) The regulation of trypanosome gene expression by RNA-binding proteins. PLoS Pathog 9:e1003680
3. Glisovic T, Bachorik JL, Yong J, Dreyfuss G (2008) RNA-binding proteins and post-transcriptional gene regulation. FEBS Lett 582:1977–1986
4. Lee FCY, Ule J (2018) Advances in CLIP technologies for studies of protein-RNA interactions. Mol Cell 69:354–369
5. Ule J, Jensen KB, Ruggiu M et al (2003) CLIP identifies Nova-regulated RNA networks in the brain. Science 302:1212–1215
6. König J, Zarnack K, Rot G, Curk T, Kayikci M, Zupan B, Turner DJ, Luscombe NM, Ule J (2010) iCLIP reveals the function of hnRNP particles in splicing at individual nucleotide resolution. Nat Struct Mol Biol 17:909–915
7. Dixit S, Müller-McNicoll M, David V, Zarnack K, Ule J, Hashimi H, Lukeš J (2017) Differential binding of mitochondrial transcripts by MRB8170 and MRB4160 regulates distinct editing fates of mitochondrial mRNA in trypanosomes. mBio 8:e02288-16
8. Dixit S, Lukeš J (2018) Combinatorial interplay of RNA-binding proteins tunes levels of mitochondrial mRNA in trypanosomes. RNA 24:1594–1606
9. Huppertz I, Attig J, D'Ambrogio A, Easton LE, Sibley CR, Sugimoto Y, Tajnik M, Konig J, Ule J (2014) iCLIP: protein–RNA interactions at nucleotide resolution. Methods 65:274–287

Chapter 20

In Vivo Tethering System to Isolate RNA-Binding Proteins Regulating mRNA Decay in *Leishmania*

Hiva Azizi and Barbara Papadopoulou

Abstract

RNA-binding proteins (RBPs) play key roles in many aspects of RNA metabolism. In *Leishmania*, a unicellular eukaryote that favors the posttranscriptional mode of regulation for controlling gene expression levels, the function of RBPs becomes even more critical. However, due largely to limited in vivo approaches available for identifying RBPs in these parasites, there have been no significant advances to our understanding of the role these proteins play in posttranscriptional control through binding to cis-acting elements in the 3′ untranslated region (3′UTR) of mRNAs. Here we describe an optimized in vivo RNA tethering approach using the bacteriophage MS2 coat protein combined to immunoprecipitation and mass spectrometry analysis to identify RBPs specifically interacting with 3′UTR short interspersed degenerated retroposon elements (SIDERs). Members of the SIDER2 subfamily were shown previously to promote mRNA degradation through a novel mechanism of mRNA decay. Using this modified MS2 tethering approach, we have identified candidate RBPs specifically interacting with SIDER2 elements and contributing to the decay mechanism.

Key words Tethering systems, MS2 coat protein, MS2 binding site, SIDER2 retroposons, mRNA decay, RNA-binding proteins, Co-immunoprecipitation, Mass spectrometry

1 Introduction

Leishmania spp. are unicellular protists of the Trypanosomatidae family that unlike other eukaryotes undergo polycistronic transcription in the absence of conventional RNA polymerase II promoters. Thus, regulation of gene expression in these parasites relies predominantly on posttranscriptional control [1, 2]. Lack of transcriptional regulation along with the existence of unusually long 3′-untranslated regions (3′UTRs) have pointed out the fundamental role of *cis*-acting elements in the 3′UTR of trypanosomatid mRNAs. One such class of 3′UTR elements belong to the large family of SIDERs (SIDER1/SIDER2) (short interspersed degenerate retroposons) shown to be key players of posttranscriptional regulation in *Leishmania* [3–6]. We have shown that members of

Paul A. M. Michels et al. (eds.), *Trypanosomatids: Methods and Protocols*, Methods in Molecular Biology, vol. 2116,
https://doi.org/10.1007/978-1-0716-0294-2_20,

the SIDER2 subfamily promote rapid mRNA decay that is initiated by endoribonucleolytic cleavage as opposed to the default decay process by deadenylation in other eukaryotes [4]. This is a novel mechanism of regulated mRNA decay in trypanosomatids, which has not been well studied in other eukaryotic cells. To gain a better insight into this novel regulatory network, we have to identify the trans-acting factors contributing to mRNA decay with emphasis on the endoribonuclease(s) and associated RNA-binding proteins (RBPs).

Powerful "tethering" approaches have been used successfully to isolate proteins regulating mRNA turnover in human cells [7–9] but also in parasites [10]. The specific and robust binding of the bacteriophage MS2/R17, MS2 coat protein (MCP), to a stem-loop aptamer termed MS2 stem-loop aptamer (MS2 SL) or MS2 binding sequence (MBS) [11–14] has been exploited successfully for studying mRNA localization and capturing of RBPs by attracting them to any RNA of interest [15, 16]. In addition to MS2, lambda N peptide which binds to its cognate RNA, box B sequences, has also been widely utilized in many organisms including *Trypanosoma* species to tether RBPs to a particular RNA of interest [17–23]. Similarly, the spliceosomal U1A protein has been used successfully in tethering assays [24–26]. Both MS2 CP and lambda N peptide are ideal choices for tethering assays due to their strong and specific binding to their cognate RNA. Also, due to their small size (~14 kDa and 22 amino acids, respectively) generally cause no interference with trans-acting factors interacting with the reporter mRNA. However, in contrast to lambda N peptide, MS2 CP requires dimerization in order to bind to a single MS2 SL, making it a suitable choice when a higher amount of tethered protein is required for binding to the reporter mRNA [27].

Recently, we have developed a bipartite MS2 tethering system to attract SIDER2-specific RBPs regulating mRNA decay. This system consists of the bacteriophage MS2 coat protein and a luciferase (LUC) reporter gene whose expression is driven by a 3′UTR harboring two MS2 binding sites and an active or a truncated SIDER2 element [28] (Fig. 1a). Using this tethering approach in combination with immunoprecipitation (IP) and LC-MS/MS studies, we identified a number of RBPs, some with known functions in mRNA decay [28]. A member of the Pumilio-family (PUF6), shown previously to bind to 3′UTRs of various eukaryotic mRNAs and to enhance turnover or repressing translation [29], was shown to increase SIDER2-mediated mRNA degradation upon tethering to a SIDER2-harboring reporter mRNA. Moreover, its genetic inactivation resulted in mRNA accumulation [28], suggesting a role of PUF6 in the decay process. RBPs interacting with PUF6 are currently under investigation to assess their role in SIDER2-mediated decay using tethering assays, among other approaches.

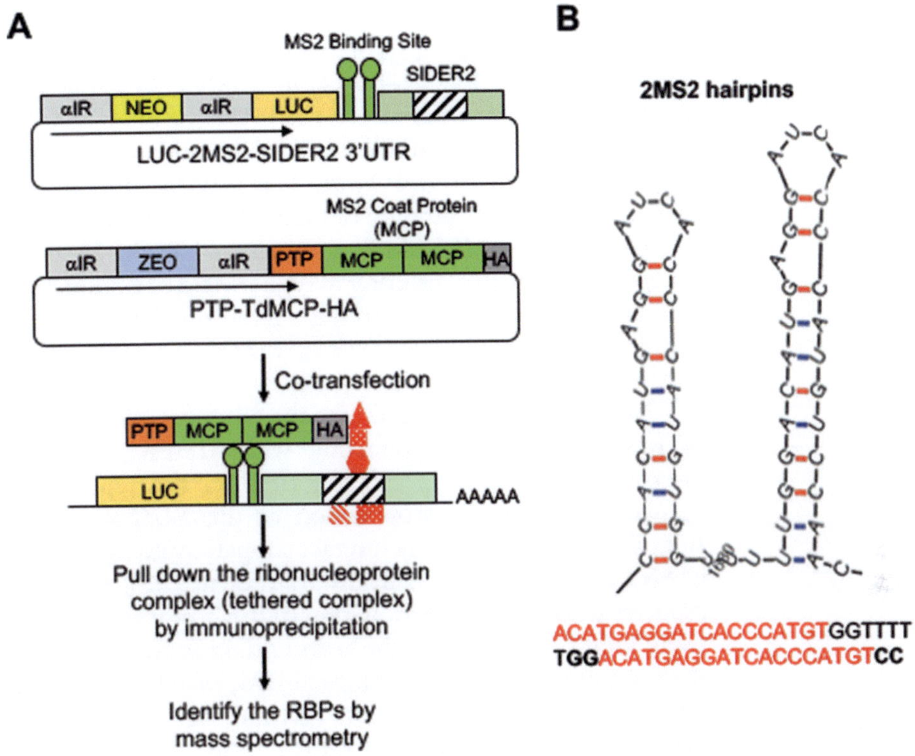

Fig. 1 Schematic diagram of the constructs used for the optimized MS2 tethering system and pull-down approach. (**a**) *Leishmania* promastigotes are cotransfected with two plasmids, one expressing two tandem copies of the MS2 coat protein tagged with PTP at the N-terminus and the HA epitope at the C-terminus (PTP-tdMCP-HA) and the other expressing the reporter LUC-2MS2-SIDER2 3′UTR mRNA. The tandem MS2 coat protein recognizes and binds to the tandem MS2 binding sequences (2MS2 hairpins) on the reporter mRNA. Trans-acting factors, preferentially those involved in SIDER2-mediated mRNA decay will be tethered to the SIDER2 RNA and coimmunoprecipitated together with the PTP-tdMS2-HA protein (an-anti HA Ab or an anti-MCP Ab can be used for IP). This protein complex could then be identified by mass spectrometry. (**b**) We used the mFold RNA secondary structure prediction software to determine the most suitable flanking sequences required to form a MS2 stem-loop structure in the context of the LinJ.36.4000 SIDER2-bearing 3′UTR. In red are the two MS2 binding sites and in black the linker sequence used here to optimize the formation of the MS2 hairpin

In our efforts to optimize the MS2 tethering system for use in *Leishmania*, we made the following modifications. First, we improved expression levels and binding efficiency of MCP. In our hands, a single copy of MCP was not well expressed (data not shown). In the absence of an effective inducible protein expression system in *L. infantum*, we opted for an episomal expression system to obtain higher levels of MCP and consequently sufficient binding to the MS2 SL RNA. It has been shown previously that fusing two MCP copies from head to tail through a linker sequence results in a dimer which has an affinity to MBS similar to the wild type protein [30]. Therefore, we generated a vector expressing a tandem MCP protein (tdMCP) that was tagged at the N-terminus with a PTP (**P**rotC-**T**EV-**P**rotA) tag [31] and at the C-terminus with an HA epitope (Fig. 1a). Expression of this tdMCP in *Leishmania* substantially increased protein levels [28]. The use of tandem MCP has also been shown in mRNA localization studies to improve the signal when fused to GFP [32]. This artificial dimerization may also increase efficient binding of the tdMCP protein to the reporter mRNA harboring MS2 binding sequences and the SIDER2 regulatory element, hence resulting in higher yield of ribonucleoprotein complex pull down. Interestingly, because MCP binds the MS2 hairpin as preformed dimers, it can recruits two copies of the fused RBP of interest to the tethering site.

Second, in order to minimize the potential occupational effect of tdMCP on RBPs interacting with SIDER2 sequences, we inserted only two MS2 binding sites on the reporter mRNA, immediately after the stop codon of the *LUC* gene (Fig. 1a). Bound coat protein dimers interact cooperatively with one another when tandem arrays of hairpins are present [33]. Given that the reporter mRNA controlled by the SIDER2-bearing 3′UTR is relatively long (~3.6 kb) and the surrounding sequences could affect the formation of MS2 stem loops in vivo, we used the mFold RNA secondary structure prediction software to determine the best flanking sequences required to form a MS2 stem–loop structure. By testing different flanking sequence combinations, we were able to find the most suitable sequence allowing the tandem MS2 hairpin to form in silico (**ACATGAGGATCACCCATGT**GGTTTTTGG**ACATGAGGATCACCCATGT**CC, in bold are the two MS2 binding sites; *see* also Fig. 1b). Insertion of two MS2 hairpin structures downstream of the *LUC* reporter mRNA and their interaction with tdMCP did not alter decay rates of the *LUC*-SIDER2 reporter transcript [28]. Since MCP binds specifically to the loop sequence of its cognate RNA, engineering the sequences of the MBS stem that we found necessary for its in vivo structure assembly, should not interfere with binding to the MCP [34].

To identify proteins contributing to SIDER2-mediated mRNA decay that are attracted to the SIDER2 RNA using our bipartite MS2 tethering system, we followed up with immunoprecipitation (IP) and LC-MS/MS studies. *Leishmania infantum* transfectants co-expressing the tdMCP-HA protein and the LUC-2MS2-SIDER2 reporter mRNA were subjected to immunoprecipitation using magnetic beads coupled to the HA antibody under native conditions. To exclude nonspecific binding, we used as a control a *Leishmania* strain expressing only the tdMCP protein without any reporter RNA. The presence of tdMCP-HA protein prior and after co-IP studies was verified by western blotting (Fig. 2). One tenth of

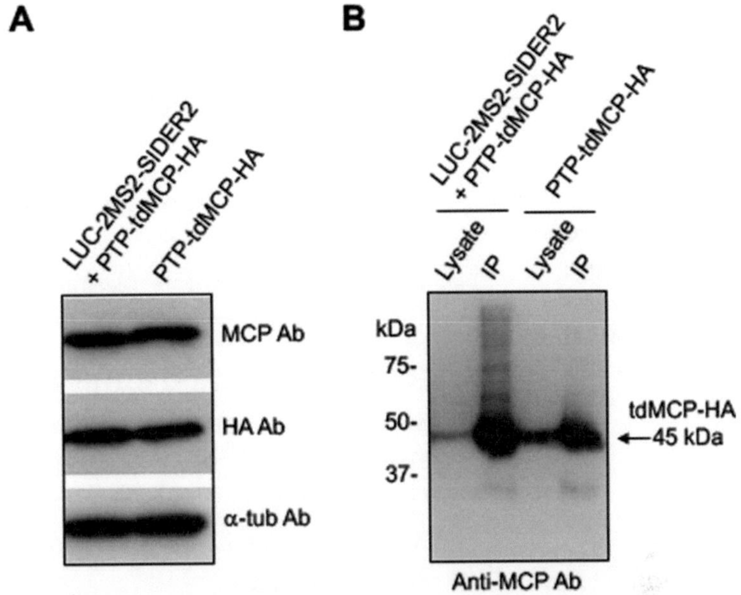

Fig. 2 The tandem MS2 coat protein is well expressed when episomally transfected in *Leishmania infantum*. (**a**) Western blot analysis of total protein lysates from *L. infantum* promastigotes co-transfected with PTP-tdMCP-HA and LUC-2MS2-SIDER2 3′UTR (the SIDER2 element present in the LinJ.36.4000 3′UTR was used here) or transfected only with PTP-tdMCP-HA. The membranes were hybridized with both anti-HA and anti-MCP antibodies in order to confirm suitable expression of the tdMCP protein in both transfectants. The α-tubulin Ab was used to normalize against the input protein material. (**b**) Following immunoprecipitation of PTP-tdMS2-HA in *L. infantum* promastigotes cotransfected with PTP-tdMCP-HA and LUC-2MS2-SIDER2 3′UTR or transfected only with PTP-tdMCP-HA, one tenth volume of the co-IP samples was resolved on SDS-PAGE and analyzed by western blot using an anti-MCP antibody, before proceeding to protein identification by mass spectrometry

the immunoprecipitated particles were used to confirm the efficacy of IP by western blotting before proceeding with mass spectrometry analysis (Fig. 2b). Finally, the remaining eluate-magnetic beads were sent to mass spectrometry. Several RBP candidates have been identified as mentioned above and are currently under study.

In conclusion, our optimized MS2 tethering system was applied successfully for the first time in trypanosomatids to capture RBPs bound to cis-acting 3′UTR elements. Compared to other in vitro and in vivo approaches to isolate RNA-binding proteins, our method is robust and provides reliable results and could be applied in both small and medium scale experiments while also being very cost effective.

2 Materials

2.1 Generating Leishmania Stable Transfectants Co-expressing the MS2 Coat Protein and the Reporter LUC-2MS2-SIDER2 3′UTR or the MS2 Coat Protein Alone

1. *Leishmania infantum* promastigotes grown in mid-exponential phase.
2. *Leishmania* expression plasmid for the tandem MS2 coat protein construct (PTP-tdMCP-HA); pSP72-αIR-HYG-αIR-PTP-tdMCP-HA.
3. *Leishmania* expression plasmid for the luciferase reporter *(LUC)* fused to two MS2 binding sequences and a SIDER2-harboring 3′UTR (from LinJ.30.4000 gene); pSP72-αIR-NEO-αIR-LUC-2MS2-SIDER2 3′UTR.
4. SDM-79 medium supplemented with 10% heat-inactivated fetal calf serum (FCS) (Wisent) and 5 μg/mL hemin.
5. Gene Pulser electroporation cuvettes (Bio-Rad).
6. Bio-Rad Gene Pulser II Electroporation System.
7. Cell culture flasks.
8. 15 and 50 mL Falcon tubes.
9. CO_2 incubator at 25 °C for *Leishmania* promastigote culture.
10. Cooling table centrifuge.
11. PBS (Phosphate Buffered Saline) 1× (pH 7.4).
12. Ultraviolet cross-linker.
13. 10 cm^2 petri dish.
14. Liquid nitrogen tank.
15. Spectrophotometer.
16. Sterile transfection buffer: 21 mM HEPES,150 mM NaCl, 120 mM KCl, 0.7 mM NaH_2PO_4, 6 mM glucose (pH 7.05).
17. Drugs against selection markers.

2.2 Confirmation of the MS2 Coat Protein Expression by Western Blotting

1. *Leishmania* promastigotes stably transfected with the tdMCP-HA expressing plasmid.
2. Hematocytometer.
3. Laemmli 2× lysis/loading buffer: 4% SDS, 10% 2-mercaptoethanol, 20% glycerol, 0.004% bromophenol blue, 0.125 M Tris–HCl (pH 6.8).
4. 100 °C heat block.
5. SDS-PAGE gel and electrophoresis system.
6. SDS-PAGE protein transfer system.
7. Running buffer: 25 mM Tris base, 190 mM glycine, 0.1% SDS; adjust the pH to 8.3.
8. Transfer buffer: 25 mM Tris base, 190 mM glycine, 20% methanol.

9. PVDF (polyvinylidene fluoride) membrane.
10. Wash buffer: PBS–Tween 20, 0.1%.
11. Blocking buffer: 5% milk in PBS–Tween.
12. Anti-HA primary antibody (abmgood, Canada).
13. Anti-MCP rabbit polyclonal antibody (EMD Millipore).
14. Mouse anti-alpha tubulin antibody (Sigma).
15. Anti-mouse HRP-conjugated, anti-rabbit HRP-conjugated or anti-goat HRP-conjugated secondary antibodies.
16. Rocker or rotator.
17. Protein marker.
18. Chemoluminescence with an ECL+ western blotting detection kit (GE Healthcare).

2.3 Coimmunoprecipitation of the MS2 Coat Protein Complex Upon Tethering to the Reporter LUC-2MS2-SIDER2 3′UTR mRNA

1. *Leishmania* transfectant tdMCP-HA promastigotes and cotransfectants with LUC-2MS2-SIDER2 3′UTR cultures in exponential stage.
2. Dounce homogenizer.
3. 1.5 mL sterile microcentrifuge tubes.
4. Refrigerated centrifuge.
5. Magnetic stand.
6. End-over-end rotator.
7. Anti-HA protein G magnetic beads.
8. Protein G magnetic beads (Thermo Scientific).
9. Coimmunoprecipitation lysis buffer: 25 mM Tris–HCl pH 7.4, 100 mM NaCl, 1.5 mM $MgCl_2$, 1 mM EDTA, 0.5% NP40, 5% glycerol, 1 mM PMSF supplemented with protease inhibitors (Roche).
10. Wash Buffer: Tris-buffered saline containing 0.05% Tween 20 Detergent (TBS-T).
11. 50 mM ammonium bicarbonate.

3 Methods

3.1 Generating *Leishmania* Stable Transfectants Co-expressing the MS2 Coat Protein and the Reporter LUC-2MS2-SIDER2 3′UTR or the MS2 Coat Protein Alone

1. Culture *Leishmania* promastigotes in SDM-79 medium supplemented with 10% fetal calf serum (FCS) and 5 μg/mL hemin at 25 °C in a CO_2 atmosphere until they reach late-log phase.
2. Measure the optical density (O.D.) of a late-log *Leishmania* culture at 600 nm using a spectrophotometer.
3. All cultures should have O.D. values of 0.4–0.5, which corresponds to approximately 5×10^7 promastigotes.

4. Spin 10 mL of *Leishmania* culture in a 15 mL tube at 3000 × *g* for 5 min; 5 mL of culture is needed for each transfection.
5. Remove the supernatant and wash the parasites using HEPES–NaCl buffer.
6. Resuspend the parasites and then spin again for another 5 min at 3000 × *g*.
7. Remove the supernatant and then add to the pellet 800 μL of HEPES-NaCl buffer.
8. Resuspend parasites by gently pipetting a few times up and down.
9. Prechill two transfection cuvettes on ice.
10. Add 10 μg of plasmid DNA (max. volume of 40 μL) expressing either the tandem MS2 coat protein (*see* **Note 1**) or the luciferase (*LUC*) reporter gene fused to a tandem of MS2 binding sequences (*see* **Note 2**) and to a SIDER2-bearing 3′UTR (LUC-2MS2-SIDER2 3′UTR) or a combination of both plasmids to each transfection cuvette.
11. As a negative control, transfect another 5 mL of *Leishmania* culture without any plasmid DNA.
12. Carefully pipet 350 μL of *Leishmania* promastigotes to each transfection cuvette and gently pipet up and down for a few times so that the plasmid DNA is mixed well.
13. Incubate the transfection cuvettes on ice for 10 min.
14. Follow with electroporation using Bio-Rad Gene Pulser II Electroporation System or a similar instrument by applying one electrical pulse at 450 V and capacitance at 500 μF (microfarads).
15. Add immediately 1 mL of fresh SDM-79 medium to each electroporation cuvette.
16. Incubate on ice for 10 min.
17. Transfer the transfection mix from each cuvette to a culture flask containing 5 mL fresh SDM-79 medium.
18. Place the culture flasks in the 25 °C cell culture incubator and allow the parasites to recover for 24 h.
19. Add 5 mL fresh SDM-79 medium to each flask.
20. Preselect the transfected promastigotes by adding half amount of the corresponding drug to be used for selection. Similar amount of drug should be added to the control flask (−DNA).
21. At 48 h post-transfection, start selecting transfectants with the appropriate dose of the drug.
22. For each dose of drug, inoculate 1 mL of transfected cells into a new flask containing 9 mL of fresh SDM-79 medium.

23. Incubate the cultures at 25 °C, allowing stable transfectants to emerge within 7–14 days or rarely more, depending on the species of *Leishmania* or the selective drug pressure. The negative control (−DNA) should not grow in the presence of drug selection.
24. Once stable transfectants grow, subculture them in the desired volume of SDM-79 medium (*see* **Note 3**).
25. Use 5 mL culture of single transfectants for the second round of transfection to obtain double transfectants coexpressing tdMCP-HA and LUC-2MS2-SIDER2 3′UTR. Continue the procedure from **step 1** (*see* **Note 4**).
26. Prepare sufficient cultures of transfectants for coimmunoprecipitation (co-IP) studies.
27. Use 100 mL of exponential phase promastigotes for co-IP.
28. Centrifuge the parasites for 5 min at 4 °C.
29. Remove the supernatant and wash twice with ice-cold PBS.
30. Resuspend the cell pellet in 5 mL ice-cold PBS 1× and transfer it to a 10 cm^2 petri dish while on ice.
31. Apply 400 mJ/cm^2 UV irradiation on the cultures (*see* **Note 5**).
32. Immediately transfer the parasites to a 15 mL Falcon tubes and centrifuge for 5 min at 4 °C.
33. Discard the supernatant and snap-freeze the pellet in liquid nitrogen.
34. At this point the parasites could be stored at −80 °C for the short term or in liquid nitrogen for the longer term.

3.2 Confirmation of the MS2 Coat Protein Expression by Western Blotting

1. Count 2×10^7 cells from exponentially grown *Leishmania* promastigotes expressing the MS2 coat protein and from wild type cells using a hematocytometer and centrifuge them for 5 min at 3000 × *g*.
2. Remove the supernatant and wash the cells once with HEPES-NaCl or PBS.
3. Centrifuge again for 5 min at 3000 × *g*.
4. Discard the supernatant and add 200 μL of freshly prepared 2× Laemmli lysis buffer.
5. Resuspend well and heat the sample for 5 min at 95–100 °C.
6. Set up the SDS-PAGE gel in the electrophoresis system.
7. Add the running buffer.
8. Load 30 μg of protein lysates from the transfected and control samples into the SDS-PAGE gel by keeping at least one well empty between the replicates along with a suitable protein marker.

9. Allow the samples to resolve on the gel until the marker bands corresponding to the tdMCP and housekeeping control proteins reach the desired position.
10. Add the freshly prepared transfer buffer to the transfer system and continue with protein transfer to the PVDF membrane at 100 V for 1 h at 4 °C.
11. Place the membrane immediately in the blocking buffer and incubate at room temperature for 1 h.
12. Cut the membrane from the separation line, so that each part will by hybridized with either an anti-HA or an anti-MCP antibody in blocking buffer for 1 h at room temperature (*see* **Note 6**).
13. Wash the membranes 3× for 5 min each with wash buffer.
14. Add the appropriate secondary antibodies in blocking buffer on a rocker or a rotator for 1 h.
15. Wash 3× for 5 min each with wash buffer.
16. Dry the membranes.
17. Quickly add the substrate and proceed with chemoluminescence detection of signals as per the manufacturer's instructions.

3.3 Co-immunoprecipitation of the MS2 Coat Protein Complex Upon Tethering to the Reporter LUC-2MS2-SIDER2 3′UTR mRNA

1. Remove the frozen pellets from −80 °C or from liquid nitrogen and immediately resuspend them into 1–2 mL of ice-cold co-IP lysis buffer.
2. Lyse the cells by applying 20–30 strokes using a Dounce homogenizer while on ice.
3. Take 10 μL from each sample to evaluate lysis efficiency on a counting slide. If more than 10% of the parasites are not lysed yet, proceed with another 5–10 strokes.
4. Transfer the lysate to a prechilled microcentrifuge tube on ice.
5. Centrifuge the lysate for 30 min at 10,000 × *g* at 4 °C to remove cell debris, genomic DNA, and other insoluble material.
6. Add 25 μL of protein G magnetic beads into a 1.5 mL microcentrifuge tube (*see* **Note 7**).
7. Add 175 μL of 0.05% TBS-T to the beads and gently vortex.
8. Place the tubes into a magnetic stand to collect the beads against the side of the tube.
9. Discard the supernatant.
10. Add 1 mL of TBS-T to the tube.
11. Invert the tube several times.
12. Collect beads with magnetic stand.

13. Remove and discard the supernatant.
14. Transfer the cleared lysate to the beads.
15. Invert the tube several times or gently vortex to mix.
16. Place the sample on an end-over-end rotator.
17. Allow the samples to mix for 30 min at 4 °C.
18. Place 50 μL of protein G anti-HA magnetic beads in a microcentrifuge tube (*see* **Note 8**).
19. Add 450 μL TBS-T to the tube and gently mix for 30 s.
20. Collect the beads with the magnetic stand and then discard the supernatant.
21. Wash the anti-HA magnetic beads with 1 mL TBS-T.
22. Collect the beads and discard the supernatant.
23. Place the tubes containing the cleated lysate incubating with protein G magnetic beads on the magnetic stand.
24. Carefully transfer the cleared lysate to the anti-HA magnetic beads from **step 21** and gently mix.
25. Place the tubes on an end-over-end rotator and allow the samples to mix for 4 h at 4 °C.
26. Collect the beads with the magnetic stand, remove and discard the unbound sample.
27. Add 1 mL TBS-T to the tube and gently mix for 30 s.
28. Collect the beads and discard the supernatant.
29. Repeat the washing step twice more.
30. Wash the beads once with 1 mL of 50 mM ammonium bicarbonate. From each tube, take 100 μL and put in a separate tube (tube B).
31. Collect the beads and remove any traces of wash buffer from all tubes.
32. Place the tubes containing the co-IP beads on ice.
33. Store the samples at −20 °C.
34. Proceed with western blotting on the samples collected in tubes B as described in Subheading 3.2 (**steps 4–16**) (*see* **Note 9**).
35. Proceed with protein identification by mass spectrometry (LC-MS/MS).

4 Notes

1. To increase expression of the MS2 coat protein and to consequently improve tethering to the tandem array of MS2 hairpins, it is important to use a tandem MCP construct (tdMCP). Bound coat protein dimers interact cooperatively with one another when are present [33].
2. Optimizing the sequence environment surrounding the MS2 binding hairpins can increase the likelihood of bona fide MS2 hairpin structures in vivo. This is particularly important when inserting few MS2 binding sites on large transcripts. Thus, the linker and surrounding nucleotides should be designed and optimized for each individual mRNA (*see* our example in Fig. 1b).
3. Following confirmation of single or double transfectants by Southern blot and western blot, store several aliquots in liquid nitrogen. This is an important provision particularly when working with episomally transfected parasites as plasmid copy number variations could occur from one passage to another, leading to differences in expression levels.
4. It is possible to obtain double transfectants coexpressing the MS2 coat protein and the *LUC* reporter gene fused to the MS2 binding sequences and to a SIDER2-containing 3′UTR by simultaneously transfecting both plasmids and selecting for two drugs. Alternatively, the reporter LUC-2MS2–3′UTR construct could be integrated as linear fragment into its corresponding 3′UTR chromosomal location. We have shown that a single copy of MCP was not expressed sufficiently (data not shown). It is thus preferable to express the MS2 coat protein in tandem episomally in order to obtain higher protein levels.
5. RNA-protein interactions could be potentially disrupted throughout the sample processing. UV irradiation converts the transient electrostatic interaction of RNA-protein complexes to permanent covalent bonds [35]. Therefore, a 400 mJ/cm^2 UV irradiation of the parasites is recommended prior to freezing the *Leishmania* cells. This will help stabilizing the RNA–protein complex(es) formed in vivo.
6. It is important to carry out western blots to validate tdMCP expression in the double transfectants. In addition, a Northern blot hybridization experiment needs to be done to test whether in vivo tethering of the tdMCP to the reporter mRNA could affect its regulation.

7. Incubation of the cleared lysate with protein G magnetic beads is not necessary, however, it greatly reduces the nonspecific interaction of the *Leishmania* proteins following incubation with protein G anti-HA magnetic beads.
8. The tdMCP protein is tagged with a PTP (ProtC-TEV-ProtA) tag (useful for tandem affinity purification, if needed; [31]) at the N-terminus and with an HA epitope at the C-terminus. PTP is a small tag that enables users to apply affinity purification using Protein A or C resins to purify the RNA-protein complex. As a provision, we also wanted to exploit this approach, however, in our hands immunoprecipitation of the ribonucleoprotein complex using anti-HA magnetic beads generated satisfactory results. Nevertheless, a tdMCP construct without a PTP tag could also be used.
9. Note that at this step it is not necessary to hybridize the membrane with both anti-HA and anti-MCP antibodies. However, as the anti-HA antibody can detect the IgG heavy and light chains (if a mouse anti-HA Ab is used), it is recommended to use an anti-MCP Ab for western blotting to confirm the efficacy of the co-IP (Fig. 2).

Acknowledgments

This work was supported by the Canadian Institutes of Health Research Grant MOP-12182 awarded to B.P.

References

1. Haile S, Papadopoulou B (2007) Developmental regulation of gene expression in trypanosomatid parasitic protozoa. Curr Opin Microbiol 10(6):569–577
2. Clayton CE (2016) Gene expression in kinetoplastids. Curr Opin Microbiol 32:46–51
3. Bringaud F, Müller M, Cerqueira GC et al (2007) Members of a large retroposon family are determinants of post-transcriptional gene expression in Leishmania. PLoS Pathog 3 (9):1291–1307
4. Müller M, Padmanabhan PK, Rochette A et al (2010) Rapid decay of unstable Leishmania mRNAs bearing a conserved retroposon signature 3′-UTR motif is initiated by a site-specific endonucleolytic cleavage without prior deadenylation. Nucleic Acids Res 38 (17):5867–5883
5. Müller M, Padmanabhan PK, Papadopoulou B (2010) Selective inactivation of SIDER2 retroposon-mediated mRNA decay contributes to stage- and species-specific gene expression in Leishmania. Mol Microbiol 77(2):471–491
6. Azizi H, Romao TP, Charret SK et al (2017) RNA secondary structure and nucleotide composition of the conserved hallmark sequence of Leishmania SIDER2 retroposons are essential for endonucleolytic cleavage and mRNA degradation. PLoS One 12(7):e0180678
7. Clement SL, Lykke-Andersen J (2008) A tethering approach to study proteins that activate mRNA turnover in human cells. Methods Mol Biol 419:121–133
8. Park E, Gleghorn ML, Maquat LE (2013) Staufen2 functions in Staufen1-mediated mRNA decay by binding to itself and its paralog and promoting UPF1 helicase but not ATPase activity. Proc Natl Acad Sci U S A 110 (2):405–412
9. Yokoshi M, Li Q, Yamamoto M et al (2014) Direct binding of Ataxin-2 to distinct elements in 3′ UTRs promotes mRNA stability and protein expression. Mol Cell 55(2):186–198
10. Erben ED, Fadda A, Lueong S et al (2014) A genome-wide tethering screen reveals novel potential post-transcriptional regulators in

Trypanosoma brucei. PLoS Pathog 10(6): e1004178

11. Bernardi A, Spahr PF (1972) Nucleotide sequence at the binding site for coat protein on RNA of bacteriophage R17. Proc Natl Acad Sci U S A 69(10):3033–3037
12. Carey J, Lowary PT, Uhlenbeck OC (1983) Interaction of R17 coat protein with synthetic variants of its ribonucleic acid binding site. Biochemistry 22(20):4723–4730
13. Bardwell VJ, Wickens M (1990) Purification of RNA and RNA-protein complexes by an R17 coat protein affinity method. Nucleic Acids Res 18(22):6587–6594
14. LeCuyer KA, Behlen LS, Uhlenbeck OC (1996) Mutagenesis of a stacking contact in the MS2 coat protein-RNA complex. EMBO J 15(24):6847–6853
15. Keryer-Bibens C, Barreau C, Osborne HB (2008) Tethering of proteins to RNAs by bacteriophage proteins. Biol Cell 100(2):125–138
16. Buxbaum AR, Haimovich G, Singer RH (2015) In the right place at the right time: visualizing and understanding mRNA localization. Nat Rev Mol Cell Biol 16(2):95–109
17. Jha BA, Fadda A, Merce C et al (2014) Depletion of the Trypanosome Pumilio domain protein PUF2 or of some other essential proteins causes transcriptome changes related to coding region length. Eukaryot Cell 13(5):664–674
18. Singh A, Minia I, Droll D et al (2014) Trypanosome MKT1 and the RNA-binding protein ZC3H11: interactions and potential roles in post-transcriptional regulatory networks. Nucleic Acids Res 42(7):4652–4668
19. Droll D, Minia I, Fadda A et al (2013) Post-transcriptional regulation of the trypanosome heat shock response by a zinc finger protein. PLoS Pathog 9(4):e1003286
20. Wurst M, Seliger B, Jha BA et al (2012) Expression of the RNA recognition motif protein RBP10 promotes a bloodstream-form transcript pattern in Trypanosoma brucei. Mol Microbiol 83(5):1048–1063
21. Delhi P, Queiroz R, Inchaustegui D et al (2011) Is there a classical nonsense-mediated decay pathway in trypanosomes? PLoS One 6 (9):e25112
22. Gehring NH, Hentze MW, Kulozik AE (2008) Tethering assays to investigate nonsense-mediated mRNA decay activating proteins. Methods Enzymol 448:467–482
23. Jha BA, Gazestani VH, Yip CW et al (2015) The DRBD13 RNA binding protein is involved in the insect-stage differentiation process of Trypanosoma brucei. FEBS Lett 589 (15):1966–1974
24. Finoux AL, Seraphin B (2006) In vivo targeting of the yeast Pop2 deadenylase subunit to reporter transcripts induces their rapid degradation and generates new decay intermediates. J Biol Chem 281(36):25940–25947
25. Brodsky AS, Silver PA (2002) Identifying proteins that affect mRNA localization in living cells. Methods 26(2):151–155
26. Brodsky AS, Silver PA (2000) Pre-mRNA processing factors are required for nuclear export. RNA 6(12):1737–1749
27. Witherell GW, Wu HN, Uhlenbeck OC (1990) Cooperative binding of R17 coat protein to RNA. Biochemistry 29(50):11051–11057
28. Azizi H, Dumas C, Papadopoulou B (2017) The Pumilio-domain protein PUF6 contributes to SIDER2 retroposon-mediated mRNA decay in Leishmania. RNA 23 (12):1874–1885
29. Quenault T, Lithgow T, Traven A (2011) PUF proteins: repression, activation and mRNA localization. Trends Cell Biol 21(2):104–112
30. Peabody DS, Lim F (1996) Complementation of RNA binding site mutations in MS2 coat protein heterodimers. Nucleic Acids Res 24 (12):2352–2359
31. Schimanski B, Nguyen TN, Gunzl A (2005) Highly efficient tandem affinity purification of trypanosome protein complexes based on a novel epitope combination. Eukaryot Cell 4 (11):1942–1950
32. Wu B, Chao JA, Singer RH (2012) Fluorescence fluctuation spectroscopy enables quantitative imaging of single mRNAs in living cells. Biophys J 102(12):2936–2944
33. Johansson HE, Liljas L, Uhlenbeck OC (1997) RNA recognition by the MS2 phage coat protein. Semin Virol 8:176
34. Dertinger D, Dale T, Uhlenbeck OC (2001) Modifying the specificity of an RNA backbone contact. J Mol Biol 314(4):649–654
35. Sei E, Conrad NK (2014) UV cross-linking of interacting RNA and protein in cultured cells. Methods Enzymol 539:53–66

Chapter 21

Forward Genetics in African Trypanosomes

Sebastian Hutchinson and Lucy Glover

Abstract

Forward genetic screens in *Trypanosoma brucei* have enabled researchers to move from a candidate-gene based approach to one where we are able to studying all genes required for a single process simultaneously. In this protocol, we describe how to generate RNAi library strains in bloodstream form trypanosomes, run a screen by selecting for drug resistance or using a reporter gene and process the high-throughput sequencing data for a genome scale RNAi library screen.

Key words *Trypanosoma brucei*, Forward genetics, RNAi, Phenotypic screen, High-throughput sequencing

1 Introduction

Genome-scale genetic phenotypic screens have the potential to uncover novel biology, making it an invaluable tool considering that 65% of the *Trypanosoma brucei brucei* (T. brucei) genes is classed as hypothetical conserved [1]. Genetic tools such as RNAi have long been available to study the gene function in trypanosomes, but establishing high-throughput RNAi library screens in bloodstream form parasites was hampered by relatively low transfection efficiency. This was solved through combining Lonza Nucleofection and I-*Sce*I meganuclease technology [2], resulting in a 250-fold increase in transfection efficiency or approximately 250,000 transformants per electroporation, which allows researchers to generate million-clone RNAi libraries in a facile manner. Access to in-house or commercial sequencing platforms now allows for the routine application of high-throughput sequencing to genome scale RNAi libraries.

Here we describe how genome-scale RNAi libraries are set up to ensure high coverage, and the steps taken to reduce false positives. Generating a high coverage library where multiple RNAi fragments target the same gene and are maintained during selection ensures high-confidence hits and reduces the risk of false positive

Paul A. M. Michels et al. (eds.), *Trypanosomatids: Methods and Protocols*, Methods in Molecular Biology, vol. 2116, https://doi.org/10.1007/978-1-0716-0294-2_21,

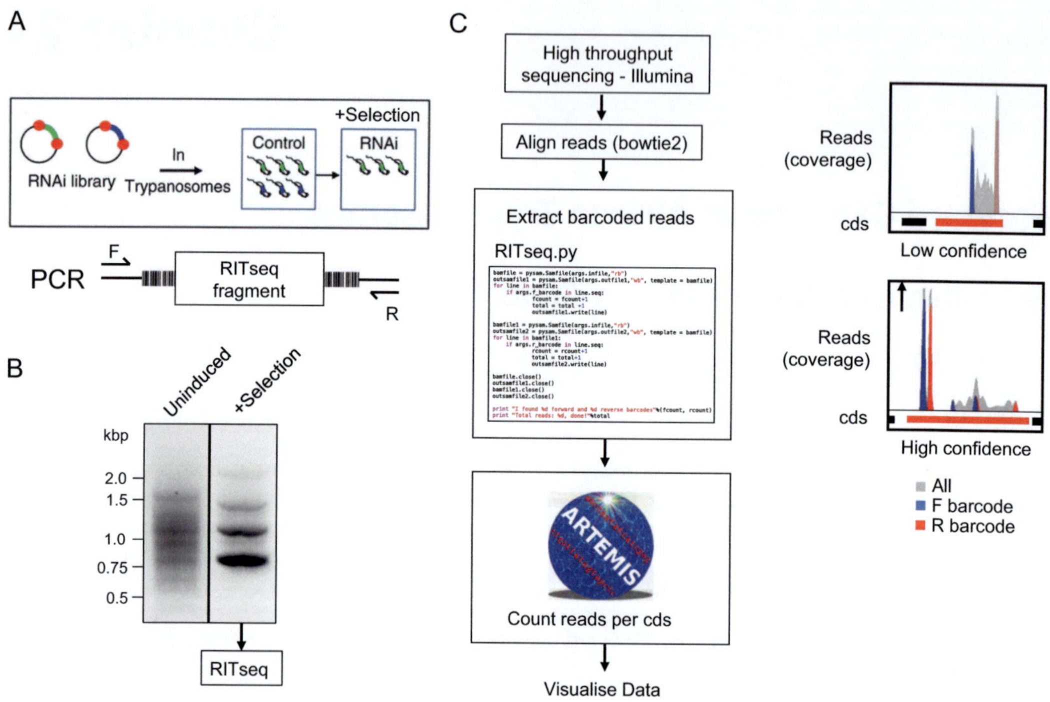

Fig. 1 RITseq pipeline. (**a**) Schematic of RITseq. Above, the library strain is selected for RNAi fragments that confer resistance to a selectable agent. Below, RITseq fragments are PCR amplified from extracted DNA using primers outside of unique 14-b barcode sequences (indicated as barcodes). (**b**) Gel image of DNA amplified from either uninduced or a selected library. Following PCR amplification, DNA is sequenced on the Illumina pipeline. (**c**) RITseq analysis pipeline. Reads are generated on the Illumina platform, and aligned to the T. brucei genome sequence. Reads containing barcodes are extracted using a custom script [2], the number of reads per cds calculated, and "hits" visualized and assessed for complexity in Artemis [16]. Examples of high and low confidence hits are shown

hits (Fig. 1a and b). Observing multiple RNAi targets on the same gene shows that multiple cells in the screen displayed the same phenotypic response to selection (Fig. 1c). Each RNAi target fragment serves as an individual barcode within a complex population, and library selection results in enrichment of individual RNAi clones within that population, while identification of these barcodes in high-throughput sequencing data further rules out false positives from PCR amplification (Fig. 1a–c). Robust selection, using a toxin, drug, or reporter, is therefore paramount as it reduces background noise from cells that survive the selection process. Given the nature of RNAi, gene knockdown that results in lethality or loss of fitness will not be reported in this assay. Thus far, RNAi libraries in trypanosomes have been successfully used to link genotype to phenotype for fitness [3], drug action and resistance [4], cAMP signaling [5], quorum sensing [6, 7], human serum resistance [8], DNA damage [9], and antigenic variation [10].

2 Materials

2.1 T. brucei *Culturing*

1. T. brucei cell line 2T1 [11]. All T. brucei cell lines described in this protocol are derived from *Trypanosoma brucei brucei* strain Lister 427.
2. HMI-11 culturing medium: To prepare 5 l of HMI-11 medium, add 1 pot of HMI-9 powder (*see* **Note 1**) to 4 l of sterile distilled water in a large beaker with continuous stirring. Weigh 15 g of sodium bicarbonate ($NaHCO_3$) and transfer to the beaker. Add 70 μl of β-mercaptoethanol and 25 ml of penicillin/streptomycin, 10,000 U/ml/10,000 μg/ml and mix fully. Check pH and adjust to pH 7.6 if necessary. Make up to 4.5 l with water. Filter 450 ml medium into sterile bottles using a 0.22 μm filter and store at 4 °C. Before use, add 50 ml of non–heat-inactivated fetal bovine serum to complete the medium.
3. Culture flasks with vented caps, 25 cm^2, 75 cm^2, 175 cm^2.
4. Antibiotic stock solutions: G418 (10 mg/ml), hygromycin b (5 mg/ml), phleomycin (10 mg/ml), puromycin (2.5 mg/ml), blasticidin S (10 mg/ml), penicillin/streptomycin (10,000 U/ml/10,000 μg/ml), tetracycline (1 mg/ml).
5. Other culturing reagents: Resazurin sodium salt 0.125 mg/ml in PBS.

2.2 T. brucei *Library Strain Setup*

1. High transformation efficient electrocompetent DH5α *Escherichia coli* (E. coli) cells.
2. Luria broth (LB): Dissolve 10 g tryptone, 5 g yeast extract, 10 g sodium chloride in 1 l of distilled water (dH_2O).
3. Ampicillin: Dissolve 2.5 g ampicillin powder in 50 ml 70% ethanol for a 50 mg/ml stock solution. Store in a 50 ml Falcon tube wrapped in foil at −20 °C.
4. LB plates with 50 μg/ml ampicillin: 1.5% (w/v) Bacto Agar added to 1 l LB medium. Ampicillin added to a final concentration of 50 μg/ml.
5. Plasmids: pZJM-660 RNAi library (obtained from Jim Morris and Paul Englund [12], available from the author on request), pT7Pol-BLA ([2] available from the author on request), pRPaSce∗ ([2] available from the author on request, and on signing a material transfer agreement from the Institut Pasteur).
6. Cytomix: 2 mM EGTA pH 7.6, 120 mM KCl, 0.15 mM $CaCl_2$, 10 mM $^1K_2HPO_4/KH_2PO_4$ pH 7.6, 25 mM HEPES pH 7.6, 5 mM $MgCl_2{\cdot}6H_2O$, 0.5% glucose (dextrose), 100 μg/ml BSA, 1 mM hypoxanthine, adjust to pH 7.6 with

KOH, and store at 4 °C. [1]Prepare 10× K_2HPO_4/KH_2PO_4 pH 7.6 stock solution by mixing 8.66 ml 1 M K_2HPO_4 with 1.34 ml 1 M KH_2PO_4 in 90 ml H_2O (adapted from [13]).

7. Amaxa nucleofector and Lonza human T cell Nucleofector kit.

2.3 Library Sequencing and Mapping

1. UNIX based computer system (Mac OSX or Linux).
2. Bowtie2 short read aligner [14].
3. SAMtools [15].
4. Artemis pathogen genome browser [16].
5. Pysam htslib interface for python [15].
6. RITseq.py script [2].
7. *Trypanosoma brucei* genome sequence FASTA file and accompanying genome feature file (gff).
8. Microsoft Excel.

3 Methods

All steps are done at room temperature, unless otherwise specified.

3.1 Preparation of Plasmid DNA for RNAi Library Strain Setup

1. Transformation of E. coli with pZJM-660 plasmid DNA should be done in triplicate. Mix 0.1 μg of plasmid DNA with high transformation efficient electrocompetent DH5α E. coli cells and transform the cells according to manufacturer's instructions. Pool the three samples and add to 1 l of LB with 50 μg/ml ampicillin. Swirl LB to mix. To check the transformation efficiency, remove and plate out 80 μl and 16 μl, for a 1/10,000 and 1/50,000 dilution, respectively, on LB + amp plates and place in a 37 °C incubator overnight. Grow the bacteria in the 1 l of inoculated LB overnight in a shaking incubator at 37 °C and 4 × *g*.
2. The following morning, count the colonies on the two plates. In order to maintain a high complexity library of at least 1 million transformants, there should be a minimum of 80 and 16 colonies per plate, respectively. Do not proceed further if fewer colonies are counted.
3. Extract plasmid DNA using 4x maxi-prep columns and quantify the plasmid DNA. The DNA should be dissolved to 1 μg/μl in distilled water and stored at −20 °C.
4. Digest the plasmids overnight according to Table 1. Digest 10 μg of DNA per transfection for pT7POL1-Bla and pRPaSce∗ and 40 μg of pZJM-660 library DNA.

Table 1
Plasmids and corresponding digests required for RNAi library strain setup

Plasmid	μg to digest	Transfection digest	Drug selection
pT7Pol-BLA	10	*Nsi*I and *Eco*RV	Blasticidin
pRPaSce∗	5	*Asc*I	Hygromycin
pZJM-660	50	*Not*I	Phleomycin

5. In parallel, digest pRPaSce∗ with recombinant I-*Sce*I to ensure that the Sce site is still present in the plasmid. I-*Sce*I should linearize the plasmid.
6. The following day, run 0.5 μg of digested DNA alongside 0.5 μg of undigested DNA to check for complete linearization of the plasmids.
7. Clean the DNA using phenol–chloroform–isoamyl alcohol (25:24:1). Add an equal volume of phenol–chloroform–isoamyl alcohol to the digest and vortex to mix. Microcentrifuge for 1 min at 18407 × *g*. Remove the top layer being careful not to disturb the bottom layer and place in a clean 1.5 ml microcentrifuge tube. Add three volumes of ice cold 100% ethanol and gently agitate to mix. A white DNA precipitate may be visible at this point. Place at either −20 °C or −80 °C for 20 min. Spin for 5 min at 18407 × *g* and remove supernatant. Add 250 μl of 70% ethanol and spin for a further 5 min. Remove 950 μl of the supernatant and spin for a further 1 min. Remove the remaining supernatant being careful not to disturb the pellet. Air-dry in a laminar flow hood to keep DNA sterile. Once dry, resuspend in sterile distilled water to 1 μg/μl and store at −20 °C until ready to use.

3.2 T. brucei RNAi Library Strain Setup

1. Generating $2T1^{T7}$ cell line: This method is for one transfection. This step is to remove the phleomycin drug resistance cassette and replace it with blasticidin and integrate T7 into the cell line. Expression of the RNA fragment in pZJM-660 is driven by a T7 promoter, and the plasmids contain a phleomycin resistance cassette [12]. Grow (*see* **Note 2**) 2T1 cells in HMI-11 medium with 1 μg/ml phleomycin and 1 μg/ml puromycin. 24 h prior to transfection, spin the cells for 10 min at 1000 × *g* at room temperature and discard the supernatant. Resuspend the cell pellet in fresh medium with 1 μg/ml puromycin only. Transfection with pT7Pol1-BLA replaces the bleomycin resistance gene with blasticidin resistance. For the transfection, spin down 2.5 × 10^7 cells for 10 min at 1000 × *g* at room temperature in a 50 ml centrifuge tube. During the spin, prepare one 25 cm^2 culture flask per

transfection with 36 ml warmed HMI-11 medium only. For the linearized pT7POL1-BLA, add 100 μl of cytomix to the prepared DNA and place it in a 37 °C water bath to warm up. Pour off the medium and then invert the centrifuge tube over paper towel to remove excess medium. Resuspend the cell pellet in the warmed DNA–cytomix solution and place 100 μl in a 0.2 cm gap cuvette, and nucleofect using the X-001 program. Immediately place the transfected cells into the prepared flasks and place in an incubator to allow the cells to recover for approximately 6 h. After 6 h, for each transfection flask, prepare solutions for limiting dilution by preparing 1/25 and 1/5 dilutions of the culture in a total volume of 48 ml medium with 1 μg/ml puromycin and 10 μg/ml blasticidin and distribute into 48 well plates. Add 1 μg/ml puromycin and 10 μg/ml blasticidin to the remaining transfection culture and distribute into a 48 well plate, this is the "neat plate." Place the plates into the incubator. After 4 days, check the plates for positive wells. Pick positive wells from plates where less that 30% of the wells are positive. Clones with the correct integration of the construct should be resistant to puromycin and blasticidin and sensitive to phleomycin.

2. Screening clones for correct integration: To identify the correct clones, split each clone into two wells of a 48-well plate. To one well add medium with 1 μg/ml puromycin and 1 μg/ml blasticidin and in the second well add medium with 1 μg/ml phleomycin. After 24 h screen the well for clones that are sensitive to phleomycin but grow in blasticidin and puromycin. Expect 10–20% of the clones to be sensitive. Pick 2–3 clones and freeze for future use.
3. Making frozen stabilates: Expand T. brucei clones to 1×10^6 cells/ml. Add 0.5 ml of culture to 0.5 ml of a 20% glycerol solution in HMI-11 medium in a 1 ml cryovial and mix gently by pipette 2–3 times. Place at −80 °C immediately. Cryostocks are stable at −80 °C for up to 6 months and in liquid nitrogen indefinitely.
4. Generating $2T1^{T7}$Sce∗ cell line: Follow the protocol for transfection as set out in **step 1** with the following modifications. Grow the $2T1^{T7}$ cell line in HMI-11 medium with 1 μg/ml blasticidin and 1 μg/ml puromycin. 24 h prior to transfection, spin the cells for 10 min at 1000 × *g* at room temperature and discard the supernatant. Resuspend the cell pellet in fresh medium with 1 μg/ml blasticidin only. Transfect with digested pRPaSce∗. Plate out the transfection as before but selecting with 2 μg/ml hygromycin and 1 μg/ml blasticidin. After 4 days, check the plates for positive wells. Pick positive wells from plates where less that 30% of the wells are positive. Clones with the correct integration of the construct should be resistant to hygromycin and blasticidin and sensitive to puromycin [11].

5. Screening clones for correct integration: To identify the correct clones, split each one into two wells of a 48 well plate. To one well add medium with 1 μg/ml hygromycin and 1 μg/ml blasticidin and in the second well add medium with 1 μg/ml puromycin. After 24 h check the wells for clones that are sensitive to puromycin but grow in blasticidin and hygromycin. Expect 10–20% of the clones to be sensitive. Once correct clones have been identified, proceed directly to **step 6** (*see* **Note 3**).
6. Generating $2T1^{T7}$Lib cell line: This protocol is for 4 library transfections. Grow the appropriate $2T1^{T7}$Sce∗ cell line, for each library transfection 5×10^7 cells are used, therefore ensure you have a total of 2×10^8 cells on the morning of the transfection. Add 1 μg/ml tetracycline to the $2T1^{T7}$Sce∗ cells and place in the incubator for 3 h (*see* **Note 4**). After 3 h, split the culture into 4 × 50 ml centrifuge tubes and spin the cells for 10 min at 1000 × *g* at room temperature. Pour off the supernatant and replace with 20 ml fresh medium without drugs and spin as before (this step removes the tetracycline from the medium and prevents RNAi induction following transfection with the library DNA). During the spin, prepare the 2 × 175 cm^2 flasks with 300 ml HMI-11 medium of 37 °C. Pour off the medium and invert the centrifuge tubes onto a paper towel to remove any excess medium. Resuspend the cells in 100 μl Human T-cell Nucleofector solution (Lonza) and 10 μg of prepared pZJM-660 library DNA (Subheading 3.1, **step 4**) and immediately place 100 μl of the solution into a 0.2 cm gap electroporation cuvette and transfect using the X-001 Nucleofector setting. Immediately place the transfected cells into the prepared flasks, 2 transfections per flask and rinse out the cuvettes with medium to ensure maximum recovery of cells. Place the flasks in an incubator to recover for 6 h. Following 6 h of recovery, add 2 μg/ml phleomycin and 1 μg/ml blasticidin to the flasks. Do not add hygromycin as the gene is replaced by integration of the RNAi library constructs. Before placing the flask in the incubator, remove 100 μl from each of the 300 ml transfection cultures and add to 2.4 ml of HMI-11 medium with 2 μg/ml phleomycin and 1 μg/ml blasticidin for **step 7**. Place flasks in the incubator for 48 h.
7. Determining library complexity: Prepare a flat bottomed 96 well plate for threefold dilution series by leaving columns 1 and 7 empty, adding 200 μl of HMI-11 medium with 2 μg/ml phleomycin and 1 μg/ml blasticidin to columns 2–5 and 8–11 and 100 μl to columns 6 and 12 using a multichannel pipette. Add 300 μl of the cell culture (100 μl + 2.4 ml HMI-11) from flask 1 into lane 1. Using a multichannel pipette, remove 100 μl from lane 1 and add to lane 2, pipet

up and down gently to mix and repeat up to lane 6. Repeat this with cells from flask 2 starting from column 7–12. Place the plate in an incubator for 5 days. After 5 days determine the number of wells with healthy dense population of cells in each column. For a library complexity of more than 1×10^6 clones, the number of positive wells in columns 4–6 (for flask 1) and 10–12 (flask 2) should exceed 16 combined for each flask.

8. Freezing RNAi library strain: After 48 h, pellet the cells from flask 1 by centrifuging for 10 min at $1000 \times g$. Pour off the supernatant and resuspend the cells in the remaining medium. Add this cell suspension to flask 2, rinsing out the centrifuge tube with a small amount of medium to ensure maximum recovery. Gently swirl the flask to fully mix the cells. Count the cells using a hemocytometer or cell counter to determine the cell density. 48 h is adequate time to allow for selection by phleomycin. A cell density of 1×10^8 cells/ml or higher indicates that $\geq 1 \times 10^6$ cells were transformed. Do not proceed with running a screen or freezing down the RNAi library strain if you have $<5 \times 10^7$ cells. To maintain library complexity, freeze down 1×10^7 RNAi library cells per cryovial in 10% glycerol and place at −80 °C for overnight to 6 months before placing in liquid nitrogen for indefinitely storage. We suggest freezing down as many aliquots as possible to allow for multiple screens to be run from a single RNAi library.

3.3 Running an RNAi Library Screen—Selection by Drug Resistance

1. Determining the EC_{50} of a drug by Alamar blue assay [17]: For this assay use wild-type bloodstream form T. brucei cells. Prepare a flat-bottomed 96 well plate by adding 200 μl of HMI-11 medium to the wells in rows 1–4 of column 1. Add 100 μl of HMI-11 to the wells in rows 1–4 of columns 2–11. Add 200 μl of HMI-11 medium with 2× the highest concentration of your drug of choice to the wells in rows 1–4 of column 12. Establish a twofold dilution gradient across the plate by removing 100 μl of HMI-11 with drug from rows 1–4 of column 12 and adding it to the wells in column 11. Repeat this procedure up to the rows in column 3. Therefore, column 1 is the medium-only control; column 2 is the no-drug control, and columns 3–12 drug dilution gradient. Each row represents one experiment; therefore, the assay is done in quadruplicate. Add 100 μl of HMI-11 medium with 4×10^3 T. brucei cells/ml to rows 1–4 in columns 2–12. Place the plate in an incubator for approximately 66 h. Following this, add 20 μl of 0.125 mg/ml resazurin to each well and place the plates in an incubator for 6 h. Set up a plate reader as follows: excitation, 530 nm; emission, 585 nm; filter cut off, 570 nm to determine the cell viability by color change.

2. Alamar blue assay data analysis: Microsoft Excel and GraphPad Prism software (or equivalent) are required. Subtract values from columns 2–12 from medium-only control in column 1 to get "% inhibition" / "% growth" and express as a percentage proportion of the cell-only reading (column 2). Import the data into GraphPad to generate EC_{50} curves by carrying out nonlinear regression analysis using the "Sigmoidal dose-response (variable slope)" function. Derive the EC_{50} of your chosen drug from the curve.
3. Thawing the RNAi library: Use RNAi library cells generated in Subheaidng 3.2, **step 6** or thaw a frozen stock. Place the RNAi library cryovial in a 37 °C water bath for 1–2 min until completely thawed (do not leave in the water bath for an extended period). Place the cells into a 10 ml centrifuge tube with 9 ml of fresh HMI-11 at 37 °C. Rinse out the cryovial to ensure maximal recovery of the cells. Centrifuge for 10 min at 1000 × *g*. Pour off the supernatant, this step removes the excess glycerol and allows for faster recovery of the library. Place the cells in 100 ml HMI-11 medium with 1 μg/ml phleomycin and 1 μg/ml blasticidin and allow them to recover for 6 h. After 6 h count the cells, and check for more than 80% recovery. Expand the RNAi library strain in HMI-11 medium with 1 μg/ml phleomycin and 1 μg/ml blasticidin, maintain cell density below 1×10^6 cells/ml. Excess cells can be frozen down. In order to prevent loss of complexity, cells expanded from a frozen stock should be labeled as "Library 2" to indicate one round of freeze-thaw. If running a screen from a "Library 2" stock, we suggest thawing and mixing two vials per screen. To prevent long-term loss of complexity, do not exceed more than two freeze thaw cycles.
4. Running a RNAi library screen: Multiple drug screens can be run in parallel. This following protocol is to test one drug. Set up four 175 cm^2 flasks containing 150 ml HMI-11 medium with 1 μg/ml phleomycin and 1 μg/ml blasticidin and 2×10^7 cells in total. Flask 1 is the uninduced control; flask 2 is the induced control and flasks 3 and 4 drug selection screens. To flasks 2, 3 and 4 add 1 μg/ml tetracycline. After 24 h, count the cells from flasks 1–4 and split back to 2×10^7 cells/150 ml HMI-11 medium. Add $2 \times EC_{50}$ of your drug to flasks 3 and 4. Throughout the duration of the screen the cultures should be maintained on 1 μg/ml phleomycin and 1 μg/ml blasticidin. Fresh tetracycline should be added to flasks 3 and 4 when split or every 3 days as tetracycline is photolabile. Count the cells daily to generate a growth curve, splitting and adding fresh drug where necessary. Depending on the efficacy of the selectable drug, selection should result in a reduction in the number of cells between days 2 and 5. Maintain the cell number at

2×10^7 cells/150 ml HMI-11, splitting only when necessary, to ensure library complexity. Following library selection, a resistant population outgrowth is typically seen between days 5 and 8. Aim to obtain a minimum of 3 orders of magnitude difference in cellular growth between unselected and selected flasks to obtain a high signal-to-noise ratio. Following 2–3 days of exponential growth, extract DNA from 1×10^8 cells from flasks 1–4, and freeze down two vials of cells from flasks 2, 3, and 4 (*see* Subheading 3.2, **step 8**).

5. RNAi library PCR reaction mix: Per 50 μl reaction, add 10 μl 10× Taq reaction buffer, 1 μl dNTPs (10 mM stock), 5 μl $MgCl_2$ (25 mM stock), 1 μl Lib2 Forward primer (10 mM stock; TAGCCCCTCGAGGGCCAGT), 1 μl Lib2 Reverse primer (10 mM stock; GGAATTCGATATCAAGCTTGGC), 0.1 μg T. brucei RNAi library DNA, 1.25 units Taq DNA Polymerase, dH_2O up to 50 μl.
6. RNAi library reaction conditions: 1 cycle for 2 min at 95 °C; 30 cycles of 30 s at 95 °C, 30 s at 57 °C, 130 s at 72 °C; 1 cycle of 10 min at 72 °C. Final hold at 4 °C.
7. Gel Purification of PCR products: Run 5 μl of the PCR product in a 1% agarose gel and visualize the bands with a DNA stain. The uninduced (flask 1) and induced (flask 2) PCRs should produce a "smear" from approximately 250–1500 bp, due to the number and complexity of products, whereas the selected RNAi libraries should produce discrete bands. Gel-purify the bands from the RNAi library PCR and Sanger sequence using the Lib2 forward and reverse primers for initial identification of RNAi target sequences using BLAST. The gel-purified bands can also be ligated into a vector such as pGEM-T Easy if sequencing directly from a PCR product gives sub-optimal results.
8. Validation of hits: From the low-throughput sequencing, genes of interest can be validated using an RNAi and native tagging for localization. Multiple systems are available for both RNAi and gene tagging in T. brucei (these include, but are not limited to [11, 18, 19]).

3.4 Running a RNAi Library Screen-Selection by Toxin

1. RNAi library screens can be run using selection with a toxin such as human serum [8] or methyl methanesulfonate (MMS) [9].
2. Follow **steps 1–8** of Subheading 3.2 to generate the $2T1^{T7}$Lib cell lines. Determine the EC_{50} of your toxin using protocol in **steps 1–2** of Subheading 3.3 or use published data to determine the selection. Follow **steps 3–7** of Subheading 3.3.

3.5 Running an RNAi Library Screen—Selection by Reporter Construct

1. Generating a reporter cell line: For a reporter construct, use a neomycin drug resistance cassette. Follow **steps 1–3** of Subheading 3.2 to generate the $2T1^{T7}$ cell line. Transfect with your reporter construct and screen for transformants. Select clones and determine the EC_{50} of G418 using protocol in **steps 1–2**, Subheading 3.3. Follow the remaining protocol as set out in Subheading 3.2, **steps 4–8** and Subheading 3.3, **steps 3–7**.

3.6 High-Throughput Sequencing—RIT-Seq

1. There are a number of different options available for high-throughput sequencing, including in-house sequencing platforms and external services. Ion Torrent, Illumina and BGI (Beijing Genomics Institute) sequencing protocols have been successfully used [6, 7, 9, 10]. The protocol detailed here follows a standard PCR free library construction protocol with <800 bp fragments.
2. Library PCR: Run the library PCR as detailed in Subheading 2.3, **steps 5–6**. Pool the PCRs so that you have at least 10 μg of DNA. Do not gel-purify these samples. Quantify the samples using a NanoDrop or Qubit Fluorometer (Invitrogen). We suggest sequencing both the uninduced and induced libraries. The uninduced libraries will allow you to assess coverage.
3. Library construction using an Illumina DNA library preparation kit: Fragment 10 μg of DNA using an ultrasonicator (e.g., Covaris ultrasonicator). Check the fragmentation on a 1% agarose gel. Purify the fragmented DNA using a PCR Purification Kit. Using a DNA End-repair kit, combine the fragmented DNA and End Repair Mix; incubate reaction for 30 min at 20 °C and then purify the end-repaired DNA with a PCR Purification Kit. Using an A-tailing kit, combine the end-repaired DNA and A-Tailing Mix; incubate the A-Tailing reaction for 30 min at 37 °C. Ligate the adaptors to the A-tailed DNA by combining the Adenylate 3′Ends DNA, PCR Free index adapters and T4 DNA Ligase Mix, mix well by pipetting. Incubate the ligate reaction for 16 h at 16 °C. Purify the end-repaired DNA with a PCR Purification Kit.
4. Library size-selection and purification: Size select the ligated products by running a 2% agarose gel purifying products centered between 150 and 600 bp with a gel Extraction kit.
5. Library validation: Determine the average length of the DNA library using the Agilent 2100 bioanalyzer instrument (Agilent DNA 1000 Reagents), and quantify the library by real-time quantitative PCR (QPCR) (TaqMan Probe).
6. Library sequencing: Amplify the libraries within the cBot instrument flow cell for cluster generation (Hiseq 4000 PE Cluster Kit Illumina). Load the clustered flowcell onto the Hiseq 4000 Sequencer for paired-end sequencing (Hiseq 4000 SBS Kit, Illumina) with recommended read lengths 100 bp or 150 bp.

3.7 Analyzing Sequence Data

Analysis of high-throughput sequencing data requires basic understanding of command line tools, readers with little bioinformatics experience are strongly recommended to read a primer on using the UNIX terminal.

1. Prepare a bowtie2 index of the T. brucei genome using the command `bowtie2-build [options]* <reference_in> <bt2_base>`
2. Align RITseq reads in fastq files to the bowtie2 index using the command: `bowtie2 --very-sensitive-local -p <n> -x <T. brucei Index> -1 <Read1.fq.gz> -2 <Read2.fq.gz> | samtools view -bS - | samtools sort -T temp.bam -O BAM -o <RITseq_alignments.bam>`
3. Create a BAM index file using `samtools index <RITseq_alignments.bam>`
4. Extract RNAi target barcoded reads using the RITseq.py script. Use the command: `python RITseq.py -i <RITseq_alignments.bam> -1 RITseq_forward.bam -2 RITseq_reverse.bam -f GTGAGGCCTCGCGA -r TCGCGAGGCCTCAC`.
5. Create BAM index files for the two RITseq files created using `samtools index <RITseq_[forward/reverse].bam`.
6. Open the T. brucei genome FASTA file and load the genome feature file in Artemis.
7. Open the three aligned read files in BAM format from **step 4**.
8. Select all CDS features in Artemis and right-click in the BAM viewer and click Analyze > Read count of selected features. Save the resulting file as a ".txt" file.
9. Open the file from **step 8** in Microsoft Excel. Sum the forward and reverse barcoded read counts and rank order from highest to lowest.

4 Notes

1. HMI-11 powder is prepared once a year by Life Technologies for the Trypanosome community.
2. Cell growth: Bloodstream form trypanosomes are sensitive to high density. The strains described here divide approximately every 6–7 h and should be split when cell density reaches 1×10^6 cells/ml. Media should be warmed to 37 °C before use and cells grown in an incubator with 5% CO_2. All culturing should be done in sterile hood.

3. Due to leaky expression the $2T1^{T7}Sce*$ cell line is unstable. Expression on the I-*Sce*I gene and cutting of the Sce recognition site leads to loss of the site in the cell line and subsequent loss of transfection efficiency. We therefore do not recommend freeze-thawing this cell line. It should be remade for each new library cell line.
4. The 3-h induction with tetracycline allows for expression of I-*Sce*I and cleavage of the Sce site prior to transfection with the library DNA.

References

1. El-Sayed NM, Hegde P, Quackenbush J, Melville SE, Donelson JE (2000) The African trypanosome genome. Int J Parasitol 30:329–345
2. Glover L, Alsford S, Baker N, Turner DJ, Sanchez-Flores A, Hutchinson S, Hertz-Fowler C, Berriman M, Horn D (2015) Genome-scale RNAi screens for high-throughput phenotyping in bloodstream-form African trypanosomes. Nat Protoc 10:106–133
3. Alsford S, Turner DJ, Obado SO, Sanchez-Flores A, Glover L, Berriman M, Hertz-Fowler C, Horn D (2011) High-throughput phenotyping using parallel sequencing of RNA interference targets in the African trypanosome. Genome Res 21:915–924
4. Alsford S, Eckert S, Baker N, Glover L, Sanchez-Flores A, Leung KF, Turner DJ, Field MC, Berriman M, Horn D (2012) High-throughput decoding of antitrypanosomal drug efficacy and resistance. Nature 482:232–236
5. Gould MK, Bachmaier S, Ali JA, Alsford S, Tagoe DN, Munday JC, Schnaufer AC, Horn D, Boshart M, de Koning HP (2013) Cyclic AMP effectors in African trypanosomes revealed by genome-scale RNA interference library screening for resistance to the phosphodiesterase inhibitor CpdA. Antimicrob Agents Chemother 57:4882–4893
6. Rico E, Ivens A, Glover L, Horn D, Matthews KR (2017) Genome-wide RNAi selection identifies a regulator of transmission stage-enriched gene families and cell-type differentiation in Trypanosoma brucei. PLoS Pathog 13: e1006279
7. Mony BM, MacGregor P, Ivens A, Rojas F, Cowton A, Young J, Horn D, Matthews K (2014) Genome-wide dissection of the quorum sensing signalling pathway in Trypanosoma brucei. Nature 505:681–685
8. Alsford S, Currier RB, Guerra-Assuncao JA, Clark TG, Horn D (2014) Cathepsin-L can resist lysis by human serum in Trypanosoma brucei brucei. PLoS Pathog 10:e1004130
9. Stortz JA, Serafim TD, Alsford S, Wilkes J, Fernandez-Cortes F, Hamilton G, Briggs E, Lemgruber L, Horn D, Mottram JC et al (2017) Genome-wide and protein kinase-focused RNAi screens reveal conserved and novel damage response pathways in Trypanosoma brucei. PLoS Pathog 13:e1006477
10. Glover L, Hutchinson S, Alsford S, Horn D (2016) VEX1 controls the allelic exclusion required for antigenic variation in trypanosomes. Proc Natl Acad Sci U S A 113 (26):7225–7230
11. Alsford S, Kawahara T, Glover L, Horn D (2005) Tagging a T. brucei RRNA locus improves stable transfection efficiency and circumvents inducible expression position effects. Mol Biochem Parasitol 144:142–148
12. Morris JC, Wang Z, Drew ME, Englund PT (2002) Glycolysis modulates trypanosome glycoprotein expression as revealed by an RNAi library. EMBO J 21:4429–4438
13. van den Hoff MJ, Moorman AF, Lamers WH (1992) Electroporation in 'intracellular' buffer increases cell survival. Nucleic Acids Res 20:2902
14. Langmead B, Trapnell C, Pop M, Salzberg SL (2009) Ultrafast and memory-efficient alignment of short DNA sequences to the human genome. Genome Biol 10:R25
15. Li H, Handsaker B, Wysoker A, Fennell T, Ruan J, Homer N, Marth G, Abecasis G, Durbin R, Genome Project Data Processing, S (2009) The sequence alignment/map format and SAMtools. Bioinformatics 25:2078–2079
16. Carver T, Harris SR, Berriman M, Parkhill J, McQuillan JA (2012) Artemis: an integrated platform for visualization and analysis of high-throughput sequence-based experimental data. Bioinformatics 28:464–469

17. Raz B, Iten M, GretherBuhler Y, Kaminsky R, Brun R (1997) The Alamar blue(R) assay to determine drug sensitivity of African trypanosomes (T-b-rhodesiense and T-b-gambiense) in vitro. Acta Trop 68:139–147
18. Alsford S, Horn D (2008) Single-locus targeting constructs for reliable regulated RNAi and transgene expression in Trypanosoma brucei. Mol Biochem Parasitol 161:76–79
19. Dean S, Sunter J, Wheeler RJ, Hodkinson I, Gluenz E, Gull K (2015) A toolkit enabling efficient, scalable and reproducible gene tagging in trypanosomatids. Open Biol 5:140197
20. Yang Y, Ko TP, Chen CC, Huang G, Zheng Y, Liu W, Wang I, Ho MR, Hsu ST, O'Dowd B et al (2016) Structures of trypanosome vacuolar soluble pyrophosphatases: antiparasitic drug targets. ACS Chem Biol 11:1362–1371

Chapter 22

Analysis of Base Excision and Single-Strand Break Repair Activities in Trypanosomatid Extracts

Daria M. Kania, Michael L. Ginger, and Sarah L. Allinson

Abstract

Cellular DNA is inherently unstable, subject to both spontaneous hydrolysis and attack by a range of exogenous and endogenous chemicals as well as physical agents such as ionizing and ultraviolet radiation. For parasitic protists, where an inoculum of infectious parasites is typically small and natural infections are often chronic with low parasitemia, they are also vulnerable to DNA damaging agents arising from innate immune defenses. The majority of DNA damage consists of relatively minor changes to the primary structure of the DNA, such as base deamination, oxidation, or alkylation and scission of the phosphodiester backbone. Yet these small changes can have serious consequences, often being mutagenic or cytotoxic. Cells have therefore evolved efficient mechanisms to repair such damage, with base excision and single strand break repair playing the primary role here. In this chapter we describe a method for analyzing the activity from cell extracts of various enzymes involved in the base excision and single strand break repair pathways of trypanosomatid parasites.

Key words AP endonuclease, Base excision repair, Cell extracts, DNA repair, Glycosylase, In vitro repair assay, *Leishmania*, Polynucleotide kinase/phosphatase, Single-strand break repair, *Trypanosoma*

1 Introduction

Trypanosomatid parasites—*Trypanosoma*, *Leishmania*, *Phytomonas* species—cause a broad spectrum of pathologies and diseases in susceptible mammals and plants [1–4]. Unsurprisingly, the greatest degree of experimental investigation has been for the etiological agents of the serious tropical diseases: visceral, mucocutaneous, and cutaneous leishmaniasis, Chagas disease (caused by *T. cruzi*), and African sleeping sickness (caused by T. brucei) plus veterinary relevant animal trypanosomiases (caused by a variety of *Trypanosoma* species of perceived "African" and "American" origins).

DNA-damaging and mutagenic agents continue to be considered for their potential application as novel antitrypanosomatid drugs. Base excision, single-strand break, and other pathways of DNA repair have been identified and partially characterized in

Paul A. M. Michels et al. (eds.), *Trypanosomatids: Methods and Protocols*, Methods in Molecular Biology, vol. 2116, https://doi.org/10.1007/978-1-0716-0294-2_22, © Springer Science+Business Media, LLC, part of Springer Nature 2020

several trypanosomatid parasites [5]. From these studies roles for DNA damage response and repair pathways in T. brucei in response to innate immunity-induced insults have also emerged e.g., [6] and differences in DNA repair activities have been identified in different life cycle stages of the same trypanosomatid species (T. brucei [7]) and between species (e.g., *T. cruzi* and *Leishmania major* [8]). Such differences potentially reflect involvement of some DNA repair enzymes, if not entire pathways, in processes central to the tissue-specific trophisms particular to different trypanosomatid life cycles (e.g., antigenic variation in African trypanosomes [9, 10] or the recently discovered role(s) for large-scale gene amplifications during *Leishmania* life cycles [11, 12]). However, despite recent advances we know little about the interplay between the different pathways of DNA repair in trypanosomatids or the potential importance of specific repair pathways at different points of cell cycle control (e.g., during S-phase or G2/M transitions). With cell cycle synchronization by elutriation now possible [13] and a wide array of reverse genetics tools available including CRISPR/Cas9 [14, 15] the stage is well set for continued investigation and comparative analyses of DNA repair in trypanosomatids.

Here, we describe how to assay the activities of DNA repair enzymes associated with the base excision and single strand break repair pathways within trypanosomatid cell extracts. The preparation of extract and assay of enzyme activities can be readily applied to other microbial eukaryotes; for instance, we have recently used similar methods to assay repair activities in *Giardia*, *Naegleria*, and *Spironucleus* cell-free extracts (unpublished data). Moreover, although in this chapter we focus on the base excision and single strand break repair pathways, the extracts could be combined with appropriately designed substrates to assay for other DNA metabolism activities such as topoisomerase cleavage activity [16] or flap cleavage [17].

2 Materials

All solutions should be made using molecular biology-grade reagents and ultrapure, sterile distilled water.

2.1 Preparation of Whole Cell Extracts

1. Buffer I: 10 mM Tris–HCl, pH 7.8, 200 mM KCl.
2. Buffer II: 10 mM Tris–HCl, pH 7.8, 600 mM KCl, 2 mM EDTA, 40% glycerol, 0.2% Nonidet P-40, 2 mM dithiothreitol (DTT).
3. Dialysis buffer: 25 mM HEPES, pH 7.5, 5 mM $MgCl_2$, 200 mM NaCl, 1 mM EDTA, 15% glycerol, 1 mM DTT (*see* **Note 1**).

2.2 Preparation of Oligonucleotide Substrates

1. TE buffer: 10 mM Tris–HCl, pH 8.0, 1 mM EDTA.
2. Fluorescently labeled oligonucleotides (*see* **Note 2**).
3. 10× TBE buffer: 890 mM Tris, 890 mM boric acid, 20 mM EDTA.
4. Acrylamide solution: 40% acrylamide (19:1 acrylamide–bisacrylamide). We purchase this ready-prepared (National Diagnostics AccuGel™).
5. 8% nondenaturing polyacrylamide gel: 10 ml acrylamide solution, 5 ml 10× TBE, 35 ml deionized water, 300 μl 10% ammonium persulfate (*see* **Note 3**), 30 μl *N*,*N*,*N*′,*N*-′-tetramethylethylenediamine (TEMED). This prepares sufficent for an 18 cm × 20 cm 1 mm thick gel. Use a wide well (e.g., 2.5 cm) comb.

2.3 DNA Repair Activity Assays

1. 20× BER buffer: 800 mM HEPES, pH 7.5, 100 mM $MgCl_2$, 20 mM DTT, 2 mM EDTA.
2. 2 mM NAD^+: A 1 M stock solution can be readily prepared from β-nicotinamide adenine dinucleotide sodium salt solid powder. Stock solutions can be stored frozen at −80 °C for up to 2 years.
3. 1 mM ATP: A 1 M stock solution can be readily prepared from adenosine 5′-triphosphate disodium hydrate solid powder. Stock solutions can be stored frozen for up to 1 year.
4. 1 mM ddNTP: a mixture of ddATP, ddCTP, ddGTP, and ddTTP (*see* **Note 4**).
5. 1 mg/ml creatine kinase (CK): 1 mg/ml (Roche) in 10 mM HEPES, pH 7.5, 50 mM NaCl, 50% glycerol. If prepared in this way, aliquots of creatine kinase will maintain activity for up to 2 years in the −80 °C freezer (*see* **Note 5**).
6. 100 mM phosphocreatine (PC): aliquots of the prepared solution can be stored frozen for at least 1 year.
7. 1 mg/ml bovine serum albumin (BSA): molecular biology grade BSA (e.g., New England Biolabs) must be used. The BSA should be diluted to the appropriate concentration in deionized water.
8. 100 μM nonspecific oligonucleotide: we use 35–40 nt random sequence oligonucleotides (e.g., leftover primers) for this purpose.
9. FA buffer: 10 mM EDTA, 98% formamide, 10 mg/ml blue dextran (*see* **Note 6**).
10. FA/NaOH buffer: 10 mM EDTA, 10 mM NaOH, 98% formamide, 10 mg/ml blue dextran.

2.4 Denaturing Polyacrylamide Gel Electrophoresis

1. TBE buffer: 89 mM Tris, 89 mM boric acid, 2 mM EDTA.
2. Denaturing acrylamide gel solution: 25% acrylamide (19:1 acrylamide–bisacrylamide), 7.5 M urea. We purchase this ready prepared (National Diagnostics UreaGel™).
3. 5× denaturing PAGE buffer: 445 mM Tris, 445 mM boric acid, 10 mM EDTA, 8 M urea. This can be prepared by dissolving 480 g of urea in 250 ml of 10× TBE solution and making up the final volume to 500 ml.

3 Methods

We recommend wearing gloves at all times. Use nuclease-free microcentrifuge tubes and tips to avoid nuclease contamination of your samples. We recommend thawing reagents on ice, mixing them thoroughly before use, keeping them on ice during the assembly of reactions and returning them immediately to the freezer after being used. Multiple freeze-thaw cycles of reagents, particularly cell extracts is not recommended. Reactions are typically 10 μl but can be scaled up if required.

3.1 Preparation of Cell Extracts

1. Allow the frozen cell pellet to thaw on ice. Pulse-spin the tube to collect the cells at the bottom of the tube.
2. Estimate the volume of the cell pellet. This is the packed cell volume (PCV). Resuspend cells in one PCV of ice-cold Buffer I containing protease inhibitors (e.g., *c*Omplete, Mini, EDTA-free from Roche) and transfer the cell suspension into a 1.5 ml microcentrifuge tube.
3. Add one PCV of ice-cold Buffer II to the suspension.
4. To facilitate cell lysis place the tube on a rotator for 2 h at 4 °C.
5. Remove insoluble cell debris by centrifugation in a microfuge at 13,000 rpm (16,600 × *g*) for 20 min at 4 °C.
6. Collect the cleared cell lysate and start dialysis in 500 ml of freshly prepared ice-cold dialysis buffer at 4 °C using dialysis membrane with a 2 kDa molecular weight cut-off. We use Slide-A-Lyzer Dialysis cassettes.
7. After 2 h, exchange the dialysis buffer with 500 ml of fresh ice-cold dialysis buffer. Allow the dialysis to continue overnight at 4 °C.
8. Remove the dialyzed cell lysate from the membrane and centrifuge in a microfuge at 13,000 rpm (16,600 × *g*) for 10 min at 4 °C to remove any precipitated material.

9. Collect the soluble cell extracts. Determine the protein concentration using the Bradford assay [18].
10. Snap-freeze aliquots of cell extracts in liquid nitrogen and store at −80 °C (*see* **Note 7**).

3.2 Preparation of Oligonucleotide Substrates

A wide range of modified bases and 3′ and 5′ end modifications are available from commercial oligonucleotide suppliers, enabling many DNA repair activities to be measured. Examples of activities that can be measured using simple oligonucleotide substrates of this type include glycolytic removal of a damaged base, endo- or exonucleolytic cleavage of the DNA backbone or removal of a 5′ or 3′ end moiety (*see* references [19–21] for examples). Where AP endonuclease activity is being assayed, the most convenient substrate to use is the abasic site analogue tetrahydrofuran (often referred to as "dSpacer") due to the low stability of true AP sites to hydrolysis.

The use of fluorescently labeled substrates offers several advantages over ^{32}P, which is still often used in many reported studies. These include improved user safety, increased substrate longevity, and the possibility of measuring more than one activity at a time. In the examples shown in Fig. 1, the 5′ end of the substrate oligonucleotide has been labeled with a fluorescent dye but 3′-end labeling can be used instead depending on the particular activity that is being studied. If two activities need to be measured simultaneously (e.g., both 5′ and 3′ end-processing) then two complementary fluorescent dyes can be used at either end of the substrate (see reference [22] for an example of this).

1. If the oligonucleotides have been supplied lyophilized, redissolve them in TE buffer to a concentration of 100 μM (i.e., 100 pmol/μl) (*see* **Note 8**).
2. Mix 1000 pmol of fluorescently labeled oligonucleotide (s) with 1100 pmol unlabeled complementary oligonucleotide in a microcentrifuge tube.
3. Add sufficient 5 M NaCl to give a final concentration of 200 mM. Mix gently. If needed, pulse-spin the tube to collect the solution at the bottom of the tube.
4. Place the tube in a thermoblock at 95 °C. Switch off the thermoblock and allow it to cool down slowly to room temperature to anneal the oligonucleotides (*see* **Note 9**).
5. Add 1/5 volume of 50% glycerol to the annealed oligonucleotides. Load the annealed oligonucleotides onto a prerun 8% nondenaturing polyacrylamide gel and carry out the electrophoresis at the constant voltage of 150 V for 2 h (*see* **Note 10**).

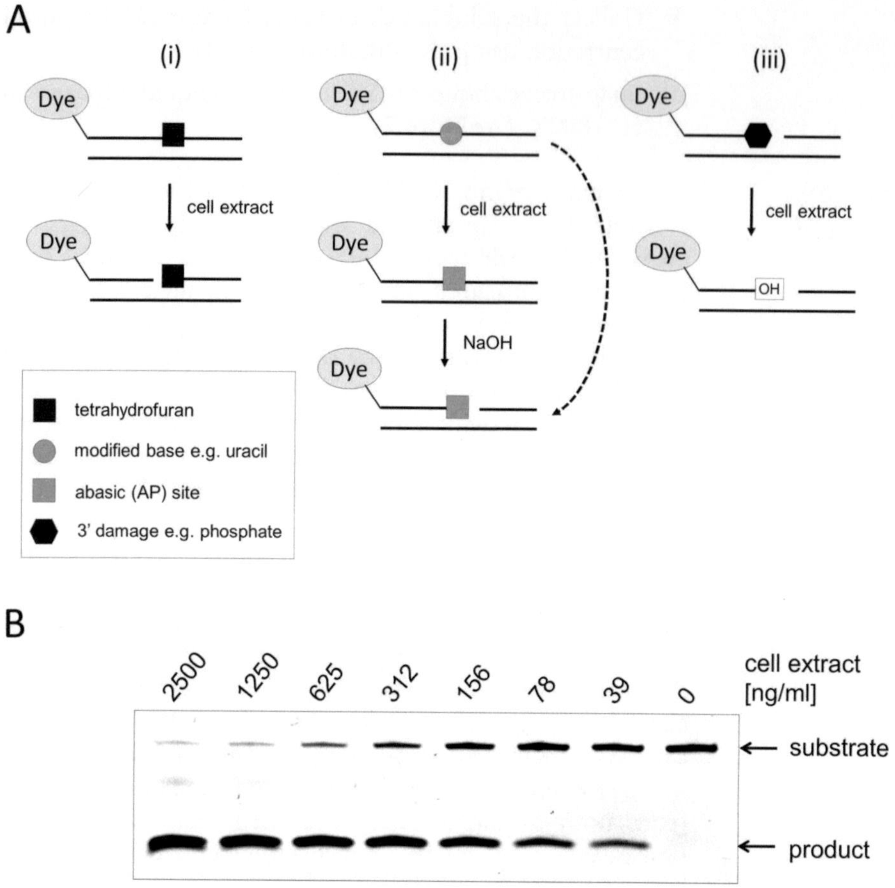

Fig. 1 In vitro base excision repair and single strand break repair assays. (**a**) Schematic representation of the processing of various oligonucleotide substrates by cell extracts. The upper (dye-labeled) strand is shown in 5′–3′ orientation in each case. (1) Substrate containing a site-specifically located tetrahydrofuran (dSpacer, AP site mimic) moiety is cleaved by an AP endonuclease immediately 5′ to the modified site. (2) Removal of a damaged base by a glycosylase in the cell extract results in the formation of an AP site. In the case of a monofunctional glycosylase, the removal of the base can be revealed by subsequent heating of the stopped reaction in the presence of NaOH, which will drive the hydrolytic cleavage of the phosphodiester backbone at the AP site. Bifunctional glycosylases have an associated AP lyase activity (dotted line) which results in enzymatic cleavage of the backbone. (3) The assay can also be used to measure DNA end-processing activities. In the example shown here, the removal of a terminal phosphate would result in slightly decreased mobility through a denaturing PAGE gel. (**b**) Example repair assay results. A 39-nucleotide double stranded oligonucleotide substrate (25 nM), containing a dSpacer at position 18 on one strand labeled at the 5′-end with Cy5, was incubated for 30 min at 37 °C with the indicated concentrations of cell extracts prepared from procyclic *T. brucei brucei* strain 427. Following addition of FA loading/stop buffer, the reaction mixtures were loaded onto a prerun 20% denaturing PAGE gel (minigel format) and run at 210 V for 1 h. The gel was imaged on a Bio-Rad ChemiDoc system, where the 39-nucleotide substrate could be readily discerned from the 17-nucleotide product

6. Once the electrophoresis is complete, open the glass plates carefully and cut out the band corresponding to oligonucleotide duplex with a clean razor blade (*see* **Note 11**).
7. Place the piece of gel containing the DNA in a clean microcentrifuge tube. Add 300 μl of TE buffer ensuring that the whole piece of gel is covered with buffer and leave at 4 °C overnight.
8. Apply the supernatant from **step** 7 to a Spin-X centrifuge tube filter (with cellulose acetate membrane of 0.22 μm membrane pore size). This essential step removes any small particles of polyacrylamide that may have carried over from the microcentrifuge tube.
9. Add 11 μl of 3 M sodium acetate and 900 μl of 100% cold ethanol to the filtered supernatant and leave at −80 °C for 20 min.
10. Centrifuge at 13,000 rpm (16,600 × *g*) in a microfuge for 20 min at 4 °C.
11. Remove and discard the supernatant carefully, taking care to avoid disturbing the pellet.
12. Wash the pellet twice with ice-cold 70% ethanol.
13. Air-dry the pellet for 5–10 min and then redissolve the oligonucleotide duplex in a suitable volume of TE buffer containing 200 mM NaCl.
14. Determine the DNA concentration by UV spectrophotometry at 260 nm (*see* **Note 12**).
15. Store aliquots of the substrate at −80 °C. The substrate can be stored for several years under these conditions with no loss of fluorescence or other degradation.

3.3 In Vitro DNA Repair Assays

A schematic of the repair assays and an example of the types of results that can be expected can be seen in Fig. 1. When first beginning experiments to assay for a particular activity, it is advisable to begin by titrating cell extracts across a wide range of concentrations (i.e., varying by several orders of magnitude) to determine the optimum amount of cell extract to include.

1. Prepare the appropriate reaction mastermix as shown below, where $n =$ the number of samples +1:

   Composition of glycosylase activity assay reaction:

20× BER buffer: 0.5 n μl

BSA (1 mg/ml): 1 n μl.

DNA substrate (500 nM): 0.5 n μl.

100 mM EDTA: 1 n μl

Nuclease-free water: 5 n µl.

Composition of phosphatase/kinase/endonuclease activity assay reaction:

20× BER buffer: 0.5 n µl

NAD^+ (2 mM): 1 n µl.

ATP (1 mM): 1 n µl.

ddNTPs (1 mM): 1 n µl.

CK (1 mg/ml): 1 n µl.

PC (200 mM): 1 n µl.

BSA (1 mg/ml): 1 n µl.

Oligonucleotide substrate (500 nM): 0.5 n µl.

Nonspecific single-stranded oligonucleotides (0.1 mg/ml): 1 n µl.

2. Dilute the cell extracts in dialysis buffer using the serial dilution method to the desired concentration(s).
3. Label the required number of the microcentrifuge tubes for all reactions and control.
4. Add 2 µl from each dilution of cell extracts into the correct tube and 2 µl of dialysis buffer for the control reaction.
5. Add 8 µl of mastermix into each microcentrifuge tube.
6. Mix gently by pipetting and pulse-spin in the microfuge to collect the solution at the bottom of the tube.
7. Incubate in a thermoblock at 37 °C for the appropriate time. We find that 15–30 min is a good starting point.
8. Stop the reactions by adding 10 µl of either FA or FA/NaOH buffer, as appropriate (*see* **Note 13**). Mix gently by pipetting.
9. Place the samples in a thermoblock at 95 °C for 5 min. At this step you can load the samples immediately onto a preheated 8 M urea 20% denaturing polyacrylamide gel or store the samples at −20 °C for later electrophoresis. If choosing the second option, remember to heat the samples in the thermoblock at 95 °C for 5 min again prior to loading the samples onto the gel.

3.4 Denaturing Polyacrylamide Gel Electrophoresis

The instructions provided here are for a 38 cm × 20 cm × 0.4 mm gel. The amounts can be scaled down if using minigel format. The choice of which size of gel to use is determined in part by the nature of the substrate and product (*see* **Note 14**).

1. Assemble the set of glass-plates including the 0.4 mm spacers on each side and tape together carefully, reinforcing the bottom corners with extra tape to prevent leaking.

2. Mix 40 ml of the denaturing acrylamide gel solution with 10 ml of 5× denaturing PAGE buffer.
3. Add 250 μl of 10% ammonium persulfate (*see* **Note 3**). Mix gently.
4. Add 25 μl of TEMED. Mix gently.
5. Immediately pour the gel solution between the glass plates avoiding the introduction of air bubbles.
6. Insert the comb (we typically use a 12-well comb) and allow the gel to set for approximately 10–15 min.
7. Remove the comb and immediately wash the wells with deionized water. Remove the tape from the bottom of the glass plates. Assemble the glass plates with the electrophoresis equipment. Add 1× TBE buffer in the top and bottom buffer reservoirs.
8. Run the gel at a constant power of 42 W for 40–50 min to preheat it.
9. Flush the wells with TBE buffer before loading 10 μl of each sample. Run the gel for a further 2.5 h at 42 W.
10. Image the gel using either a laser scanning fluorimager, such as a Typhoon FLA7000, or a gel documentation system equipped with fluorescence imaging (e.g., Bio-Rad ChemiDoc). The gel can be left within the glass plates for this step.

4 Notes

1. Dialysis buffer can be prepared ahead of time and stored at 4 °C but the DTT should always be added just before use. Stocks of 1 M DTT can be stored in the freezer for this purpose. Aliquots of dialysis buffer can also be stored in the freezer for use in diluting cell extracts for assays.
2. For achieving the best signal-to-noise ratio, we recommend selecting fluorescent dyes that emit in the far red range (Cy5, Alexa Fluor 633, Atto 655, etc.). The option to have oligonucleotides HPLC-purified during manufacture should be selected. In most cases, we find that this results in oligonucleotides of sufficient purity that they can be used directly in the preparation of double-stranded substrates. In some cases, the oligonucleotides supplied by the manufacturer are insufficiently pure, evidenced by additional bands (failure sequences) visible on denaturing PAGE. In this case, the oligonucleotide can be purified by denaturing PAGE beforehand. To do this, the oligonucleotide should be mixed with an equal volume of FA buffer (Subheading 2.3, **item 9**) for loading, heated to 95 °C for 5 min and then loaded onto a 20 cm × 20 cm × 1 mm

20% denaturing PAGE gel (prepared as in Subheading 3.4) that has been prerun at 800 V for 1 h. The wells should be flushed with TBE before loading. The gel should then be run at 800 V for 1 h. The protocol thereafter is the same as **steps 6–14** of Subheading 3.2.

3. A preprepared solution of 10% ammonium persulfate can be stored in the refrigerator for up to 2 weeks.
4. Dideoxynucleoside triphosphates are included in standard reactions for glycosylase and AP endonuclease activity to prevent primer extension, potentially completing repair and resulting in the formation of a product that would be indistinguishable from the substrate by denaturing PAGE.
5. Creatine kinase and phosphocreatine are included in the reaction mixtures to provide an ATP-recycling system. This is particularly important if assaying for DNA kinase or ligase activities.
6. Blue dextran is included to allow the samples to be visualized when loading onto the gel. The blue dextran will remain in the well throughout the electrophoresis. We do not recommend the use of migratory dyes such as xylene cyanol or bromophenol blue, as they give a high background on fluorescence imaging.
7. If liquid nitrogen is not readily available, label the required number of microcentrifuge tubes, leave them open in a rack in a −80 °C freezer for an hour and subsequently pipet 50–100 μl of cell extracts into each tube, close the tubes and place them immediately back in the −80 °C freezer. Avoid multiple freeze–thaw cycles as this can affect protein integrity and therefore decrease DNA repair activity.
8. The concentration of the oligonucleotides should be accurately measured after dissolution in TE. The extinction coefficient for each particular oligonucleotide can be obtained using an online tool such as OligoCalc (http://biotools.nubic.northwestern.edu/OligoCalc.html).
9. An alternative method that can be used to anneal the oligonucleotides is to heat a beaker of water to boiling, place a float containing the microcentrifuge tube of oligonucleotide mixture in the water and allow to cool to room temperature.
10. There is no need to add any loading dyes to this sample as the fluorescent label will allow it to be visualized.
11. The use of an excess of unlabeled complementary strand should mean that there is only one band visible. However, if more than one band is visible then the duplex is the upper of these.

12. Again, an online tool such as OligoCalc should be used to calculate the extinction coefficient of the oligonucleotide duplex. Note that base-stacking effects mean that the extinction coefficient of double-stranded DNA is lower than that of single-stranded DNA. Accordingly, the "dsDNA" option should be selected in OligoCalc.
13. In the majority of cases, FA buffer should be used for this step which serves to stop the reaction and also add loading buffer. However, when measuring the activity of glycosylases, particularly monofunctional DNA glycosylases such as UDG, the samples need to be heated under basic conditions to allow strand cleavage at the abasic site generated to occur. In this case FA/NaOH buffer should be used.
14. The best resolution of substrate and product is achieved on 38 cm long "sequencing" gels and this is essential for separating species that differ in size by three nucleotides or less. Where the substrate and product differ more extensively in size, a smaller gel, such as the size commonly used in the laboratories for SDS-PAGE, can be used. A pair of glass plates 7 cm × 10 cm with 1 mm spacer requires 7.5 ml of gel solution. Smaller gels should be prerun for 30–45 min at a constant voltage of 30 V/cm and run for 60 min at a constant voltage of 30 V/cm.

Acknowledgments

D.M.K. is in receipt of a PhD studentship from the Faculty of Health and Medicine, Lancaster University.

References

1. Bern C (2015) Chagas' disease. N Engl J Med 373:456–466
2. Rao SPS, Barrett MP, Dranoff G et al (2019) Drug discovery for kinetoplastid diseases: future directions. ACS Infect Dis 5:152–157
3. Ponte-Sucre A, Gamarro F, Dujardin JC et al (2017) Drug resistance and treatment failure in leishmaniasis: a 21st century challenge. PLoS Negl Trop Dis 11:e0006052
4. Jaskowska E, Butler C, Preston G, Kelly S (2015) *Phytomonas*: trypanosomatids adapted to plant environments. PLoS Pathog 11: e1004484
5. Genois MM, Paquet ER, Laffitte MC et al (2014) DNA repair pathways in trypanosomatids: from DNA repair to drug resistance. Microbiol Mol Biol Rev 78:40–73
6. Yagüe-Capilla M, Garcia-Caballero D, Aguilar-Pereyra F et al (2019) Base excision repair plays an important role in the protection against nitric oxide- and in vivo-induced DNA damage in *Trypanosoma brucei*. Free Radic Biol Med 131:59–71
7. Vieira-da-Rocha JP, Passos-Silva DG, Mendes IC et al (2019) The DNA damage response is developmentally regulated in the African trypanosome. DNA Repair 73:78–90
8. Garcia JB, Rocha JP, Coasta-Silva HM et al (2016) *Leishmania major* and *Trypanosoma cruzi* present distinct DNA damage responses. Mol Biochem Parasitol 207:23–32
9. Castillo-Acosta VM, Aguilar-Pereya F, Bart J-M et al (2012) Increased uracil insertion in DNA is cytotoxic and increases the frequency of mutation, double strand break formation and VSG switching in *Trypanosoma brucei*. DNA Repair 11:986–995

10. McCulloch R, Cobbold CA, Figueiredo L et al (2018) Emerging challenges in understanding trypanosome antigenic variation. Emerg Top Life Sci 1:585–592
11. Laffitte MN, Leprohon P, Papadopoulou B, Ouellette M (2016) Plasticity of the *Leishmania* genome leading to gene copy number variations and drug resistance. F1000Res 5:2350
12. Bussotti G, Gouzelou E, Côrtes Boité M et al (2018) *Leishmania* genome dynamics during environmental adaptation reveal strain-specific differences in gene copy number variation, karyotype instability and telomeric amplification. MBio 9:e01399–e01318
13. Benz C, Dondelinger F, McKean PG, Urbaniak MD (2017) Cell cycle synchronization of *Trypanosoma brucei* by centrifugal counterflow elutriation reveals the timing of nuclear and kinetoplast replication. Sci Rep 7:17599
14. Beneke T, Madden R, Makin L et al (2017) A CRISPR Cas9 high-throughput genome editing toolkit for kinetoplastids. R Soc Open Sci 4:170095
15. Lander N, Li ZH, Niyogi S, Docampo R (2015) CRISPR/Cas9-induced disruption of paraflagellar rod protein 1 and 2 genes in *Trypanosoma cruzi* reveals their role in flagellar attachment. MBio 6:e1012
16. Das BB, Sen N, Roy A, DesGupta SB, Ganguly A, Mohata BC, Dinda B, Majumder HK (2006) Differential induction of *Leishmania donovani* bi-subunit topoisomerase I-DNA cleavage complex by selected flavones and camptothecin: activity of flavones against camptothecin-resistant topoisomerase I. Nucleic Acids Res 34:1121–1132
17. Ponce I, Aldunate C, Valenzuela L, Sepúlveda S, Garrido G, Kemmerling U, Cabrera G, Galanti N (2017) A flap endonuclease (TcFEN1) is involved in *Trypanosoma cruzi* cell proliferation, DNA repair and parasite survival. J Cell Biochem 118:1722–1732
18. Bradford MM (1976) A rapid and sensitive method for the quantitation of microgram quantities of protein utilizing the principle of protein-dye binding. Anal Biochem 72:248–254
19. Peña-Diaz J, Akbari M, Sundheim O, Farez-Vidal ME, Andersen S, Sneve R, González-Pacanowska D, Kroka HE, Slupphaug G (2004) *Trypanosoma cruzi* contains a single detectable uracil-DNA glycosylase and repairs exclusively *via* short patch base excision repair. J Mol Biol 342:787–799
20. Charret KS, Requena CE, Castillo-Acosta VM, Ruiz-Pérez LM, González-Pacanowska D, Vidal AE (2012) *Trypanosoma brucei* AP endonuclease 1 has a major role in the repair of abasic sites and protection against DNA-damaging agents. DNA Repair 11:53–64
21. Ormeño F, Barrientos C, Ramirez S, Ponce I, Valenzuela L, Sepúlveda S, Bitar M, Kemmerling U, Machado RM, Cabrera G, Galanti N (2016) Expression and the peculiar enzymatic behavior of the *Trypanosoma cruzi* NTH1 DNA glycosylase. PLoS One 11: e0157270
22. Dobson CJ, Allinson SL (2006) The phosphatase activity of mammalian polynucleotide kinase takes precedence over its kinase activity repair of single strand breaks. Nucleic Acids Res 34:2230–2237

Part IV

Cell Biology

Chapter 23

Light Microscopy in Trypanosomes: Use of Fluorescent Proteins and Tags

Samuel Dean and Jack Sunter

Abstract

Fluorescence microscopy enables the localization of proteins to specific structures within a cell which have either been fused to a fluorescence protein or detected by immunofluorescence. Here, we describe the various procedures that can be used to prepare both the procyclic form and bloodstream form of the human pathogen *Trypanosoma brucei* for fluorescence microscopy. The choice of procedure to be used is determined by various parameters, including protein characteristics and the scientific question being investigated.

Key words Light microscopy, Trypanosomes, Live cell, Fluorescent proteins, Cytoskeletons

1 Introduction

Light microscopy enables images of cells to be acquired; however, unstained cells have little inherent contrast, meaning phase contrast [1] or differential interference contrast (DIC) [2] microscopy is required to visualize cellular features, and these techniques are the foundation on which cellular imaging is based. As informative as these simple phase contrast/DIC images are, they do not provide any information about the localization of specific proteins.

The localization of a protein to a structure or organelle within a cell is informative when considering the function of that protein. The highly structured and polarized cell architecture of *Trypanosoma brucei* makes them an ideal cell type for defining protein localization as each cell has the same pattern of organelle positioning [3]. Fluorescence molecules absorb light of one wavelength and emit light of a longer wavelength. Numerous fluorescent reagents are available to study the localization of a protein, including specific stains, lectins, antibodies, and genetically encoded protein tags including both fluorescent proteins and epitopes [4–8]. Historically, microscopy was performed on fixed cells; however, with the development of fluorescent proteins and other reporters there has

Paul A. M. Michels et al. (eds.), *Trypanosomatids: Methods and Protocols*, Methods in Molecular Biology, vol. 2116, https://doi.org/10.1007/978-1-0716-0294-2_23,

been a switch to imaging live cells, which has opened up a wide range of experimental possibilities including fluorescence recovery after photobleaching, tracking moving fluorescent particles, and measuring intracellular calcium fluctuations [9–11].

T. brucei has a complex life cycle with many developmental forms; however, only the procyclic form (insect midgut) and the bloodstream form (mammal) are readily culturable and imaging protein localizations in these stages will be the focus of this chapter. The quality of the image acquired during microscopy is dependent on the preparation of the cells for microscopy with poorly handled and prepared samples giving poor quality and inconsistent data. Therefore, we have detailed the protocols we use for preparing trypanosome cells for microscopy and highlighted which approach is most appropriate for which type of protein and which application. This chapter focuses on *T. brucei*, the organism in which these protocols were developed; however, with minor modifications these techniques will be applicable to the other trypanosomatid parasites.

2 Materials

Prepare all solutions using ultrapure water and analytical grade chemicals at room temperature. Store solutions at room temperature, unless indicated otherwise.

1. Phosphate buffered saline (PBS): 137 mM NaCl, 2.7 mM KCl, 10 mM Na_2HPO_4, 1.8 mM KH_2PO_4. For a 10× stock, add approximately 100 mL of water to a 1 L measuring cylinder. Weigh 80 g NaCl, 1 g KCl, 14.4 g Na_2HPO_4 and 2.4 g KH_2PO_4 and transfer to the measuring cylinder. Add water to make volume up to 1 L. Store at room temperature and dilute as necessary.
2. Voorheis modified PBS (vPBS) [12]: 137 mM NaCl, 3 mM KCl, 16 mM Na_2HPO_4, 3 mM KH_2PO_4, 46 mM sucrose. For a 1× stock, add approximately 100 mL of water to a 1 L measuring cylinder. Weigh 8 g NaCl, 0.22 g KCl, 2.27 g Na_2HPO_4, 0.41 g KH_2PO_4, and 15.7 g sucrose and transfer to the measuring cylinder. Add water to make up to 1 L and then sterile filter through a 0.22 μm filter. Always transfer vPBS from the stock bottle in a sterile environment.
3. 1 mg/mL Hoechst 33342 solution: Weigh 50 mg Hoechst 33342 and transfer to a 100 mL measuring cylinder. Add water to a volume of 50 mL and mix well. Transfer solution to a 50 mL Falcon tube and store at 4 °C. This is a 1000× stock solution.

4. 4% (w/v) formaldehyde in PBS solution: Add 4 mL of formaldehyde 16% (w/v) solution, methanol free (TAAB, F017/3) to 10.4 mL water and 1.6 mL of 10× PBS stock.
5. 1% (w/v) glycine in PBS solution: Weigh 0.5 g glycine and add to 50 mL PBS.
6. 10% (v/v) IGEPAL CA-630 (Sigma-Aldrich, I8896) solution: Measure 5 mL of IGEPAL CA-630 into a 50 mL measuring cylinder and then add water to make up to 50 mL. Mix thoroughly.
7. 0.1% (v/v) IGEPAL CA-630 in PBS solution: Add 500 μL 10% (v/v) IGEPAL CA-630 solution to 50 mL PBS.
8. 1 M piperazine-*N,N′*-bis(2-ethanesulfonic acid) (PIPES)–NaOH pH 6.9: Add approximately 300 mL of water to a 500 mL measuring cylinder. Weigh 151 g PIPES and transfer to the measuring cylinder. Adjust the pH to 6.9 with NaOH and then make up the volume to 500 mL. Sterile filter through a 0.22 μm filter and always transfer PIPES–NaOH from the stock bottle in a sterile environment.
9. 100 mM $MgSO_4$: Add approximately 150 mL of water to a 250 mL measuring cylinder. Weigh 3 g $MgSO_4$ and transfer to the measuring cylinder. Add water to make up to 250 mL.
10. 200 mM ethylene glycol-bis(β-aminoethyl ether)-*N,N,N′,N′*-tetraacetic acid (EGTA) pH 8: Add approximately 150 mL of water to a 250 mL measuring cylinder. Weigh 19 g EGTA and transfer to the measuring cylinder. Adjust the pH to 8 with NaOH and then make up the volume to 250 mL.
11. 200 mM ethylenediaminetetraacetic acid (EDTA) pH 8: Add approximately 150 mL of water to a 250 mL measuring cylinder. Weigh 14.6 g EGTA and transfer to the measuring cylinder. Adjust the pH to 8 with NaOH and then make up the volume to 250 mL.
12. PEME buffer: 100 mM PIPES–NaOH pH 6.9, 1 mM $MgSO_4$, 2 mM EGTA, 0.1 mM EDTA. For a 1x stock add approximately 50 mL of water to 100 mL measuring cylinder. Then add 10 mL 1 M PIPES–NaOH pH 6.9, 1 mL $MgSO_4$, 1 mL 200 mM EGTA pH 8, 50 μL 200 mM EDTA pH 8. Make up the volume to 100 mL with water.
13. Fetal calf serum free HMI-9 [13]: Add approximately 400 mL of water to a 500 mL measuring cylinder. Weigh 9 g HMI-9 powder (Gibco), 1.5 g $NaHCO_3$, and 1.7 μL 2-mercaptoethanol. Adjust the pH to 7.5 with NaOH. Make up the volume to 500 mL with water and then sterile filter through a 0.22 μm filter. Always transfer FCS free HMI-9 from the stock bottle in a sterile environment.

14. 1% (w/v) bovine serum albumin in PBS solution: Weigh 500 mg bovine serum albumin and dissolve in 50 mL PBS. Split into 1 mL aliquots and store at −20 °C.
15. 1 M Na_2HPO_4 solution: Add approximately 50 mL water to a 100 mL measuring cylinder. Weigh 14.2 g Na_2HPO_4 and transfer to the measuring cylinder. Make the volume up to 100 mL with water.
16. 1 M NaH_2PO_4 solution: Add approximately 50 mL water to a 100 mL measuring cylinder. Weigh 12 g NaH_2PO_4 and transfer to the measuring cylinder. Make the volume up to 100 mL with water.
17. Mounting medium: Add 448 μL 1 M Na_2HPO_4 solution and 52 μL 1 M NaH_2PO_4 solution to 500 μL water. Then add 9 mL glycerol and mix thoroughly. Split into 1 mL aliquots and store at 4 °C.
18. Slides—high quality, plain glass or poly-L-lysine.
19. Coverslips No. 0.
20. DAKO pen (Agilent, S2002).

3 Methods

3.1 Procyclic Form Cell Preparation

For procyclic form trypanosomes we generate the endogenously tagged protein cell lines using the long primer PCR tagging methodology we have previously described (*see* **Notes 1** and **2**) [4, 14].

Imaging should always be performed on cells that have been in log phase growth for 48 h. It is best to maintain procyclic form cells at between 2×10^6 and 1×10^7 cells/mL. Example images in Fig. 1.

3.1.1 Preparation of Live Procyclic Form Trypanosomes for Imaging

1. Pipet 1 mL of culture into a 1.5 mL microcentrifuge tube and centrifuge at 800 × *g* for 3 min (*see* **Note 3**).
2. After centrifugation carefully aspirate the medium without disturbing the cell pellet and resuspend the cells in 1 mL of vPBS containing 1 μg/mL Hoechst 33342 (*see* **Notes 4** and **5**), then centrifuge again at 800 × *g* for 3 min.
3. After centrifugation carefully aspirate the vPBS/Hoechst 33342 solution and resuspend the cell pellet in 1 mL vPBS, then centrifuge again at 800 × *g* for 3 min.
4. After the final centrifugation carefully aspirate the vPBS and resuspend the cell pellet in vPBS to give a cell density of ~1×10^8 cells/mL (*see* **Note 6**).
5. Spray a glass microscope slide with 70% (v/v) ethanol and wipe clean. Pipet 3 μL of cell solution onto the glass slide and carefully place a No. 0 coverslip (50 × 22 mm) on top of the cell solution.

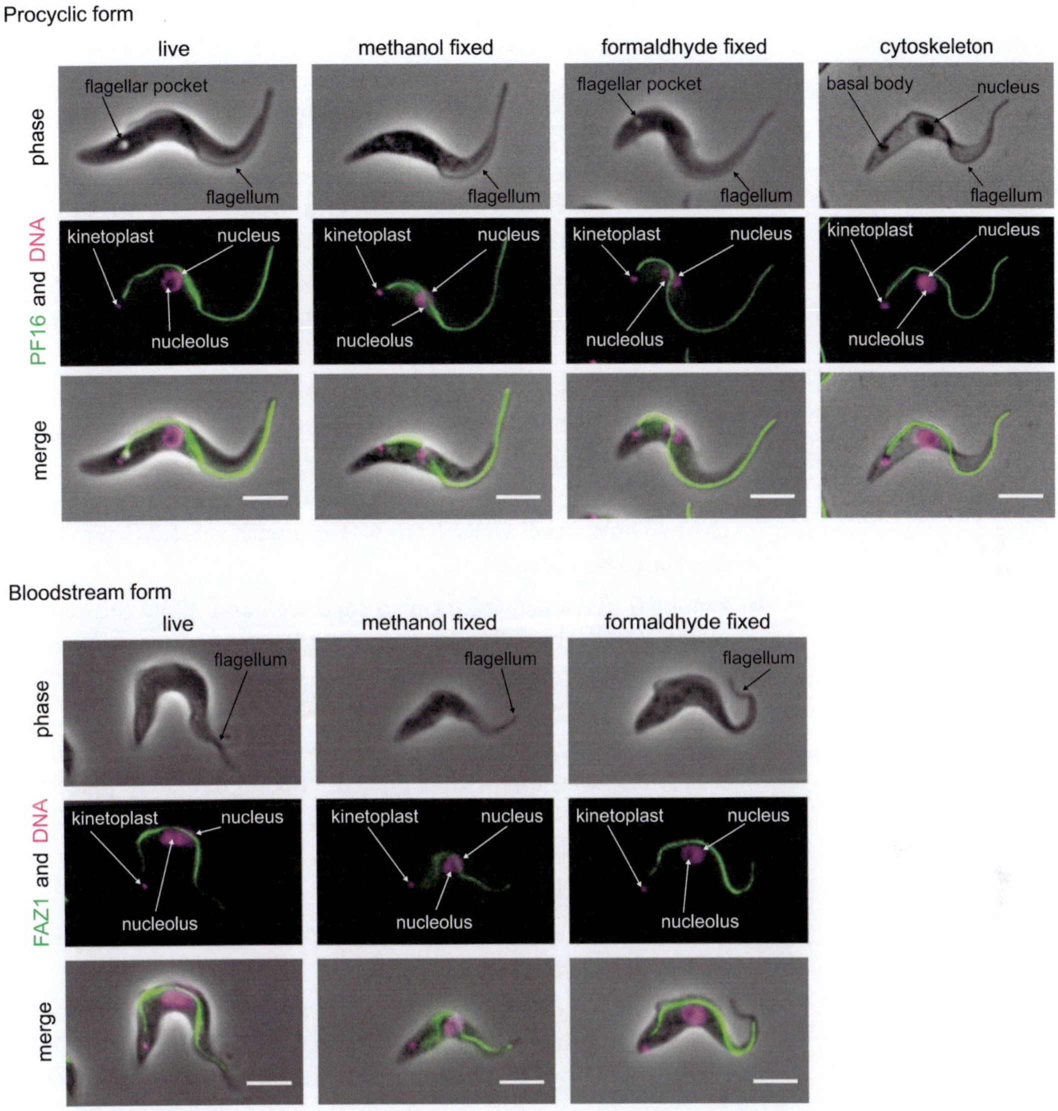

Fig. 1 Representative micrographs of procyclic and bloodstream form *T. brucei* either imaged live or after fixation. Procyclic cells are expressing PF16::mNeonGreen [15] and bloodstream form cells are expressing mNeonGreen::FAZ1 [16]. In the phase channel key cellular structures (flagellum, flagellar pocket) that should be seen if the cell preparation was good are highlighted (black arrows). DNA is stained with Hoechst 33342 and the nucleolus is observable (white arrow) indicating that this channel is not overexposed. Scale bar is 5 μm

6. Check the slide on an inverted microscope using a 20× objective to ensure that the cells are well immobilized on the slide (*see* **Note 7**).
7. Transfer the slides to a microscope suite, ensuring that the transfer is done using the appropriate local health and safety rules for moving pathogens. For imaging instructions *see* Subheading 3.4 below.

3.1.2 Preparation of Methanol Fixed Procyclic Form Trypanosomes for Imaging

Before starting this protocol ensure that there is a Coplin jar in a −20 °C freezer filled with fresh methanol chilled to −20 °C.

1. Pipet 1 mL of culture into a 1.5 mL microcentrifuge tube and centrifuge at 800 × *g* for 3 min (*see* **Note 3**).
2. After centrifugation carefully aspirate the medium without disturbing the cell pellet and resuspend the cells in 1 mL of vPBS (*see* **Note 4**), then centrifuge again at 800 × *g* for 3 min.
3. After centrifugation carefully aspirate the vPBS and resuspend the cell pellet in 1 mL of vPBS, then centrifuge again at 800 × *g* for 3 min.
4. After the final centrifugation carefully aspirate the vPBS and resuspend the cell pellet in vPBS to give a cell density of ~1 × 10^7 cells/mL.
5. Spray a glass microscope slide with 70% (v/v) ethanol and wipe clean. Draw small wells 1 cm × 1 cm with a DAKO pen onto the slide (*see* **Note 8**).
6. Pipet 40 μL of cell solution to each well and allow the cells to settle. Watch the cells adhere to the glass on an inverted microscope using a 20× objective until the adhered cells occupy ~80% of the surface in the field of view (*see* **Note 7**).
7. When the correct density of adhered cells is achieved remove excess cell solution with a pipette and immediately place the slide into the Coplin jar containing the methanol at −20 °C and return to the freezer.
8. Incubate at −20 °C for 20 min.
9. Transfer the slide to a Coplin jar containing PBS and rehydrate cells at room temperature for 5 min.
10. The slide is now suitable for processing by immunofluorescence (*see* Subheading 3.3) or simply staining with a DNA stain, mounting, and imaging (*see* Subheading 3.3, **step 10**).

3.1.3 Preparation of Formaldehyde Fixed Procyclic Form Trypanosomes for Imaging

Before starting this protocol ensure that there is one Coplin jar containing PBS with 1% (w/v) glycine and another Coplin jar containing PBS with 0.1% (v/v) IGEPAL CA-630.

1. Pipet 1 mL of culture into a 1.5 mL microcentrifuge tube and centrifuge at 800 × *g* for 3 min (*see* **Note 3**).
2. After centrifugation carefully aspirate the medium without disturbing the cell pellet and resuspend the cells in 1 mL of vPBS (*see* **Note 4**), then centrifuge again at 800 × *g* for 3 min.
3. After centrifugation carefully aspirate the vPBS and resuspend the cell pellet in 1 mL of vPBS, then centrifuge again at 800 × *g* for 3 min.

4. After the final centrifugation carefully aspirate the vPBS and resuspend the cell pellet in vPBS to give a cell density of ~1×10^7 cells/mL.
5. Spray a glass microscope slide with 70% (v/v) ethanol and wipe clean. Draw small wells 1 cm × 1 cm with a DAKO pen onto the slide (*see* **Note 8**).
6. Pipet 40 μL of cell solution to each well and allow the cells to settle. Watch the cells adhere to the glass on an inverted microscope using a 20× objective until the adhered cells occupy ~80% of the surface in the field of view (*see* **Note** 7).
7. When the correct density of adhered cells is achieved, remove excess cell solution with a pipette. Then pipet 40 μL of a 4% (v/v) formaldehyde solution in vPBS into each well and incubate at room temperature for 5 min (*see* **Note 9**).
8. Remove formaldehyde solution with a pipette and immediately place the slide into a Coplin jar containing PBS with 1% (w/v) glycine to block unreacted aldehyde groups. Incubate at room temperature for 5 min.
9. Transfer slide to a Coplin jar containing PBS and incubate at room temperature for 2 min to rinse off glycine solution.

   Steps 10 and **11** are only required if the cells will be processed for immunofluorescence.
10. Transfer slide to a Coplin jar containing PBS with 0.1% (v/v) IGEPAL CA-630 and incubate at room temperature for 5 min to permeabilize the cells.
11. Transfer slide to a Coplin jar containing PBS and incubate at room temperature for 2 min to rinse off IGEPAL CA-630 solution.
12. The slide is now suitable for processing by immunofluorescence (*see* Subheading 3.3) or simply staining with a DNA stain, mounting, and imaging (*see* Subheading 3.3, **step 10**).

3.1.4 Preparation of Methanol Fixed Procyclic Form Cytoskeleton for Imaging

A high quality cytoskeleton is indicated by the kinetoplast and nuclear DNA remaining as discrete structures when visualized using a DNA stain. Before starting this protocol ensure that there is one Coplin jar containing methanol at −20 °C.

1. Pipet 1 mL of culture into a 1.5 mL microcentrifuge tube and centrifuge at 800 × *g* for 3 min (*see* **Note 3**).
2. After centrifugation carefully aspirate the medium without disturbing the cell pellet and resuspend the cells in 1 mL of vPBS (*see* **Note 4**), then centrifuge again at 800 × *g* for 3 min.
3. After centrifugation carefully aspirate the vPBS and resuspend the cell pellet in 1 mL of vPBS, then centrifuge again at 800 × *g* for 3 min.

4. After centrifugation carefully aspirate the vPBS and resuspend the cell pellet at 1×10^7 cells/mL
5. Spray a glass microscope slide with 70% (v/v) ethanol and wipe clean. Draw small wells 1 cm × 1 cm with a DAKO pen onto the slide (*see* **Notes 8** and **10**).
6. Pipet 40 μL of cell solution to each well and allow the cells to settle. Watch the cells adhere to the glass on an inverted microscope using a 20× objective until the adhered cells occupy ~80% of the surface in the field of view (*see* **Note** 7).
7. When the correct density of adhered cells is achieved, remove excess cell solution with a pipette and replace with 50 μL of vPBS.
8. If unbound cells are still apparent by microscopy, remove vPBS with a pipette and replace with 50 μL of vPBS.
9. Remove vPBS and add 30 μL of 1% (v/v) IGEPAL CA-630 in PEME solution for 10 s (*see* **Note 10**).
10. Remove IGEPAL CA-630 /PEME solution and transfer the slide to the Coplin jar containing methanol at −20 °C and return to the freezer, incubating for 20 min (*see* **Note 11**)
11. Transfer the slide to a Coplin jar containing PBS and rehydrate cells at room temperature for 5 min.
12. The slide is now suitable for processing by immunofluorescence (*see* Subheading 3.3) or simply staining with a DNA stain, mounting and imaging (*see* Subheading 3.3, **step 10**).

3.2 Bloodstream Form Cell Preparation

For the generation of bloodstream form trypanosome cell lines expressing endogenously tagged proteins we use the CRISPR based method described by Beneke et al. [17] (*see* **Notes 1** and **2**).

Imaging should always be performed on cells that are in log phase growth and have been in log phase growth for the previous 48 h. It is best to maintain bloodstream cells at between 1×10^5 and 1×10^6 cells/mL. Example images in Fig. 1.

3.2.1 Preparation of Bloodstream Trypanosomes for Live Cell Imaging

1. Pipet 8 mL of culture into a 15 mL Falcon tube and centrifuge at 800 × *g* for 7 min (*see* **Note 3**).
2. After centrifugation carefully aspirate the medium without disturbing the cell pellet and resuspend the cells in 1 mL of FCS-free HMI-9 containing 1 μg/mL Hoechst 33342 (*see* **Notes 5** and **12**).
3. Transfer cells to a 1.5 mL microcentrifuge tube and centrifuge at 800 × *g* for 3 min.
4. Carefully aspirate the medium without disturbing the cell pellet and resuspend the cells in 20 μL of FCS free HMI-9.

5. Lightly fix cells by adding 20 μL of 0.04% (v/v) formaldehyde in FCS free HMI-9 (*see* **Notes 13** and **14**).
6. Remove 2.4 μL with a pipette and place on a clean glass slide and put a No. 0 (50 × 22 mm) coverslip on top.
7. Transfer the slides to a microscope suite, ensuring that the transfer is done using the appropriate local health and safety rules for moving pathogens. For imaging instructions *see* Subheading 3.4 below.

3.2.2 Methanol Fixed Bloodstream Form

Before starting this protocol ensure that there is a Coplin jar in a −20 °C freezer filled with fresh methanol chilled to −20 °C.

1. Pipet 8 mL of culture into a 15 mL centrifuge tube and centrifuge at 800 × *g* for 3 min (*see* **Note 3**).
2. After centrifugation carefully decant the medium without disturbing the cell pellet and resuspend the cells in 1 mL of vPBS (*see* **Note 4**), transfer to a 1.5 mL microfuge tube then centrifuge again at 800 × *g* for 3 min.
3. Aspirate the supernatant and resuspend the cell pellet in 1 mL of vPBS, then centrifuge again at 800 × *g* for 3 min.
4. After the final centrifugation carefully aspirate the vPBS and resuspend the cell pellet in vPBS to give a cell density of ~1 × 10^7 cells/mL.
5. Spray a poly-L-lysine microscope slide (*see* **Note 16**) with 70% (v/v) ethanol and wipe clean. Draw small wells 1 cm × 1 cm with a DAKO pen onto the slide (*see* **Note 8**).
6. Pipet 40 μL of cell solution into each well and allow the cells to settle for 10 min. Check the slide on an inverted microscope using a 20× objective to ensure that there is a "good" density of cells settled onto the slide (*see* **Note 7**).
7. Carefully remove excess cell solution with a pipette and immediately place the slide into the Coplin jar containing the methanol at −20 °C and return to the freezer.
8. Incubate at −20 °C for 20 min.
9. Transfer the slide to a Coplin jar containing PBS and rehydrate cells at room temperature for 5 min.
10. The slide is now suitable for processing by immunofluorescence (*see* Subheading 3.3) or simply staining with a DNA stain, mounting, and imaging (*see* Subheading 3.3, **step 10**).

3.2.3 Preparation of Formaldehyde Fixed Bloodstream Form Trypanosomes for Imaging

Before starting this protocol ensure that there is a Coplin jar containing PBS with 1% (w/v) glycine.

1. Pipet 8 mL of culture into a 15 mL Falcon tube and centrifuge at 800 × *g* for 8 min (*see* **Note 3**).

2. After centrifugation carefully aspirate the medium without disturbing the cell pellet and resuspend the cells in 10 mL vPBS, then centrifuge again at 800 × *g* for 8 min.
3. After centrifugation carefully aspirate the medium without disturbing the cell pellet and resuspend the cells in 1 mL vPBS.
4. Pipet 1 mL of 8% formaldehyde (v/v) in vPBS into the cell solution and mix by inverting the tube several times. Incubate at room temperature for 10 min to fix the cells (*see* **Note 9**)—during this period occasionally invert the tube to avoid the cells settling.
5. Pipet 20 μL of 10% (v/v) IGEPAL CA-630 into the cell solution and mix by inverting the tube four times. Incubate at room temperature for 10 min.
6. Pipet 12 mL of vPBS into cell solution and invert the tube several times. Then centrifuge at 800 × *g* for 8 min.
7. After centrifugation carefully aspirate the medium without disturbing the cell pellet and resuspend the cells in 500 μL vPBS.
8. Spray a poly-L-lysine microscope slide (*see* **Note 16**) with 70% (v/v) ethanol and wipe clean. Draw small wells 1 cm × 1 cm with a DAKO pen onto the slide (*see* **Note 8**).
9. Pipet 50 μL of cell solution to each well and allow the cells to settle for 15 min in a humid chamber (*see* **Note 15**). Check the slide on an inverted microscope using a 20× objective to ensure that there is a "good" density of cells have settled onto the slide (*see* **Note 7**).
10. Place the slide into a Coplin jar containing PBS with 1% (w/v) glycine to block unreacted aldehyde groups. Incubate at room temperature for 5 min.
11. Transfer slide to a Coplin jar containing PBS and incubate at room temperature for 2 min to rinse off glycine solution.
12. The slide is now suitable for processing by immunofluorescence (*see* Subheading 3.3) or simply staining with a DNA stain, mounting, and imaging (*see* Subheading 3.3, **step 10**).

3.3 Immunofluorescence of Fixed Trypanosomes

If using the fixation procedures described above (Subheadings 3.1.2–3.1.4, 3.2.2, 3.2.3) the slides will be in a Coplin jar containing PBS (*see* **Note 3**).

1. Remove the slide from the Coplin jar and carefully dry the back of the slide and between the wells with paper towel. Place the slide within the humid chamber with the lid off (*see* **Note 15**).
2. Pipet 50 μL of 1% BSA (w/v) in PBS (*see* **Note 17**) onto each well on the slide to block nonspecific protein binding sites. Replace the lid of the humid chamber and incubate for 1 h at room temperature.

3. Remove block solution with a pipette and then pipet 50 μL of primary antibody diluted to the appropriate concentration in 1% BSA (w/v) in PBS and incubate for 1 h at room temperature in a humid chamber.
4. Remove the primary antibody solution with a pipette and place the slide into a Coplin jar containing PBS and incubate for 5 min at room temperature.
5. Remove the slide and place into another Coplin jar containing PBS and incubate for 5 min at room temperature (*see* **Note 18**). Repeat this process until the slide has been washed four times in total.
6. Remove the slide from the Coplin jar and carefully dry the back of the slide and between the wells with paper towel. Place the slide within the humid chamber with the lid off.
7. Pipet 50 μL of secondary antibody diluted to the appropriate concentration in 1% BSA (w/v) in PBS and incubate for 1 h at room temperature in a humid chamber.
8. Remove the secondary antibody solution with a pipette and place the slide into a Coplin jar containing PBS and incubate for 5 min at room temperature.
9. Remove the slide and place into another Coplin jar containing PBS and incubate for 5 min at room temperature (*see* **Note 18**).
10. Remove the slide and place into another Coplin jar containing PBS with 0.1 μg/mL Hoechst 33342 (*see* **Note 19**) and incubate for 5 min at room temperature.
11. Remove the slide and place into another Coplin jar containing PBS and incubate for 5 min at room temperature (*see* **Note 18**).
12. Remove the slide from the Coplin jar and carefully dry the back of the slide and between the wells with paper towel.
13. Place the slide onto a clean and dry sheet of paper towel and pipet 3 μL of mounting medium (*see* **Notes 20** and **21**) onto each well.
14. Carefully place a coverslip onto the slide. Invert the slide and press down, squeezing any excess mounting medium onto the paper towel.
15. Invert the slide and carefully wipe any excess mounting medium off the slide.
16. Secure the coverslip in place by adding a drop of nail varnish to each of the 4 corners of the coverslip. The slide is now ready to be imaged (see Subheading 3.4).

3.4 Microscopy of Trypanosomes (See Notes 22–25)

1. Set up Köhler illumination on the microscope (*see* **Note 26**).
2. Focus on the cells using the camera and the transmitted light channel (*see* **Notes 27** and **28**).

3. Optimize the exposure times such that the signal from each channel is maximised but there are no saturated pixels (*see* **Notes 29** and **30**).
4. Capture at least ~100 cells (usually ~3 fields using a 63x objective) to ensure that cells in each stage of the cell cycle are represented.
5. Save the data in the native microscope format or as stacked tiffs that do not discard the data.

4 Notes

1. Development of PCR based methods to generate transgenic cell lines has enabled the localization of proteins using a genetically encoded tag (e.g., fluorescent protein, epitope tag, HaloTag) to be rapidly assessed. Fluorescent proteins are our preferred tool of choice for this. There are a wide variety of fluorescent proteins available that have dramatically different characteristics. mNeonGreen is by far the best choice for most applications because it is bright, stable and very fast folding. Red proteins still lag behind but we find that mScarlet-I works well for most applications. Currently, blue and far red proteins are not bright enough to be useful for imaging in trypanosomes. "Timer" fluorescent proteins and tags (SNAP and HaloTag) that can be labeled with fluorescent ligands offer intriguing experimental possibilities. A comprehensive list of fluorescence proteins and their properties can be found here: http://www.fpvis.org. Fluorescent proteins normally provide simple steady-state information about protein localization and so the dynamics of protein localization is missed. Techniques such as fluorescence recovery after photobleaching can be used to assess this using fluorescent proteins [10]; however, this requires an expensive microscope setup and generally only provides data over a short timescale. We have found the genetically encoded HaloTag can provide information about protein dynamics over a much longer timescale [15].
2. A key experimental consideration when beginning to design an approach for determining the localization of a protein is to examine the characteristics of the protein. A simple bioinformatic analysis of the protein will reveal whether it has any predicted transmembrane domains or targeting signals and this will influence the type of tag used and terminus on which the tag should be fused to the protein [18]. For example, if a signal peptide is predicted it is best to tag on the protein on the C-terminus. Obviously, tagging approaches come with caveats that should be borne in mind such as interfering with protein folding or targeting. If this is a concern, then an antibody

specific to the protein of interest can be used as the basis for an immunofluorescence approach. However, immunofluorescence requires the use of fixatives (formaldehyde and methanol), which can cause fixation artifacts and careful controls are required to show that the antibody signal is specific to the protein of interest. Methanol fixation is not suitable for imaging proteins that localize to membranous structures, such as the mitochondrion or cell-surface membrane, but works well for imaging proteins that localize to the cytoskeleton, such as the flagellum or subpellicular microtubules. However, formaldehyde fixation may reduce the antigenicity of the epitope that the immunofluorescence antibody binds to, meaning that different formaldehyde concentrations and incubation times may need to be trialed. Our initial approach to defining the localization of a protein would be to tag the N and C termini of the protein of interest with mNeonGreen and perform live cell fluorescence microscopy as this usually gives high quality data and can be done rapidly and with high throughput.

3. All steps should be carried out at room temperature unless otherwise stated.
4. We prefer to use vPBS for imaging; however, this does starve the cells of amino acids and will stress the cells leading to the formation of RNA stress granules. As an alternative medium without fetal calf serum can be used for the washing steps as a direct replacement for vPBS; however, we have found there is an issue with imaging in red channel as a background endocytic signal appears due to accumulation of phenol red in the cells especially if the signal from the tagged protein is weak.
5. Hoechst 33342 is used as this DNA stain is cell permeable.
6. When examining cells by live cell microscopy this density of cells gives a good number of evenly spaced cells in each field of view.
7. Tissue culture facilities routinely have a microscope of this nature for monitoring cell cultures. This quick check ensures that only slides with cells suitable for imaging at higher resolutions are used and allows for an assessment of cell density on the slide, ensuring the cells are evenly spaced and not overlapping on the slide but of sufficient density for efficient imaging. In our system using an ORCA-Flash4.0 Digital CMOS camera, we would aim to capture for 20–30 cells per image with a 100× objective and 40–50 cells per image for a 63× objective.
8. Ensure that the hydrophobic boundary of the well has completely dried before adding the cell solution as the solvent will lyse the cells at the edge of the well.
9. We prefer to use electron microscopy grade formaldehyde as this means we do not have to prepare the solution from

paraformaldehyde powder. This is our standard initial fixation conditions when using formaldehyde; however, if this does not give acceptable results then we recommend that the user titers the concentration of formaldehyde from 2 to 4% and time from 5 to 30 min.

10. Small wells are critical for the rapid detergent extraction that is necessary to get high quality cytoskeletons. When drawing the wells, it is convenient to use the holes in a 0.5 mL microfuge tube rack as a template.
11. Extended storage in methanol (~1 week) will quench fluorescent proteins and increase autofluorescence of the nucleus and kinetoplast.
12. For bloodstream form cells washing and resuspending in HMI-9 without FCS helps to maintain the viability of the cells. Bloodstream form cells are very sensitive to changes in osmotic potential and it is therefore important to ensure that the buffers used are at the correct osmolarity.
13. The low concentration of formaldehyde stops flagellum movement but does not initially kill the cell. Moreover, the trapping of the cells between the slide and the coverslip helps to "flatten" the cells.
14. For bloodstream form cells the time for imaging is very short (5–10 min) so only fix and visualize one sample at a time.
15. We construct our humid chambers using square plastic dishes covered in aluminum foil with a piece of damp paper towel in the bottom.
16. Unlike procyclic form cells, bloodstream form cells do not adhere well to glass due to the presence of the glycosylated surface coat. The poly-L-lysine surface will cross-link to the formaldehyde fixed cells ensuring that the cells attach to the slide. Moreover, methanol dehydration will both attach and flatten cells to the glass slide.
17. This is our general purpose blocking solution; however, for specific applications we have found using a 10% serum solution in PBS also to be effective. Especially if the serum is from the same species in which the secondary antibody was raised.
18. We recommend transferring slides between Coplin jars rather than pouring out contents of Coplin jar and refilling with the slide in situ as this will disturb the cells settled on the slide.
19. Other DNA stains such as DAPI or Hoechst 33258 would also work.
20. We normally use our home-made mounting medium, which is simply a phosphate buffer with glycerol; however, commercially available mounting media are also suitable but the user

should test to make sure these do not introduce any background signal.

21. We recommend that microscope slides with fixed cells/cytoskeletons are mounted just before imaging as this reduces the level of background fluorescent signal. This is especially important when imaging with cytoskeletons.

22. For trypanosome imaging we use a widefield epifluorescence microscope and both an upright and an inverted microscope are suitable. However, an upright microscope is preferable as the condenser has a much higher numerical aperture (NA), which gives a higher phase contrast resolution and a reduced depth of field. Generally, we have found that confocal microscopes are not effective for imaging trypanosomes. The resolution of the final image will depend on the magnification and numerical aperture of the objective, and the camera pixel size. We find that a 63× NA1.4 objective combined with a camera pixel size of 6.5 μm ensures Nyquist sampling, which gives optimal resolution over a large field of view.

23. Mercury vapor bulbs, metal halide bulbs and modern LEDs all give high power illumination suitable for fluorescence. Most mercury vapor bulbs need to be replaced every 300 h of usage, whereas metal halide bulbs should be replaced annually regardless of usage. Mercury bulbs need to be aligned upon installation to ensure an evenness of fluorescent illumination.

24. Ensure that the microscope has the appropriate filter sets for each fluorescent protein or fluorophore that you want to image. The standard microscope filter sets for fluorescence microscopy are not well optimized for working with fluorescence proteins and can dramatically reduce the signal–noise ratio of the fluorescence and the subsequent quality of the final dataset. Investing in bespoke filter-sets will therefore reap significant dividends. We use Thorlabs MDF-GFP2 for mNeonGreen and MDF-TOM for mScarlet fluorescence.

25. We recommend that sCMOS cameras are used for acquisition because they have excellent sensitivity, a large field of view and 16-bit linear range.

26. Köhler illumination should be set up at the beginning of each session to ensure high quality transmitted light images—if the microscope is old or needs servicing, it may be necessary to repeat the setup or Köhler illumination mid-session, but it only takes a few seconds once you know how to do it. If DIC is used, adjust the DIC such that the detail of the cells is preserved but the background of the slide remains smooth (nongranular). In our hands, a value of −600 works well, but this will vary depending upon the microscope.

27. A transmitted light (phase contrast or DIC) image should always be acquired so that the quality of the sample can be assessed and as a reference for the fluorescence. Bright field should not be used because the cells do not have enough contrast to be easily visible.
28. If the location of the fluorescent protein is unknown within the cell we focus either on the flagellar pocket, which appears as a bright circle of signal in the phase channel in cells with one flagellum or the flagellum. By focusing on these structures one can ensure a consistent plane of focus between different images (Fig. 1).
29. For general fluorescence imaging, it is best to use the most intense illumination available in your system. However, some fluorescence proteins (e.g., mScarlet) are rapidly bleached at high illumination intensities and superior results are achieved by reducing the illumination to 50% of maximum. Additionally, for time-lapse fluorescence microscopy, reducing the intensity may allow for longer imaging than would be possible using maximum light intensity. Fluorescent channels should be collected longest-wavelengths first (i.e., from red to blue) to ensure that the unimaged fluorescent proteins/labels are not bleached.
30. We find that 3 s is optimal for imaging most proteins tagged with a fluorescent protein, but exposure times when imaging immunofluorescent signals can be much shorter. The nucleolus should be clearly visible in the DAPI/Hoechst-stained nucleus as a less well stained area. Assess the data using captured images as the camera is more sensitive and has better linear range than your eye.

Acknowledgments

We thank colleagues past and present for their discussions as these protocols have been developed and refined. We would especially like to thank Karen Billington and Clare Halliday, Ross Madden and Philip Dyer of the TrypTag project for their extensive testing of this protocol. Work in the Gull lab is supported by the Wellcome Trust [108445/Z/15/Z, 104627/Z/14/Z], and the support and advice of Professor Keith Gull have been invaluable.

References

1. Zernike F (1942) Phase contrast, a new method for the microscopic observation of transparent objects. Physica 9(7):686–698
2. Nomarski G (1955) Microinterféromètre différentiel à ondes polarisées. J Phys Radium 16:9S–11S
3. Dean S, Sunter JD, Wheeler RJ (2017) TrypTag.Org: a trypanosome genome-wide protein localisation resource. Trends Parasitol 33 (2):80–82
4. Dean S, Sunter J, Wheeler RJ et al (2015) A toolkit enabling efficient, scalable and

reproducible gene tagging in trypanosomatids. Open Biol 5(1). https://doi.org/10.1098/rsob.140197

5. Woods A, Sherwin T, Sasse R et al (1989) Definition of individual components within the cytoskeleton of Trypanosoma brucei by a library of monoclonal antibodies. J Cell Sci 93 (Pt 3):491–500
6. Bastin P, Bagherzadeh Z, Matthews KR, Gull K (1996) A novel epitope tag system to study protein targeting and organelle biogenesis in Trypanosoma brucei. Mol Biochem Parasitol 77(2):235–239
7. Balber AE, Frommel TO (1988) Trypanosoma brucei gambiense and T. b. rhodesiense: concanavalin a binding to the membrane and flagellar pocket of bloodstream and procyclic forms. J Protozool 35(2):214–219
8. Vassella E, Straesser K, Boshart M (1997) A mitochondrion-specific dye for multicolour fluorescent imaging of Trypanosoma brucei. Mol Biochem Parasitol 90(1):381–385
9. Santi-Rocca J, Chenouard N, Fort C et al (2015) Imaging intraflagellar transport in trypanosomes. Methods Cell Biol 127:487–508
10. Vincensini L, Blisnick T, Bertiaux E et al (2018) Flagellar incorporation of proteins follows at least two different routes in trypanosomes. Biol Cell 110(2):33–47
11. Huang G, Bartlett PJ, Thomas AP, Moreno SNJ, Docampo R (2013) Acidocalcisomes of Trypanosoma brucei have an inositol 1,4,5-trisphosphate receptor that is required for growth and infectivity. Proc Natl Acad Sci U S A 110(5):1887–1892
12. Subramaniam C, Veazey P, Redmond S et al (2006) Chromosome-wide analysis of gene function by RNA interference in the African trypanosome. Eukaryot Cell 5(9):1539–1549
13. Hirumi H, Hirumi K (1991) In vitro cultivation of Trypanosoma congolense bloodstream forms in the absence of feeder cell layers. Parasitology 102 Pt 2:225–236
14. Dyer P, Dean S, Sunter J (2016) High-throughput gene tagging in Trypanosoma brucei. J Vis Exp JoVE 114. https://doi.org/10.3791/54342
15. Dean S, Moreira-Leite F, Varga V, Gull K (2016) Cilium transition zone proteome reveals compartmentalization and differential dynamics of ciliopathy complexes. Proc Natl Acad Sci U S A 113(35):E5135–E5143
16. Sunter JD, Varga V, Dean S, Gull K (2015) A dynamic coordination of flagellum and cytoplasmic cytoskeleton assembly specifies cell morphogenesis in trypanosomes. J Cell Sci. https://doi.org/10.1242/jcs.166447
17. Beneke T, Madden R, Makin L et al (2017) A CRISPR Cas9 high-throughput genome editing toolkit for kinetoplastids. R Soc Open Sci 4 (5):170095
18. Aslett M, Aurrecoechea C, Berriman M et al (2010) TriTrypDB: a functional genomic resource for the Trypanosomatidae. Nucleic Acids Res 38(Database issue):D457–D462

Chapter 24

ImageJ for Partially and Fully Automated Analysis of Trypanosome Micrographs

Richard J. Wheeler

Abstract

Trypanosomes and related parasites such as *Leishmania* are unicellular parasites with a precise internal structure. This makes light microscopy a powerful tool for interrogating their biology—whether considering advance techniques for visualizing the precise localization of proteins within the cell or simply measuring parasite cell shape. Methods to partially or fully automate analysis and interpretation are extremely powerful and provide easier access to microscope images as a source of quantitative data. This chapter provides an introduction to these methods using ImageJ/FIJI, free and open source software for scientific image analysis. It provides an overview of how ImageJ handles images and introduces the ImageJ macro/scripting language for automated images, starting at a basic level and assuming no previous programming/scripting experience. It then outlines three methods using ImageJ for automated analysis of trypanosome micrographs: Semiautomated cropping and setting image contrast for presentation, automated analysis of cell properties from a light micrograph field of view, and example semiautomated tools for quantitative analysis of protein localization. These are not presented as strict methods, but are instead described in detail with the intention of furnishing the reader with the ability to "hack" the scripts for their own needs or write their own scripts for partially and fully automated quantitation of trypanosomes from light micrographs. Most of the methods described here are transferrable to other types of microscope image and other cell types.

Key words Trypanosome, Microscopy, Image analysis, Automation, High content analysis

1 Introduction

Microscope images are an incredibly rich data source. Light microscopy is undergoing an ongoing revolution, with the development of genetically encoded fluorescent markers [1], the refinement of digital cameras [2], accessible super resolution light microscopy [3] and most recently the ongoing developments in selective plane illumination (SPIM) methods [4]. Computational analysis of microscope images is a necessity for much modern research which

---

Electronic supplementary material: The online version of this chapter (https://doi.org/10.1007/978-1-0716-0294-2_24) contains supplementary material, which is available to authorized users.

Paul A. M. Michels et al. (eds.), *Trypanosomatids: Methods and Protocols*, Methods in Molecular Biology, vol. 2116,
https://doi.org/10.1007/978-1-0716-0294-2_24, © The Author(s) 2020

may involve an extremely large number of images [5]. For example, microscopy-based screens and the nascent field of genome-wide sub-cellular protein localization [6–9]. Alternatively, it may involve three dimensional imaging of large volumes (such as SPIM or electron tomography) or precise image analysis (such as super resolution image analysis). Automation makes these analyses more accessible, scalable, and repeatable.

This chapter focuses on accessible methods for partial or full automation of image analysis of trypanosomes, particularly *Trypanosoma brucei*, *T. cruzi*, and *Leishmania* spp. Automated image analysis is a flexible tool, therefore these methods have been designed to both be methods and accessible introductions to fundamentals of automated image analysis. The methods cover principals which are applicable to many pieces of image analysis software but the specific examples are written in the ImageJ macro language. Similarly, the image analysis principles are explained using trypanosomatids, but are transferrable to many nontrypanosomatid systems.

ImageJ (https://imagej.nih.gov/ij/) is the leading free and open source scientific image analysis software and includes a powerful and accessible scripting language [10, 11]. ImageJ has recently ceased active development, with a complete reimplementation (called ImageJ2) now spearheading development [12, 13]. A distribution of ImageJ2 packaged with community-derived plugins is called FIJI (FIJI is just ImageJ) and is very popular (https://fiji.sc/) [14]. ImageJ2 and FIJI also use the ImageJ macro language, but also have several other scripting languages. For these methods the use of ImageJ is described, as the ImageJ macro language is simple and ImageJ has debugging tools which help learning. However FIJI and ImageJ2 are better suited for more complex applications.

The methods here can be followed using only a copy of ImageJ or FIJI along with example phase contrast and fluorescence micrographs. To this end, example micrographs of a procyclic form *T. brucei* cell line expressing Histone H3 (Tb927.1.2430) N terminally tagged with mNeonGreen (mNG) [15] are included as supplemental material for this chapter. These images are taken from the TrypTag project, the ongoing project on track to determine the subcellular localization of every protein encoded in the trypanosome genome [6]. These are micrographs typical of a modern epifluorescence microscope, and include phase contrast, green fluorescence (mNG) and blue fluorescence (Hoechst 33342, a DNA stain) channels.

This chapter is not an overview of how to use ImageJ; there are many tutorials for basic image handling in ImageJ (for example, https://imagej.nih.gov/ij/docs/guide/user-guide.pdf). Instead it focuses on scripting for full and partial automation. This is of particular advantage for trypanosomatids, as existing automated tools are typically optimized for use with mammalian cells, restricting the options for using existing scripts and plugins. Relative to mammalian cells, *Trypanosoma* and *Leishmania* pose particular challenges. This is particularly because of their vermiform shape and the two DNA-containing organelles, the kinetoplast and nucleus—both of these features are fundamentally unlike typical mammalian cells. However, the precisely defined morphology of these parasites means micrographs are particularly data rich; cell-to-cell variation of an asynchronous population encodes cell cycle information [16] and subcellular localization of a protein is particularly informative for function through the precise positioning of many organelles [17]. The methods are built on concepts from several pieces of work using automated analysis. However, the concepts here are related and transferrable to automated high-content image based screening—an important topic for trypanosomatid drug development [18–24].

There are a great range of computational image analysis methods of value for trypanosomatid biology, many more that can be summarized in this chapter. Valuable methods include image corrections (camera readout noise correction, correction of illumination unevenness and chromatic aberration correction), video corrections (photobleaching correction, image stabilization), *z* stack corrections (chromatic offset, post-capture autofocus), particle tracking (cell swimming behaviors, subcellular particles), and quantitative analysis of microscopy techniques (fluorescence recover after photobleaching (FRAP), ratiometry). I hope that the methods described here give a useful introduction to the toolkit available for these approaches.

These methods are written assuming no programming experience. It is possible to perform automated image analysis by only making use of previously published tools, however the ultimate value of automated analysis is customizability—these methods aim to confer the reader some scripting ability to achieve this. The chapter begins with a quick introduction of how image data is handled by computers and an overview of the ImageJ macro language syntax (which falls in the "curly-bracket" group along with languages like C and javascript). This is followed with an explanation of how ImageJ handles multidimensional image stacks. Three experimental methods are then covered: Firstly, partial automation of the preparation of images for figures, secondly, methods for automating the analysis of protein expression level and cell cycle stage of trypanosomes, then, finally, two methods for quantitative image analysis. The intention is to introduce sufficient concepts, starting with simple examples, so that automated image analysis methods published with primary research papers will be accessible to people who have followed the examples in this chapter. Readers with some programming experience may want to jump straight to the later examples.

When using the scripts in the methods it is heavily recommended to type them out, rather than copying and pasting. Please also be aware that typesetting can wrap long lines which may introduce incorrect new lines when copying and pasting. Recognizing errors in syntax in handwritten code and interpreting the errors reported when trying to execute invalid code are important for understanding how to write scripts.

2 Materials

2.1 Software

1. ImageJ (https://imagej.nih.gov/ij/) or FIJI (https://fiji.sc/): Both are free and open source, and can be downloaded and run on Windows, Mac, or Linux.
2. ImageJ reference guides: The ImageJ User Guide (for new ImageJ users) https://imagej.nih.gov/ij/docs/guide/user-guide.pdf and the Macro Reference Guide https://imagej.nih.gov/ij/docs/macro_reference_guide.pdf.
3. LOCI Bio-Formats plugin: If using ImageJ with images in proprietary formats, for example saved from light microscope software (*see* **Note 1**), this plugin is required. Download the jar file (http://www.openmicroscopy.org/bio-formats/downloads/) and copy it to the plugins folder of your ImageJ directory. You will have to restart ImageJ for it to be recognized.

2.2 Images

High bit-depth images with separate images for each imaging channel: merged images are not suitable and compressed image formats (e.g., jpg/jpeg) or image formats for day-to-day use (e.g., png) should be avoided wherever possible (*see* **Notes 2** and **3**). Similarly, for videos, compressed formats (avi, mp4, etc.) should be avoided wherever possible—a series of uncompressed still images is more suitable. For any quantitative analysis images must be captured with great care (*see* **Note 4**). Problems with the images will cause systematic errors in any downstream analysis and can prevent automated analysis entirely. Example images are provided in the supplemental material. These are good examples of the quality of image suitable for quantitative image analysis.

3 Methods

3.1 Loading and Running ImageJ Macros

ImageJ scripts are called macros and are simply text files. They can be saved as a text (file extension txt) but are often saved with the file extension ijm. To open a macro simply use File>Open... in ImageJ and it will open as a new window showing the macro text. The macro can also be opened by dragging the file from a file explorer window to the ImageJ window.

Once open, the macro can be run using Macros>Run Macro in the window showing the macro text, or by selecting the macro window and using the keyboard shortcut it Ctrl+R. Macros can also be run in debug mode (*see* **Note 5**).

3.1.1 ImageJ Macro Syntax

At the basic level, an ImageJ script/macro is a set of commands to run in order. Almost every menu option can be used as a command in a macro and ImageJ provides the means to record the commands you enter using the Macro Recorder (Plugins>Macros>Record...). There are also many functions specific to the scripting language, these can be found in the macro reference documentation (https://imagej.nih.gov/ij/docs/macro_reference_guide.pdf) or by the search box in the main window (only in ImageJ2/FIJI).

```
//The command recorded for File>New>Image... then entering some
values
newImage("Untitled", "16-bit black", 256, 256, 1);
```

This function takes 5 parameters: image name (a string), image type (one of several options) then three integers: width, height, and number of slices. It generates a new blank image with these properties. This particular function can be found by using the macro recorder and creating a new image or by looking up the function in the reference material.

The semicolon at the end of the line indicates that that is the end of this line of code; new lines in this scripting language are cosmetic, ImageJ looks for the semicolon. Comments can be included in the code: Any text on a line following // is a comment is not interpreted as code. Similarly, blocks of text between /* and */ are comments.

The simplest scripts are simply a series of ImageJ commands or functions.

```
//Makes a new image with a white rectangle in the centre
newImage("Untitled", "16-bit black", 256, 256, 1);
makeRectangle(64, 64, 128, 128);
setColor(65535);
fill();
run("Select None");
```

This script first makes a new image and makes a rectangular selection in the centre of the image. These first two functions are "recordable." It then sets the current working color (an internal variable in ImageJ) and fills the selection with that color. These functions are not recordable and have to be looked up in the macro guide. Finally, it unselects all current selections.

Variables are script-defined names for values which can be used at multiple places in the script. The values of these variables can have different types: a Boolean (true or false), a number (an integer or real number) or a string (a line of text). These variables can be handled by standard string and mathematical functions.

```
//Starting variables
//The base and channel names are strings
baseName="NewImage";
channelName="Red";
//The base dimension is an integer
baseDimension=128;
//Variables derived from the starting variables
//Concatenating strings (image name)
finalName=baseName+"_"+channelName;
//Mathematics using numbers (image dimensions)
width=baseDimension;
height=baseDimension*2;
newImage(finalName, "16-bit black", width, height, 1);
```

This will generate a new image called NewImage_Red with a width of 128 pixels and a height of 256 pixels. If you are new to programming, mathematical functions (*see* **Note 6**) will be quite intuitive. String functions (*see* **Note 7**), Boolean algebra functions (*see* **Note 8**), and Boolean comparisons (*see* **Note 9**) will likely be new but are important to understand.

Variables can also be an array, which is a list of Booleans, numbers, and/or strings.

```
//Make a new array
values=newArray(10, "red", true);
print(values[0]);
print(values[1]);
print(values[2]);
```

Here, the array values has three values within it. These values can be accessed by specifying the index within the array, specified using a value in square brackets immediately following the array variable name: values[n] means the nth entry in the array (*see* **Note 10**).

Commands/functions in ImageJ may have one of several effects: Immediately running a command, doing a calculation and returning a single value, or setting multiple variables. This can be a little confusing.

```
//This immediately makes a new image using these parameters
newImage("Image1", "16-bit black", 100, 150, 1);

//This runs the ImageJ pow() exponent function
//It returns a number, and the variable a is set to the result
a=pow(2, 16);

//This runs the ImageJ getSelectionCoordinates() function
//The variables x and y are both set to equal two different parts of
```

```
the result
getSelectionCoordinates(x, y);
```

Here, newImage() immediately runs an ImageJ command, pow is a script function which returns a value (a number in this case) and getSelectionCoordinates() sets two variables.

Within a script the basic script flow controls are available: Conditional code statements (if, else if, and else) and looped statements (for and while). Custom functions can also be defined which take parameters and can be called within a script. Combining these with recorded commands provides an easy route to powerful image handling.

The syntax for any of these tools for controlling the flow of the program use braces (curly brackets: {}) to delineate the chunks of code which are within the function, loop, conditional statement, and so on. For ease of reading a script, it is recommended to indent the contents of braces using tab or a consistent number of spaces. However, like new lines, this is purely cosmetic.

The syntax of each of these flow control tools is different. if, while and for use the contents of the brackets immediately following the command to define their function. Functions differ, with the parameters in the brackets representing variables to be specified when the function is called.

```
//Conditional statements
a=10;
b=4;
if (a>b) {
 //Code to run if the comparison a>b is true
 print("a is larger than b");
} else if (b>a) {
 //Code to run if the comparison b>a is true and a>b was not true
 print("b is larger than a");
} else {
 //Code to run if neither b>a or a>b were true
 print("a is equal to b");
}

//While statements
a=0;
b=10;
while (a<b) {
 //Code to loop while the comparison a>b is true
 print("This block of code has run "+(a+1)+" times");
 //a++ is the same as writing a=a+1
 a++;
}

//For loops
```

```
//Three statements are needed for a for loop:
// 1) A start condition (here, set i=0)
// 2) A continuation test (here, loop again if i<10 is true)
// 3) A command to run every loop (here, increment i by 1, ie. i=i+1)
for (i=0; i&lt;10; i++) {
 print("This block of code has run "+(i+1)+" times");
}

//Functions
customFunction("Hello", "world!");
//The function is not called by itself, only when called, as above.
function customFunction(parameter1, parameter2) {
 print("First parameter is: "+parameter1);
 print("Second parameter is: "+parameter2);
}
```

Finally, sub-macros can be defined. This essentially allows for multiple macros within a single file, and they can appear as menu or toolbar entries. This format allows for a second method of running the script; they can be installed to the Plugins menu in ImageJ using Plugins>Macros>Install....

```
//This script can be installed using Plugins>Macros>Install...
//When installed it will appear under Plugins>Macros>Save and
close all images
macro "Save and close all images" {
 //Display a directory select dialog and record the path in the
variable path
 path=getDirectory("");
 //Call the custom function saveImagesToPath
 saveImagesToPath(path);
}

//A custom function which could also be used elsewhere in the script
function saveImagesToPath(path) {
 //A while loop which continues until no images are open
 while (nImages()>0) {
  //Select the first image, save it and close it
  selectImage(1);
  saveAs("TIFF", path+getTitle());
  close();
 }
}
```

When installed, this macro appears under the Plugins>Macros menu in ImageJ as an entry called Save and close all images. The macro calls a custom function (called saveImagesToPath), which itself uses a while loop to continue looping while the logical test nImages()>0 (there is still at least one image open) gives the value true.

3.1.2 Image Handling

ImageJ best handles multichannel, multi-focal plane and multi-timepoint images as a "hyperstack"—a multislice image stack where the individual images are mapped to a channel, focal plane, and timepoint. This is then displayed one of three ways: Greyscale (where only the selected image is shown), Color (where only the selected image is shown, but pseudocolored), and Composite (where all the channels for the current focal plane and time point are combined with their pseudocolors to a single display image). In general, the Color and Composite modes are for peoples' convenience viewing images, while image processing commands may only function reliably in Greyscale mode. To make sure ImageJ understands the "structure" of the image, the number of channels, focal planes, and timepoints this can be set via Image>Hyperstack>Stack to Hyperstack.... New images can also be created as hyperstacks using the newImage function. When loaded correctly it is easy to access the different images in the hyperstack for analysis.

```
//Create a new hyperstack
newImage("HyperStack", "16-bit composite-mode label", 400, 300,
3, 1, 5);

//Set the display mode to greyscale
Stack.setDisplayMode("grayscale");
//Set the displayed image to channel 2 of the 5th timepoint
Stack.setChannel(2);
Stack.setFrame(5);
```

3.2 Semiautomated Image Preparation for Presentation or Publication

When displaying micrographs it is important to recognize that they are primary data and treated as such [25]. Useful guidelines are: Firstly, to aid interpretation, showing cells in images cropped to a consistent size and in a consistent orientation helps side-by-side comparison. Secondly, to give a fair representation of the data, the mapping of the raw data to image intensity in the final image (i.e., the brightness and contrast) should be selected which do not saturate detail or clip the background. Finally, to avoid artificial enhancement of structures, no filtering should be used which alter some areas of the image but not others.

This method outlines three ImageJ macros which help follow these guidelines and streamline image preparation for presentation. Firstly cell cropping, secondly automatic setting of contrast, and finally saving of raw and composite images. These examples assume a composite image with three channels (phase contrast, a green fluorescent protein and a DNA stain) and just one focal plane and time point. This is an excellent example of how simple sequential commands can do very useful functions.

3.2.1 Semiautomated Cell Rotation and Cropping

Trypanosomes (and related organisms like *Leishmania*) are highly polarized, so it is simple to identify a preferred orientation. This script rotates and crops a cell in a larger field of view to a standard orientation and image size. This is semiautomated, and the cell orientation must be specified manually. In this case, the user must draw a line, using the line selection tool in ImageJ, along the cell anterior to posterior axis (*see* **Note 11**).

```
//Two variables to define the output image size in pixels
width=323;
height=162;

//Check if the current selection type is 5 (a line selection)
if (selectionType()!=5) {
//Exit and display an error if the selection is missing or is
not a line
exit("Error: No line selection found!");
}
//Get the coordinates of the user-specified line
//This sets x and y to arrays which describe the x and y coordinates of
the selection
getSelectionCoordinates(x, y);
//Calculate the orientation and center of the line
angle=-180*atan2(y[1]-y[0], x[1]-x[0])/PI;
centerX=(x[1]+x[0])/2;
centerY=(y[1]+y[0])/2;
print("Center: "+centerX+"px, "+centerY+"px Orientation: "+angle+"
degrees");

//Start the cropping process
//First, calculate a temporary image width
//This will allow subsequent rotation of the image without clipping
tempWidth=pow(width*width/4+height*height/4, 0.5);
//Make a rectangle of twice the temporary width around the cell
makeRectangle(centerX-tempWidth, centerY-tempWidth, temp-
Width*2, tempWidth*2);
//Duplicate this region of the image to a new image
run("Duplicate...", "duplicate");
//Rotate by the angle
run("Rotate... ", "angle="+angle+" grid=1 interpolation=Bicu-
bic stack");
//Crop to the outut image size
makeRectangle(tempWidth-width/2, tempWidth-height/2, width,
height);
run("Crop");
```

3.2.2 Automated Contrast

The cropped image can then be prepared for display. ImageJ has a useful built-in function for automatically setting image brightness and contrast to clip/saturate a specified percentage of pixels. This script uses this function to quickly set the contrast and display color of the phase contrast, green, and DNA stain channels.

```
//The phase contrast and DNA stain images are set to have 0.1% clipped
pixels
//This gives good contrast for easy viewing
//The Green fluorescence image is set to have 0% clipped pixels
//This ensures no image data is lost in saturated bright or clipped
dark pixels
//Phase contrast
Stack.setChannel(1);
run("Grays");
run("Enhance Contrast", "saturated=0.1");
//Green fluorescence
Stack.setChannel(2);
run("Green");
run("Enhance Contrast", "saturated=0");
//DNA stain
Stack.setChannel(3);
run("Magenta");
run("Enhance Contrast", "saturated=0.1");
```

For some applications it is more important to show images with the same contrast for direct comparison, for example green signal intensity before and after induction of an inducible cell line. In these cases, it is likely better to specify the specific contrast to use, for example replacing line 12 with:

```
setMinAndMax(1000, 15000);
```

This function sets the display of the image such that values of 1000 map to black (0 on your 8-bit screen) and 15,000 maps to white (255 on your 8-bit screen). The particular values suitable for any set of images require careful consideration.

3.2.3 Automated Saving of Raw and Composite Images

Finally, it is convenient to automate the saving of the image with the raw data (as a tiff) and composite images for display (as png) (*see* **Note 12**). This script asks the user for a directory, then saves the raw data as a tiff and png images of the overlay and the green fluorescent channel alone.

```
//Bring up a window for the user to select a directory
path=getDirectory("");
//Save the raw data as a tiff
name=getTitle();
saveAs("TIFF", path+name+".tif");
```

```
//Set the display to all three channels in composite mode and save as a
png
Stack.setDisplayMode("composite");
Stack.setActiveChannels("111");
saveAs("PNG", path+name+"_overlay.png");
//Set the display to the green channel only in greyscale mode and save
as a png
Stack.setDisplayMode("grayscale");
Stack.setActiveChannels("010");
saveAs("PNG", path+name+"_gfp.png");
//Rename the image back to its starting name (it gets modified when
saved)
rename("name");
```

These are deliberately written to be minimal scripts, specific to this particular combination of image channels. For example, these do not check that the image has the expected number of channels or that they are in the correct order. Adjusting these to a particular data set is intentionally left as a challenge for the reader.

3.3 Automated Cell Cycle Analysis

Micrographs of cells at random cell cycle stages encode information about the cell cycle of the cell [16]. This is particularly true in *T. brucei* where the precise series of cell cycle events can be analyzed [26]. This is also readily accessible by automated analysis, by mixing ImageJ commands with basic flow control. Automated analysis ensures unbiased repeatable analysis, important for any cell profiling [5].

This method shows a basic measurement of green fluorescence signal intensity for a field of view of multiple trypanosomes. If using the example images this is a measurement of Histone H3 (green fluorescence signal intensity) in trypanosomes as a proxy for cell cycle stage. There are two steps to analyzing the particles (the cells) in the image: Firstly, identifying them and isolating them from the background. Secondly, measuring the properties of interest. In this method, this is extended to a third step, which outlines a method for counting the number of kinetoplasts and nuclei in cells.

3.3.1 Thresholding Trypanosomes from Phase Contrast

Phase contrast images (*see* **Note 13**) can be prefiltered to allow intensity thresholding to generate a simplified image where particles (assuming it has all worked correctly, cells) are white (255) and the background is black (0). However, depending on the precise sample preparation method (*see* **Note 14**) and the particular microscope (*see* **Note 15**) these will need some adaptation, particularly of the radii of the unsharp masks and the background subtraction.

```
//Select the phase contrast image
Stack.setChannel(1);
run("Select None");
```

```
//Switch to grayscale display mode, as thresholding only works in
this mode
Stack.setDisplayMode("grayscale");

//Filter the phase image to highlight particles the size of
trypanosomes
run("Unsharp Mask...", "radius=10 mask=0.60 slice");
run("Unsharp Mask...", "radius=20 mask=0.60 slice");
run("Subtract Background...", "rolling=25 light slice");

//Threshold the image
setOption("BlackBackground", true);
setAutoThreshold("Default");
//Next we manually convert this image to a binary image (either
black 0 or white 255)
//This is a little more manual than the built-in ImageJ tools
to handle the 16-bit image
getThreshold(min, max);
changeValues(0, max, 0);
changeValues(max, pow(2, 16)-1, 255);
run("Macro...", "code=v=255-v slice");

//Filter and re-threshold the binary image
//This helps separate closely-spaced cells
run("Gaussian Blur...", "sigma=3 slice");
changeValues(0, 192, 0);
changeValues(192, 255, 255);
```

In this example the process of converting the phase contrast image to a binary thresholded image is a little complex. When working with a single image the ImageJ command run("Convert to Mask") can be used to generate the binary image. However, this command is not compatible with processing only a single slice of a hyperstack made of 16-bit images, forcing the more convoluted approach here. Making the thresholded image as part of the stack simplifies the following steps.

3.3.2 Quantitation of Fluorescence Intensity

To analyze these particles a list of coordinates of particles can be retrieved then looped through, selecting the particle at each coordinate with the "wand" tool for automated analysis. At this point, we can check the area of the particle to determine if it is likely to be a cell and analyze the integrated signal intensity in the green fluorescence image to get a measure of expression of Histone H3 tagged with mNG.

```
//Variables setting the minimum and maximum area that looks like a
single cell
minimumArea=2500;
maximumArea=8000;
```

```
//Use a built-in tool to make a point selection of all the thresholded
particles
Stack.setChannel(1);
run("Select None");
run("Find Maxima...", "noise=10 output=[Point Selection]");
//Record the list of coordinates of the particles as two arrays, x and y
getSelectionCoordinates(x, y);
//Loop through the list of coordinates to analyse the particles
for (i=0; i&lt;lengthOf(x); i++) {
 //Select the thresholded phase contrast image
 Stack.setChannel(1);
 //Use the wand selector to select the particle
 doWand(x[i], y[i]);
 //Get the particle area (in pixels)
 getRawStatistics(area);
 if (area>minimumArea && area<maximumArea) {
  //Only analyse particles large enough to be a cell
  //Check the bounds of the selection
  getSelectionBounds(sx, sy, sw, sh);
  if (sx&gt;0 && sy&gt;0 && sx+sw&lt;getWidth()-1 &&
sy+sh&lt;getHeight()-1) {
  //Only analyse if the particle is not touching the image edge
  //Get the image intensity from the DNA stain channel
  Stack.setChannel(3);
  getRawStatistics(area, mean);
  //Output the result
  print(x[i], y[i], area, mean*area);
  } else {
  //'Delete' particles which should not be analysed
  setColor(0);
  fill();
  }
 } else {
  //'Delete' particles which should not be analysed
  setColor(0);
  fill();
 }
}
```

This script will output a tab-delimited data table in the log window with four columns: *X* coordinate, *Y* coordinate, area (in pixels), and sum signal intensity in the green fluorescence channel.

3.3.3 Kinetoplast and Nucleus Counts

This approach can be extended to threshold both the phase contrast and DNA stain image, then loop through the particles in the phase contrast image and count the number of DNA particles within the bounds of the phase contrast particle. This is simplified by the behavior of the run("Find Maxima...") tool which only identifies particles within the area of the current selection—in this case finding thresholded particles in the DNA stain image within the bounds of the cell as identified in the phase contrast image. These particles can then be classified based on area, yielding a count of the number of kinetoplasts and nuclei in the cell. The following script takes the analyzed image resulting from the previous script (i.e., with cells already identified in a binary image), and reanalyzes it to look at the number of kinetoplasts and nuclei per cell.

```
//The area threshold to count as a kinetoplast or nucleus
knAreaCutoff=100;

//Set the DNA stain channel
Stack.setChannel(3);
run("Select None");
//Do a small blur then thresholding, similar to the phase
contrast image
run("Gaussian Blur...", "sigma=1 slice");
setAutoThreshold("Otsu dark");
getThreshold(min, max);
changeValues(0, min, 0);
changeValues(min, pow(2, 16)-1, 255);

//Repeat the cell detection as before
//The cells have already been filtered to be within the necessary
size range
Stack.setChannel(1);
run("Find Maxima...", "noise=10 output=[Point Selection]");
getSelectionCoordinates(x, y);
for (i=0; i&lt;lengthOf(x); i++) {
 Stack.setChannel(1);
 doWand(x[i], y[i]);
 //Do the kinetoplast and nucleus count
 countKN(knAreaCutoff);
}

function countKN(knAreaCutoff) {
 //Setup variables to record the count of Ks and Ns
 kCount=0;
 nCount=0;
 Stack.setChannel(3);
 //Analyse the particles using the same strategy as for the cells
 run("Find Maxima...", "noise=10 output=[Point Selection]");
 getSelectionCoordinates(x2, y2);
 for (i=0; i&lt;lengthOf(x2); i++) {
  //Select the current DNA particle
  doWand(x2[i], y2[i]);
```

```
    getRawStatistics(area);
   //If the area is larger than the cutoff count as N, otherwise K
    if (area>knAreaCutoff) {
    nCount++;
    } else {
    kCount++;
    }
  }
  //Print the resulting K and N count
  print(kCount+"K"+nCount+"N");
}
```

The limit in the quality of an approach such as this is the accuracy of thresholding the phase contrast and DAPI images and the accuracy of classifying phase contrast particles as cells and DAPI particles as kinetoplasts or nuclei. Careful analysis of the output will reveal a tendency to split some nuclei into multiple particles and miss some kinetoplasts. More advanced thresholding methods can be used, and more classifiers just area can be used (circularity, maximum length dimension, signal properties), but ultimately more information may be required.

Use of additional DNA stains, with a differing preference for AT or GC rich DNA is one such approach [27]. This is a powerful approach, allowing for unambiguous analysis of the kinetoplasts and nuclei of candidate *T. brucei* gametes [28] and diverse kinetoplastids and related organisms [29]. The example images with this chapter have an mNeonGreen fusion of Histone H3 along with the DNA stain; it is a challenge to the reader to adapt this approach to use that additional information for a more accurate kinetoplast/nucleus count.

3.4 Automated Quantitative Analyses

Computational image analysis has access to the raw numerical data which defines the image and can therefore carry out quantitative analyses that are not possible by eye. Two example methods selected here are quantitative colocalization and very precise localization of the center of signal from a diffraction limited particle, both of which exploit the built-in curve fitting functions in ImageJ.

3.4.1 Quantitative Colocalization

Quantitative measures of colocalization are valuable in many biological contexts. Using the example images provided it can be used to quantitatively compare Histone H3 and DNA stain signal and compare the result for nuclei and kinetoplasts.

Every pixel in a fluorescence microscope image is a proxy for the local concentration of the fluorescent marker, therefore colocalization of two molecules visualized in two different fluorescence channels should manifest as correlation of the pixel values in one channel versus the other. When plotted as a scatter plot a strong colocalization is manifested as a linear positive correlation in pixel values with a small Pearson's correlation coefficient (R^2) [30].

```
if (selectionType!=0) {
 exit("Error: Needs a rectangular selection!");
}
//Get the bounds of the current selection
getSelectionBounds(x, y, w, h);
//Sets up two arrays to contain green (v1) and blue (v2) pixel values
v1=newArray(w*h);

v2=newArray(w*h);
//Loop through x and y coordinates to record values from the green
channel
Stack.setChannel(2);
//For values of a between 0 and the width of the selection
for (a=0; a&lt;w; a++) {
 //And values of b between 0 and the height of the selection
 for (b=0; b&lt;h; b++) {
  //Record the value of the pixel in the corresponding array entry
   //The pixel value at (x+a, y+b) is recorded as array entry [a+b*w]
 v1[a+b*w]=getPixel(x+a, y+b);
 }
}
//Loop through x and y coordinates to record values from the blue
channel
Stack.setChannel(3);
for (a=0; a&lt;w; a++) {
 for (b=0; b&lt;h; b++) {
  v2[a+b*w]=getPixel(x+a, y+b);
 }
}
//Do a linear regression analysis
//A positive linear correlation indicates co-localisation
//Carries out the actual fit
Fit.doFit("Straight Line", v1, v2);
//Plots the fit as a graph
Fit.plot();
//Prints the return values
print("R squared: "+Fit.rSquared()+" Gradient: "+Fit.p(1));
```

This script uses several approaches. Firstly, it reads image information in the form of pixel values (using getPixel()) and records it as entries in an array, mapping the 2D pixel data (relative coordinates a and b) into a 1D array (index a + b × w). Secondly, it analyzes this data by automated use of the built-in graph plotting and curve fitting functions in ImageJ.

Using the example images, if this is run with a rectangular selection covering a nucleus then it will return a high R^2, a positive gradient and a plot showing a positive linear correlation of nuclear

DNA stain signal with Histone H3 signal. If the selection covers a kinetoplast then it will show a very low R^2, near-zero gradient, and no correlation of the two signals.

3.4.2 Point Spread Function Fitting for Superresolved Analysis

Precise determination of the center of a signal is a powerful tool whenever considering structures which are very small. Its particular power is in measuring distances between small structures. If the structures are sparse or in separate fluorescent channels then this is a non–diffraction-limited measurement. Repeated imaging of sparse single fluorophores is the basis for the PALM/STORM class of superresolution microscopy, while comparison between two channels can allow the reconstruction of molecule position in very small structures [31]. This is normally achieved by 2D Gaussian (a good approximation for the Airy disk point spread function) fitting of near-point sources [32, 33].

This method uses an example macro to take a user-selected point, then measures the signal distribution at that point to refine that point to the precise center of the signal. Specifically, it fits a Gaussian in X and then Y and the center of those Gaussian distributions are used to shift the initially selected coordinate to the signal center.

```
//Distance in pixels to use for Gaussian fitting
r=6;

//Call the custom refinePoints function
//This refines every point in a user-specified selection
refinePoints(r);

function refinePoints(r) {
 //Get the coordinates of the point selection
 if (selectionType()!=10) {
  exit("Error: Point selection needed!");
 }
 getSelectionCoordinates(x, y);
 //Setup output arrays for the corrected x and y coordinates
 ox=newArray(); oy=newArray();
 for (i=0; i&lt;lengthOf(x); i++) {
  //For every point, make a point selection
  //Round the coordinates to the nearest pixel
  makePoint(round(x[i]), round(y[i]));
  //Call the custom refinePoint function to do the Gaussian fitting
  refinePoint(r);
  //Check if a selection exists
  //(if the refinePoint function can't fit the Gaussian)
  if (selectionType!=-1) {
  //Record the refined location for output
  getSelectionCoordinates(cx, cy);
```

```
   ox=Array.concat(ox, cx); oy=Array.concat(oy, cy);
   }
  }
 //Make a point selection of the refined points
 makeSelection("points", ox, oy);
}

function refinePoint(r) {
 //Record the ID of the original image
 src=getImageID();
 //Get the coordinates of the point to refine
 getSelectionCoordinates(x, y);
 x=x[0]; y=y[0];
 if (x>=r && y>=r && x<getWidth()-r && y<getHeight()-r) {
  //Only continue if the point is not too close to the image
edge
  xo=x; yo=y;
  //Duplicate a rectangle around the point to refine
  makeRectangle(x-r, y-r, r*2, r*2);
  run("Duplicate...", " ");
  tmp=getImageID();
  //Do the Gaussian fitting
   //This part of the code needs to be run in the X and Y
direction
   //By using a for loop the code can avoid unnecessary
duplication
  for (o=0; o&lt;2; o++) {
  //Select the image and get the signal intensity profile
  makeRectangle(0, 0, r*2, r*2);
  vy=getProfile();
  //Setup an array of horizontal pixel positions
  vx=newArray(lengthOf(vy));
  for (i=0; i&lt;lengthOf(vx); i++) {
  //The offset of 0.5 is due to the handling of pixel data
  //The distances are from the top left corner of the pixel
  vx[i]=i-r+0.5;
  }
  //Do the gaussian fit
  Fit.doFit("Gaussian", vx, vy);
  if (Fit.rSquared()>0.9) {
  //If a good fit is achieved
  if (Fit.p(2)>-r/2 && Fit.p(2)<r/2) {
  //And the centre of the Gaussian reasonable
  //Correct either the X or Y coordinate
  if (o==0) {
  x+=Fit.p(2);
  } else if (o==1) {
  y+=Fit.p(2);
```

```
    }
    } else {
    //Failure to fit returns an invalid number
    if (o==0) {
    x=0/0;
    } else if (o==1) {
    y=0/0;
    }
    }
    } else {
    //Failure to fit returns an invalid number
    if (o==0) {
    x=0/0;
    } else if (o==1) {
    y=0/0;
    }
    }
    if (o==0) {
    //After the first (X) loop rotate the image for Y
    run("Rotate 90 Degrees Left");
    } else if (o==1) {
    //After the second loop close the temporary image
    selectImage(tmp);
    close();
    }
    }
  } else {
   //Return an invalid number if too close to the image edge
         x=0/0; y=0/0;
  }
  //Make a selection of the corrected point location in
  the source image
  selectImage(src);
  if (!isNaN(x) && !isNaN(y)) {
   makePoint(x, y);
  } else {
   run("Select None");
  }
  setBatchMode(false);
}
```

This script uses two custom functions, refinePoints() and refinePoint(), to carry out the analysis. This modularity in the design of the script is deliberate, and allows easy reuse or adaptation of all or part of the script in a future analysis. It also makes use of setting a variable to equal 0/0 (which has no defined value and recorded in ImageJ as "NaN" or not a number) when an analysis is not possible, then later checking for this internal error using the function is NaN().

The example images do not provide a valuable use case for this method, but the function of the script can be readily tested on kinetoplasts. *T. brucei* kinetoplasts are very small and, although they are not a diffraction limited point, their position can be analyzed by this method. Running this script with a point selection in the DNA stain channel close to the center of a kinetoplast will refine the point location to the precise fitted center of signal. In the case of kinetoplasts this allows, for example, precise measurement of kinetoplast separation in 2 K cells.

4 Notes

1. Microscopes may save images in a proprietary format, for example, czi files (Zeiss), lif files (Leica), nic files (Nikon), and oir files (Olympus). These normally record the image data in a similar way to high bit-depth TIFF files (*see* **Note 3**), but potentially pack multiple images or more metadata into the file. Most can be opened using the LOCI Bio-Formats plugin.
2. It is important to understand the different types of image data. Most images in day-to-day life are RGB images, where each pixel has a red, green and blue value between 0 and 255 (2^8-1, 8-bit), and are typically compressed, where the image data has been compressed (with some loss of information) to reduce the file size. Example formats are jpg, png, and gif. Scientific images are often not colored (although may be artificially pseudocolored), are either uncompressed or losslessly compressed and often have a higher bit-depth (*see* **Note 3**). Scientific images with multiple imaging modes of colors of fluorescence normally exist as a set of independent images. "Merged" images (combining multiple fluorescence or other images using pseudocolors) are useful for our interpretation, but unusable for a computational analysis.
3. Bit-depth refers to the number of bits used to store intensity values per pixel, and a higher bit depth corresponds to the ability to store a larger range of values. Scientific images often have pixel values from 0 to 65,535 (2^{16}-1, 16-bit). While our eyes cannot easily perceive this additional graduation of intensity it is important data.
4. Microscope images must be high quality and captured with care. If an image is in any way tricky to analyze by eye then it is not suitable for automated image analysis: Your eye and brain represent hundreds of millions of years of evolution of image analysis, a computer will not be as good. Key things to consider during image capture are: eliminate dirt on the slide, contamination of the sample and damage or death of any cells. Optimize sample preparation to minimize background fluorescence. Do not over-expose the image (saturate pixels)

but also pick a suitably long exposure time to avoid image noise in balance with avoiding photobleaching. Ensure the illumination is uniform, realign the Kohler illumination and fluorescence light sources if necessary, and critically assess any offset between channels (e.g., chromatic aberration or stage instability).

5. The macro can also be run line by line by starting it in debug mode: Debug>Debug Macro or the keyboard shortcut Ctrl +D. Once in debug mode it can be run line by line (Debug> Step or Ctrl+E), and the current line being executed is highlighted. When running in debug mode an additional window showing the values of each variable is also shown. This is extremely useful for understanding how the macro runs.
6. The normal functions of + addition, – subtraction or negation, / division, and * multiplication. Exponents must be written using the pow() function.
7. Two strings can be joined together (concatenated) using +. The opposite of concatenation is extracting a subportion of a string using substring().
8. Boolean algebra functions allow the combination of true and false values using logic functions (sometimes called logic gates). The three common functions are: ! not, || or, && and. For example !true equals false, true || false equals true.
9. Logical comparators give a value of true or false depending on the values being compared. These include the > greater than, < less than, >= greater or equal to and <= less or equal to. For example 1>2 equals false, 3<=3 equals true. Equality is tested using == (double equals sign). Using a single equals sign in a logical comparison will generally be reported as a syntax error, but can give unexpected behaviors.
10. Entries in arrays are numbered from zero, which is a common programming convention.
11. The line selection tool is on the normal ImageJ toolbar—simply select the tool then click on the start and endpoint for the line in the image. Note there are several line selection tools available (straight line, polyline, etc.) which can be switched between by right clicking on the line selection tool.
12. All multichannel high bit-depth information can be preserved by saving images as tiff files (the default ImageJ format). These are noncompressed and preserve all the image data. Here, we will be analyzing images of this format: A collection of 16-bit images of different channels aligned with each other in a multislice image stack. To save an image for presentation (in a figure or talk), it will normally need to be converted to an 8-bit or RGB color image and saved in a more widely used format—png is widely compatible and has lossless compression.

13. Phase contrast is preferred to either bright field or differential interference contrast (DIC) for the automated identification of cells. Phase contrast provides much higher image contrast than bright field illumination and the directional pseudo-shadow of DIC leads to minimal image contrast perpendicular to the interference contrast axis.
14. The recommended sample preparations for high quality phase contrast images of trypanosomes are either live cells or cells fixed with formaldehyde. Drying, methanol fixation and/or detergent treatment can reduce contrast (by extracting material) or alter cell morphology. For detailed protocols concerning sample preparation for light microscopy see Chapter 23 by Dean and Sunter.
15. The microscopes used for optimization of this approach were Leica DM550b (upright), Zeiss Axio Scope.A1 (upright) and Zeiss Axio Observer.A1 (inverted) widefield epifluorescence microscopes, using standard halogen or LED transillumination and 40×, 63×, or 100× phase-contrast objectives.

Acknowledgments

I would like to thank the members of the Gull, Gluenz, Vaughan, and Sunter labs, interaction with whom have helped select the contents of this chapter. I would also like to thank the TrypTag project team; the TrypTag data set has demanded the refinement of many of the approaches outlined here. Research underlying the methods described here was supported by the Wellcome Trust [103261/Z/13/Z, 104627/Z/14/Z, 108445/Z/15/Z, 211075/Z/18/Z].

References

1. Cranfill PJ et al (2016) Quantitative assessment of fluorescent proteins. Nat Methods 13 (7):557–562
2. Stuurman N, Vale RD (2016) Impact of new camera technologies on discoveries in cell biology. Biol Bull 231(1):5–13
3. Sahl SJ, Hell SW, Jakobs S (2017) Fluorescence nanoscopy in cell biology. Nat Rev Mol Cell Biol 18(11):685–701
4. Power RM, Huisken J (2017) A guide to light-sheet fluorescence microscopy for multiscale imaging. Nat Methods 14(4):360–373
5. Caicedo JC et al (2017) Data-analysis strategies for image-based cell profiling. Nat Methods 14 (9):849–863
6. Dean S, Sunter JD, Wheeler RJ (2017) TrypTag.Org: a trypanosome genome-wide protein localisation resource. Trends Parasitol 33 (2):80–82
7. Huh W-K et al (2003) Global analysis of protein localization in budding yeast. Nature 425 (6959):686–691
8. Thul PJ et al (2017) A subcellular map of the human proteome. Science 356(6340): eaal3321
9. Werner JN et al (2009) Quantitative genome-scale analysis of protein localization in an asymmetric bacterium. Proc Natl Acad Sci 106 (19):7858–7863
10. Collins TJ (2007) ImageJ for microscopy. BioTechniques 43(1 Suppl):25–30
11. Schneider CA, Rasband WS, Eliceiri KW (2012) NIH image to ImageJ: 25 years of image analysis. Nat Methods 9:671–675

12. Rueden CT et al (2017) ImageJ2: ImageJ for the next generation of scientific image data. BMC Bioinformatics 18(1):529
13. Schindelin J, Rueden CT, Hiner MC, Eliceiri KW (2015) The ImageJ ecosystem: an open platform for biomedical image analysis. Mol Reprod Dev 82(7–8):518–529
14. Schindelin J et al (2012) Fiji: an open-source platform for biological-image analysis. Nat Methods 9(7):676–682
15. Shaner NC et al (2013) A bright monomeric green fluorescent protein derived from Branchiostoma lanceolatum. Nat Methods 10 (5):407–409
16. Wheeler RJ (2015) Analyzing the dynamics of cell cycle processes from fixed samples through ergodic principles. Mol Biol Cell 26 (22):3898–3903
17. Halliday C et al (2018) Cellular landmarks of Trypanosoma brucei and Leishmania mexicana. Mol Biochem Parasitol. https://doi.org/10.1016/j.molbiopara.2018.12.003
18. Alonso-Padilla J et al (2015) Automated high-content assay for compounds selectively toxic to trypanosoma cruzi in a myoblastic cell line. PLoS Negl Trop Dis 9(1):e0003493
19. Dagley MJ, Saunders EC, Simpson KJ, McConville MJ (2015) High-content assay for measuring intracellular growth of leishmania in human macrophages. Assay Drug Dev Technol 13(7):389–401
20. Engel JC et al (2010) Image-based high-throughput drug screening targeting the intracellular stage of Trypanosoma cruzi, the agent of Chagas' disease. Antimicrob Agents Chemother 54(8):3326–3334
21. Eren RO et al (2018) Development of a semi-automated image-based high-throughput drug screening system. Front Biosci Elite Ed 10:242–253
22. Moon S et al (2014) An image-based algorithm for precise and accurate high throughput assessment of drug activity against the human parasite trypanosoma cruzi. PLoS One 9(2). https://doi.org/10.1371/journal.pone.0087188
23. Siqueira-Neto JL et al (2012) An image-based high-content screening assay for compounds targeting intracellular Leishmania donovani amastigotes in human macrophages. PLoS Negl Trop Dis 6(6):e1671
24. Sykes ML, Avery VM (2015) Development and application of a sensitive, phenotypic, high-throughput image-based assay to identify compound activity against Trypanosoma cruzi amastigotes. Int J Parasitol Drugs Drug Resist 5(3):215–228
25. Cromey DW (2013) Digital images are data: and should be treated as such. Methods Mol Biol 931:1–27
26. Woodward R, Gull K (1990) Timing of nuclear and kinetoplast DNA replication and early morphological events in the cell cycle of Trypanosoma brucei. J Cell Sci 95(1):49–57
27. Wheeler RJ, Gull K, Gluenz E (2012) Detailed interrogation of trypanosome cell biology via differential organelle staining and automated image analysis. BMC Biol 10(1):1
28. Peacock L, Bailey M, Carrington M, Gibson W (2014) Meiosis and haploid gametes in the pathogen Trypanosoma brucei. Curr Biol 24 (2):181–186
29. Lukeš J, Wheeler R, Jirsová D, David V, Archibald JM (2018) Massive mitochondrial DNA content in diplonemid and kinetoplastid protists. IUBMB Life 70(12):1267–1274
30. Zinchuk V, Zinchuk O (2008) Quantitative colocalization analysis of confocal fluorescence microscopy images. Curr Protoc Cell Biol 4:19
31. Haase J et al (2013) A 3D map of the yeast kinetochore reveals the presence of core and accessory centromere specific histone. Curr Biol 23(19):1939–1944
32. Deschout H et al (2014) Precisely and accurately localizing single emitters in fluorescence microscopy. Nat Methods 11(3):253–266
33. Small A, Stahlheber S (2014) Fluorophore localization algorithms for super-resolution microscopy. Nat Methods 11(3):267–279

Chapter 25

Motility Analysis of Trypanosomatids

Timothy Krüger and Markus Engstler

Abstract

Motility analysis of microswimmers has long been limited to a few model cell types and broadly restricted by technical challenges of high-resolution in vivo microscopy. Recently, interdisciplinary interest in detailed analysis of the motile behavior of various species has gained momentum. Here we describe a basic protocol for motility analysis of an important, highly diverse group of eukaryotic flagellate microswimmers, using high spatiotemporal resolution videomicroscopy. Further, we provide a special, time-dependent tomographic approach for the proof of rotational locomotion of periodically oscillating microswimmers, using the same data. Taken together, the methods describe part of an integrative approach to generate decisive information on three-dimensional in vivo motility from standard two-dimensional videomicroscopy data.

Key words Trypanosome, Microswimmer, Flagellum, Motility, Spatiotemporal resolution, In vivo microscopy, Time-dependent tomography, Procyclic, Flagellar beat

1 Introduction

Trypanosomatids are a highly diverse group of eukaryotic uniflagellate parasites with a very broad host range [1]. During their life cycle they typically develop many distinct morphotypes that are largely versatile microswimmers. As such, they navigate manifold microenvironments in their host animals, but there is still scant knowledge about most of these parasites' motile behavior [2–7]. Thorough motility analyses have been performed with prokaryotes, on the one hand, which swim using a disparate rotary flagellar apparatus or other mechanisms [8, 9]. On the other hand, analysis of eukaryotic cells has historically concentrated on sperm cells [10, 11]. These important reproductive cells possess a single, long and free flagellum whose central structure, the axoneme, oscillates due to force-producing dyneins. In this way a traveling wave is generated along the flagellum that propels the sperm head efficiently through viscous fluids [12–14].

The sperm cell with its free propulsive flagellum represents only one morphotype of several adopted by parasitic uniflagellates.

Paul A. M. Michels et al. (eds.), *Trypanosomatids: Methods and Protocols*, Methods in Molecular Biology, vol. 2116, https://doi.org/10.1007/978-1-0716-0294-2_25,

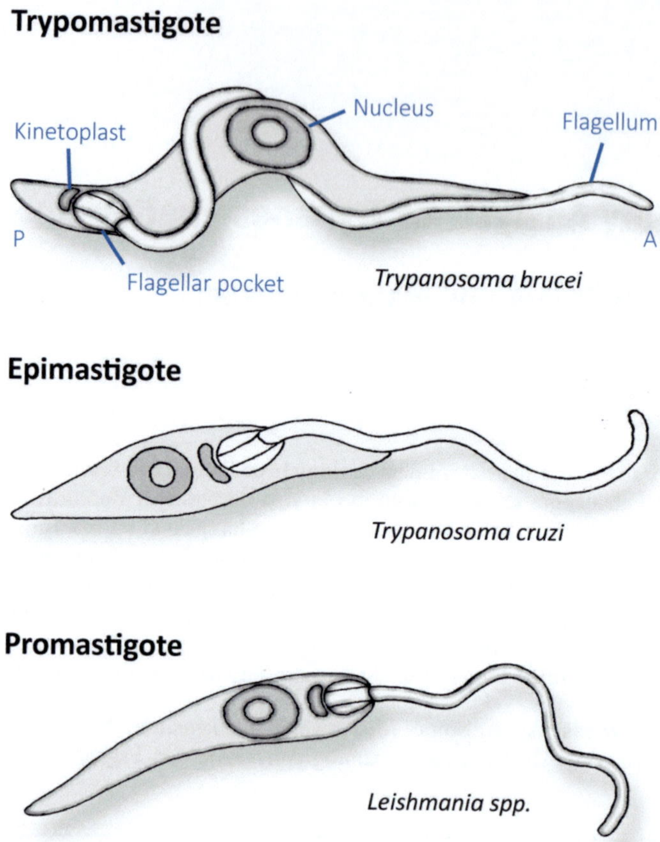

Fig. 1 Morphotypes of trypanosomatid microswimmers. Examples of selected developmental stages of different trypanosomatid species, representing the main morphotype categories of motile flagellates. Top: Trypomastigote cell of *T. brucei* bloodstream forms. The flagellum emanates from the flagellar pocket located at the posterior end, and runs along a flagellar attachment zone along the cell body to and beyond the anterior end. Middle: Epimastigote cell of *T. cruzi*. The flagellum is attached to the anterior part of the cell body. Bottom: Promastigote morphotype from *Leishmania* spp. with a free flagellum

Among trypanosomatids, cells with a free flagellum belong to the category of promastigotes, whereas cells that have varying portions of the flagellum attached to the cell body are called epimastigotes, when the basal body is positioned on the anterior side of the nucleus and trypomastigotes when the basal body lies on the posterior side [15] (Fig. 1). The extraordinary case of a flagellate microswimmer that has its cell body firmly attached to the greater part of the force generating axonemal structure warrants a detailed description of the methods of motility analyses.

As recent studies have shown, the principles of the well-established sperm motility analyses can also be applied to the trypo- or epimastigote versions of flagellates, with the extended challenge of considering the elastic and rotational three-dimensional movement of the complete cell body [4, 5, 16] (*see* [17] for analysis of promastigote trypanosomatid species). Therefore we will describe here, a basic and generally applicable method of motility analyses for high spatiotemporal resolution data of these uniflagellate cell types and additionally describe a special tomography method used for analyzing the rotational modus of trypanosome swimming.

For a better understanding of the methodological aspects, some background information on the actual swimming mechanism of trypanosomes might be useful. The details are probably not entirely common knowledge yet, and deliberation thereof discloses several interesting cell biological, as well as physical aspects and problems [2–5, 16, 18].

Trypanosomes are propelled through fluids with the force generated by dynein motors in the flagellar axoneme. The periodic alternating bending of the flagellum, orchestrated by the axonemal machinery, can begin at the distal, free tip of the flagellum or at the proximal, flagellar pocket based end. The bend is propagated along the flagellum to produce a traveling wave that is generally sustained until it reaches the other end. Under most conditions, the wave more frequently runs from the free flagellar tip along the attached cell body and the resulting movement of the cell in the opposite direction is thus called forward swimming. The flagellar wave initiated at the anterior tip is planar and symmetrical. It reaches the mass of the spindle-shaped cell body and is propagated helically around it, as the flagellum is firmly attached in a 180° turn, ending at the flagellar pocket [16]. Through the tight connection with the cell body, the generated wave bends the elastic cell body and produces a hydrodynamically effective "cellular waveform" [4, 5]. This dynamic chiral arrangement results in the regular rotation around the longitudinal cell axis, producing the eponymous auger-like appearance of swimming trypanosomes.

Forward swimming by "tip-to-base" flagellar beats is frequently interrupted by "base-to-tip" beats, which initiate reverse traveling waves. Single reverse waves will interfere with forward waves, slow down the cell and initiate a change of swimming direction, as the regular cellular waveform is distorted and the opposing forces cause the cell to rotate around transverse body axes. Higher frequency reverse waves will interrupt the regular succession of forward waves and bring the cell to a halt. Periodic switching between forward and reverse waves results in minimal net translocation and the cell tumbling [16]. Cell populations have been subclassified, defining persistent swimmers, tumblers, and intermediate or switching swimmers [5, 19]. The frequency of reversal can be highly variable between cell populations, individual cells, and also between successive points in time of single-cell trajectories. Thus, this classification depends on the time frame of observation, as any persistent swimmer can enter a tumbling phase at time-points outside of the observation window. Importantly, we have shown that motility behavior is strongly dependent on the environment. Mechanical resistance, in high viscosity media, tissue or synthetic microchannels, for example, increases swimming persistency, forward or backward [4, 5, 16].

The general classification of motility behavior by swimming direction and persistency can be performed with data of any spatiotemporal resolution, as long as the optical magnification is sufficient to identify the orientation of the cell, and the speed of acquisition is sufficient to continuously track single cells at speeds of several tens of μm/s [5, 19–21]. However, if the aim is to precisely characterize motility behavior certain minimum requirements for spatiotemporal resolution apply. In order to resolve flagellar beats, images should be acquired with at least 200 frames per second as beat frequencies range from around 10–40 Hz, yielding a minimum of 5 images per beat. Wave propagation can reach well over 100 μm/s, so recording with an acquisition time of 5 ms allows for following the traveling wave with a resolution of ~0.5 μm. This is sufficient to identify single waves of persistently swimming cells, but in the case of irregular events and waves in opposing directions, the temporal resolution buffer might be spent quickly.

The importance of analyzing cells in this detail lies in the fact that any microswimmer in the size and speed range of trypanosomes is a moving object for which inertia is irrelevant. Viscous forces are all the swimming cell experiences [22]. This means that every external physical influence has an immediate impact on cell motility, that is, the parasites will keep on moving for less than a microsecond after the propulsive force stops [5]. The rotational swimming mode further complicates the analyses [16]. Although the rotation frequency is usually lower than beat frequency (~3 Hz for BSF), the helical movement turns the flagellar wave plane periodically, which renders only a part of the original images useful for certain detailed analysis, that is, measurement of wavelength, amplitude, and wave speed. What ′makes up for′ the necessity of high frame rates, is the fact that the mode of regular locomotion is repetitive, making it easy to characterize a cell with relatively short recordings. A persistently swimming cell has fairly constant beat and rotation frequencies and maximum swimming speeds, depending on morphotype. It will also react immediately to any perturbances, making rapid quantitative analysis feasible.

Bearing these facts in mind, the high resolution analysis of motility could be valuable in order to discriminate between environments, cell types and mutants that exhibit minor variations of motility phenotype. For example, only major effects of drastic motility phenotypes have been analyzed in greater detail so far, that is, the complete detachment of the flagellum, or the inhibition of forward flagellar waves which result in obvious swimming deficits [23–28]. Most motility phenotypes, however, will be subtle, with changing ratios of beat directionality or variations of beat frequency. Likewise, the reaction to obstacles can be hampered, a phenotype that can easily escape observation, if the analysis is not done with high accuracy.

2 Materials

Only material used for the specific example shown in this protocol is listed. Please refer to the text and notes for the discussion of general applications.

Pleomorphic *Trypanosoma brucei brucei* strain EATRO 1125 (AnTat1.1) were cultivated in SDM-79.

Microscope: Leica DMI6000B with 63× glycerin immersion objective and differential interference contrast (DIC) optics.

pco edge sCMOS.camera.

Fiji (ImageJ) [29].

Amira 3D Visualization & Analysis Software (ThermoFisher Scientific).

3 Methods

3.1 Motility Analysis

1. Grow cultured *T. brucei* cells to maximum density of exponential growth phase (i.e., 5×10^5 cells/ml for bloodstream forms (BSF), 1×10^7 cells/ml for procyclic culture forms (PCF) or extract in high density (~10^7 cells/ml) from infected hosts.
2. Pipette 3 μl of trypanosome containing fluid (cell culture medium, compatible buffers, wet blood film, or other host fluids) onto a glass slide and cover with a 24 × 60 mm coverslip (*see* **Note 1**).
3. Place directly onto microscope stage (*see* **Note 2**). Examine under microscope using 60×–100× objective and contrast method of choice (*see* **Note 3**).
4. Acquire image series with at least 200 fps (*see* **Note 4**). Record continuously until cells of interest have crossed the field of view in the focal plane. Alternatively, if available, use custom automated tracking and autofocus software to simplify the acquisition of adequately focused and longer trajectories. Here, we focus on the detailed analysis of single, repetitive motion patterns, on the time scale of the cells rotational frequency (0.5–3 Hz). This means that for one cycle of a free persistent swimmer, a recording of maximally 2 s will be necessary. Continuous recording with these framerates requires a computer system with sufficient RAM, or sufficiently high transfer and writing speeds (*see* **Note 5**).

5. Assess recorded trajectories by slow motion playback, select, crop and save adequate recordings as TIF stacks (note the amount of possibly accumulating data, **Note 5**).
6. Analyze single cell motility by loading TIF stacks with Fiji (Image J) [29]. Choose a starting frame where the flagellar beating plane is on the horizontal (x, y) imaging plane and the flagellar tip is in focus (Fig. 2a). With a temporal resolution of 4 ms, it should be possible to determine the switching point where the flagellar tip changes the bending direction to produce a new half-wave (Fig. 2b, d, h). In the next couple of frames, the flagellum will form the first arc of a sinusoidal wavelength, switch bending direction and complete the second arc (Fig. 2g). The second half cycle will be almost symmetrical to the first half cycle, if the free flagellar end is as long as a complete wavelength. For cell types with shorter free ends, the waveform will be altered, depending on the specifics of the attached cell body.
7. The traveling wave produced by the flagellar beat will travel further along the flagellum and deform the elastic cell body while being damped. It will also follow a chiral path around the cell body, if a chiral attachment of the flagellum exists, and run on to the flagellar pocket underneath which the basal body is located. The traveling wave will have moved the cell in the opposite direction (anterior) while rotating the cell around its longitudinal axis by a specific angle. Following the trajectory of the cell, count the number of flagellar beats and note the number of beats performed until the cell has rotated 360°, and thus reached the starting position again. This image should be almost identical to the starting image, depending on the angle of the recorded trajectory relative to the horizontal plane (Fig. 3).
8. Calculate the beat and rotational frequencies in Hz (*see* legend to Fig. 3). These values are valid for unperturbed series of successive beats where relatively constant beat frequencies can be expected. Any interruption by reverse beats or obstacles must be taken into account individually.
9. Measure swimming distances and calculate swimming speeds. Determine the longitudinal midline of the cell in each frame and draw an orthogonal line marking the posterior end of the cell body (Fig. 3). Measure the distance between successive frames in the translocation direction in order to calculate the instantaneous speed, or between other equally spaced frames in order to calculate an average speed. Distance measurements covering at least one complete cell axis rotation will yield a straight-line velocity (VSL). Finer resolution measurement results in the curvilinear velocity (VCL) along the oscillating

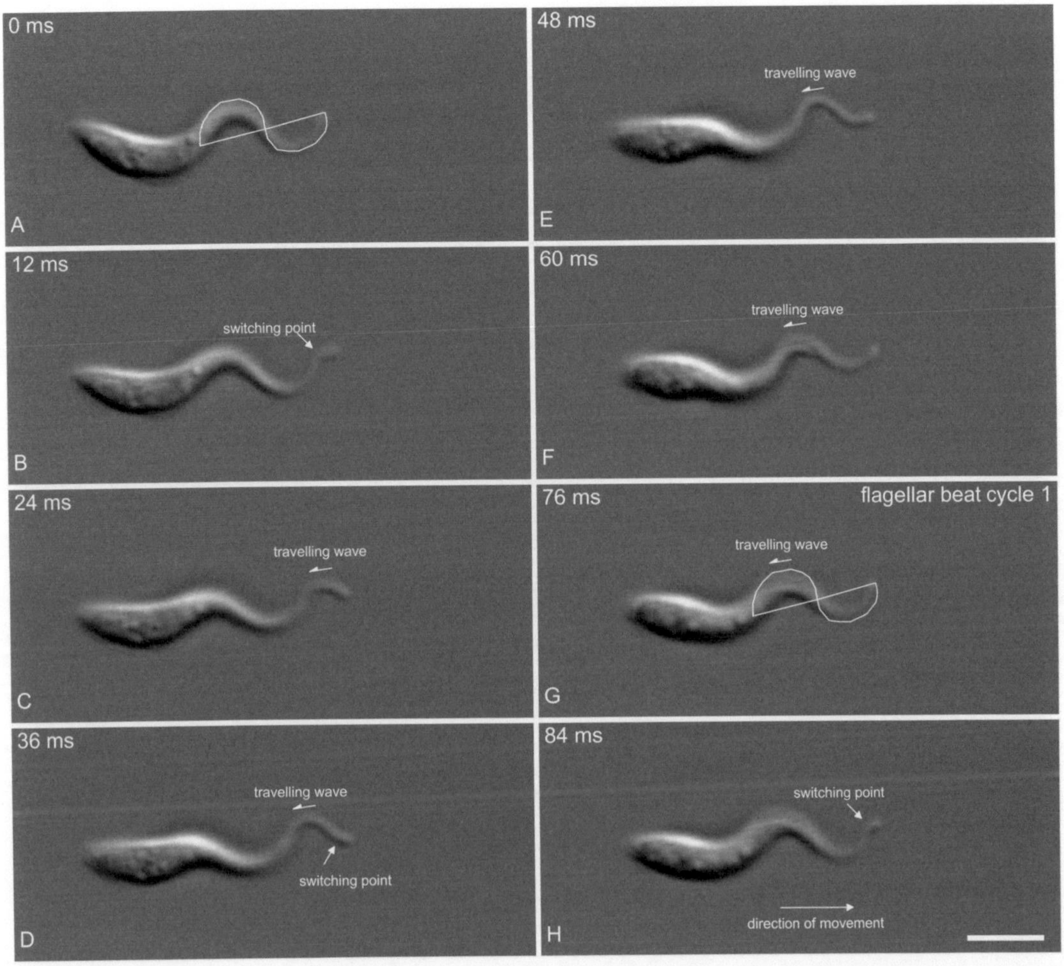

Fig. 2 Description of a single flagellar beat cycle. (**a**) Trypanosome with its longitudinal axis aligned horizontally. The anterior part of the flagellum forms a planar sinusoidal wave, recorded in the *xy*-plane. (**b**) During the following milliseconds, the bending of the flagellar tip can be clearly followed. (**c**) The bending flagellum has developed the crest of a traveling wave. (**d**) The flagellar tip switches bending direction again. (**e**) The flagellar tip forms an opposing wave-crest while the posterior part of the cell has rotated due to the previous wave running chirally across and around the cell body. (**f**) The second arc of the wavelength has almost been completed. The cell has rotated to a position where the anterior end of the cell body and the free overhang of the flagellum are visible (~ half a wavelength in this case). (**g**) The first beat cycle is complete. A new wavelength has been developed whose plane has rotated around the longitudinal axis of the cell (compare with A). (**h**) The next flagellar beat begins with another switch of bending direction. The cell has moved in the opposite direction of the traveling wave and its velocities can be measured as described in the text and illustrated in Fig. 3. Scale bar: 5 μm (*see* **Note 13**)

trajectory of the cell body. The posterior end will be the most reliable position marker in transmission light microscopy or labeling of the cell surface, because of unambiguous localization. Using fluorescence microscopy, a labeled structure (e.g., the nucleus) can also be used to perform tracking of a position closer to the centroid of the cell (*see* **Note 6**).

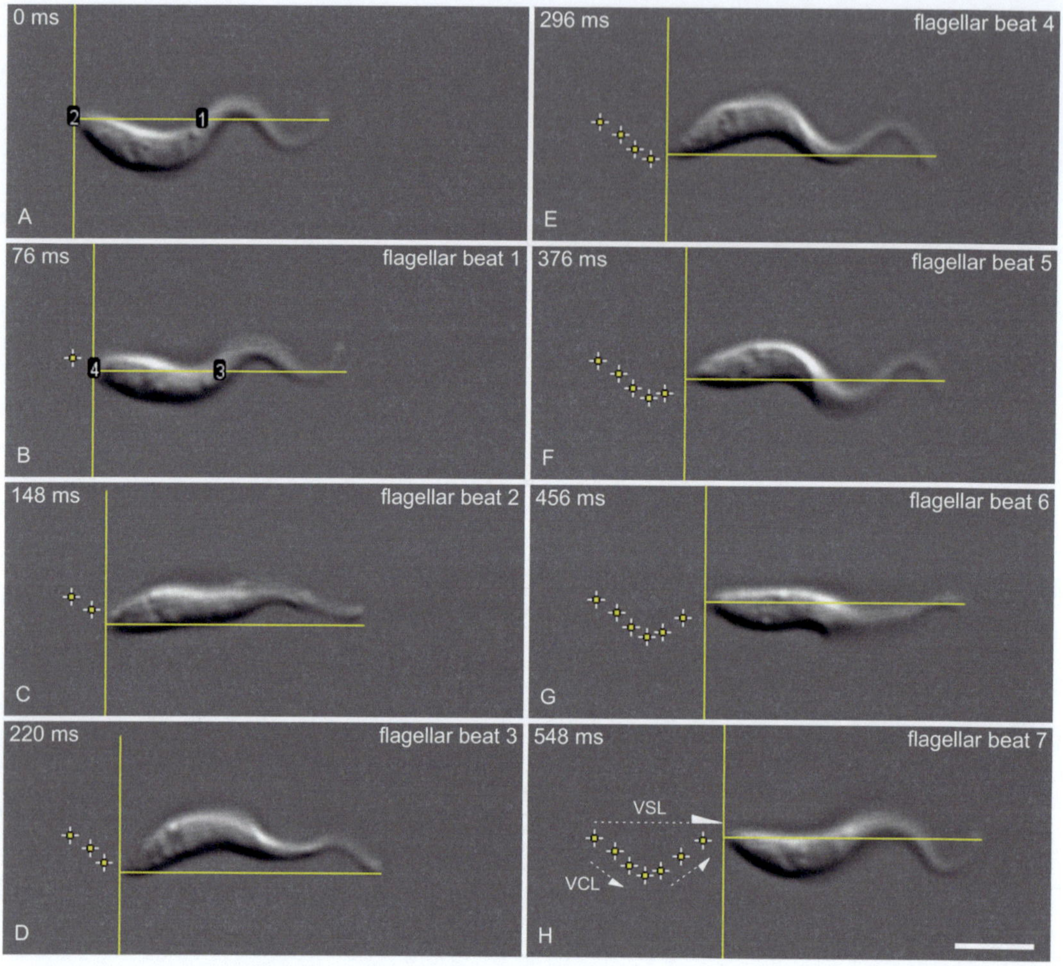

Fig. 3 High resolution motility analysis during one rotational cycle. (**a**) Trypanosome at the beginning of a beat cycle, with a planar waveform of the anterior part of the flagellum (the frame shown is the same as in Fig. 2a). A horizontal line is drawn from the posterior to the anterior tip along the *x*-axis (the image stack had previously been rotated in order to align the *x*-axis with the averaged velocity path). (**b**) The first flagellar beat has been completed (the frame shown is the same as in Fig. 2g). The position of the posterior tip in A is marked by the point selection. (**c**) The second flagellar beat has been completed. The cell has rotated approximately 90° around the longitudinal axis (*see* Fig. 4). Posterior tip positions of the previous time points are shown. (**d**, **e**) During flagellar beats 3 and 4, in sum, the cell rotates around the *x*-axis approximately 180°, thus showing a vertical mirror image of the cell (compare **a** and **e**). (**f–h**) The cell completes the 360° turn around its longitudinal axis, in order to assume the same position as in A, translocated by a distance of 8.43 μm along the *x*-axis (0.9–1.5 μm per beat) in 548 ms. This computes to a straight line velocity (VSL) of 15.38 μm/s. The curvilinear or instantaneous speed /VCL) as measured by translocation of the posterior tip is 17.38 μm/s. The flagellar beat frequency is 12.8 Hz (7/548 ms). The rotational frequency is 1.8 Hz. Scale bar: 5 μm

10. Analyze averaged curvilinear or straight line velocities, beat frequencies, wave amplitudes or wave speeds of persistently swimming, unobstructed cells under defined environmental conditions (temperature, cell density, viscosity, etc.). Register

inherent variety of specific cell culture types (i.e., monomorphic or pleomorphic cells) and determine characteristic, independent criteria (i.e., maximal speed, constant beat frequency, wave amplitude and symmetry) (*see* **Note 7**). These data will allow the best possible comparability between different cell types on one side, and between microenvironments or mutant phenotypes of one cell type on the other.

11. Analyze single frame, high resolution data of obstructions to persistent forward swimming, either internal, that is, interrupting base-to-tip beats causing changes of swimming direction, reversal or tumbling, or external, that is, mechanical hindrance of material or obstacles (*see* **Note 8**).

3.2 Time-Dependent Tomography

1. Record, select, and analyze data as described in Subheading 3.1, **steps 4–6**. Select a recorded sequence covering one rotational cycle of a persistently forward swimming cell. Select the first image of every successive flagellar beat cycle, that is, for a cell performing seven flagellar beats per 360° longitudinal axis rotation, select eight images (Fig. 3). The last image should show the cell at the beginning of the first beat of the next rotational cycle and therefore be almost identical to the first image (i.e., Fig. 3a and h). A cell beating persistently with a constant frequency will exhibit relatively equable rotation angles per flagellar wave, that is, 51° in our example.
2. Import images with 3D analysis software [e.g., Amira (Thermo Scientific)]. Trace the outline of the visible cell shape in each image to create filled binary contours, using the segmentation module (Fig. 4a).
3. In the 3D viewer, align all contours on a common longitudinal axis (*see* **Note 9**).
4. Rotate each image by the calculated angle around the *x*-axis (label 2 by 51°, label 3 by 102°, etc., Fig. 4a), using the transform editor (*see* **Note 10**).
5. Extrude each contour by expanding the binary image in the *z*-plane (the *z*-dimension needs to be adjusted to the height (*y*-dimension) of the original image volume). The expanded contour creates a volume that can be visualized by a volume or an isosurface model (Fig. 4b).
6. Calculate the sum of the overlapping data by using the arithmetic "logical AND" (&&) expression (*see* **Note 11**).
7. Visualize the result as a volume or surface rendering model (Fig. 4b). The result will only be a realistic approximation of the 3D cell morphology if the assumption of constant unidirectional rotation was correct (*see* **Note 12**).

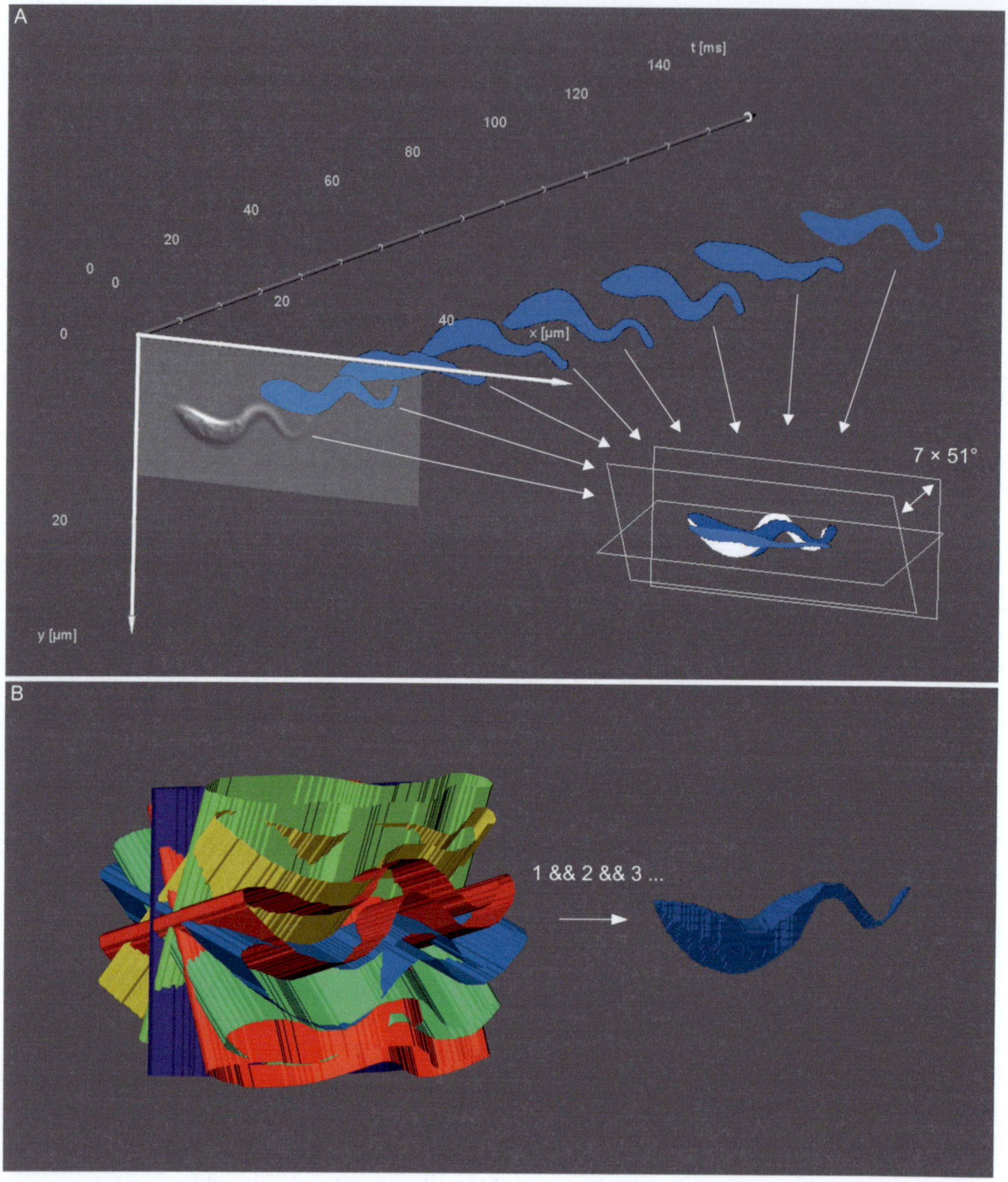

Fig. 4 Time dependent tomography. (**a**) The DIC image at $t = 0$ ms shows the trypanosome at the beginning of the first beat cycle (the frame shown in Figs. 2a and 3a). The images behind are filled binary outlines of the light microscopic images at the starting time points of the successive flagellar beats (Figs. 3b–h). These images are at the original positions in the xyt space. Bottom right. The binary image labels are aligned longitudinally and rotated around their corresponding *x*-axes (*see* **Note 9**). Only three label planes are shown for clarity. (**b**) Left: The extruded contours of the aligned and rotated cells are represented as surface models. Right: The arithmetic combination of the binary data results in a realistic 3D model (compare with DIC image in A, *see* **Note 12**). The rotation of the created model allows a comparison of every two-dimensionally recorded view in the original image stack

4 Notes

1. This simple setup is routinely used to record freely swimming trypanosomes. The fluid spreads between the glass surfaces to result in a layer of ~8–10 μm. This is sufficient for the cells (thickness 2–4 μm) to swim freely in the horizontal plane without constant surface interference. The trajectories of persistent and intermediate swimmers can thus be recorded reliably across the field of view, using 60×–100× objectives. In order to compare free motility in three dimensions, any spacers or microchambers can be used for volumes of 25–50 μl (e.g., μ-Slides, h = 100 or 200 μm (ibidi), Gene Frame chambers, h = 250 μm (Thermo Fisher Scientific)). Here the free three-dimensional rotation of tumblers or cells swimming along the vertical axis can be recorded, albeit most of the recording will be outside the focus plane. In order to record free 3D trajectories completely, holographic methods must be used, which are technically elaborate and have only recently become readily applicable for very high spatiotemporal resolution [19, 30–34]. Persistent motility analyzed by us so far, showed no significant differences between swimmers in chamber heights of 10–250 μm.
2. Motility analyses have typically been performed at room temperature or slightly above, to match the standard culture temperature of PCF trypanosomes (27 °C). The effect of temperature differences on motility behavior has been systematically analyzed for BSF cells. There was a slight increase of swimming persistency at the standard culture temperature for BSF cells (37 °C) compared to analysis at room temperature, but the absolute swimming speed was unchanged, especially maximum swimming speeds, which are a good value to compare (*see* Subheading 3.1, **step 9**). Standard incubation chambers, commonly available for all microscope setups, regulate temperatures around 37 °C and 5% CO_2.
3. Any imaging technique can be used for basic motility analysis. Bright field or dark field illumination, phase contrast methods (Phase contrast, differential interference contrast (DIC, aka. Nomarski), modulation contrast) are ideal in order to analyze wild type cells or any cell type without need for extraneous manipulation. Among these methods, DIC is best suited to discern the movement of the attached flagellum. Of importance are clearly focused images of the beating flagellar tip and the posterior end, at least during the beating phase of the planar flagellum lying in the *x*–*y* plane (which is repeatedly the case following the cell's helical trajectory, *see* Introduction). Fluorescent protein expressing cell lines can be used, as long as the complete cell is detectable (cytoplasmic signal or staining

of the entire surface membrane). In this case the analysis might be developed into a fully automated tracking and analysis routine with more ease than the transmitted light data. Staining the entire cell surface, including the flagellum is one of the rare possibilities to unequivocally and directly show the rotational character of the swimming cell (*see* Subheading 3.2). Note that fluorescence imaging at speeds of 200 fps and more requires a fast and very light sensitive camera (i.e., sCMOS, scientific Complementary Metal-Oxide Semiconductor).

4. Standard CCD (charged coupled device) cameras will record at maximum speeds of 20–30 fps. With flagellar beat frequencies in the same range and higher (>40 Hz), the cell movement is significantly undersampled. The high beat frequencies and especially high wave speeds the flagellates thus reach, necessitate recording speeds of 200 fps and higher (*see* Introduction; note that the Nyquist–Shannon theorem for correctly recording a beat frequency (e.g., 40 Hz) requires sampling at twice that frequency (e.g., 80 Hz), but to account for rotational out of plane image data and irregular reverse flagellar waves, the Nyquist frequency should be multiplied by a factor of around 3). These speeds are reached by several CMOS chip based cameras (e.g., Phantom (Vision Research, USA) and scientific CMOS (sCMOS) cameras).
5. Camera control will allow the acquisition of images until the RAM of the computer is full in sequential mode, or use a "ring buffer" mode overwriting the first recorded data, filling memory until the acquisition is stopped by the user. Direct recording to hard drive requires a system with sufficient high transfer (i.e, "camera link" protocol) and writing speeds as well as ample disk space (recording a 1 min video with 800 × 800 pixels resolution and 16 bit, at 250 fps will result in 19.2 GB of data).
6. Note that the deflection of the posterior end will be more pronounced in cells with the basal body located further away from the posterior end (e.g., procyclic forms). Generally, any part of the cell body will follow a more or less asymmetric, helical trajectory around the longitudinal axis, that depends on the combined morphology of the rotating cell body and attached flagellum, and which cannot be resolved by two-dimensional microscopy. Although the different trypanosome morphotypes with their variant flagellum attachment complicate analyses, the principles of three-dimensional swimming apply as in well-studied sperm cells. For these microswimmers, motility analysis has been standardized (CASA, Computer assisted sperm analysis, [35]). For a detailed description of sperm helical motility, *see* [10]).

7. As stated in **Note 6**, sperm motility analysis is routinely performed and there are several attempts to standardize and (semi) automate the image analysis (e.g., SpermQ, [36]). Note that these methods rely on the nonvariant morphology of a sperm cell of one species. In these cases, parameters like the longitudinal rotation of the sperm head can be inferred from two-dimensional microscopic data. The variety of trypanosomatid morphotypes does not allow for this straightforward kind of automatization, but machine learning approaches should make similar approaches feasible in the near future, where detailed knowledge of 3D morphology can be "fed," in order for algorithms to recognize motility patterns of specific cell-types.
8. Because inertia is irrelevant for microswimmers in viscous surroundings (conditions are characterized by low Reynolds numbers [22]), every impact on the cells will have an immediate effect on swimming behavior. In reverse, every change in motile force production can be measured instantaneously, making the high spatiotemporal resolution analysis invaluable for the evaluation of subtle effects of phenotype or external physical impact, especially in the light of the apparent interdependence of morphotype and environment.
9. Assuming the cell body is reversibly deformed, that is, oscillates precisely as dictated by the flagellar wave, the cell body will adopt exactly the same confirmation after completion of each flagellar beat. This means that the only difference between the aligned images (forward translocation subducted) is the viewer's point around the longitudinal cell axis (i.e., now defined as x-axis). The careful alignment is paramount for the generation of a meaningful 3D model. This step has to be performed manually. Existing registration algorithms will only allow an approximate first alignment of cell shapes. Note that this problem belongs to the set of general issues with the automatization of complex three-dimensional movement addressed in **Note 8**.
10. This tomography method relies on the inherent rotation of the cell to identify different view angles on one morphological state. Instead of tilting the probe or the recording apparatus in conventional tomography, the snapshot of the cell at defined timepoints yields the 2d slices to be used for the 3D reconstruction. Hence the term "time-dependent tomography."
11. The process can be viewed as a simple filtered backprojection method as known from computer tomography reconstruction [37]. The extruded cell contours of cell morphology positioned in 3D space corresponding to the original viewing angles at defined timepoints (start of flagellar beat), are projected back to one original location of the cell on its helical trajectory. The binary conversion of the cell contours counts as a simple filter to obtain a relatively well defined 3D model.

12. The filtered backprojection method in conventional computer tomography depends on a large number of view angles to obtain results as close as possible to the original object. The method described here is naturally restricted to as many view points as the longitudinal rotation of the cell performs per beat. Thus, this method is not suitable for reconstructing precise 3D models of cells, it is only useful for the showing the regular rotational swimming mechanism of a cell. Any irregular movements not accountable for adjusting the unidirectional rotation (i.e., by simply adjusting the rotation angle) will not result in the meaningful reconstruction of a complete cell.
13. Figures 2–4 were assembled and annotated using the ImageJ plugin ScientiFig [38].

References

1. Krüger T, Engstler M (2015) Flagellar motility in eukaryotic human parasites. Semin Cell Dev Biol 46:113–127. https://doi.org/10.1016/j.semcdb.2015.10.034
2. Krüger T, Schuster S, Engstler M (2018) Beyond blood: African trypanosomes on the move. Trends Parasitol 34:1056–1067. https://doi.org/10.1016/j.pt.2018.08.002
3. Krüger T, Engstler M (2016) Trypanosomes – versatile microswimmers. Eur Phys J Spec Top 225:2157–2172. https://doi.org/10.1140/epjst/e2016-60063-5
4. Schuster S, Krüger T, Subota I et al (2017) Developmental adaptations of trypanosome motility to the tsetse fly host environments unravel a multifaceted in vivo microswimmer system. elife 6:e27656. https://doi.org/10.7554/eLife.27656
5. Bargul JL, Jung J, McOdimba FA et al (2016) Species-specific adaptations of trypanosome morphology and motility to the mammalian host. PLoS Pathog 12:e1005448. https://doi.org/10.1371/journal.ppat.1005448
6. Sunter J, Gull K (2017) Shape, form, function and *Leishmania* pathogenicity: from textbook descriptions to biological understanding. Open Biol 7:170165. https://doi.org/10.1098/rsob.170165
7. Andrade LO, Andrews NW (2005) The Trypanosoma cruzi–host-cell interplay: location, invasion, retention. Nat Rev Microbiol 3:819–823. https://doi.org/10.1038/nrmicro1249
8. Son K, Brumley DR, Stocker R (2015) Live from under the lens: exploring microbial motility with dynamic imaging and microfluidics. Nat Rev Microbiol 13:761–775. https://doi.org/10.1038/nrmicro3567
9. Jarrell KF, McBride MJ (2008) The surprisingly diverse ways that prokaryotes move. Nat Rev Microbiol 6:466–476. https://doi.org/10.1038/nrmicro1900
10. Gray J (1955) The movement of sea-urchin spermatozoa. J Exp Biol 32:775–801
11. Gray J, Hancock GJ (1955) The propulsion of sea-urchin spermatozoa. J Exp Biol 32:802–814
12. Lindemann CB, Lesich KA (2016) Functional anatomy of the mammalian sperm flagellum: mammalian sperm mechanics. Cytoskeleton 73:652–669. https://doi.org/10.1002/cm.21338
13. Ishimoto K, Gadêlha H, Gaffney EA et al (2018) Human sperm swimming in a high viscosity mucus analogue. J Theor Biol 446:1–10. https://doi.org/10.1016/j.jtbi.2018.02.013
14. Miller DJ (2018) Review: the epic journey of sperm through the female reproductive tract. Animal 12:s110–s120. https://doi.org/10.1017/S1751731118000526
15. Hoare CA (1972) The trypanosomes of mammals. A zoological monograph. Blackwell Scientific Publications, Oxford, Edinburgh
16. Heddergott N, Krüger T, Babu SB et al (2012) Trypanosome motion represents an adaptation to the crowded environment of the vertebrate bloodstream. PLoS Pathog 8:e1003023. https://doi.org/10.1371/journal.ppat.1003023
17. Gadelha C, Wickstead B, Gull K (2007) Flagellar and ciliary beating in trypanosome motility. Cell Motil Cytoskeleton 64:629–643. https://doi.org/10.1002/cm.20210
18. Alizadehrad D, Krüger T, Engstler M, Stark H (2015) Simulating the complex cell design of

trypanosoma brucei and its motility. PLoS Comput Biol 11. https://doi.org/10.1371/journal.pcbi.1003967

19. Weiße S, Heddergott N, Heydt M et al (2012) A quantitative 3D motility analysis of Trypanosoma brucei by use of digital in-line holographic microscopy. PLoS One 7:e37296. https://doi.org/10.1371/journal.pone.0037296
20. Uppaluri S, Nagler J, Stellamanns E et al (2011) Impact of microscopic motility on the swimming behavior of parasites: straighter trypanosomes are more directional. PLoS Comput Biol 7:e1002058. https://doi.org/10.1371/journal.pcbi.1002058
21. Wheeler RJ (2017) Use of chiral cell shape to ensure highly directional swimming in trypanosomes. PLoS Comput Biol 13:e1005353. https://doi.org/10.1371/journal.pcbi.1005353
22. Purcell EM (1977) Life at low Reynolds number. Am J Phys 45:3. https://doi.org/10.1119/1.10903
23. Branche C, Kohl L, Toutirais G et al (2006) Conserved and specific functions of axoneme components in trypanosome motility. J Cell Sci 119:3443–3455. https://doi.org/10.1242/jcs.03078
24. Broadhead R, Dawe HR, Farr H et al (2006) Flagellar motility is required for the viability of the bloodstream trypanosome. Nature 440:224–227. https://doi.org/10.1038/nature04541
25. Engstler M, Pfohl T, Herminghaus S et al (2007) Hydrodynamic flow-mediated protein sorting on the cell surface of trypanosomes. Cell 131:505–515. https://doi.org/10.1016/j.cell.2007.08.046
26. Hutchings NR, Donelson JE, Hill KL (2002) Trypanin is a cytoskeletal linker protein and is required for cell motility in African trypanosomes. J Cell Biol 156:867–877. https://doi.org/10.1083/jcb.200201036
27. Ralston KS, Lerner AG, Diener DR, Hill KL (2006) Flagellar motility contributes to cytokinesis in *trypanosoma brucei* and is modulated by an evolutionarily conserved dynein regulatory system. Eukaryot Cell 5:696–711. https://doi.org/10.1128/EC.5.4.696-711.2006
28. Baron DM, Kabututu ZP, Hill KL (2007) Stuck in reverse: loss of LC1 in Trypanosoma brucei disrupts outer dynein arms and leads to reverse flagellar beat and backward movement. J Cell Sci 120:1513–1520. https://doi.org/10.1242/jcs.004846
29. Schindelin J, Arganda-Carreras I, Frise E et al (2012) Fiji: an open-source platform for biological-image analysis. Nat Methods 9:676–682. https://doi.org/10.1038/nmeth.2019
30. Wilson LG, Carter LM, Reece SE (2013) High-speed holographic microscopy of malaria parasites reveals ambidextrous flagellar waveforms. Proc Natl Acad Sci 110:18769–18774. https://doi.org/10.1073/pnas.1309934110
31. Jikeli JF, Alvarez L, Friedrich BM et al (2015) Sperm navigation along helical paths in 3D chemoattractant landscapes. Nat Commun 6. https://doi.org/10.1038/ncomms8985
32. Muschol M, Wenders C, Wennemuth G (2018) Four-dimensional analysis by high-speed holographic imaging reveals a chiral memory of sperm flagella. PLoS One 13: e0199678. https://doi.org/10.1371/journal.pone.0199678
33. Daloglu MU, Luo W, Shabbir F et al (2018) Label-free 3D computational imaging of spermatozoon locomotion, head spin and flagellum beating over a large volume. Light Sci Appl 7:17121. https://doi.org/10.1038/lsa.2017.121
34. Flewellen JL, Zaid IM, Berry RM (2019) A multi-mode digital holographic microscope. Rev Sci Instrum 90:023705. https://doi.org/10.1063/1.5066556
35. Gallagher MT, Smith DJ, Kirkman-Brown JC (2018) CASA: tracking the past and plotting the future. Reprod Fertil Dev 30:867. https://doi.org/10.1071/RD17420
36. Hansen J, Rassmann S, Jikeli J, Wachten D (2018) SpermQ–a simple analysis software to comprehensively study flagellar beating and sperm steering. Cell 8:10. https://doi.org/10.3390/cells8010010
37. Smith SW (2002) Digital signal processing: a practical guide for engineers and scientists. Newnes, Boston
38. Aigouy B, Mirouse V (2013) ScientiFig: a tool to build publication-ready scientific figures. Nat Methods. 10:1048–1048. https://doi.org/10.1038/nmeth.2692

Chapter 26

Electron Microscopy Techniques Applied to Symbiont-Harboring Trypanosomatids: The Association of the Bacterium with Host Organelles

Maria Cristina M. Motta and Carolina M. C. Catta-Preta

Abstract

In this chapter we describe different electron microscopy techniques such as freeze fracture, deep etching, and three-dimensional reconstruction, obtained by electron tomography or focused ion beam scanning electron microscopy (FIB-SEM), combined with quick-freezing methods in order to reveal aspects of the cell structure in trypanosomatids. For this purpose, we chose protists that evolve in a mutualistic way with a symbiotic bacterium. Such cells represent excellent models to study the positioning and distribution of organelles, since the symbiotic bacterium interacts with different organelles of the host trypanosomatid. We demonstrate that the employment of such techniques can show the proximity and even the interaction of the symbiotic bacterium with different structures of the protist host, such as the nucleus and the glycosomes. In addition, the quick-freezing approach can reveal new aspects of the gram-negative bacterial envelope, such as the presence of a greatly reduced cell wall between the two membrane units.

Key words Quick freezing, Freeze fracture, Deep etching, Freeze substitution, FIB-SEM, Electron tomography, Three-dimensional reconstruction, Symbiont-harboring trypanosomatids

1 Introduction

Protists are interesting models for ultrastructural studies, since they retain unique characteristics of primitive beings that diverged very early from the last eukaryotic common ancestor (LECA) [1, 2]. Trypanosomatids have been widely studied because they cause diseases to men and to animals and plants of economic interest. However, most protists in this family are not pathogenic and among them, there are seven species, namely, *Angomonas deanei*, *Angomonas desouzai*, *Angomonas ambiguus*, *Strigomonas oncopelti*, *Strigomonas culicis*, *Strigomonas galati*, and *Kentomonas sorsogonicus*, that harbor a single symbiotic bacterium of Gram-negative origin in their cytoplasm [3, 4]. The relationship between the prokaryote and the protist is mutualistic, thus permitting exciting and revealing investigations about cell evolution and the bacterial origin of organelles.

Paul A. M. Michels et al. (eds.), *Trypanosomatids: Methods and Protocols*, Methods in Molecular Biology, vol. 2116, https://doi.org/10.1007/978-1-0716-0294-2_26,

This symbiotic association is characterized by intense metabolic changes and the bacterium is seen in close association with various structures of the protist such as the nucleus, with which it maintains division synchrony throughout the cell cycle, in such a way that each new trypanosomatid generated contains only one prokaryote [5–8]. In addition, the symbiont has high proximity to glycosomes and to the single and branched mitochondrion, which is related to the influence of the bacterium on the energy metabolism of the host protist [9, 10]. The endosymbiosis in trypanosomatids represents a very interesting model to study the association between cellular structures, since the permanent integration between two different microorganisms resulted in a single being with unique characteristics in nature.

In this chapter we present different techniques of electron microscopy that were used in order to show the association of the symbiotic bacterium with different organelles of the trypanosomatid host. Among these techniques is the freeze fracture, where samples are frozen, fractured, and then metallized. When cells are frozen and then fractured, an opening of the lipid bilayer occurs in the hydrophobic region of biological membranes, thus separating their two leaflets (Fig. 1). Such technique generates cellular replicas that allows for mainly the observation of intramembranous particles (IMPs), also referred as membrane-associated particles, that correspond to integral proteins that are not fractured during this process and remain inserted in either the inner or the outer leaflet of the lipid bilayer. IMPs may be integrated into the protoplasmic face (P face) that corresponds to the outer face of the plasma membrane's inner leaflet, or to the external face (E face) that is equivalent to the inner face of the outer membrane's leaflet. The images obtained by freeze-fracture offer a three-dimensional visual impression; the P face of the membrane is convex, while the E face is concave. The fracture plane can also reach the cytoplasm revealing IMPs present in membranes that delimit structures and organelles. However, in this case the inner leaflet of the membrane is directed toward the cytosol, while the outer leaflet is facing the matrix of the organelle. Thus, an inversion occurs and the P face is concave while the E face is convex (Figs. 2 and 3). The deep-etching method can also be applied to samples, but in this case, a prolonged sublimation of the frozen surface and a reduced angle of the metallization are employed, thus enhancing the three-dimensional (3D) appearance of cell membranes and cytosolic structures (Fig. 4) [11]. The quick-freeze, freeze-fracture and deep-etching techniques were applied in the study of trypanosomatids and other protists, revealing important ultrastructural aspects of these microorganisms [12–16].

In general, conventional electron microscopy requires the water to be exchanged by inorganic solvents, which allows for the observation of cells in the vacuum environment of the microscope. Water removal implies missing important in vivo information, such

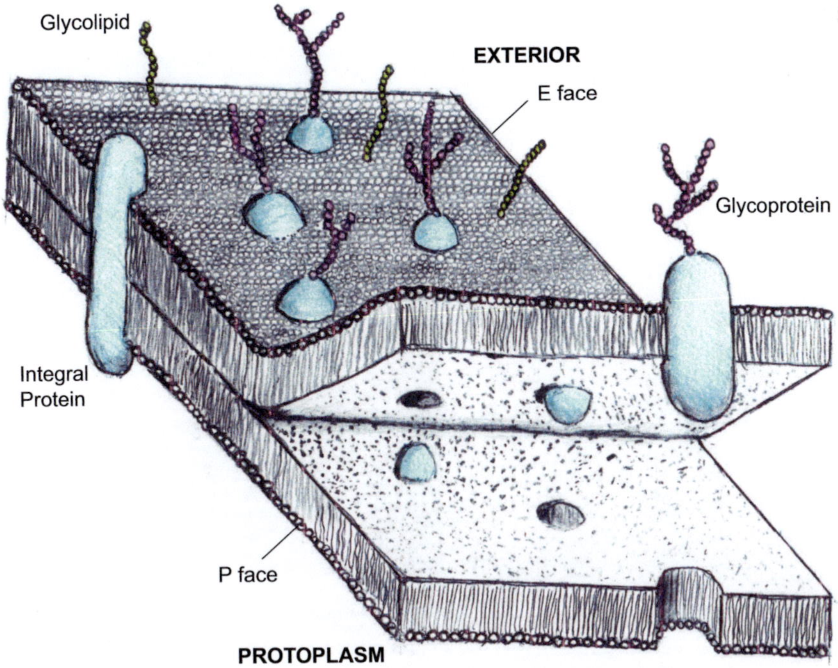

Fig. 1 Plasma membrane fracture plane in cells submitted to freeze-fracture. Scheme by Alexandre Gonçalves de Souza

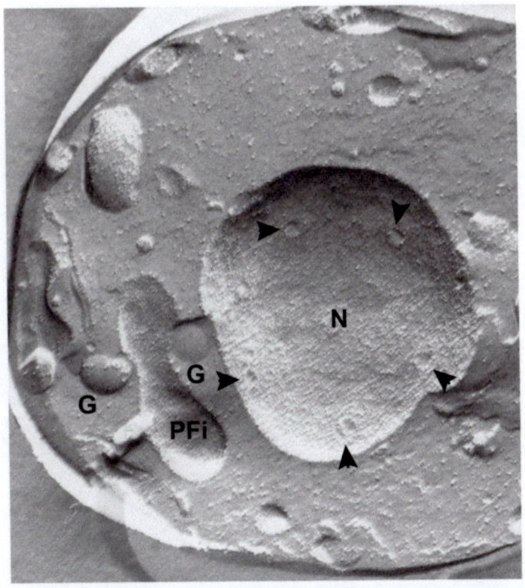

Fig. 2 A freeze-fracture view of the *Angomonas desouzai* cytoplasm showing the symbiotic bacterium close to the host trypanosomatid nucleus. Note the pore complex distribution in the nucleus (arrow heads). PFi – Protoplasmic face of the symbiont inner membrane, N - nucleus, G - glycosomes. Negative 20.000X

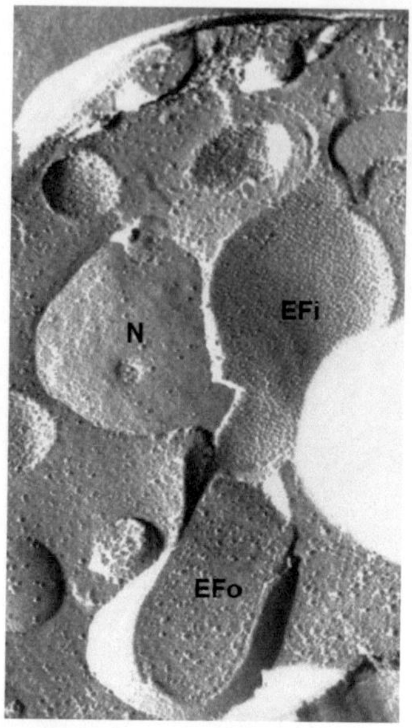

Fig. 3 A freeze-fracture image showing a close association between a dividing endosymbiont and the *Angomonas desouzai* nucleus. As previously described, in symbiont-bearing trypanosomatids, the bacterium lies down over the host cell nucleus that represents a topological reference during the prokaryote division process. EFi – Extracellular face of the symbiont inner membrane, EFo – Extracellular face of the symbiont outer membrane, N - nucleus. Negative 20.000X

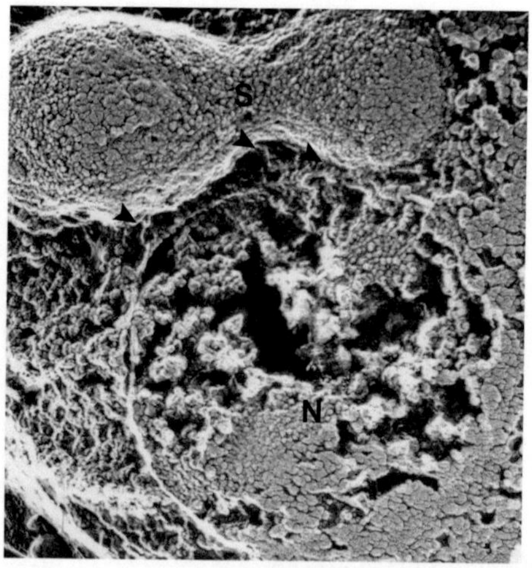

Fig. 4 A deep-etching view of the *Angomonas deanei* symbiont in great proximity to the nucleus. At some points filamentous structures seems to link the bacterium and the DNA containing organelle (arrow head). N – nucleus, S - symbiont. Negative 50.000X

as misplacement of soluble proteins and altered organization of subcellular structures. In order to obtain a good preservation of organelles and avoid artifacts caused by chemical fixation, an ideal procedure is to immobilize the water by freezing the cells. It is important to keep in mind that water must not crystallize, but rather reach a vitreous, amorphous state, characterized by the total absence of crystals. Vitrification of biological hydrated samples is not an easy task and requires high-speed freezing and/or alteration of normal pressure. Thus, a number of methods are available using different cryogens such as Liquid Nitrogen (LN_2), Propane and Freon 22. In this chapter we will describe methods of choice that are routinely used to study the cell's ultrastructure, as the high-pressure freezing (HPF), which increases the depth of freezing up to 200 μm [17]. This technique uses a high pressure (2100 bar in 20 ms), thus reducing the freezing point of a biological material to −22 °C and the speed of freezing necessary for vitrification in 200×. Either a commercial or an in-house built prototype is required to pressurize samples in such conditions, while LN_2 jets are directed to the sample holder. Although efficient to maintain the structure of the cells, this method produces a sample without contrast, thus impairing an accurate observation of the cell structure, as for example the proximity and fusion of organelle membranes. The freeze-substitution is a procedure that avoids the crystallization of the immobilized water, while cells are dehydrated under low temperatures to circumvent artifacts observed in dehydration performed at room temperature (25 °C). The principle of this technique is to dilute slowly the immobilized water with an organic solvent containing chemical fixatives, followed by a stepwise increase of the temperature before proceeding to resin inclusion. The embedded samples can be observed by conventional transmission electron microscopy (TEM) or by state-of-the-art methods such as the focused ion beam scanning electron microscopy (FIB-SEM) and electron tomography (ET). Such methods have been used in biological sciences to resolve high volume structures and even to reconstruct the whole cell [18–20].

One may want to determine relative volumes of cellular structures, their position through the cell cycle or if organelles are somehow associated. Methods of 3D reconstruction often involve problems such as to obtain a series of images to reconstruct the volume of a cell or tissue, without discontinuities, correctly aligned and free of variations of thickness and heating caused by the uneven radiation of the sections. FIB-SEM allows for direct three-dimensional imaging and superior z-axis resolution, by combining a Scanning Electron Microscopy Field Emission Gun (FEG-MEV)

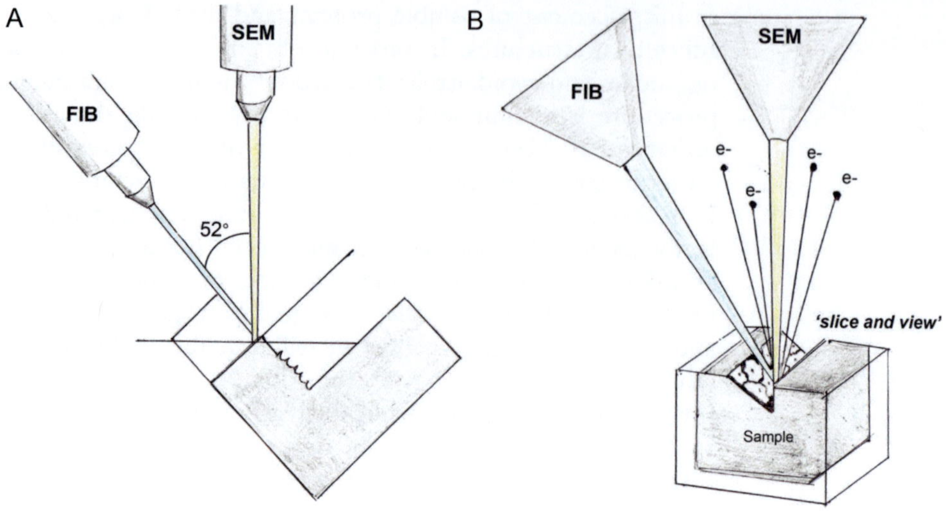

Fig. 5 Scheme of FIB-SEM working principle. A – The equipment works with a focused ion beam (FIB) positioned at 52° of the electron beam scanning the sample (SEM). B – During image acquisition the ion beam mills the sample ('slice'), while the electron beam performs the reading ('view'). Scheme by Alexandre Gonçalves de Souza

and a milling instrument using an ion beam (FIB) (Fig. 5). This technique associates high-resolution imaging of larger volumes with an automated system that allows for rapid and efficient data collection, the "slice and view," and generate a series of images that can be aligned and reconstructed using specific software, as described below. Another technique used to resolve volumes is the Electron Tomography (ET), which allows for the observation of thicker sections (0.2–2 μm) tilted on their own *Y* axis, varying angles perpendicular to the electron beam, with acquisition of projected views. Reconstruction of the 3D volume consists of calculation of back-projection profiles to be shown as stacked aligned sections. To reconstruct the 3D volume, the projection images are smeared out to the reconstruction volume along their viewing directions to form back-projection profiles. Then, the final volume is calculated by summation of all the back-projection profiles and is represented as a series of stacked thin slices (Fig. 6). Those techniques were recently applied to trypanosomatids to understand biological process involving ultrastructure modifications during cell division, as well as to better describe morphology and content of intracellular structures [5, 7, 21–23]. Here we also show images of the reduced peptidoglycan layer from *Angomonas*'s symbionts, which is only visualized when applying freezing fixation, as well as details of the association between the nucleus and the bacterium (Figs. 7 and 8).

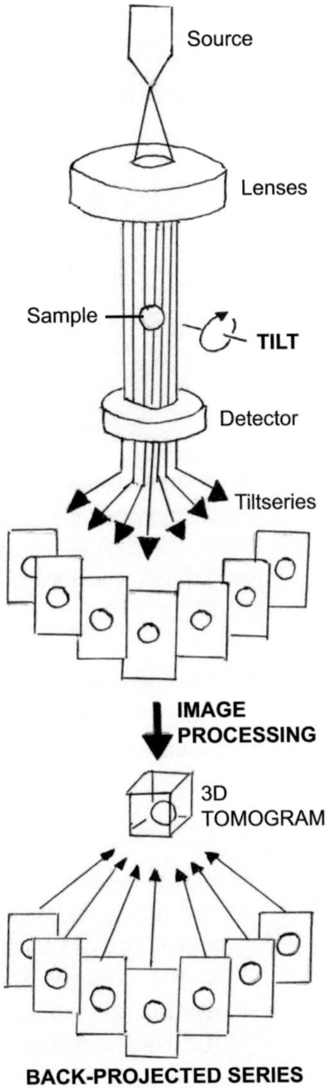

Fig. 6 Electron tomography principle. The three-dimensional sample when crossed by the electron beam projects two-dimensional images for each angulation that, when back projected, recompose the initial volume. Scheme by Alexandre Gonçalves de Souza

2 Materials

Several techniques described here use LN_2. Please wear personal protective equipment (PPE), such as gloves, goggles or protective face shields, as well as oxygen monitors that must be worn at all times while manipulating LN_2. Please always refer to local regulations.

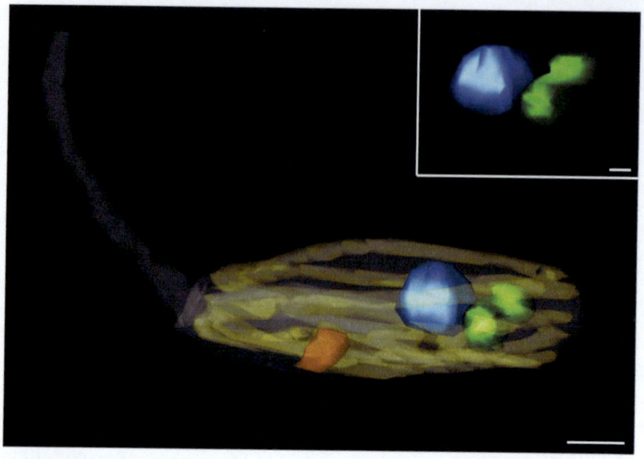

Fig. 7 Three-dimensional model of *Angomonas deanei* whole-cell obtained by manual segmentation FIB-SEM slice-and-view series. Cell body in gray, nucleus in blue, mitochondrion in yellow, symbiont in green, kinetoplast in orange. Scale bar: 2.5 mm. Insert showing close association of nucleus and symbiont. Scale bar: 0.25 mm.

2.1 Freeze Fracture and Deep Etching

2.1.1 Equipment

Balzers apparatus or equivalent commercial equipment available.

Zeiss 900 electron microscope operated at 80 kV or similar microscopes available.

2.1.2 Sample Processing

1. Ultrapure water.
2. 0.1 M cacodylate buffer (pH 7.2): prepare a solution of 0.2 M sodium cacodylate (MW: 160) diluted in ultrapure water and adjust the pH with 0.2 M HCl dropwise. To obtain the buffer at the concentration of 0.1 M, dilute in ultrapure water to double the initial volume (1:1 v/v). The recommended salt for the preparation of the cacodylate buffer contains three molecules of water [$Na(CH_3)2AsO_4{\cdot}3H_2O$]. Since this buffer contains arsenic, it cannot be used while processing live cells. Please respect local regulations for disposal of arsenic waste.
3. 2.5% glutaraldehyde type I: the commercial glutaraldehyde is 25% concentrated. Dilute tenfold in 0.1 M cacodylate buffer. Protect the solution from light using foil paper.
4. Sulfuric or chromic acid P.A.
5. Sodium hypochlorite 5%.
6. 30% glycerol ≥99%: 30% solution in ultrapure water.

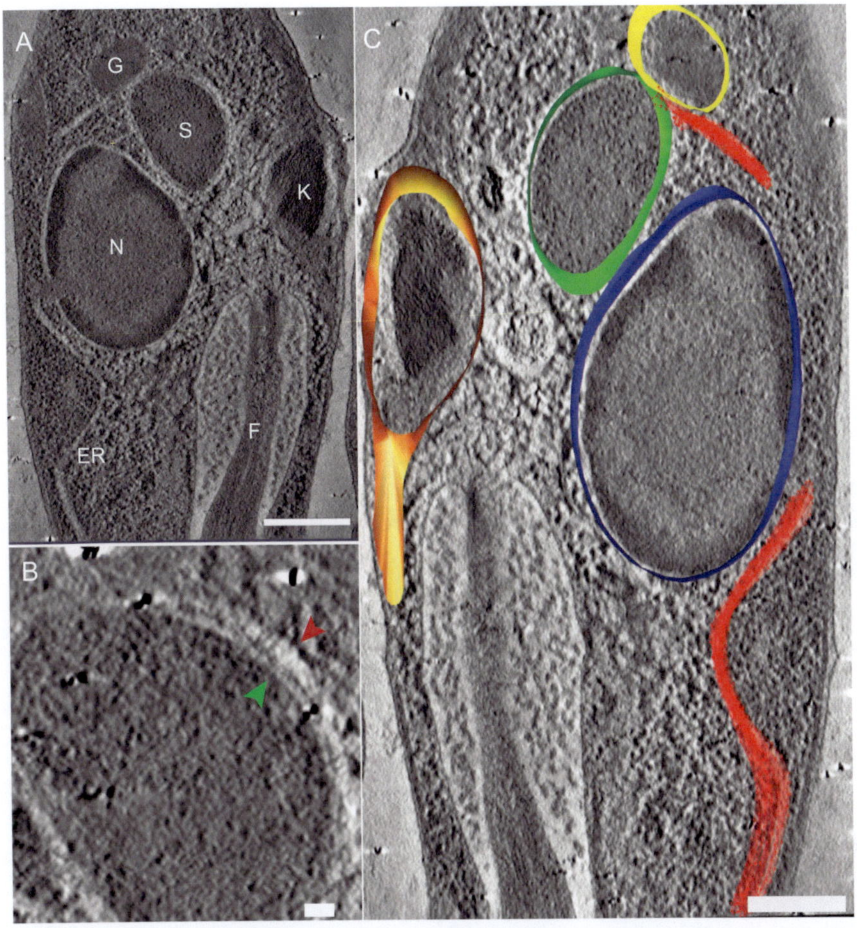

Fig. 8 Electron tomography of high-pressure freezing (HPF) and freeze substitution (FS) of *Angomonas deanei*. A - The symbiont is always observed in close association with the nucleus and glycosomes. N – nucleus, S – symbiont, G, glycosome, K, kinetoplast, ER – endoplasmic reticulum, F – flagellum. B - Internal (green arrow head) and external (red arrow head) as well as the reduced peptidoglycan wall are easily distinguished using HPF and FS. Black beads are fiducial markers (colloidal golden) used on series alignment. C – Digital slice and 3D model representing the kinetoplast (orange), symbiont (green), glycosome (yellow), nucleus (blue) and endoplasmic reticulum (red). Scale bar: A and C – 2 mm; B – 0.25 mm

2.2 High-Pressure Freezing

2.2.1 Equipment

High Pressure Freezer Leica EM ICE. Other equivalent commercial equipment are available, as well as the option to build in-house prototypes.

2.2.2 Sample Processing

1. Liquid Nitrogen (LN_2) (90 L: 85 L for HPF equipment; 5 L for sample transport and maintenance).
2. Stereo microscope for mounting capillaries on capillaries and specimen carrier.
3. Cellulose capillary tubes—cut capillary with a scalpel to about 2 mm.

4. Scalpel n° 22.
5. Tweezers to hold capillary tubes.
6. Petri dishes covered with plastic paraffin film (Parafilm) for mounting capillary tubes with cells.
7. Phosphate-buffered saline, pH 7.4.
8. Specimen carrier (1.5 mm in diameter; depths 100 or 200 μm).
9. 1-Hexadecene, ≥98.5%.
10. HPM010 Abra Fluid adaptor and HMP100 Leica adaptor (or equivalent).
11. Antistatic tweezers.
12. CryoCooler for sample transport.

2.3 Freeze–Substitution

2.3.1 Equipment

Freeze Substitution and Low Temperature Embedding System for Light and Electron Microscopy Leica EM AFS2 equipment. Please see Subheading 2 for an option using LN_2, −80 °C freezer, −20 °C freezer, and refrigerator.

2.3.2 Sample Processing

1. LN_2: 50 L for the equipment.
2. Substitution media (*see* **Note 1**).
3. 1 Recipe for improvement of *membrane staining*
   (a) 0.5% (v/v) glutaraldehyde 70%, aqueous EM grade
   (b) 2% (w/v) osmium tetroxide (OsO_4)
   (c) 0.2% (w/v) uranyl acetate
   (d) 1% (v/v) ultrapure water
   (e) q.s.p. acetone P.A.
4. 2 Recipe for *immunolabeling*
   (a) 2% (w/v) Formaldehyde
   (b) 0.05% (v/v) Glutaraldehyde 70%, aqueous EM grade
   (c) 0.5% (w/v) Uranyl acetate
   (d) q.s.p. acetone P.A.

   Prepare solutions in dry-ice, using prechilled identified vials in a chemical fume hood.

   Aliquot substitution media in cryo-vials and keep in LN_2 until use.

   Please be aware OsO_4 fumes are extremely toxic. It is important to dispose of any contaminated waste as proposed by local regulation. Usually use of mineral or vegetable oil is suggested to immobilize OsO_4 followed by disposal in cat litter to absorb.
5. Acetone P.A.
6. 1.5 mL Safe Lock microcentrifuge tubes.

7. Epon resin. Prepare resin by slowly mixing 12.5 mL of Embed 812 and 7.5 mL of Araldite 502. Add 27 mL DDSA to the mixture and finally 1.3 mL BDMA dropwise (*see* **Note 2**).

2.4 Focused Ion Beam

2.4.1 Equipment and Software

1. High-resolution scanning electron microscope with field emission cannon and focused ion beam (FIB-SEM), equipped with secondary and backscattered electron detectors. Optional: scanning transmission electron microscope (STEM) detector. Several models are commercially available.
2. Alignment and reconstruction software package. There are a number of commercial and free access packages with good performance available. Two commonly used packages:
   (a) IMOD (Free access) [24]: http:/bio3d.colorado.edu/imod/

      Please refer to tutorials available for download and sample examples for training. It is also helpful to subscribe to IMOD forum.

   (b) Amira (commercial): https://www.fei.com/software/amira-for-life-sciences/

      There is a trial available upon request from the website.

2.4.2 Sample Processing

1. Razor blades for trimming Epon block.
2. Diamond knife.
3. Ultramicrotome.
4. Ultrapure water.
5. SEM stub.
6. Conductive silver paint.

2.5 Electron Tomography

2.5.1 Equipment and Software

1. Transmission electron microscope with Field emission gun (FEG) electron source, operating at least at 200 kV, equipped with a tomography holder to obtain images in Y axis, angular range −70° to +70°.
2. 4 k × 4 k pixel CCD camera.
3. Software package IMOD [24]:
   (a) R-weighted back-projection: ETOMO command file.
   (b) Joining serial tomograms: JOIN command file.
   (c) Segmentation and 3D reconstruction: 3DMOD command file.

2.5.2 Sample Processing

1. Razor blades for trimming Epon block.
2. Diamond knife.
3. Ultramicrotome.

4. Ultrapure water for ultramicrotomy.
5. Formvar solution: Prepare the solution by measuring 0.5 g of formvar in 100 mL chloroform. Slowly stir solution overnight at room temperature, protected from light.
6. Copper or golden slot grids coated with Formvar film (see Methods for homemade protocol. There is a range of pre-coated grids available commercially).
7. Antistatic grid tweezers.
8. Filter paper.
9. Plastic paraffin film (Parafilm).
10. Lead citrate solution: boil 100 mL of ultrapure water, and chill it in ice before preparing solutions: (I) 15 mL of 133 mM lead (III) nitrate solution; (II) 15 mL of 223 mM sodium citrate; (III) 5 mL 1 M NaOH. Mix solution I and II in a 50 mL volumetric balloon or flask and add, dropwise, solution III until transparent (pH 12). Complete volume to 50 mL with boiled ice-chilled water and aliquot in small volumes (100 μL). The solution is stable when protected from contact with air, since lead precipitates in the presence of CO_2 (*see* **Note 3**).
11. Filtered ultrapure water (to wash grids).
12. Colloidal gold beads (10 nm)—Fiducial marker for tilt series alignment.

3 Methods

3.1 Freeze-Fracture (Fig. 9)

1. Fix in 2.5% glutaraldehyde diluted in 0.1 M sodium phosphate or sodium cacodylate buffer (pH 7.2), for 1 h at room temperature.
2. Wash the sample twice by centrifugation at 100 × *g* for 5 min in a clinical centrifuge with 0.1 M sodium cacodylate buffer.
3. Resuspend cells in a small volume of 0.1 M sodium cacodylate buffer or dip the sample in this buffer if it has a reduced size, such as pieces of tissue (*see* **Note 4**). The buffer volume depends on the sample quantity.
4. Infiltrate with glycerol, a cryoprotectant that prevents the formation of ice crystals, by dropping 30% glycerol diluted in this same buffer for 30 min at 5 min intervals.
5. Cryoprotect the samples in 30% glycerol for a minimum period of 3 h to a maximum of overnight (or ~18 h) (*see* **Note 5**).
6. Freeze samples, that are mounted on support disks, for 10–12 s in liquid Freon 22 (−150 °C) cooled by liquid nitrogen (−196 °C) and then to liquid nitrogen, where they can be stored until fractured (*see* **Note 6**).

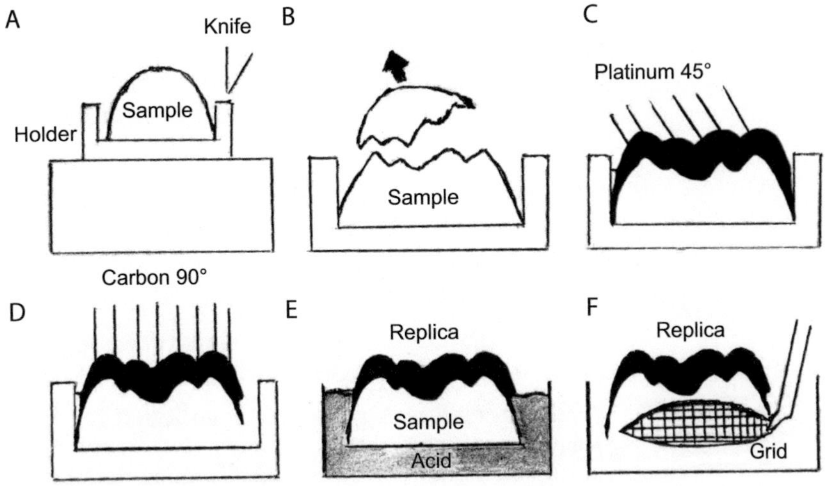

Fig. 9 Simplified scheme of the freeze-fracture process. A - Sample is placed in the freeze-fracture equipment, B - Sample fracture, C - Platin shade (Pt) at 45°, D - Carbon deposition at 90°, E - Replica cleaning for removal of organic the material that served as mold, F - Replica wash in water and gather in the grid. Scheme by Alexandre Gonçalves de Souza

7. Fracture samples at −115 °C in a Balzers apparatus with high vacuum (10^{-6}–10^{-7} Torr) using a steel blade similar to a razor (*see* **Note 7**).
8. Shadow the fracture surface by vaporizing platinum at 45° angle, in relation to the sample surface, and then applying carbon evaporation at a 90° angle to give resistance to the metal replica (*see* **Note 8**).
9. Clean the replica with sulfuric or chromic acid overnight. The next day, wash in distilled water (3×) and incubate for 3 h in 5% sodium hypochlorite solution (the commercial solution can be used). Then rinse again in distilled water (3×) (*see* **Note 9**).
10. Mount the replica on 200–300 mesh grids for observation in a transmission electron microscope (*see* **Note 10**).

3.2 Quick Freeze and Deep Etching

1. Rinse cells in distilled water and concentrate by centrifugation. Tissues should be cut as previously mentioned (*see* **Note 4**).
2. Place the pellet containing cells or the small pieces of tissues on a support disk, that has been designed for the Balzers freeze-etch apparatus, containing a 3 mm × 3 mm × 0–8 mm cushion of gelatine or rat lung (*see* **Note 11**).
3. Fix samples in 15% methanol diluted in distilled water or in 2.5% glutaraldehyde in 0.1 M cacodylate buffer (pH 7.2). This step can be omitted, but if applied, cells should be washed four times in distilled water after fixation (*see* **Note 12**).

4. Affix the support disk containing the specimen disks to the plunger of a Med-Vac rapid freezing device assembled for impact freezing against a copper block which is cooled by liquid helium to −270 °C or by liquid nitrogen to −196 °C (*see* **Note 13**).
5. Store samples in liquid nitrogen before freeze-fracturing at −115 °C in a vacuum of 2.10^{-6} Torr (*see* **Note 14**).
6. Etch the samples by raising the temperature to −100 °C for 5–10 min (*see* **Note 15**).
7. Evaporate platinum onto the specimen at an angle of 15° while it is rotating, then evaporate carbon at an angle of 90°.
8. Clean the replicas as previously mentioned for freeze-fracture procedures (*see* **Note 9**).
9. Mount the replica on 200–300 mesh grids for observation in a transmission electron microscope.
10. Acquire stereo pairs by tilting the sample through ±10° and then examine micrographs in negative contrast by photographically reversing them (*see* **Note 16**).

3.3 High-Pressure Freezing

Please wear hearing protectors, since during freezing sound level exceeds 85 decibels.

1. Centrifuge cells to concentrate in a loose pellet. Do not wash cells.
2. Run a first test using an appropriate holder that does not contain a sample and check if pressure and temperature curves are correct, reaching 2100 bar in 20 ms followed by a quick (30 ms) change in temperature to −196 °C. Pressure must be released in a maximum of 0.5 s.
3. Cut cellulose capillary tubes in pieces of approx 2 mm under the stereoscope.
4. Place a drop of concentrated cells on a petri dish covered with Parafilm.
5. On the side, fill a specimen carrier at the 2 mm side with 12 μL of 1-Hexadecene (*see* **Note 17**).
6. Holding one end of the capillary with a tweezers, touch the other side of the tube into the drop and watch it fill.
7. Transfer the capillary to the 1-hexadecene prefilled carrier. Fit up to 3 capillaries in one carrier and close it, like a sandwich, using the flat side of another carrier. Clean the 1-hexadecene excess, transfer the closed carrier to the adaptor, turn it clockwise to safely close it and attach to the equipment holder.

8. Lock the high-pressure freezing chamber and run a freezing cycle with the sample holder. Check if pressure and temperature behaved as expected (*see* **Note 18**).
9. Transfer the holder into the CryoCooler filled with LN_2 and transfer carrier into cryovials with the lid pierced to allow for samples to be immersed in LN_2. Transfer it as soon as possible to a stable LN_2 container or proceed to Freeze substitution immediately (Subheading 3.4).
10. Warm up the holder and adaptor until it is dry and mount a new sample to continue the process.

3.4 Freeze Substitution

3.4.1 Using a Commercial Freeze Substitution System

1. Transfer cryovial containing the substitution medium to the equipment metal support previously equilibrated to −90 °C. Wait until substitution medium becomes liquid (*see* **Note 19**).
2. Dip antistatic tweezers in LN_2 and transfer the specimen carrier containing frozen capillaries with cells into −90 °C precooled liquid substitution medium.
3. Set equipment for the following gradient:
   (a) Increase temperature stepwise (1 °C/2 h) and maintain at −80 °C for 72 h (*see* **Note 20**).
   (b) Increase temperature stepwise (5 °C/h) and maintain at −20 °C for 16 h (*see* **Note 21**).
   (c) Increase temperature stepwise (10 °C/h) and maintain at 4 °C for 3 h.
4. Remove samples from the equipment and wait until it equilibrates to room temperature (20–25 °C). Keep samples in a chemical fume hood for about an hour protected from light.
5. Carefully remove the substitution medium from cryovials avoiding capillaries that may have been detached from the specimen carriers. Both samples and solution must be dark as a result of OsO_4 reaction. Treat all waste as OsO_4 disposal as recommended above (Subheading 2.3.2).
6. Transfer capillaries (also the specimen carrier if sample is still attached) to a new 1.5 mL Safe Lock Microcentrifuge Tube containing 500 μL of acetone P.A.
7. Wash five times by changing acetone P.A. every 10 min. At this step all capillaries should be removed from specimen carries, and only samples are taken for embedding.
8. Prepare silicon molds by filling the tile wells by half with Epon and leave to polymerize for 72 h while embedding samples (*see* **Note 22**).
9. Start slowly embedding samples for substitution of acetone (solvent) by Epon (resin using the following schedule:
   – 10% Epon/90% acetone P.A. for 3 h at room temperature

- 25% Epon/75% acetone P.A. for 12 h at room temperature
- 50% Epon/50% acetone P.A. for 12 h at room temperature
- 75% Epon/25% % acetone P.A. for 12 h at room temperature
- 100% Epon for 12 h at room temperature
- 100% Epon for 3 h at room temperature.

10. Using the Epon supports place a capillary at 90° facing the block face and leave to polymerase for 72 h.

*3.4.2 Using a Homemade System (see **Note 23**)*

1. Use a metal support as a rack for cryovials. It is important to have a tight fit for the cryovials since direct contact with the cold metal will guarantee heat exchange. If possible, use an ultra-low temperature thermometer to monitor variations.
2. Leave the metal support at −80 °C in a freezer for at least 2 h to equilibrate the temperature.
3. Transfer cryovials containing substitution medium to a dry-ice bath to transport them to the cold metal support. Keep them in the −80 °C freezer for 1 h until the medium reaches the liquid phase.
4. Transfer the metal support to a dry-ice bath and transfer specimen carriers to cryovials with liquid substitution medium using antistatic tweezers prechilled in LN_2.
5. Transport the metal support back to the −80 °C freezer and leave it for 72 h.
6. Transport the metal support to a −20 °C freezer and leave it overnight (approx 18 h).
7. Transfer the metal support to a 4 °C (refrigerator) and leave it for 4 h.
8. Transfer the metal support to a chemical fume hood and wait until it reaches room temperature (20–25 °C).
9. Continue the sample processing as described above for the "Freeze substitution system" (from **step 5**).

3.5 Focused Ion Beam (Fig. 5)

1. Trim the face of the resin block to reach the cellulose capillary tube using a razor blade. Remove as much resin as possible from around the sample shaping it as a trapezoid form.
2. Proceed to routine ultramicrotomy and collect sections to evaluate the quality of the preservation and membrane staining of the sample.
3. Cut the top of the block containing the sample and glue it to a SEM stub using silver paint, with the sample facing to the microscope column.

4. Insert sample into the microscope and coat the surface of the sample with a layer of 3 nm of platinum using the coater system located in the main specimen chamber. If the equipment does not have a sputter device do it prior to inserting the sample into the chamber.
5. Tilt the specimen stage to 52° to place it parallel to the FIB.
6. Insert a first course cut using a high beam current (7–20 nA) and accelerating voltage 30 kV digging a 50–150 μm trench in order to expose the cross section of the sample.
7. Smooth the surface of the block using a current of 3–7 nA.
8. Adjust the slice step considering the resolution needed to resolve structures of interest, how many views from the sample will be acquired, and the total acquisition time. Start tests with 15 nm milling step size.
9. Adjust magnification (e.g., for a wide-field start with 15 K and 8.0 nm pixel size).
10. Record images using a backscattered electron detector, accelerating voltage of 1–5 kV and a beam current of 4000–8000 pA using the immersion lens mode.
11. Transfer images to a computer capable of processing images and invert the contrast of the images to resemble conventional TEM images.
12. Align slice-and-view series using the automatic tool of XfAlign command in IMOD.
13. Perform a second alignment using the MIDAS command in IMOD (*see* **Note 24**). Save final alignment as a 3D volume.
14. Draw structures to generate three-dimensional models using the 3dmod command in IMOD. For correct morphometrical analysis and modeling insert pixel size and milling step size for the series.

3.6 Electron Tomography (Fig. 6)

1. Trim the face of the resin block to reach the cellulose capillary tube using a razor blade. Remove as much resin as possible from around the sample making a trapezoid form (*see* **Note 25**).
2. Prepare slot grids coated with formvar (*see* **Note 26**).
3. Proceed to ultramicrotomy to collect ribbon of serial sections. Collect 200 nm sections and allow to dry on filter paper. Make sure the ribbon is centralized in the slog grid and carefully manipulate it to avoid ripping the formvar film.
4. Incubate grids in a drop of lead citrate for 5 min and wash by transferring the grid into three sequential drops of deionized water. Dry on filter paper.

5. Incubate grids in a drop colloidal gold for 20 min and dry on filter paper. Keep protected from dust until taking grids to the microscope.
6. Carefully transfer the grid to the microscope holder and insert it in the chamber.
7. Follow specific TEM software commands to set angle range and increment. For software packages with automated acquisition plugin it is possible to select a cell of interest in all sections (for serial tomography) and run a batch tomography command (*see* **Note 27**).
8. Set electron dose for acquisition to approx. 4.0×10^4 e/nm^2 and acquire the tilt series.
9. Flip grids manually to acquire tilt series on both sides for dual-axis electron tomography. Repeat **steps 7** and **8**. If acquiring single-axis tomography proceed to **step 9**.
10. Transfer tilt series to a computer capable of processing images and perform the back projection and alignment using the ETOMO command in IMOD.
11. Align tilt series by running the Beadtrack command to generate a fiducial model and the Tiltalign command for a fine alignment. Final alignment stack and tomogram will be generated using commands Newstack and Tilt. For full details on the process and a complete tutorial please access https://bio3d.colorado.edu/imod/doc/tomoguide.html.
12. Draw structures to generate three-dimensional models using the 3dmod command in IMOD (*see* **Note 28**).

4 Notes

1. Prepare a substitution media batch using OsO_4 crystals, uranyl acetate powder, and glutaraldehyde 70% stock to minimize water in solution, which would increase chances of crystallization of water. Cells must be totally dehydrated when reaching room temperature. The low percentage of water added to the solution helps with the infiltration of staining agents.
2. The combination of Araldite 502 and Embed812 allows for taking advantage of the thermal stability of araldite and best contrast for images from samples embedded in Epon.
3. To avoid lead citrate precipitation during incubations add a couple of NaOH pearls/pellets around lead citrate drops containing grids. Keep protected under a petri dish cover.
4. Tissues should be cut to approximately 2 mm in size to ensure better penetration of the cryoprotectant, which will be used in a next step, and also to obtain satisfactory results during the freezing process.

5. When freezing samples, it is always desirable to achieve a vitrified or crystal-free state, since ice crystals can cause cellular deformations, protein denaturation and loss of osmotic balance, culminating in the breakdown of cell membranes. Cryoprotectors interfere with the physical properties of water, reducing the chance of crystal formation. Glycerol has often been chosen in ultrastructural studies, but when used it is always necessary to fix the sample first in order to facilitate its penetration into the cells.
6. During the freezing process two cryogenic liquids are used: first the Freon, which is placed in a small container that is cooled by liquid nitrogen. Prior to sample immersion, a metal rod must be inserted into the receptacle containing Freon so that it passes from the frozen state to the liquid phase. Although Freon is at a higher temperature than LN_2, it remains liquid when in contact with the sample to be frozen, while the nitrogen forms a gaseous cloud, which impairs the quality of the freezing.
7. The freeze-fracture equipment should be properly cooled. The support containing the sample is placed in an area of the equipment called "table" where the temperature is held at −196 °C. When the high vacuum is reached, the sample is heated to −115 °C for fracture, which is done with a steel blade. This blade is attached to a rotating arm that advances toward the sample. The blade then scrubs the frozen surface of the sample, whose surface becomes smooth. This fracture procedure may be interrupted by the operator at any time considered appropriate.
8. Replicas are obtained by vaporizing heavy metals on the surface of the fractured material. They must be thin enough to allow the electron beams to pass through the transmission electron microscopy: the platinum film must have 2 nm and the carbon film must have 20 nm. This procedure generates a Pt/C replica with good contrast for observation.
9. The purpose of this step is to clean the replica digesting the biological material that served as a template. For this, the support containing the sample is inserted into a petri dish containing distilled water at an angle of 30°. Thus, the replica remains on the surface of the water and can be manipulated with the help of a platinum handle so that it can pass through the different cleaning solutions.
10. Images should be presented with the dark area of the particles, which was shaded by the platinum, positioned downward (Figs. 2 and 3).
11. The cushion is used to reduce the impact of the material during freezing, which will be described below.

12. As the freezing method used is extremely fast, there is no need to fix the samples or use cryoprotectors.
13. There are several commercially available quick-freeze equipment based on the model proposed by Heuser and colleagues [25]. The copper block on which the sample collides should not present any irregularities, must be extremely clean and should not contain condensed water on its surface. The ideal freezing depends on the perfect contact of the sample with the cooled metal.
14. During fracture, only one pass with the knife is made in the sample, so that the fracture plane will be within 10–20 μm of the surface of impact to the copper block. This detail is very important because in this quick-freeze procedure only the most superficial layer of the sample will present an ideal freezing without the formation of crystals.
15. The sublimation time of the sample may vary; the longer it is, the greater is the thickness of the fractured space; this can be cytosolic or within organelles.
16. When adopting this procedure, differently from images obtained by freeze fracture, the platinum deposits look white and the background look dark [25]. This contrast-reversal enhances the three-dimensional aspect of the images (Fig. 4).
17. The 1-Hexadecene is used to optimize the heat and pressure transfer to the sample, has a low surface tension and does not interfere with osmotic balance of the sample. 1-hexadecene is not a cryoprotectant, since it does not interfere with the physical properties of the water. It also removes the water and air from surroundings of the sample.
18. The sample is frozen in approximately 30 ms, although the temperature reaches −50 °C in 10 ms, and the pressure must normalize in less than 1 s (usually 500 ms) in order to avoid distortions or even destruction of the material.
19. The equipment must be adjusted to the lowest temperature at which fixative/dehydrating agents reach the liquid stage and the material is still frozen without crystals.
20. The slower the dehydration, the better will be the preservation of the material, with minimum chances of ice crystal nucleation.
21. During this step, the ideal temperatures for inclusion of fixative and staining agents are the following: −70 °C for uranyl acetate; between −40 °C and −30 °C for glutaraldehyde.
22. Having a resin support will make it easier to place the capillaries at 90°, facing the block face that will be trimmed and prepared for ultramicrotomy. Identification tags for the Epon bloc can also be added to this support, using paper and pencil or laser printed tags.

23. We found that this homemade protocol produces well preserved material, with excellent contrast that was reproduced several times. It is most important to carefully manipulate samples at appropriate temperature for each step, in order to avoid water crystallization, especially during the dehydration step (−80 °C).
24. The alignment is based on the sequential overlapping of image pairs, the top one being used as a reference for the next one. The software makes the images transparent in a way that aligned regions appear in gray, as a regular TEM image without distortions.
25. To produce serial section ribbons, the ideal is to carve a trapezium with a face wider and lower than normally used for ultramicrotomy routine, in order to fit more sections in the same grid.
26. To prepare formvar-coated grids, dip a clean glass slide into a burette filled with formvar solution to cover 2/3 of the slide area. Open the burette tap to slowly drain the liquid and wait for it to dry for 5 min. Scrape the limits of the slide using a scalpel, warm the slide with your breath and slowly sink it in a beaker filled with deionized water. Immersion must be performed positioning the slide at −15° angle in order to make the film float over the water mirror. The film must be gray or silver for perfect thickness. To recover the formvar film use a piece of paper or Parafilm to gently touch it and bring it out of the water. Let it dry protected from dust and lay clean grids on top of the film.
27. There is a limit for the range of tilts that can be collected, usually −70°/+70° in 200–300 kV microscopes, which is translated in loss of information when building the tomogram. This is known as missing edge. There are strategies to help with this limitation, as combining serial sectioning with tomography (serial tomography) and the dual axis tomography, which consist in acquiring tomograms for the same sample in both orthogonal axes. Those are time-consuming strategies, but will certainly increase the resolution of the final tomogram. Recent versions for software packages available, as IMOD, already include an option for dual-axis tomogram alignment and assembly of serial tomograms.
28. Electron tomography, as well as TEM, of freeze-substituted samples will appear with an inverted contrast compared to samples observed in room temperature processing. Figure 8 (a–b) provides examples of samples where membranes (lipids) appear electron-lucent and the cytoplasm (proteins) electron-dense.

References

1. Philippon H, Brochier-Armanet C, Perrière G (2015) Evolutionary history of phosphatidylinositol- 3-kinases: ancestral origin in eukaryotes and complex duplication patterns. BMC Evol Biol 15:226. https://doi.org/10.1186/s12862-015-0498-7
2. Harmer J, Yurchenko V, Nenarokova A et al (2018) Farming, slaving and enslavement: histories of endosymbioses during kinetoplastid evolution. Parasitology 145:1311–1323. https://doi.org/10.1017/S0031182018000781
3. Teixeira MMG, Borghesan TC, Ferreira RC et al (2011) Phylogenetic validation of the genera *Angomonas* and *Strigomonas* of trypanosomatids harboring bacterial endosymbionts with the description of new species of trypanosomatids and of proteobacterial symbionts. Protist 162:503–524. https://doi.org/10.1016/j.protis.2011.01.001
4. Votýpka J, Kostygov AY, Kraeva N et al (2014) *Kentomonas* gen. N., a new genus of endosymbiont-containing trypanosomatids of Strigomonadinae subfam. N. Protist 165:825–838. https://doi.org/10.1016/j.protis.2014.09.002
5. Motta MCM, Catta-Preta CMC, Schenkman S et al (2010) The bacterium endosymbiont of *Crithidia deanei* undergoes coordinated division with the host cell nucleus. PLoS One 5: e12415. https://doi.org/10.1371/journal.pone.0012415
6. Motta MCM, Martins AC de A, de Souza SS et al (2013) Predicting the proteins of *Angomonas deanei*, *Strigomonas culicis* and their respective endosymbionts reveals new aspects of the trypanosomatidae family. PLoS One 8: e60209. https://doi.org/10.1371/journal.pone.0060209
7. Brum FL, Catta-Preta CMC, de Souza W et al (2014) Structural characterization of the cell division cycle in *Strigomonas culicis*, an endosymbiont-bearing trypanosomatid. Microsc Microanal 20:228–237. https://doi.org/10.1017/S1431927613013925
8. Catta-Preta CMC, Brum FL, da Silva CC et al (2015) Endosymbiosis in trypanosomatid protozoa: the bacterium division is controlled during the host cell cycle. Front Microbiol 6:520. https://doi.org/10.3389/fmicb.2015.00520
9. Azevedo-Martins AC, Machado ACL, Klein CC et al (2015) Mitochondrial respiration and genomic analysis provide insight into the influence of the symbiotic bacterium on host trypanosomatid oxygen consumption. Parasitology 142:352–362. https://doi.org/10.1017/S0031182014001139
10. Loyola-Machado AC, Azevedo-Martins AC, Catta-Preta CMC et al (2017) The symbiotic bacterium fuels the energy metabolism of the host trypanosomatid *Strigomonas culicis*. Protist 168:253–269. https://doi.org/10.1016/j.protis.2017.02.001
11. Bozzola JJ, Russell LD (1999) Electron microscopy: principles and techniques for biologists, illustrated. Jones & Bartlett Learning, Burlington
12. de Souza W, de Carvalho TU, Benchimol M, Chiari E (1978) *Trypanosoma cruzi*: ultrastructural, cytochemical and freeze-fracture studies of protein uptake. Exp Parasitol 45:101–115
13. Souto-Padrón T, de Souza W, Heuser JE (1984) Quick-freeze, deep-etch rotary replication of *Trypanosoma cruzi* and *Herpetomonas megaseliae*. J Cell Sci 69:167–178
14. Benchimol M, Kachar B, de Souza W (1993) The structural organization of the pathogenic protozoan *Tritrichomonas foetus* as seen in replicas of quick frozen, freeze-fractured and deep etched cells. Biol Cell 77:289–295
15. Benchimol M (2004) Mitosis in *Giardia lamblia*: multiple modes of cytokinesis. Protist 155:33–44. https://doi.org/10.1078/1434461000162
16. Cavalcanti DP, Thiry M, de Souza W, Motta MCM (2008) The kinetoplast ultrastructural organization of endosymbiont-bearing trypanosomatids as revealed by deep-etching, cytochemical and immunocytochemical analysis. Histochem Cell Biol 130:1177–1185. https://doi.org/10.1007/s00418-008-0450-7
17. Moor H (1987) Theory and practice of high pressure freezing. In: Steinbrecht RA, Zierold K (eds) Cryotechniques in biological electron microscopy. Springer Berlin Heidelberg, Berlin, Heidelberg, pp 175–191
18. de Souza W, Attias M (2018) New advances in scanning microscopy and its application to study parasitic protozoa. Exp Parasitol 190:10–33. https://doi.org/10.1016/j.exppara.2018.04.018
19. Lacomble S, Vaughan S, Gadelha C et al (2009) Three-dimensional cellular architecture of the flagellar pocket and associated cytoskeleton in trypanosomes revealed by electron microscope tomography. J Cell Sci 122:1081–1090. https://doi.org/10.1242/jcs.045740
20. Gluenz E, Povelones ML, Englund PT, Gull K (2011) The kinetoplast duplication cycle in

Trypanosoma brucei is orchestrated by cytoskeleton-mediated cell morphogenesis. Mol Cell Biol 31:1012–1021. https://doi.org/10.1128/MCB.01176-10

21. Girard-Dias W, Alcântara CL, Cunha-e-Silva N et al (2012) On the ultrastructural organization of *Trypanosoma cruzi* using cryopreparation methods and electron tomography. Histochem Cell Biol 138:821–831. https://doi.org/10.1007/s00418-012-1002-8
22. Alcantara CL, Vidal JC, de Souza W, Cunha-e-Silva NL (2014) The three-dimensional structure of the cytostome-cytopharynx complex of *Trypanosoma cruzi* epimastigotes. J Cell Sci 127:2227–2237. https://doi.org/10.1242/jcs.135491
23. Alcantara C de L, de Souza W, da Cunha E Silva NL (2018) Tridimensional electron microscopy analysis of the early endosomes and endocytic traffic in trypanosoma cruzi epimastigotes. Protist 169:887–910. https://doi.org/10.1016/j.protis.2018.09.004
24. Kremer JR, Mastronarde DN, McIntosh JR (1996) Computer visualization of three-dimensional image data using IMOD. J Struct Biol 116:71–76. https://doi.org/10.1006/jsbi.1996.0013
25. Heuser JE, Reese TS, Dennis MJ et al (1979) Synaptic vesicle exocytosis captured by quick freezing and correlated with quantal transmitter release. J Cell Biol 81:275–300. https://doi.org/10.1083/jcb.81.2.275

Chapter 27

Airyscan Superresolution Microscopy to Study Trypanosomatid Cell Biology

Jane Harmer, Asma Belbelazi, Martin Carr, and Michael L. Ginger

Abstract

The recent introduction by Carl Zeiss Ltd. of the Airyscan detector module for their LSM880 confocal laser-scanning microscope has enabled routine superresolution microscopy to be combined with the advantages of confocal-based fluorescence imaging. Resulting enhanced spatial resolution in X, Y, and Z provides tractable opportunity to derive new insight into protein localization(s), organelle dynamics, and thence protein function within trypanosomatids or other organisms. Here, we describe methods for preparing slides, cells, and basic microscope setup for fluorescence imaging of trypanosomatids using the LSM-880 with Airyscan platform.

Key words Confocal, *Crithidia*, Live-cell imaging, Immunofluorescence, *Leishmania*, *Novymonas*, Superresolution microscopy, *Trypanosoma*, Trypanosomatids

1 Introduction

Often, one of the first steps in determining the function of a protein is to ascertain its localization within a cell. To this end, cell biologists are increasingly using highly sensitive and noninvasive superresolution microscopy approaches. Superresolution microscopy (SRM) encompasses a group of techniques that enable fluorescence-based imaging of biological samples well beyond the diffraction-limited resolution (~200–300 nm in the lateral direction and 500–700 nm in the axial direction) of more conventional wide-field or confocal light microscopy approaches [1]. This diffraction limit means standard wide field epifluorescence microscopy, while preferable in terms of image acquisition speed and low phototoxicity, is limited in terms of resolution. With the resolution available, only tissue morphology and whole-cell dynamics are reliably imaged although application of deconvolution algorithms after image acquisition enhances contrast and helps limit inherent image blur. Conversely the majority of SRM techniques enable imaging of many subcellular structures down to, in some instances,

Paul A. M. Michels et al. (eds.), *Trypanosomatids: Methods and Protocols*, Methods in Molecular Biology, vol. 2116,
https://doi.org/10.1007/978-1-0716-0294-2_27,

only a few tens of nanometers apart. However, no SRM technique is ideal. For example, at the higher levels of affordable lateral resolution (~20 nm) photoactivated-localization microscopy (PALM) [2, 3] and stochastic optical reconstruction microscopy (STORM) [4] require long acquisition times (thereby inducing phototoxicity incompatible, in most instances, with live-cell imaging) and complex postacquisition processing; STORM and stimulated emission depletion (STED) microscopy (where lateral resolution can be <20 nm with 40–50 nm axial resolution) require the use of fluorophores with specialized photochemical properties [5, 6] and structured illumination microscopy (SIM) [7, 8] and STED require expensive microscope systems, an unrealistic expectation in many research laboratories where SRM may form only a part of routine experimental work.

Recently emergent superresolution microscopes have been applied in studies of trypanosomatid biology. For instance, the demonstration (by SIM) of membrane contact sites between acidocalcisomes and mitochondria in evolutionarily divergent trypanosomatids [9]; mitochondrial fission and fusion dynamics and positional insight into the structural hierarchy of a highly unusual trypanosome mitochondrial genome–basal body attachment structure (both by STED microscopy) [10, 11]; spatial positioning of neighboring, potentially interacting basal body proteins (by SIM) [12]; and dynamic trypanosomatid membrane organization [13, 14].

Confocal laser scanning microscopy (CLSM) offers several advantages compared to wide-field approaches, and is readily applicable to trypanosome microscopy e.g., [15]. Advantages of CLSM include marginal improvements in lateral and axial resolution and up to a factor of $\sqrt{2}$ spatial resolution improvement by excluding "out-of-focus" light or glare at the pinhole aperture placed directly in front of the photomultiplier. Yet further enhancing spatial resolution beyond the diffraction limit using an infinitely small pinhole is not possible; however, the recently introduced Airyscan detector enables SRM imaging using a standard confocal microscope platform [9]. Thus SRM that combines the advantages of a CLSM (controllable depth-of-field, capability to image serial optical sections from thick samples (>2 μm)) with enhanced spatial resolution, comparable with that of SIM, is now routinely available to numerous research laboratories.

The Airyscan detector is a specialized module attached to the out-coupling port of the Zeiss LSM880 CLSM. Consisting of a photomultiplier (PMT) array with 32 sensitive GaAsP (Gallium Arsenide Phosphide) detector elements, it works to increase spatial resolution by improving image signal-to-noise ratios (SNR). On a standard confocal microscope, possessing only a single detector

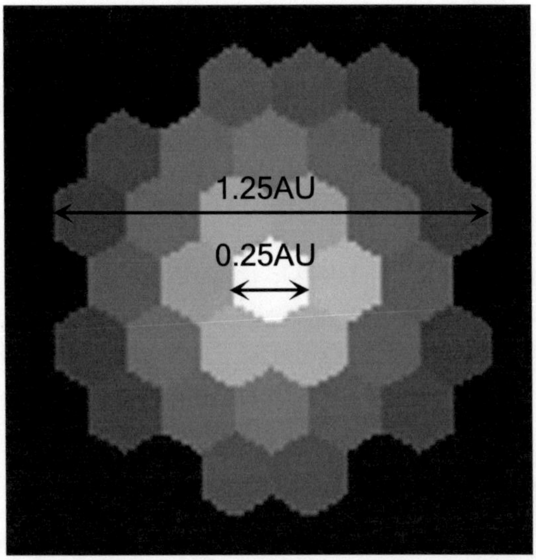

Fig. 1 The Airyscan detector. The Airyscan detector consists of an array of 32 sensitive GaAsP detector elements. By setting each individual sub-Airy pinhole to <1 AU (0.25 AU in this figure) it ensures spatial resolution is improved by a factor of 1.7 in all directions while not compromising SNR

element, decreasing the pinhole aperture to significantly <1 Airy-Unit (AU, where 1 AU corresponds to the theoretical optimal pinhole diameter where investigators collect the physical equivalent of in-focus light and reject the remaining scattered light) is not possible as resulting images tend toward critically low SNRs. Increasing illumination power increases SNR, but problems of photobleaching and phototoxicity in live-cell imaging arise. As 1–4 AU can be imaged across the diameter of the Airyscan detector array (at its greatest width the detector array is six individual elements across, Fig. 1), it is possible to set each individual sub-Airy pinhole to significantly <1 AU, while at the same time rejecting no light at the pinhole aperture. Significantly more photons are collected, thereby not compromising SNR and improving spatial resolution by up to a factor of 1.7 in all directions [16]. Summarizing, CLSM coupled to superresolution level detection has emerged as a versatile, contemporary approach for fast and gentle cell-imaging beyond the regular diffraction limit of light microscopy. Here we outline methods for the preparation of fixed trypanosomatid cells, cytoskeletons, isolated flagella and live cells for microscopy. We also outline key points for consideration and a basic setup of the Zeiss LSM880 CLSM with Airyscan for superresolution microscopy imaging.

2 Materials

Microscope slides should be high-quality plain glass or precoated with poly-L-lysine. Selected coverslips should be of the optimal thickness for the microscope objective that will be used for imaging (*see* **Note 1**).

2.1 Preparation of Poly-L-Lysine–Coated Glass Slides

1. Slide cleaning solution: 1% HCl, 70% ethanol.
2. Working poly-L-lysine Solution: 0.1% (w/v) poly-L-lysine diluted 1:10 with ultrapure water. Working solution can be stored at 4–8 °C and reused several times. It is advised to filter (0.2 μm) the solution after each use.

2.2 Preparation of Cells for Live-Cell Microscopy

1. CyGEL™ (BioStatus).
2. 1× Phosphate Buffered Saline (PBS): 137 mM NaCl, 3 mM KCl, 1 mM Na_2HPO_4, 1.5 mM KH_2PO_4, pH 7.2–7.4. Can be stored for up to 3 days at 4–8 °C.

2.3 Preparation of Fixed Cells for Microscopy

1. 1× Phosphate Buffered Saline (PBS): as in Subheading 2.2, **item 2**.
2. Paraformaldehyde stock solution (5× strength): weigh 1.8 g paraformaldehyde in approximately 6 ml 1× PBS. Add 400 μl of 1 M NaOH and heat to 65 °C until dissolved. Make up to 10 ml with 1× PBS; store 0.5 ml aliquots at −20 °C.
3. 3.7% (w/v) Paraformaldehyde in PBS: defrost a 0.5 ml 5× paraformaldehyde stock solution aliquot and add to 2 ml 1× PBS solution.
4. Methanol, cooled at −20 °C prior to use.

2.4 Preparation of Cell Cytoskeletons for Microscopy

1. 1× Phosphate Buffered Saline (PBS): as in Subheading 2.2, **item 2**.
2. PEME buffer: 100 mM PIPES, 2 mM EGTA, 0.1 mM EDTA, 1 mM $MgSO_4$, pH 6.9. Filter (0.2 μm) and store at room temperature.
3. Paraformaldehyde stock solution (5× strength): as in Subheading 2.3, **item 2**.
4. 3.7% (w/v) Paraformaldehyde in PBS: as in Subheading 2.3, **item 3**.

2.5 Preparation of Isolated Flagella for Microscopy

1. 1× Phosphate Buffered Saline (PBS): as in Subheading 2.2, **item 2**.
2. PEME buffer: as in Subheading 2.4, **item 2**.
3. Paraformaldehyde stock solution (5× strength): as in Subheading 2.3, **item 2**.

4. 3.7% (w/v) Paraformaldehyde in PBS: as in Subheading 2.3, **item 3**.

2.6 Staining Cells with MitoTracker® Deep Red

1. MitoTracker® Deep Red stock solution: dissolve lyophilized MitoTracker® Deep Red in 100% DMSO to a final concentration of 1 mM. Store at −20 °C and protect from light.

2.7 Immunofluorescence

1. 1× Phosphate Buffered Saline (PBS): as in Subheading 2.2 **item 2**.
2. Blocking Solution: 1% bovine serum albumin (BSA) in 1× PBS containing 0.05% (v/v) Tween 20.
3. Washing Solution: 1× PBS containing 0.05% (v/v) Tween 20.

2.8 Mounting of Fixed Cell Preparation Prior to Microscopy

1. VECTASHIELD® (Vector Laboratories), hard-set or liquid form.
2. Nail varnish, if using liquid form VECTASHIELD®.

3 Methods

3.1 Preparation of Poly-L-Lysine–Coated Glass Slides

Poly-L-lysine is a positively charged amino acid polymer that aids often cell adhesion to glass microscope slides (*see* **Note 1**).

1. Clean glass slides with slide cleaning solution.
2. Ensure working stock of poly-L-lysine is at room temperature, place slides into a clean rack and immerse in working poly-L-lysine solution for 5 min.
3. Drain slides and place in a 60 °C oven for 1 h or overnight at 37 °C to dry.

3.2 Preparation of Cells for Live-Cell Microscopy

CyGel™ (BioStatus) is a thermoreversible mountant used to immobilize nonadherent cells. Below 20/21 °C CyGEL™ is a liquid, forming a gel when warmed. CyGEL™ is entirely compatible with fluorescence light microscopy (RI ~1.37, no visible autofluorescence, nonquenching).

1. Thoroughly precool P1000 and P200 pipette tips at 4 °C and place Eppendorf tubes and a vial of CyGEL™ on ice.
2. Aliquot 1.0–1.5 ml (dependent upon density, ~10^5 cells are required) of cells into uncooled Eppendorf tubes and harvest by centrifugation at 3500 × *g* for 3 min at room temperature.
3. Remove supernatant and resuspend cell pellet in 1× PBS.
4. Recentrifuge at 3500 × *g* for 3 min at room temperature and resuspend cell pellet in a 10 μl 1× PBS (*see* **Note 2**).
5. Transfer resuspended cells into precooled Eppendorf tubes (*see* **step 1**) and place on ice for 2 min.

6. Add 2.56 μl of supplied 40× PBS to the precooled vial of CyGEL™ (2.5% v/v).
7. Pipet the cell suspension into the PBS-primed CyGEL™.
8. Using precooled pipette tips immediately transfer CyGEL™/cell suspension and streak along one side of the microscope slide and immediately apply coverslip.
9. Carefully place the microscope slide onto an ice pack or onto a strip of foil placed in a level bucket of ice. The CyGEL™/cell suspension should spread out across the slide, under the coverslip.
10. Remove slide from ice pack or ice bucket and allow to warm to room temperature, the CyGEL™ should set and form a gel. Visualize cells immediately (*see* **Note 3**).

3.3 Preparation of Fixed Cells for Microscopy

1. Aliquot 1.0–1.5 ml (dependent upon density, ~5×10^5 cells are required) of cells and harvest by centrifugation at 3500 × *g* for 3 min at room temperature.
2. Remove the supernatant and resuspend cell pellet in 1× PBS.
3. Recentrifuge at 3500 × *g* for 3 min at room temperature and repeat the wash with 1× PBS.
4. Remove supernatant and resuspend cell pellet in 1 ml 1× PBS.
5. Draw a well (~2 cm × 2 cm) on microscope slide with hydrophobic barrier pen and leave to dry completely (approximately 5 min).
6. Fill well completely with cells and incubate at room temperature for 5–10 min.
7. Every 2–3 min check cell density using a compound microscope. Incubate until required number of cells per field of view is immobilized on the slide surface, ensuring the slide does not dry out at any point. If required, then add a further drop of 1× PBS to the hydrophobic well.
8. To fix cells, tap excess liquid from the slide and immediately fill well with 3.7% (w/v) paraformaldehyde in 1× PBS.
9. Allow cells to fix at room temperature for 5 min.
10. Remove excess liquid and place slide immediately into an ice-cold methanol-filled Coplin jar. Incubate at −20 °C for 10 min. Where samples are not going to be analyzed for expression or localization of fluorescent proteins (e.g., eGFP-, YFP-based fusion proteins), slides can also be stored for several months immersed in methanol at −20 °C. It is also possible to fix cells directly in −20 °C methanol for 40 min, although we prefer fixation with paraformaldehyde as our default approach.

11. Prior to mounting a slide, rehydrate cells by placing the slide in a Coplin jar of 1× PBS for 10 min.
12. Proceed to Subheading 3.8 if mounting slides directly for microscopy or Subheading 3.7 for immunofluorescence.

3.4 Preparation of Cell Cytoskeletons for Microscopy

1. Follow **steps 1–7** of Subheading 3.3.
2. Tap excess liquid off the slide and immediately fill well with PEME containing 1% (v/v) NP40 and incubate for 30 s.
3. Tap excess liquid off the slide and immediately fill well with 3.7% paraformaldehyde in 1× PBS.
4. Continue and follow **steps 9–11** of Subheading 3.3.

3.5 Preparation of Isolated Flagella for Microscopy

1. Follow **steps 1–7** of Subheading 3.3.
2. Tap excess liquid off the slide and immediately fill well with PEME containing 1% (v/v) NP40; incubate for 30 s.
3. Tap excess liquid off the slide and immediately fill well with PEME to which NaCl is added at a final concentration of 1 M alongside protease inhibitors (we use cOmplete Mini Protease Inhibitor Cocktail (Roche) and PMSF (10 mM)); incubate slide for 15 min on ice. To ensure slides stay dry and flat, place them on top of a strip of foil on ice.
4. Tap excess liquid off the slide and fill well with 1× PBS.
5. Immediately tap excess 1× PBS liquid off the slide and refill well with PEME containing 1 M NaCl; incubate on ice for a further 15 min.
6. Repeat 1× PBS wash, as in **step 4**.
7. Tap excess liquid off the slide and immediately fill well with 3.7% paraformaldehyde in 1× PBS.
8. Continue and follow **steps 9–11** of Subheading 3.3.

3.6 Staining Cells with MitoTracker® Deep Red

Various dyes and other commercially available reagents are commonly used to detect organelles and subcellular or fixed/or fixed cells. Images shown here illustrate the branched mitochondrion in *Novymonas esmeraldas* and *Leishmania tarentolae* (Fig. 2). *N. esmeraldas* is a nonpathogenic trypanosomatid isolated from the scentless plant bug *Niesthrea vincentii*. It is closely related to *Leishmania* but it is an unusual trypanosomatid in that it harbors a bacterial endosymbiont. That endosymbiont is closely related to the genus *Pandoraea* [17].

1. Establish culture (10 ml) of healthy, mid-log phase trypanosomatid cells (~2×10^6 cells ml^{-1}).
2. Add MitoTracker® Deep Red to a final concentration of 250 nM and incubate for at least 30 min.

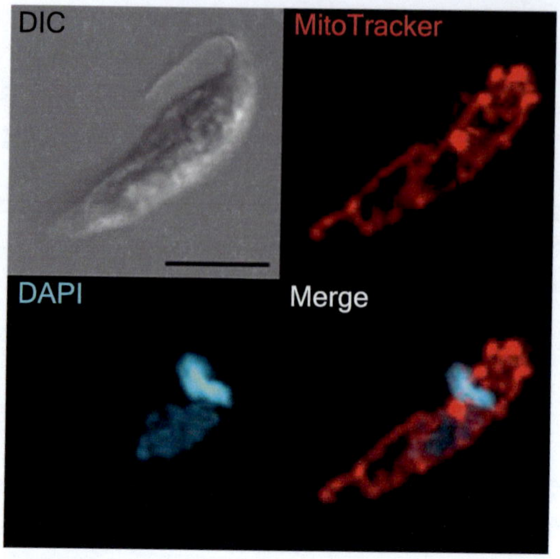

Fig. 2 Superresolution Airyscan image of a *Novymonas esmeraldas* cell. Cells were incubated with MitoTracker™ Deep Red FM and mounted with VECTASHIELD® containing 4′,6-diamidino-2-phenylindole (DAPI). Scale bar indicates 10 μm

3. Proceed to Subheading 3.2 if preparing cells for live-cell microscopy or Subheading 3.3 if fixing cells for microscopy.

3.7 Immunofluorescence

1. *See* Subheadings 3.3–3.5 for preparation of fixed cells, detergent-extracted cytoskeletons or flagella settled onto microscope slides. Slides should be immersed in ice-cold (−20 °C) methanol after fixation with paraformaldehyde for 10 min or can be stored (if there is no intention to visualize fluorescent proteins such as eGFP or YFP), immersed in methanol, at −20 °C for several months.
2. Rehydrate cells by removing slide from methanol and placing in a Coplin jar containing 1× PBS (if using uncoated glass slides) or 0.1% (w/v) glycine/1× PBS (if using poly-L-lysine–coated slides) for 10 min.
3. Place slides into a hydration chamber one at a time (ensure slides do not completely dry out) and fill well with blocking solution (*see* **Note 4**). Hydration chambers are simply vessels that can be kept loosely or tightly sealed, but where the interior environment is kept moist by the presence of water-soaked blue-roll either placed flat on the base of the chamber or rolled and placed along the sides of the chamber. The chamber interior is also protected from light.
4. Incubate for 1 h at room temperature.

5. Tap excess liquid off the slide and immediately fill well with primary antibody, diluted at the required concentration in an appropriate blocking solution.
6. Incubate in the hydration chamber for a further 1 h at room temperature.
7. Tap excess liquid off the slide and place in a Coplin jar filled with washing solution; incubate for 5 min.
8. Repeat **step** 7 twice.
9. Remove slide from Coplin jar, place into hydration chamber and fill well with secondary antibody, diluted to the correct concentration in blocking solution; incubate for 40–60 min.
10. Repeat wash **steps 7–8** and proceed to Subheading 3.8.

3.8 Mounting of Fixed Cell Preparation Prior to Microscopy

VECTASHIELD® (Vector Laboratories) is the antifade mounting medium that reduces photobleaching, which we use in our work (*see* **Note 5**).

1. Tap off excess liquid and dispense a single drop of VECTASHIELD® into the sample well.
2. Apply coverslip (ensure coverslip is correct thickness for microscope objective; we use standard No. 1.5 coverslips, with a thickness of 0.17 mm).
3. Securely pinch the top of the coverslip and slide together and, using a tissue, squeeze firmly to remove excess liquid.
4. If using hard-set VECTASHIELD®, then leave to set completely before visualizing.
5. If using liquid VECTASHIELD®, then seal coverslip completely by applying nail varnish around all edges. Leave to dry completely before visualizing.
6. Following mounting, slides can be stored in the dark at 4 °C for several weeks although we recommend viewing slides periodically to ensure fluorescence/immunofluorescence signals have not faded.

3.9 Configuring the Zeiss LSM880 with Airyscan for Superresolution Imaging

Notes 6–10 outline some general recommendations for imaging using the Airyscan detector.

1. Calibration of the Airyscan detector should be performed with a sample that has a good fluorescence signal and is uniform in staining intensity. As there is only one gain setting for all channels imaged on each track, this step should only be performed with one channel, that which has the best fluorescence signal. To limit any negative photobleaching or phototoxicity effects during detector calibration steps, select a frame size of "Optimal" or drop down to 512 × 512 pixels (depending on which is lower).

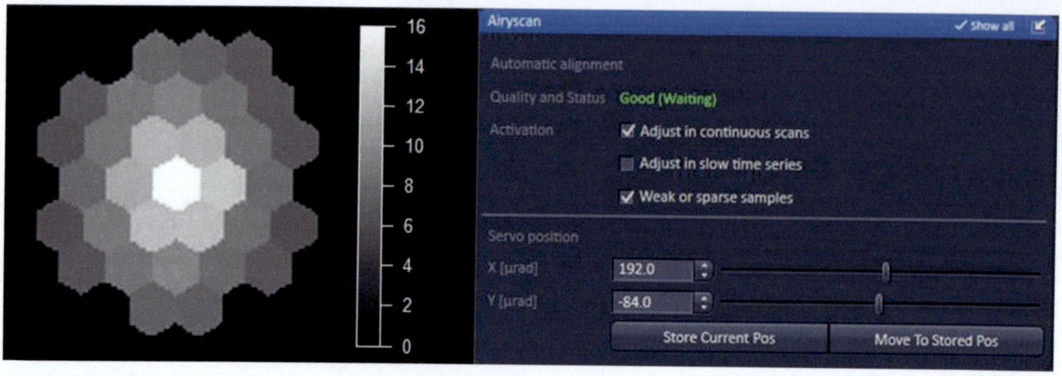

Fig. 3 Zen imaging software screenshot showing the Airyscan detector graphic and "maintain" tab indicating the quality and status of the detector alignment. The central detector on the Airyscan detector graphic should be the brightest when calibration is complete and the quality and status of the detector alignment should read "Good"

2. Select Airyscan "SR" mode.
3. Ensure zoom level is greater than 1.8.
4. Select "Continuous," focus sample and view scanning image with the "Range Indicator" tab selected—this enables visualization of oversaturated pixels and those representing a value of 0. Adjust "Laser power," "Master Gain," and "Digital Offset" to optimize images, ensuring there are no oversaturated (red) pixels.
5. Select the "Airyscan" tab. The central detector on the Airyscan Detector Graphic should be the brightest when calibration is complete (Fig. 3).
6. Select the "Maintain" tab (pull into main imaging window) check that the "Quality and Status" output is green and reads "Good." If, however, the output shows red and reads "Bad" then either try selecting another area of your sample or switch channels and retry calibration steps (Fig. 3).
7. Repeat the above calibration steps for all tracks you wish to image.
8. Once calibration is complete, reselect all tracks and select a frame size of "Optimal" to ensure Nyquist sampling in XY.
9. Common parameters for "Acquisition mode" window: Frame size: Optimal; Speed: Max; Bit Depth: 16; Zoom Factor: >1.8.
10. Common parameters for "Channels" window: Laser Power: <5%; Gain: 700–900; Digital Gain: 1; Pinhole: determined by Airyscan mode selected.
11. Click "Snap" to capture the image and ensure all raw unprocessed images are saved.

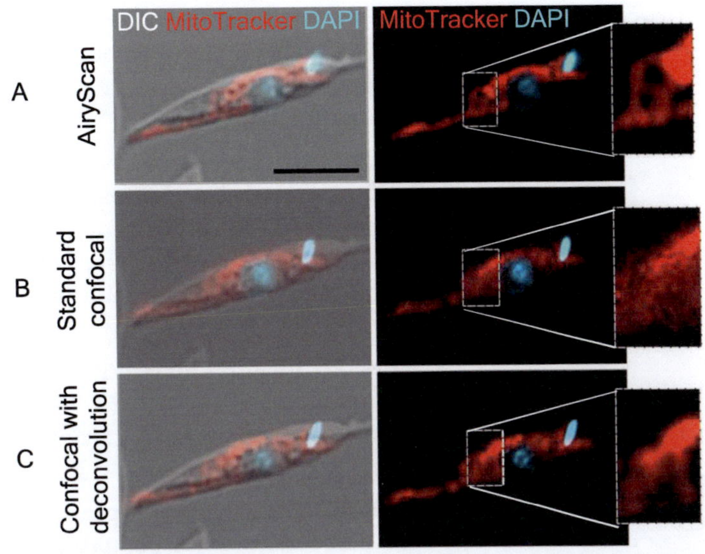

Fig. 4 Superresolution Airyscan image of a *Leishmania tarentolae* cell alongside a standard confocal image and a confocal image post-processed by deconvolution. Cells were incubated with MitoTracker™ Deep Red FM and mounted with VECTASHIELD® containing DAPI. (**a**) Airyscan superresolution image of a single *L. tarentolae* cell. (**b**) The same *L. tarentolae* cell imaged using standard confocal settings. (**c**) Panel B image postprocessed using default deconvolution settings. Scale bar indicates 10 μm

Airyscan imaging involves an element of deconvolution whereby data for all 32 individual detectors is processed to produce the final image.

12. Select the "Processing" tab.
13. Select "Airyscan Processing" under the "Method" tab and ensure selected image is the one you wish to process. Initially select the "Auto" tick-box and 2D or 3D depending upon whether a Z-stack is being processed.

Care must be taken, as with any deconvolution, that artifacts are not introduced into your image. If concerned, one could deselect the "Auto" tick-box, decrease the deconvolution strength to zero, and rerun the processing. By comparing the deconvolved (to different strengths) images side-by-side absence of artifact introduction can be ruled out (Fig. 4).

4 Notes

1. Procyclic *Trypanosoma brucei* cells will adhere to plain glass slides; insect-stage forms of other trypanosomatid species will adhere to poly-L-lysine–coated slides. Alternatively, if using

plain glass slides for other trypanosomatids, concentrate cells and drop the minimum amount of cell suspension into the slide well and leave cells to settle and adhere, ensuring the slide does not completely dry out.

2. In our hands we have found that the volumes of CyGEL™ recommended by the manufacturer exceed that which is required for a single slide. We typically use only 100 μl CyGEL™ per slide (as opposed to 500 μl) and scale the volume of priming 40× PBS and cells resuspended in 1× PBS accordingly.
3. Prior to imaging it is advisable to set the microscope-top incubation chamber to >22 °C as if the ambient room temperature is less than 21 °C CyGEL™ will transition back to a liquid.
4. If fluorescence staining appears weak or background high, then the percentage of BSA could be optimized or another protein solution (e.g., nonfat dried milk, gelatine) tested. Typical concentrations of the blocking protein are between 1 and 5%.
5. VECTASHIELD® antifade mounting medium is supplied in a liquid or hard-set form and with the option of 4′,6-diamidino-2-phentylindole (DAPI), propidium iodide (PI), or phalloidin counterstains for visualization of DNA.
6. When using a high-powered oil-immersion objection always use the correct immersion oil (Immersol 518 F ($n = 1.518$, 23 °C; Carl Zeiss). This reduces light refraction and retains the high numerical aperture value of the objective.
7. The Piezo-Z stage is recommended for superresolution imaging using the Airyscan detector.
8. For comparison purposes, it can be useful to capture a standard confocal image alongside one collected using the Airyscan detector.
9. As Airyscan imaging involves an element of deconvolution, it is crucially important to include all relevant control samples to ensure artifacts have not been introduced into your image (Fig. 4).
10. Airyscan has four different imaging options: (1) CO or "standard confocal mode," here the detector array functions as a standard GaAsP detector and resolution is governed by the size of the pinhole aperture; (2) VP or "virtual pinhole mode," here 4 AU are imaged on the detector array. Postacquisition there is the choice of which detector elements to use or bin. VP is the suggested mode to use if there is uncertainty as to whether the sample requires a boost in terms of resolution or sensitivity; (3) we use SR or "Superresolution" mode when ideal imaging conditions enable enhancement of resolution in all directions

by a factor of 1.7. The SR mode is suggested for imaging subcellular structures within 200 nm of one another; (4) R-S or "Resolution versus Sensitivity "mode is suggested for samples with critically low SNR—here, resolution is sacrificed for a boost in sensitivity.

Acknowledgments

AB is funded by a University of Huddersfield, School of Applied Sciences PhD studentship. The LSM880 confocal microscope with Airyscan used in this work is part of the Huddersfield Innovation and Incubation Project (HIIP) funded through the Leeds City Region Enterprise Partnership (LEP) Growth Deal.

References

1. Sigal YM, Zhou R, Zhuang X (2018) Visualizing and discovering cellular structures with super-resolution microscopy. Science 361 (6405):880–887
2. Hess ST, Girirajan TP, Mason MD (2006) Ultra-high resolution imaging by fluorescence photoactivation localization microscopy. Biophys J 91(11):4258–4272
3. Betzig E, Patterson GH, Sougrat R et al (2006) Imaging intracellular fluorescent proteins at nanometer resolution. Science 313 (5793):1642–1645
4. Rust MJ, Bates M, Zhuang X (2006) Sub-diffraction-limit imaging by stochastic optical reconstruction microscopy (STORM). Nat Methods 3(10):793–795
5. Hell SW, Wichmann J (1994) Breaking the diffraction resolution limit by stimulated emission: stimulated-emission-depletion fluorescence microscopy. Opt Lett 19(11):780–782
6. Schrader M, Meinecke F, Bahlmann K et al (1995) Monitoring the excited state of a fluorophore in a microscope by stimulated emission. Bioimaging 3(4):147–153
7. Bailey B, Farkas DL, Taylor DL et al (1993) Enhancement of axial resolution in fluorescence microscopy by standing-wave excitation. Nature 366(6450):44–48
8. Gustafsson MG (2000) Surpassing the lateral resolution limit by a factor of two using structured illumination microscopy. J Microsc 198(Pt 2):82–87
9. Ramakrishnan S, Asady B, Docampo R (2018) Acidocalcisome-mitochondrion membrane contact sites in Trypanosoma brucei. Pathogens 7(2):33–44
10. Jakob M, Hoffmann A, Amodeo S et al (2016) Mitochondrial growth during the cell cycle of Trypanosoma brucei bloodstream forms. Sci Rep 6:36565–36578
11. Hoffmann A, Kaser S, Jakob M et al (2018) Molecular model of the mitochondrial genome segregation machinery in Trypanosoma brucei. Proc Natl Acad Sci U S A 115(8): E1809–E1818
12. Dang HQ, Zhou Q, Rowlett VW et al (2017) Proximity interactions among basal body components in Trypanosoma brucei identify novel regulators of basal body biogenesis and inheritance. MBio 8(1):e02120–e02116
13. Wiedeman J, Mensa-Wilmot K (2018) A fixable probe for visualizing flagella and plasma membranes of the African trypanosome. PLoS One 13(5):e0197541–e0197527
14. Glogger M, Subota I, Pezzarossa A et al (2017) Facilitating trypanosome imaging. Exp Parasitol 180:13–18
15. Harmer J, Qi X, Toniolo G et al (2017) Variation in basal body localisation and targeting of trypanosome RP2 and FOR20 proteins. Protist 168(4):452–466
16. Weisshart K (2014) The basic principle of airyscanning. Techonology Note ZEISS
17. Kostygov AY, Dobáková E, Grybchuk-Ieremenko A et al (2016) Novel-trypanosomatid bacterium association: evolution of endosymbiosis in action. MBio 7: e01985–e01215

Chapter 28

All You Ever Wanted to Know About APOL1 and TLFs and Did Not Dare Ask

Joseph Verdi, Charles Schaub, Russell Thomson, and Jayne Raper

Abstract

Interest in trypanosome lytic factors (TLFs) and apolipoprotein L1, the ion channel-forming protein component of TLFs, has increased tenfold since 2010. This is due to the association of African variants of *APOL1* with kidney disease such that interest has reached circles beyond parasitology. We have extensive experience purifying and working with these proteins and protein complexes. Herein we describe our detailed purification protocols to aid the new burgeoning field by providing an opportunity for consistency in reagents used across laboratories. We emphasize that it is imperative to maintain *APOL1* protein intact (~42 kDa) to analyze the active ion channel-forming component/protein.

Key words Apolipoprotein L1, Trypanosome lytic factor, Ion channel, High density lipoprotein, Haptoglobin related protein, Kidney disease, Plasma, Serum

1 Introduction

Protein purification of native proteins from bacteria and protein complexes from blood can be rigorously assessed by an assay that follows the specific activity of the purified protein (units of activity/mg of protein). Apolipoprotein L1 (APOL1) was identified as an apolipoprotein circulating on high-density lipoprotein (HDL) complexes [1] and subsequently as the lytic component of trypanosome lytic factors [2]. Trypanosome lytic factors comprise 1–10% of the heterogeneous HDL complexes in circulation, and are defined by their ability to kill animal-infective African trypanosomes [3]. The archetypal trypanosome lytic factor is an HDL composed of apolipoprotein A-I (APOA-I), haptoglobin-related protein (HPR), and apolipoprotein L1 (APOL1) [4], known as TLF1 (~12 nm, density~1.25 g/ml). TLF1 has the highest specific activity of HDL complexes that carry APOL1 in human serum; because the haptoglobin-related protein when bound to hemoglobin (HPRHB) is a ligand for a receptor (HpHb receptor) on the parasite, which facilitates high-affinity receptor-mediated

Paul A. M. Michels et al. (eds.), *Trypanosomatids: Methods and Protocols*, Methods in Molecular Biology, vol. 2116, https://doi.org/10.1007/978-1-0716-0294-2_28,

endocytosis of TLF1 [5]. TLF2 is TLF1 noncovalently associated with polyclonal germ line IgM, which sterically blocks the ligand HPRHB from interacting with the HbHp receptor [6] resulting in reduced endocytosis and thus specific activity of TLF2 (~20 nm, density ~1.28 g/ml). A third trypanosome lytic complex in circulation is HDL composed of APOA-I and APOL1 [7], which will be taken up by fluid phase endocytosis and thus will have the lowest specific activity of all TLFs [4]. Our purification technique outlined herein will enrich for TLF1 and TLF2 that contain HPR.

APOL1 is a primate specific gene duplicated only in Old World monkeys and great apes from the ancestral *APOL3* gene [8]. Two African variants of kidney-intrinsic APOL1 are associated with nephrotic diseases [9, 10]. Most APOL1 in circulation is secreted by the liver and associated with HDL [11]. APOL1 is composed of amphipathic helices (one face is hydrophobic and the other face is hydrophilic), therefore in the absence of phospholipid (i.e., HDL) or detergent (i.e., lysophospholipids) the protein will aggregate (<600 kDa). Therefore, recombinant APOL1 protein must be detergent solubilized as outlined in our protocol to yield monomeric ~42 kDa APOL1. Furthermore, any lower molecular mass fragments are due to poor sample handling and will be inactive. The concentration of APOL1 (50–1500 mM [7]) and hence the total activity of TLFs, which carry APOL1, will vary in human serum/plasma/blood. Importantly, secreted intact functional lytic APOL1 is a ~42 kDa protein, and any doublets [12] or fragments [6] that are observed are due to proteolytic processing during sample handling. Any APOL1 protein with a molecular mass less than 42 kDa will be inactive and should be avoided by using protease inhibitors during sample collection and purification.

2 Materials

2.1 Trypanosome Lytic Factor 1 and 2 Purification

Prepare all solutions using deionized (DI) water and analytical grade reagents. Filter all solutions through a 0.22 μm membrane to remove bacterial contaminants. All solutions used in this procedure can be stored at room temperature unless otherwise specified. All solutions that will be used for size-exclusion chromatography (SEC) must be sufficiently degassed immediately prior to each use, as highlighted below. Any solutions that have come in contact with human blood products must be incubated overnight in 10% bleach prior to disposal.

2.1.1 Chemicals and solutions

1. A maximum of ~100 ml of fresh human plasma from a healthy donor. Lower starting volumes are also applicable depending on how much product is desired.
2. HALT protease inhibitor cocktail (Fisher Cat# PI78439).

3. Potassium bromide (KBr) powder (*see* **Note 1**).
4. Antibody coupling buffer: 0.2 M $NaHCO_3$, 0.5 M NaCl, pH 8.3.
5. Washing and deactivation buffer A: 0.5 M ethanolamine, 0.5 M NaCl, pH 8.3.
6. Washing and deactivation buffer B: 0.1 M sodium acetate, 0.5 M NaCl, pH 4.
7. 0.9% sodium chloride (NaCl) in water (saline). Store this at 4 °C so that it is chilled at the time of use.
8. Tris-buffered saline (TBS): 50 mM Tris, 150 mM NaCl, pH 7.4.
9. Dialysis buffer: TBS with 0.5 mM EDTA.
10. Affinity elution buffer: 100 mM glycine, 150 mM NaCl, pH 3.0.
11. Affinity neutralization buffer: 1.5 M Tris–HCl, pH 8.0.

2.1.2 Equipment

1. 37 °C water bath.
2. Beckman Coulter Quick-Seal polypropylene tubes (16 × 76 mm) (Cat#342413).
3. Beckman Coulter Centrifuge Tube Sealer (Cat#342320) and Tube Spacer (Cat#342488).
4. Beckman Coulter Near Vertical Titanium (NVTi) 65 Rotor.
5. 10 and 20 cc sterile syringes and 20 gauge needles.
6. GE HiTrap *N*-hydroxysuccinimide (NHS) activated high-performance (HP) affinity columns (Cat# 17071601).
7. Fast-performance liquid chromatography apparatus.
8. SnakeSkin Dialysis Tubing (Thermo Scientific Cat#68035).
9. Amicon 100,000 Dalton molecular weight cutoff centrifugal filter units (Fisher Cat# UFC910024). All centrifugation steps using these filter units are to be carried out at maximum speed (2775 × *g*) in a table top centrifuge at 4 °C.
10. Superose 6 size-exclusion column (1.5 × 60 cm) (or comparable column that can separate 1500 kDa and 500 kDa complexes such as HiLoad 16/600 Superose 6 pg preparative SEC column).

2.1.3 Antibodies

1. Anti-human haptoglobin mouse monoclonal IgG1 (Sigma H-6395) for affinity chromatography.
2. Anti-human immunoglobulin M peroxidase conjugate (Jackson Immuno Research Labs Cat#09-035-129) for western blotting.

3. Anti-human apolipoprotein L-1 rabbit polyclonal (Protein-Tech Group 11,486-2-AP) for western blotting.
4. Anti-human haptoglobin rabbit polyclonal (Sigma H8636) for western blotting.
5. Anti-human apolipoprotein A-I goat polyclonal (Millipore AB740) for western blotting.
6. Anti-rabbit IgG TrueBlot peroxidase conjugate (Rockland Antibodies Cat# Cat#18-8816-33) for western blotting.
7. Anti-goat IgG peroxidase conjugate (Santa Cruz Biotech Cat#SC2033) for western blotting.

2.2 Recombinant Apolipoprotein L1 Protein Purification

Prepare all solutions using ultrapure water and analytical grade reagents. All steps should be carried out at room temperature unless otherwise noted. Diligently follow all waste disposal regulations when disposing of waste materials.

2.2.1 Buffer Solutions

1. Lysis buffer: 50 mM Tris–HCl, 1 mM EDTA, pH 8.0. Weigh 3.03 g of Tris base and add to 400 ml of DI water in a 500 ml graduate cylinder. Add 1 ml of 0.5 M EDTA, mix well, and adjust pH of solution to 8.0. Make up to 500 ml with DI water. Can be stored at room temperature.
2. 10% sodium deoxycholate: Add 0.3 mg of powdered sodium deoxycholate to 2 ml of DI water in a 15 ml tube. Vortex to mix, then fill to 3 ml and vortex again. Solution must be made fresh and cannot be stored for subsequent purifications.
3. 1:5 diluted lysis buffer: Add 100 ml of lysis buffer to 400 ml of DI water in a graduated cylinder and mix well. Can be stored at room temperature.
4. 10% Zwittergent 3–14: Add 4 g of powdered detergent to 30 ml of DI water in a 50 ml Falcon tube. Vortex to mix, and fill to 40 ml. Zwittergent solution can be stored at 4 °C (*see* **Note 2**).
5. 10% Triton X-100: 10% solution in DI water (*see* **Note 3**).
6. Zwittergent running buffer: 50 mM Tris–HCl, 150 mM NaCl, 0.5% Zwittergent 3–14, pH 8.6. Weigh 3.03 g of Tris base and 4.4 g of NaCl. Add to 400 ml of DI water in a graduated cylinder. Mix well, adjust pH to 8.6 with 10 M HCl, and bring volume up to 0.5 l. Sterilize with a 0.22 μm filter, and then degas under vacuum for ~20 min. Carefully add 2.5 g of Zwittergent 3–14, and stir gently until all detergent has dissolved into solution (*see* **Note 2**).
7. Wash buffer: 50 mM Tris–HCl, pH 8.6, 150 mM NaCl, 10 mM imidazole, 0.5% Zwittergent 3–14. Weigh 3.03 g of Tris base, 4.4 g of NaCl, and 340 mg of imidazole. Add to 400 ml of DI water in a graduated cylinder. Mix well, adjust pH

to 8.6 with 10 M HCl, and bring volume up to 0.5 l. Sterilize with a 0.22 μm filter, then add 2.5 g of Zwittergent 3–14, and stir gently until all detergent has dissolved into solution (*see* **Note 2**).

8. Elution buffer: 50 mM Tris–HCl pH 8.6, 150 mM NaCl, 500 mM imidazole, 0.5% Zwittergent 3–14. Weigh 3.03 g of Tris base, 4.4 g of NaCl, and 17.02 g of imidazole. Add to 400 ml of DI water in a graduated cylinder. Mix well, adjust pH to 8.6 with 10 M HCl, and bring volume up to 0.5 l. Sterilize with a 0.22 μm filter, then add 2.5 g of Zwittergent 3–14, and stir gently until all detergent has dissolved into solution (*see* **Note 2**).
9. *n*-Dodecyl β-D-maltoside (DDM) running buffer: 50 mM Tris–HCl, 150 mM NaCl, 0.05% DDM, pH 8.6. Weigh 3.03 g of Tris base and 4.4 g of NaCl. Add to 400 ml of DI water in a graduated cylinder. Mix well, adjust pH to 8.6 with 10 M HCl, and bring volume up to 0.5 l. Sterilize with a 0.22 μm filter, and then degas under vacuum for ~20 min. Carefully add 0.25 g of DDM and stir gently until all detergent has dissolved into solution (*see* **Note 2**).
10. Overnight Express Growth medium (EMD Millipore CatN#71491-5); Luria–Bertani (LB) medium (Fisher Bioreagents Cat#BP97722).

2.2.2 Equipment

1. 37 °C water bath.
2. Temperature-controlled orbital shaker.
3. Sonic Dismembrator apparatus with microtip probe.
4. Sorvall RC-5C Plus Centrifuge (or comparable centrifuge).
5. Sorvall GSA 6 place rotor (or comparable rotor).
6. Sorvall SS-34 rotor (or comparable rotor).
7. Beckman Coulter Type 60 Ti Fixed-Angle Titanium Rotor (or comparable rotor).
8. Polycarbonate bottle with cap assembly 25 × 89 mm (Cat# 355618).
9. Fast-performance liquid chromatography apparatus.
10. GE HiLoad 16/600 Superdex 200 pg size exclusion column (or comparable column).
11. GE HisTrap HP protein purification column (Cat# 17524701).
12. Amicon Ultra-15 Centrifugal Filters 10,000 Dalton molecular weight cutoff (Fisher Cat# UFC901024).

3 Methods

3.1 Separation of TLF1 and TLF2

Keep all TLF-containing samples stored on ice whenever possible. Carry out all chromatography procedures at room temperature or 4 °C.

1. If frozen, thaw the human plasma in a 37 °C water bath. If collected fresh and processed immediately, proceed to **step 2**.
2. Add HALT protease inhibitor cocktail to the plasma and briefly mix (*see* **Note 4**).
3. Measure the density (ρ_{starting}) of the plasma by weighing exactly 1 ml in a microfuge tube. Weigh the microfuge tube first and record the weight. Then add 1 ml of plasma and weigh again. Repeat this three times to have the average density of the plasma in grams/milliliter.
4. Measure the exact volume (V_{total}) of the pooled plasma and transfer to a glass beaker.
5. Adjust the density of the plasma to 1.25 g/ml (ρ_{final}) by adding KBr according to the following formula:

$$\text{X grams of KBr to add} = V_{\text{total}} \times \left(\rho_{\text{final}} - \rho_{\text{starting}}\right) \div 0.6125$$

   Dissolve KBr by slow mixing using a magnetic stir bar. This is an endothermic reaction such that the solution will become cold. To facilitate the dissolving of the KBr be sure that the room temperature is warm. However, do not add additional heat to the sample. Once the KBr is fully solubilized, recheck the density by weighing exactly 1 ml in a microfuge tube; repeat three times (*see* **Note 5**).
6. Transfer the density-adjusted plasma to 8 Beckman Coulter Quick-Seal polypropylene tubes, adding ~12 ml to each tube using a 20 cc syringe with a long adaptor (*see* **Note 6**).
7. Seal the polypropylene tubes using the Beckman Coulter Centrifuge Tube Sealer and Tube Spacer (*see* **Note 7**).
8. Place the sealed polypropylene tubes in the NVTi65 rotor and ultracentrifuge according to the following specifications: 49,000 rpm (227,600 × *g*); 10 °C; 16 h; slow deceleration. If the tubes are not sealed they will collapse during centrifugation and disrupt the gradient. Once the run is over, be very careful collecting the tubes so as to prevent gradient disruption.
9. Remove the TLF-containing fractions of the density gradient by aspirating with 10 cc syringes and 20 gauge needles (*see* Fig. 1a). Aspirate the TLF1-containing lipoprotein fraction first by creating a needle hole in the top of the tube, and then

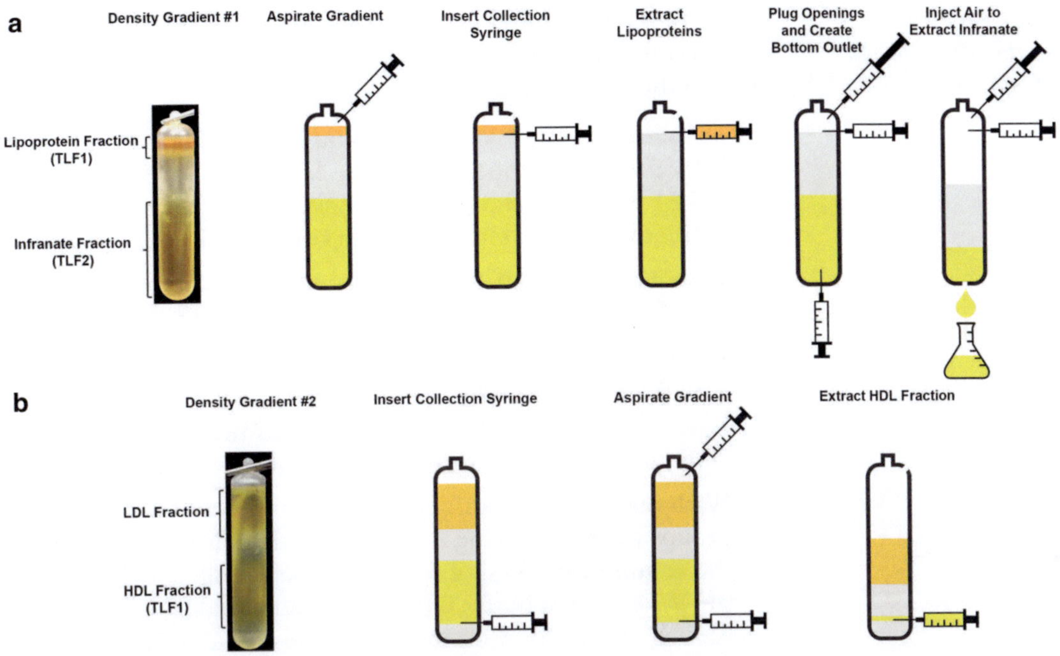

Fig. 1 (**a**) An illustration depicting the most efficient way to extract the TLFs from the first density gradient ultracentrifugation. The lipoproteins and TLF1 float to the top of the gradient when spun at 1.25 g/ml. This forms a densely packed yellow/orange layer which can be extracted using a syringe injected through the side of the tube after aspiration. The TLF2 sinks to the bottom half of the gradient, along with the majority of the serum proteins. This yellow layer can be extracted dropwise after the TLF1 has been extracted. (**b**) An illustration depicting the most efficient way to extract the TLF1 from the second density gradient ultracentrifugation. The HDL fraction, containing the TLF1, remains at the bottom of the gradient. This yellow layer can be extracted using a syringe injected through the side of the tube after aspiration. To prevent spillage, inject the collection syringe before the aspiration syringe as depicted

extracting the yellow/orange layer using a syringe injected through the side, keeping the bevel of the needle facing upward. Take care not to have fingers or hands in line with the needle on the opposing side of the tube to avoid inadvertent pricking of finger. Be sure to collect the very base of the layer as TLF1 is the densest of all lipoproteins (1.25 g/ml) and is found at the base of the yellow orange layer. Once the layer is extracted, temporarily plug the holes using needles and syringes, and then create a hole directly at the bottom of the tube to drain the TLF2-containing infranate fraction (the bottom 50% of the gradient). To prevent spillage, control the speed of draining by slowly injecting air into the top of the tube through one of the syringes that is being used to plug the previously generated holes (*see* Fig. 1a). TLF1-specific procedures will continue in Subheading 3.1, **step 3**, while TLF2 specific procedures will continue in Subheading 3.1, **step 4**.

3.2 TLF Affinity Purification Column Preparation

The anti-HP column is generated using NHS-HiTrap 1 ml columns as instructed by the manufacturer with only minor modifications to the suggested protocol.

1. Dialyze the entire vial of the anti-human HP mouse IgG1 (H6395) in antibody coupling buffer (0.2 M $NaHCO_3$, 0.5 M NaCl, pH 8.3). After dialysis, adjust the volume of the antibody to ~1 ml either through concentration or dilution.
2. Remove the top cap of the column and apply a drop of ice-cold 1 mM HCl to the column, to activate the NHS groups.
3. Remove the snap-off end at the bottom and wash the column with 6 column volumes of 1 mM HCl.
4. Inject the diluted antibody sample onto the column, seal the ends, and let it stand at room temperature for 30 min.
5. Wash out unbound antibody and deactivate excess NHS active groups by the following the manufacturer's instructions: Wash the column with 6 ml of A (0.5 M ethanolamine, 0.5 M NaCl, pH 8.3), 6 ml of buffer B (0.1 M sodium acetate, 0.5 M NaCl, pH 4), and 6 ml of buffer A. Let the column stand at room temperature for 15 min. Wash the column with 6 ml of buffer B, 6 ml of buffer A, and 6 ml of buffer B (*see* **Note 8**).
6. The ready-to-use column can be stored at 4 °C for extended periods of time. The longevity should be determined empirically (*see* **Note 9**).
7. Immediately prior to use, the column should be subjected to a "blank run," wherein no sample is loaded onto the column, while the washing and elution steps are performed exactly as they will be during the purification to remove unbound antibody.

3.3 TLF1 Purification

1. Pool the extracted TLF1-containing fractions from Subheading 3.1, **step 9** and measure both the total volume ($V2_{\text{total}}$) and density ($\rho 2_{\text{starting}}$).
2. Adjust the density to 1.3 g/ml ($\rho 2_{\text{final}}$) using more KBr and the following formula:

$$\text{X grams of KBr to add} = V2_{\text{total}} \times \left(\rho 2_{\text{final}} - \rho 2_{\text{starting}}\right) \div 0.597$$

   Dissolve KBr by slow mixing using a magnetic stir bar. Once KBr is fully solubilized, recheck the density by weighing exactly 1 ml in a preweighed microfuge tube (*see* **Note 5**).

3. Using a 20 cc syringe and a long needle adaptor (~5 in.), transfer 8 ml of ice-cold 0.9% NaCl to 6 new Beckman Coulter Quick-Seal polypropylene tubes.

4. Using a 20 cc syringe and a long adaptor, layer 4 ml of density-adjusted plasma below the 0.9% NaCl, bringing the tube to a total volume of 12 ml (*see* **Note 10**).
5. Seal the polypropylene tubes using the Beckman Coulter Centrifuge Tube Sealer and Tube Spacer (*see* **Note 7**).
6. Place the polypropylene tubes in the NVTi65 rotor (being careful to not disturb the gradient) and ultracentrifuge according to the following specifications: 49,000 rpm (227,600 × *g*); 10 °C; 3 h; slow deceleration.
7. Remove the TLF1-containing high-density lipoprotein fraction using 10 cc syringes and needles (*see* Fig. 1b). First inject a collecting needle and syringe through the side, keeping the bevel of the needle facing upward. Aspirate the top of the gradient by creating a hole with a separate needle and extract the TLF1-containing fraction (*see* **Note 11**). Pool the TLF1-containing fractions in a glass beaker.
8. Dialyze the TLF1-containing material to remove the KBr using 5 × 1-h exchanges of 1 l volumes of Tris-buffered saline with EDTA at 4 °C (*see* **Note 12**). Transfer the sample to prewetted SnakeSkin Dialysis Tubing by first sealing one end of the tubing with a knot, adding the sample, and then sealing the opposite end with another knot (*see* **Note 13**). Attach a floatation device to the tubing and dialyze with slow stirring.
9. Extract the TLF1-containing sample.
10. Concentrate the sample to <2 ml using Amicon centrifugal filter units 10 KDa MW cutoff.
11. Add an appropriate amount of HALT protease inhibitor cocktail.
12. TLF1 is among the largest of all HDLs. Separate TLF1 away from smaller HDL species and any remaining contaminating plasma-albumin by SEC on a Superose 6 column equilibrated in TBS at 1 ml/min via fast-performance liquid chromatography (FPLC) (*see* **Note 14**). Collect the TLF1 into <1 ml fractions from the size-exclusion column.
13. TLF1 quality check. Prepare SDS-PAGE gel loads for all fractions from the column (noting the TLF1-sized range (450–650 kDa)). Determine which fractions contain the majority of the TLF1 by SDS-PAGE and western blotting to specifically detect the relevant proteins of interest (APOL1, HPR, and APOA-I). If this step will take more than a day's time, the fractions should be frozen at −80 °C for the duration of the analysis (*see* **Note 15**). Do not store at 4 °C otherwise the APOL1 will degrade and TLF activity will be lost.
14. Pool the TLF1-containing sized fractions and concentrate to <1 ml using Amicon centrifugal filter units.

15. Add an appropriate amount of HALT protease inhibitor cocktail.
16. TLF1 contains HPR, which is used as a target for affinity chromatography. Load the pooled TLF1-containing sized fractions onto the anti-HP/HPR affinity column equilibrated in TBS at 1 ml/min via FPLC. Wash the column with 10 column volumes of TBS. Collect the unbound fractions and keep on ice (*see* **Note 16**). Preload the collection tubes to be used for TLF elution with 20 μl of neutralization buffer so that the eluted TLF1-containing fractions will be immediately neutralized (*see* **Note 17**). Elute the bound fraction by establishing a gradient of TBS to elution buffer that increases from 0% elution buffer to 100% elution buffer over the span of 5 ml (*see* **Note 18**).
17. Pool the unbound fractions and concentrate to <1 ml using Amicon centrifugal filter units. Repeat **steps 16** and **17** until it becomes evident that there is no longer any TLF remaining in the unbound fraction (*see* **Note 16**).
18. Pool and concentrate the eluted TLF1-containing fractions to <1 ml using Amicon centrifugal filter units.
19. Resize the purified fraction on a Superose 6 column equilibrated in TBS at 1 ml/min to isolate intact TLF1 complexes in 1 ml fractions.
20. Pool the TLF1-containing fractions and concentrate to <1 ml using Amicon centrifugal filter units.
21. Determine the total protein concentration and aliquot in suitable volumes. Store the purified TLF1 at −80 °C.

3.4 TLF2 Purification

1. Dialyze the TLF2-containing material to remove the KBr using five 1-h exchanges of 1 l volumes of Tris-buffered saline with EDTA at 4 °C (*see* **Note 12**). Transfer the sample to prewetted SnakeSkin Dialysis Tubing by first sealing one end of the tubing with a knot, adding the sample, and then sealing the opposite end with another knot (*see* **Note 13**). Attach a floatation device to the tubing and dialyze with slow stirring.
2. Extract the TLF2-containing sample.
3. Concentrate the TLF2-containing sample to <40 ml using Amicon centrifugal filter units 10 KDa MW cutoff.
4. Add an appropriate amount of HALT protease inhibitor cocktail.
5. Remove all relatively small (<700 kDa) proteins/complexes from the sample by SEC on a Superose 6 column equilibrated in TBS at 1 ml/min. Load 4 ml of TLF2-containing sample per run for a total of 10 runs (*see* **Note 19**).

6. TLF2 quality check. Prepare SDS-PAGE gel loads for all fractions within the TLF2-sized range (700–2000 kDa). Determine which fractions contain the majority of the TLF2 by SDS-PAGE and western blotting to specifically detect the relevant proteins of interest (IgM, APOL1, HPR, and APOA-I) (*see* **Note 15**). To limit freeze thaw, these gels and western blots should be performed immediately following the first SEC step, while the subsequent columns are running. The empirically determined (by western blotting) elution pattern of the first run can be used as a proxy to determine which fractions to pool from subsequent runs.
7. Pool and concentrate all TLF2-containing fractions using Amicon centrifugal filter units 10 KDa MW cutoff to <2 ml.
8. Add an appropriate amount of HALT protease inhibitor cocktail.
9. TLF2 contains HPR, which is used as a target for affinity chromatography. Perform a series of affinity chromatography steps exactly as described in Subheading 3.3, **steps 16** and **17**.
10. Pool and concentrate the eluted TLF2-containing fractions to <1 ml using Amicon centrifugal filter units 10 KDa MW cutoff.
11. Resize the purified fraction on a Superose 6 column equilibrated in TBS at 1 ml/min to isolate intact TLF2 complexes in 1 ml fractions.
12. Pool the TLF2-containing fractions and concentrate to <1 ml using Amicon centrifugal filter units 10 KDa MW cutoff.
13. Determine the total protein concentration and aliquot in suitable volumes. Store the purified TLF2 at −80 °C.

3.5 Final TLF Quality Checks

1. All fully purified TLFs must be analyzed for proteolytic digestion of the individual protein components after purification. Prepare SDS-PAGE gel loads of the purified TLFs. Analyze the TLFs by conventional SDS-PAGE and western blotting to determine whether the relevant proteins of interest (IgM, APOL1, HPR, and APOA-I) are all fully intact (Fig. 2).
2. All fully purified TLF2 samples must also be analyzed for structural integrity of the entire complex after purification (*see* **Note 20**). Prepare nondenaturing gel loads for native agarose-based protein gel electrophoresis. Prepare 0.7% agarose in TBB. Load aliquots (total amount to be empirically determined based on the success of the purification and amount of assumed degradation indicated by **step 1**) of TLF and electrophorese them at 100 mV for approximately 2 h at room temperature. Transfer the separated protein complexes from the agarose gel to a membrane for processing by capillary blotting. Determine the structural integrity of the TLFs by anti-APOL1 western blotting (Fig. 3).

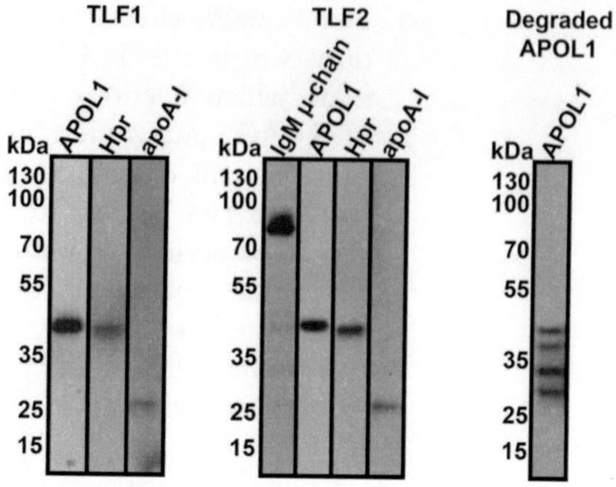

Fig. 2 Example western blots depicting the condition of the proteins of interest after TLF1 and 2 purification. Ideally, proteolysis will have been efficiently inhibited during the purification, yielding full-length proteins. The right panel shows the condition of the APOL1 after performing a purification without proper protease inhibition. The degraded fragments of APOL1 on this blot are still TLF-associated, but only the full-length protein is biochemically active. Degradation of IgM, Hpr, or APOA-I is less often observed

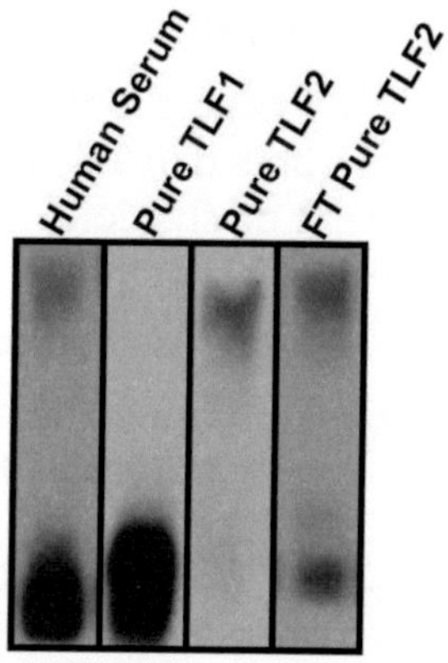

Fig. 3 Example anti-human APOL1 western blots of TLFs after native agarose gel electrophoresis. FT: Freeze thawed. TLF2 migrates slowly through the gel, while TLF1 migrates relatively fast. Normal human serum contains both TLF1 and TLF2, though the majority of the APOL1 is TLF1-associated. TLF2 samples that have been freeze-thawed or have been purified under some nonideal condition (s) will reproducibly contain TLF1. The IgM-TLF2 interaction is noncovalent and therefore the IgMs likely disassociate when the TLF2 is not handled carefully

3.6 Transformation of Bacteria with APOL1 Plasmid

Day 1

1. Bacterial expression cells: Add 10–50 ng of purified pNIC plasmid containing the APOL1 coding sequence to 50 μl of Bl21-DE3-RIPL cells under sterile conditions in a 13 ml polystyrene tube. Flick gently to mix, then let sit on ice for 30 min (*see* **Note 21**).

2. Heat-shock for 23 s at 42 °C and place back on ice for 4 min. Add 500 μl of prewarmed Luria–Bertani (LB) medium to tube and shake for 1 h at 37 °C at 300 rpm.
3. Plate 500 μl of bacterial culture on LB agar supplemented with kanamycin and incubate overnight at 37 °C.

3.7 Bacterial Growth and Protein Expression

Day 2

1. Prepare 200 ml of Overnight Express Growth medium in a 500 ml bottle and microwave with the cap loose until a slight boil to sterilize. Let cool and add kanamycin (100 μg/ml) and chloramphenicol (34 μg/ml) and mix well. Transfer 100 ml of medium into a 1 l Erlenmeyer flask under sterile conditions.
2. Examining the plates from yesterday, select 1–5 colonies and add to the flask under sterile conditions. Let shake for 16–18 h overnight at 37 °C at 300 rpm. There is no need for addition of IPTG with this protocol (*see* **Note 22**).

3.8 Isolation of Inclusion Bodies

Day 3

1. Centrifuge the bacterial milieu at 6000 × *g* for 15 min in a GSA rotor at 4 °C.
2. On ice, resuspend in 18 ml of lysis buffer and transfer to an SS34 tube (rounded cylinder). Add 10 μl 1 M DTT and 50 μl 200 mM PMSF. Lyse cells via microtip sonication using a 2 s pulse at a 40% duty cycle set to the microtip limit. Sonicate on ice for 1 min, then let stand on ice for 1 min. Repeat three times (*see* **Note 23**).
3. At room temperature, while stirring, add 20 μl of 5 mg/ml DNase1, 20 μl 5 mg/ml RNase1, and 100 μl 50 mg/ml lysozyme. Stir for 45 min. Then add 70 μl 1 M $MgCl_2$ and 40 μl 1 M $CaCl_2$ and stir for 30 min. Finally, add 1 ml 10% Triton X-100 and 1 ml 10% sodium deoxycholate (make fresh) and stir for 1 h.
4. Remove stir bars, and pellet at 26,000 × *g* (14,800 rpm in SS34 or F21S-8x50Y) for 30 min.
5. Discard supernatant and resuspend pellet in 9 ml lysis buffer. While stirring, add 1 ml 10% Triton X-100 and 0.2 ml 5 M NaCl and stir for 30 min.
6. Pellet at 17,050 × *g* (12,000 rpm) for 30 min in an SS34 rotor.
7. Discard supernatant and resuspend pellet in 10 ml lysis buffer. While stirring, add 0.2 ml 5 M NaCl. Put sample(s) back on ice, remove stir bars, and repeat sonication according to the procedure in **step 4**.

   [At this point, sample(s) can be stored overnight at 4 °C] (*see* **Note 24**).

8. Repeat centrifugation according to **step 6**.
9. Discard supernatant and resuspend pellet in 10 ml of 1:5 diluted lysis buffer.
10. Repeat centrifugation according to **step 6**.

3.9 Extraction of rAPOL1 from Inclusion Bodies

Day 3

1. Discard supernatant and resuspend pellet in 8 ml DI water. Sonicate for a continuous ~10 s to disperse. While stirring, add 2 ml 10% Zwittergent 3–14. Slowly add 100 μl 1 M NaOH (*see* **Note 25**). Wait 1 min, and add 300 μl 5 M NaCl. Wait 1 min, and slowly add 150 μl 1 M Tris–HCl, pH 7.4. Stir for 15–30 min (*see* **Note 26**).
2. Ultracentrifuge at 45,000 rpm (207,870 × *g*) for 45 min in a Ti70 rotor. Filter supernatant using a 0.45 μm filter (*see* **Note 27**).
3. [At this point, sample(s) can be stored overnight at 4 °C] (*see* **Note 28**).

3.10 Fast Protein Liquid Chromatography

Day 4

1. Concentrate sample down to ~5 ml with a centrifugal filter unit. The MW cutoff of the filter should be 10,000 Daltons to ensure rAPOL1 (~42 kDa) remains in the concentrated portion.

   Optional (ideal if highly pure yields are required). Concentrate sample down further to ~2 ml. Load the sample onto Superdex 200 16/600 column that has been equilibrated with Zwittergent running buffer. With the flow set to 1 ml/min, collect 1 ml fractions and keep tubes 45–80. APOL1 should elute around fraction ~65 ml (*see* Fig. 4a) (*see* **Note 29**).

   Optional. Run SDS-PAGE of the fractions corresponding to the anticipated APOL1 peak, and 3–4 fractions before and after. Add 1 μl of each fraction to 19 μl of 2× Laemmli sample buffer. Load 15 μl per lane and run at 150 V. Coomassie-stain and collect fractions with ideal ratios of rAPOL1 to contaminating bands. Collect no more than 5 fractions (*see* Fig. 4b) (*see* **Note 30**).
2. Load ≤5 ml of sample to a 1 ml His-Trap column. Program for a 1 ml/min flow rate and load sample onto the column. Wash column with 15 CV of wash buffer, then increase concentration of elution buffer from 0 to 60% over 20 ml. The rAPOL1 should elute during the gradient (*see* **Note 31**). After the gradient, clean the column with 5 ml of 100% elution buffer and then equilibrate with 5 ml of wash buffer. Collect 1 ml fractions, beginning with the unbound fraction that immediately elutes up until the cleaning step (*see* Fig. 5a).

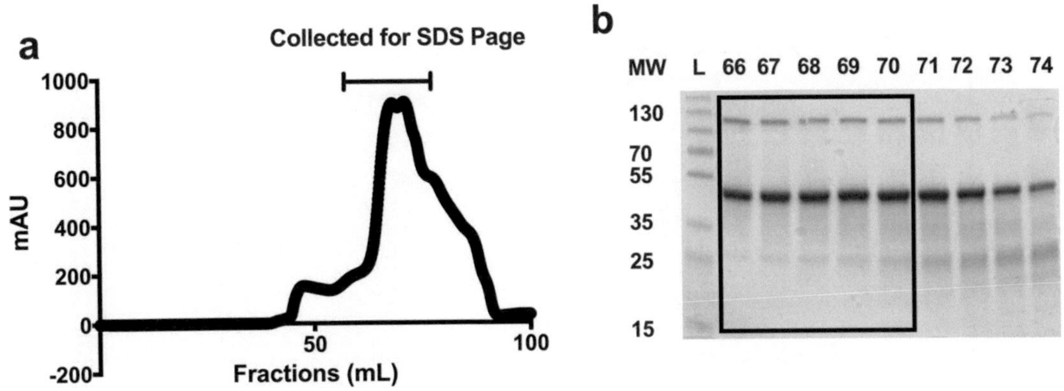

Fig. 4 rAPOL1 SEC chromatogram and accompanying SDS-PAGE after Coomassie staining. The bracket indicates the fractions run on SDS-PAGE. The box represents the fractions that should be collected for this particular purification step. *MW* Molecular weight, *L* Ladder

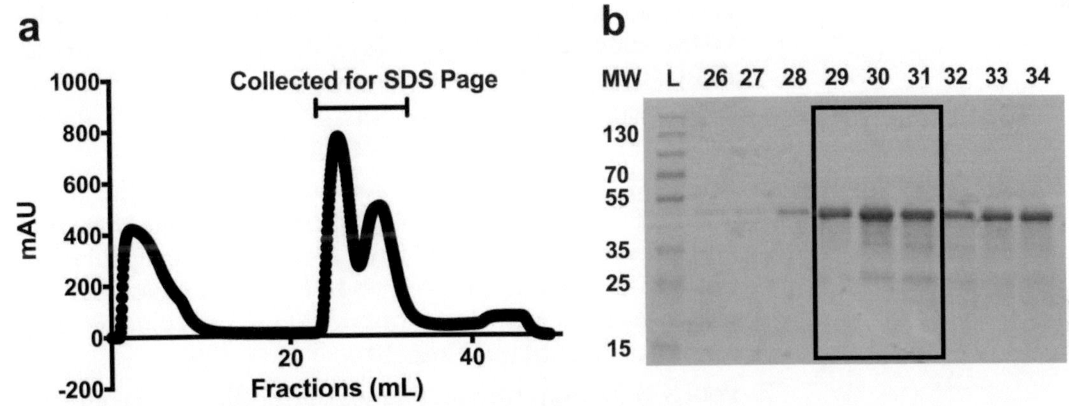

Fig. 5 rAPOL1 His-Trap affinity purification chromatogram and accompanying SDS-PAGE after Coomassie staining. The bracket indicates the fractions run on SDS-PAGE. The box represents the fractions that should be collected for this particular purification step. *MW* Molecular weight, *L* Ladder

3. Run SDS-PAGE of the fractions corresponding to the anticipated APOL1 peak, and 3–4 fractions before and after. Add 1 μl of each fraction to 19 μl of 2× Laemmli sample buffer. Load 15 μl per lane, and run at 150 V. Coomassie-stain and collect fractions with ideal ratios of rAPOL1 to contaminating bands. Collect no more than 5 fractions (*see* Fig. 5b) (*see* **Note 30**).
4. Concentrate sample down to ~2 ml with a centrifugal filter unit. The MW cutoff of the filter should be 10,000 Daltons to ensure rAPOL1 (~42 kDa) remains in the concentrated portion.

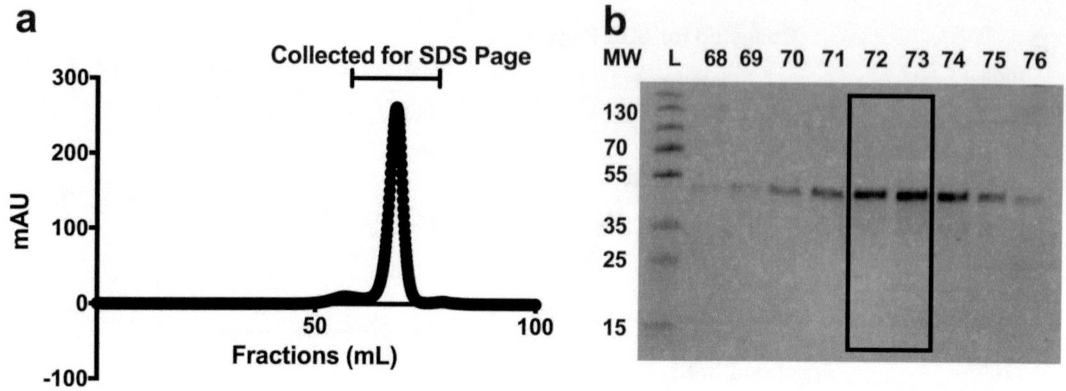

Fig. 6 rAPOL1 SEC chromatogram and accompanying SDS-PAGE after Coomassie staining. The bracket indicates the fractions run on SDS-PAGE. The box represents the fractions that should be collected for this particular purification step. *MW* Molecular weight, *L* Ladder

5. Using an equilibrated Superdex 200 16/600 column with DDM running buffer (*see* **Note 32**, load sample into an FPLC. Using DDM running buffer, flow at 1 ml/min, collect 1 ml fractions, and keep fractions 45–80 ml. APOL1 should elute around fraction ~67 ml (*see* Fig. 6a).
6. Run SDS-PAGE of the fractions corresponding to the anticipated APOL1 peak, and 3–4 fractions before and after. Add 1 μl of each fraction to 19 μl of 2× Laemmli sample buffer. Load 15 μl per lane, and run at 150 V. Coomassie-stain and collect fractions with ideal ratios of rAPOL1 to contaminating bands (*see* Fig. 6b) (*see* **Note 30**).
7. Pool 2–3 fractions with ideal ratios of rAPOL1 to contaminant bands. Mix gently by flicking or slow pipetting up and down. Aliquot into ~100 μl fractions and flash-freeze with liquid nitrogen before storage at −80 °C.

4 Notes

1. We use KBr because it is a high molecular weight salt that adjusts the density of the plasma without having to add too much solute. KBr is highly hygroscopic, however, which results in large dense clumps of salt forming in the storage bottle over time. To accelerate the process of dissolving the KBr, we crush these clumps using the blunt side of a weighing spatula.
2. Wear a mask and goggles when weighing out either Zwittergent 3–14 or DDM. Both detergents can be upper respiratory or eye irritants.
3. Surfact-Amps Triton X-100 is purchased from Thermo Scientific (Product #28314).

4. The APOL1 component of TLFs is highly sensitive to proteolytic digestion. HDLs are themselves associated with many proteases, thus juxtaposing the APOL1 to these destructive enzymes in vivo and during the lengthy purification. We add protease inhibitors at various stages throughout the procedure to ensure that the purified TLF retains maximal specific activity.
5. Calculating the appropriate amount of KBr to add to the plasma is dependent on highly accurate measurements. In the event that the rechecked adjusted density is below 1.25 g/ml, the equation can be reapplied and more KBr can be added to increase the density. If the rechecked density is above 1.25 g/ml, then a small volume deionized water can be added to the plasma to decrease the density.
6. The plasma must be added to the polypropylene tubes from the bottom using a long adaptor to decrease bubble formation in Subheading 3.1, **step 6** and Subheading 3.3, **steps 3** and **4** and from the density gradient in Subheading 3.3, **steps 3** and **4**. We use a blunted 12.5 cm needle designed to be used for lumbar punctures. Slowly eject the plasma through the needle until the volume reaches the desired fill-height of approximately 12 ml. With respect to Subheading 3.3, **steps 3** and **4**; add exactly 4 ml of density adjusted plasma to exactly 8 ml of 0.9% NaCl; otherwise the final gradient, and thus the distribution of LDL and HDL, will be disrupted.
7. Begin heating the tube sealer at the start of the procedure to bring it to the appropriate temperature by the time it is needed. To seal the tubes, place metal tube caps on the tops and depress the sealer gently until the cap is flush with the main body of the tube. Overheating the tubes will weaken them, leading to the formation of leaks. Remove the caps once they have cooled back to room temperature. The caps may need to be removed using a hemostat and slight twisting.
8. The manufacturer recommends that the experimenters measure the efficiency of antibody coupling prior to washing and deactivation, which can be performed via a variety of methods found on the product's website. We strongly encourage this as well.
9. We recommend testing the binding capacity of the column by periodically running a human HP purification. Pure human HP can be purchased from various distributors (we purchase from Millipore via Fisher Scientific Cat# 50-489-744). Once the column is no longer efficiently purifying human HP, it will also no longer be suitable for TLF purification and will require replacement.

10. This gradient cannot be reformed either before or after centrifugation. Tubes must be handled with extreme care to ensure that the gradient is properly maintained. Ideally, there will be enough material collected to fill all 6 polypropylene tubes. However, this depends on the amount of starting material and collection technique. The number of tubes used in this second density gradient may therefore vary significantly. In order to ensure that no amount of TLF-containing sample is wasted, we keep a solution of 1.3 g/ml KBr in TBS to the side which can be used to volume up the sample to a number divisible by 4.
11. In order to limit the amount of sample loss, we inject the collecting needle first. This is because the injection point is near the bottom of the tube, and if the tube is already aspirated, the fluid pressure will cause rapid leakage at the lower injection site until the needle has been completely inserted. Injecting the collecting needle first and then subsequently aspirating prevents this issue.
12. The dialysis procedure can also be completed using 2 exchanges of 5 l of the dialysis buffer with longer incubations if necessary. For example, a 3-h dialysis followed by an overnight dialysis, both at 4 °C.
13. The use of SnakeSkin tubing is preferred when operating with large sample volumes. However, if the sample volume is low enough, we will routinely instead utilize Slide-A-Lyzer dialysis cassettes with a 100,000 Dalton molecular weight cutoff. The cassettes are significantly easier to use, but also significantly more expensive.
14. SEC can be performed with any column or resin that can efficiently separate this amount of protein. Assuming that 100% of the HDL is extracted from 100 ml of a human plasma sample containing 0.5 mg/ml HDL, there can be upward of 50 mg of protein at this stage before accounting for the contaminating albumin remaining in the sample.
15. Once the protocol has been established in a laboratory, this step can be omitted purely for the purpose of accelerating the purification. Both TLF1 and TLF2 lose specific activity and APOL1 integrity with both freeze thaw and 4 °C storage for extended periods of time.
16. Yields from the affinity steps can fluctuate based on a variety of factors, including for example the condition of the affinity column itself and how much antibody was used to generate it. In this regard, we never discard the unbound fractions under the assumption that some portion of the TLF may not have bound to the column. We find that TLF1 binds with higher affinity to this anti-HP monoclonal antibody-based column,

and as such, only two rounds of affinity chromatography are usually required to isolate 99% of the TLF1. TLF2 however binds with lower affinity, and so we typically will pool, concentrate, and rerun the unbound fractions on the column 10–15 times.

17. The exact volume of neutralization buffer required to neutralize 1 ml of elution buffer will vary with each purification. The required volume should be empirically determined on the day of the experiment, prior to preloading the eluate collection tubes. Preloading the eluate collection tubes with neutralization buffer is required to limit the loss of TLF-specific activity. The complexes cannot be stored in acidic buffers for extended durations of time.
18. Gradient-based elution protocols prevent the sample from being exposed to overly harsh conditions. In our hands, the TLFs will elute roughly half way through the gradient and are therefore not fully dropped to pH 3.0.
19. This step will take a significant amount of time. Each SEC run takes approximately 1.5–2 h. In order to accelerate the process, this step should ideally be performed with multiple columns running simultaneously.
20. We consistently detect "contaminating TLF1" in purified TLF2 samples. We believe this is due to the noncovalent, and presumably low-affinity, nature of the IgM-TLF association and the stringency of the purification process. We find that nondenaturing agarose gels are the ideal way to determine the relative amounts of TLF1 and TLF2 in any given protein sample because they are quick, easy to prepare, cheap, and they allow for the comparison of multiple purifications simultaneously or use a native polyacrylamide gel 3–12%.
21. The rAPOL1 coding sequence contains a *N*-terminal 6X-His--tag followed by a TEV cleavage site. The tag allows for metal affinity purification, but can be cleaved off before beginning experiments.
22. In the event of a poor transformation efficiency, only one colony may be used for inoculation. However, several colonies help to ensure high bacterial growth and turbidity, along with high protein yields.
23. When working with two tubes, both can be brought to sonication simultaneously. While one tube is being sonicated, the other can be standing. However, you must clean the microtip between sonicating if two different proteins are being purified at once.

24. If time is a concern, the purification can be paused here until the following day. But note that storage overnight may cause proteolysis of rAPOL1 that is difficult to remove in subsequent steps. For high purity yields, it is best to continue up until Subheading 3.2, **step 2**.
25. On occasion, the solution will not go entirely clear at this point. Either there was too much rAPOL1 recovered, or the inclusion bodies were not solubilized because pH 12 was not reached. Check the pH of your solution if this is the case.
26. Adding the 1 M Tris–HCl too quickly may cause the rAPOL1 to precipitate and fall out of solution. Slowly adding and allowing the Tris-HCl to bring the pH down in a controlled manner will yield the highest amount of solubilized rAPOL1.
27. A Ti60 rotor may also be used.
28. It is best to pause the purification here. However, the remaining steps must be completed the following day for optimal purity and yield.
29. If running this additional purification step, it is important to equilibrate the column overnight from day 2 to day 3. This will save time on day 4. Run 2 column volumes of DDM size buffer through the column at 0.4 ml/min.
30. The lower, contaminating bands are often APOL1 that has been degraded by proteases during the purification process. They are difficult to remove, and every precaution must be taken when selecting fractions to avoid them. For high purity yields, it is best to choose only 1–2 ideal fractions rather than 4–5. Ideal fractions will have the highest ratio of full-length rAPOL1 to contaminating bands.
31. Often, there will be a double peak during the gradient. The second peak contains rAPOL1 aggregates that require additional imidazole to remove from the His-column. Try to avoid collecting and pooling any of these fractions before loading onto the final sizing column.
32. If running the optional Zwittergent sizing column, the column must be equilibrated before beginning **step 19**. Run 2 column volumes of DDM running buffer through the column at 1 ml/min. If not performing the optional sizing step, the column may be equilibrated overnight with DDM running buffer between days 2 and 3 at a rate of 0.4 ml/min.

References

1. Duchateau PN, Pullinger CR, Orellana RE, Kunitake ST, Naya-Vigne J, O'Connor PM, Malloy MJ, Kane JP (1997) Apolipoprotein L, a new human high density lipoprotein apolipoprotein expressed by the pancreas. Identification, cloning, characterization, and plasma distribution of apolipoprotein L. J Biol Chem 272(41):25576–25582
2. Vanhamme L, Paturiaux-Hanocq F, Poelvoorde P, Nolan DP, Lins L, Van Den Abbeele J, Pays A, Tebabi P, Van Xong H, Jacquet A, Moguilevsky N, Dieu M, Kane JP, De Baetselier P, Brasseur R, Pays E (2003) Apolipoprotein L-I is the trypanosome lytic factor of human serum. Nature 422 (6927):83–87. https://doi.org/10.1038/nature01461
3. Raper J, Fung R, Ghiso J, Nussenzweig V, Tomlinson S (1999) Characterization of a novel trypanosome lytic factor from human serum. Infect Immun 67(4):1910–1916
4. Shiflett AM, Bishop JR, Pahwa A, Hajduk SL (2005) Human high density lipoproteins are platforms for the assembly of multi-component innate immune complexes. J Biol Chem 280 (38):32578–32585. https://doi.org/10.1074/jbc.M503510200
5. Vanhollebeke B, De Muylder G, Nielsen MJ, Pays A, Tebabi P, Dieu M, Raes M, Moestrup SK, Pays E (2008) A haptoglobin-hemoglobin receptor conveys innate immunity to Trypanosoma brucei in humans. Science 320 (5876):677–681. https://doi.org/10.1126/science.1156296
6. Bullard W, Kieft R, Capewell P, Veitch NJ, Macleod A, Hajduk SL (2012) Haptoglobin-hemoglobin receptor independent killing of African trypanosomes by human serum and trypanosome lytic factors. Virulence 3 (1):72–76. https://doi.org/10.4161/viru.3.1.18295
7. Kozlitina J, Zhou H, Brown PN, Rohm RJ, Pan Y, Ayanoglu G, Du X, Rimmer E, Reilly DF, Roddy TP, Cully DF, Vogt TF, Blom D, Hoek M (2016) Plasma levels of risk-variant APOL1 do not associate with renal disease in a population-based cohort. J Am Soc Nephrol 27(10):3204–3219. https://doi.org/10.1681/ASN.2015101121
8. Smith EE, Malik HS (2009) The apolipoprotein L family of programmed cell death and immunity genes rapidly evolved in primates at discrete sites of host-pathogen interactions. Genome Res 19(5):850–858. https://doi.org/10.1101/gr.085647.108
9. Genovese G, Friedman DJ, Ross MD, Lecordier L, Uzureau P, Freedman BI, Bowden DW, Langefeld CD, Oleksyk TK, Uscinski Knob AL, Bernhardy AJ, Hicks PJ, Nelson GW, Vanhollebeke B, Winkler CA, Kopp JB, Pays E, Pollak MR (2010) Association of trypanolytic ApoL1 variants with kidney disease in African Americans. Science 329 (5993):841–845. https://doi.org/10.1126/science.1193032
10. Tzur S, Rosset S, Shemer R, Yudkovsky G, Selig S, Tarekegn A, Bekele E, Bradman N, Wasser WG, Behar DM, Skorecki K (2010) Missense mutations in the APOL1 gene are highly associated with end stage kidney disease risk previously attributed to the MYH9 gene. Hum Genet 128(3):345–350. https://doi.org/10.1007/s00439-010-0861-0
11. Shukha K, Mueller JL, Chung RT, Curry MP, Friedman DJ, Pollak MR, Berg AH (2017) Most ApoL1 is secreted by the liver. J Am Soc Nephrol 28(4):1079–1083. https://doi.org/10.1681/ASN.2016040441
12. Weckerle A, Snipes JA, Cheng D, Gebre AK, Reisz JA, Murea M, Shelness GS, Hawkins GA, Furdui CM, Freedman BI, Parks JS, Ma L (2016) Characterization of circulating APOL1 protein complexes in African Americans. J Lipid Res 57(1):120–130. https://doi.org/10.1194/jlr.M063453

Chapter 29

Isolation of *Leishmania* Promastigote Flagella

Tom Beneke, François Demay, Richard J. Wheeler, and Eva Gluenz

Abstract

Eukaryotic flagella are conserved multifunctional organelles with roles in motility, intercellular interactions, and signal transduction. *Leishmania* possess a single flagellum at all stages of their life cycle. Flagella of promastigote forms in the fly are long and motile, with a canonical 9 + 2 microtubule axoneme and an extra-axonemal paraflagellar rod (PFR). This protocol describes a simple method for the isolation of *Leishmania mexicana* promastigote flagella, optimized to yield intact flagella that retain both the cytoskeletal elements (9 + 2 axoneme and PFR) and the surrounding membrane. The isolated flagella and deflagellated cell bodies are suitable for analysis by electron microscopy, protein mass spectrometry, and lipidomics.

Key words *Leishmania*, Kinetoplastids, Flagella, Cell fractionation

1 Introduction

Eukaryotic flagella and cilia are highly conserved structures. Motile flagella typically have a 9 + 2 microtubule (MT) structure, where a ninefold symmetric cylinder of doublet microtubules surrounds a central pair of singlet MTs (CP). The coordinated activity of dynein motor proteins anchored on the doublet MTs generates a flagellar waveform, thought to be regulated by the CP and associated protein complexes. Cilia with a simpler 9 + 0 MT architecture typically perform sensory functions, which can be mediated through the interactions of external stimuli with receptors localized to the ciliary membrane [1]. Proteomic studies of diverse ciliated cell types [2–5], including trypanosomatids [6–9], have shown that flagella and cilia are composed of several hundred proteins, with a core set of evolutionarily conserved proteins and lineage-specific elaborations and losses [10]. Genetic studies and biochemical analyses of wild type and mutant flagella enabled the development of models for dynein-driven motility [11, 12] and advances in cryo-electron microscopy now help to test and refine these models

Tom Beneke and François Demay have contributed equally to this work.

Paul A. M. Michels et al. (eds.), *Trypanosomatids: Methods and Protocols*, Methods in Molecular Biology, vol. 2116, https://doi.org/10.1007/978-1-0716-0294-2_29,

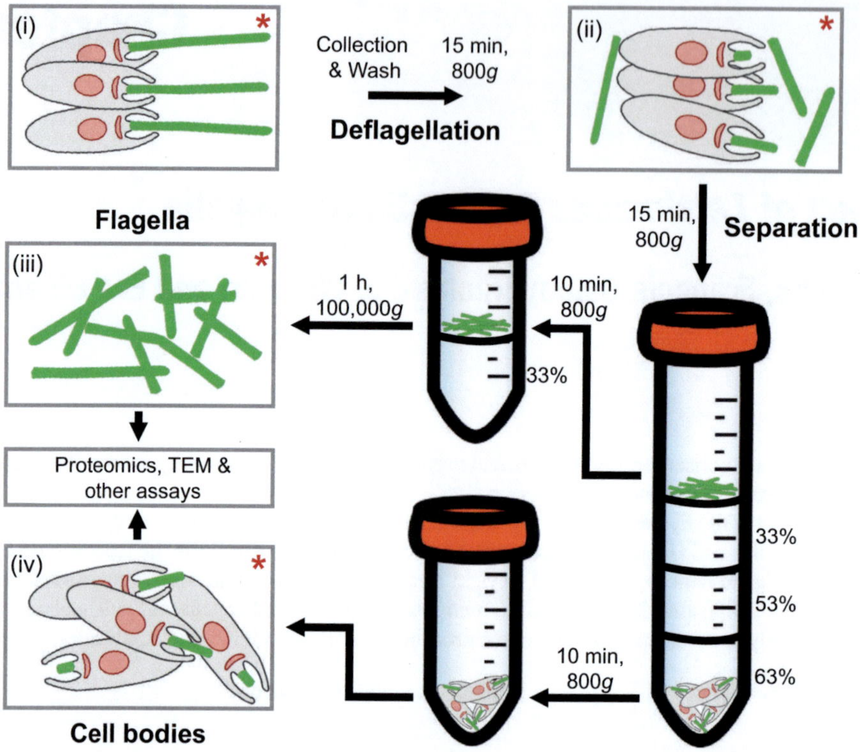

Fig. 1 Workflow of deflagellation procedure. Schematic overview of the workflow. Red asterisks (∗) indicate samples that should be examined microscopically to quantify yield and purity. Adapted from [28]

[13, 14]. Recent technological advances in gene editing have accelerated the rate at which knockout mutants can be produced [15] and offer opportunities for precision editing to alter just a few residues in a protein, for example. Further biochemical studies on wild type and mutant *Leishmania* flagella thus have the potential to yield new insights into the mechanisms underpinning the diverse functions of this fascinating organelle, which includes motility, cell morphogenesis, attachment to the insect vector and possibly sensory functions [16, 17].

Here we developed a protocol for the isolation of *Leishmania mexicana* promastigote flagella (Fig. 1), optimized to yield intact flagella that retain both the cytoskeletal elements (9 + 2 axoneme and paraflagellar rod (PFR)) and the surrounding membrane, leaving the basal body and transition zone (TZ) in the deflagellated cell body (Fig. 2a). This will enable studies both on the cytoskeletal apparatus driving motility as well as interrogation of surface and membrane-associated molecules and their potential role in adhesion and signalling.

The widespread interest in flagella and cilia produced numerous deciliation/deflagellation protocols for different cells, starting with the first reports of isolating cilia from microorganisms such as

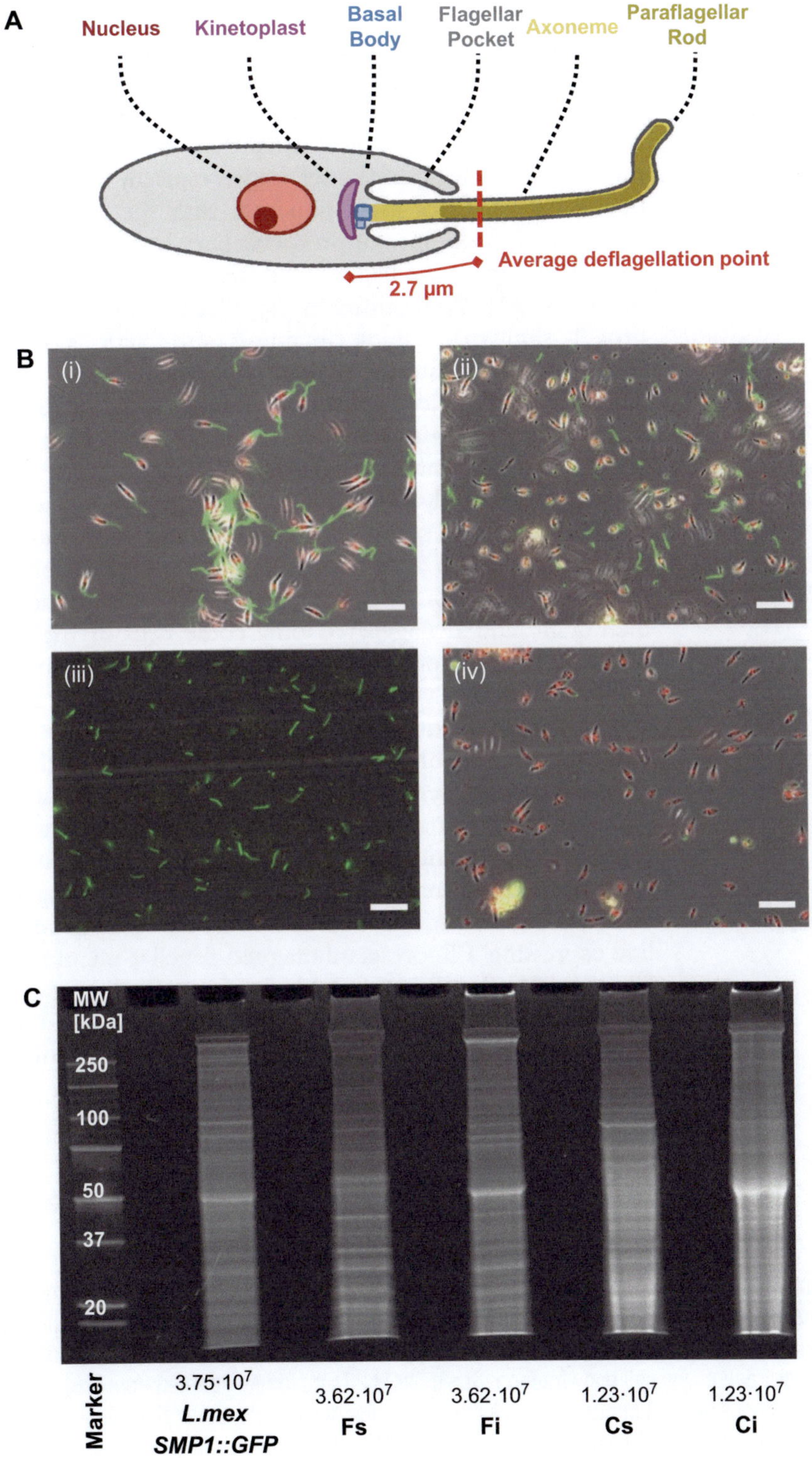

Fig. 2 Expected results. (**a**) Cartoon showing the point where flagella are severed from the cell body. The basal body and proximal part of the flagellum remain attached to the cell body, releasing the external flagellum

Tetrahymena in the 1950s and 60s [18, 19], culminating in an optimized procedure that combined a calcium shock with 2–4 shearings using a 10 ml glass syringe fitted with an 18-G needle [20]. Subsequent work, on the green alga *Chlamydomonas* and other ciliated cells, produced deflagellation methods where separation of the flagella from the cell bodies typically requires application of mechanical force in conjunction with specific chemical treatments [21]. A number of protocols have been used over the years to isolate flagella or flagellar subfractions from trypanosomatids [6, 9, 22–27]. While different flagellar isolation protocols follow broadly similar principles, obtaining pure fractions of the flagellar substructures of interest requires optimization for each cell type and species. For development of the protocol described here, a number of methods based on chemical approaches such as pH shock, ethanol treatment or drugs like dibucaine were tried and found to yield only small quantities of free *L. mexicana* flagella. Ethanol treatment combined with mechanical shearing resulted in cell fixation, while treatment with different dibucaine concentrations, incubation times or mechanical assistance permeabilized the membrane and deflagellated only some cells in the population. Shearing in a Dounce type homogenizer did result in some deflagellated cells but yielded low numbers. Passaging *L. mexicana* promastigotes through a syringe proved the most efficient at detaching the majority of flagella but this stripped the axonemes of their membranes. A combination of syringe disruption and addition of Ca^{2+} finally enabled detachment of the external flagella complete with membrane. The flagella can then be isolated away from the deflagellated cell bodies by gradient centrifugation. Analysis of the cell fractions is facilitated by using an *L. mexicana* cell line expressing a fluorescently tagged flagellar membrane protein. The resulting flagella are suitable for downstream analysis by transmission electron microscopy, protein analysis by SDS-PAGE, western blotting and mass spectrometry [28], and lipidomics.

Fig. 2 (continued) (axoneme, paraflagellar rod, and membrane). (**b**) Composite of phase contrast images and fluorescence signal from Hoechst DNA stain (red) and SMP1::GFP (green) marking the flagellar membrane, taken at different steps of the protocol: (i) whole *L. mexicana* cells before deflagellation, (ii) after deflagellation, (iii) flagellar fraction, (iv) cell body fraction. Scale bar is 20 μm. Image adapted from [28]. (**c**) The flagellar and cell body fractions were separated into 1% octylglucoside soluble (Fs, Cs) and insoluble (Fi, Ci) fractions, separated alongside whole cell lysates (*L. mex* SMP1::GFP) on a 10% polyacrylamide gel and stained with SYPRO Ruby Protein Gel Stain (Molecular Probes). Distinct banding patterns are observed for each fraction. The numbers below the gel picture indicate the cell equivalent for the amount of protein loaded

2 Materials

Follow local rules for safe handling and containment of *Leishmania* spp. and handling and disposal of hazardous chemicals.

2.1 Deflagellation and Density Gradient Centrifugation

1. Phosphate buffered saline (PBS): 137 mM NaCl, 2.6 mM KCl, 8 mM Na_2HPO_4, 1.5 mM KH_2PO_4, pH 7.2. To make a 5x concentrated solution, weigh out 40 g NaCl, 1 g KCl, 7.1 g Na_2HPO_4, and 1.35 g KH_2PO_4 and dissolve in 1 l water. Dilute 1:5 in water to make 1× PBS.
2. 10 mM PIPES (*see* **Note 1**): 10 mM NaCl, 10 mM piperazine-*N*,*N′*-bis(2-ethanesulfonic acid), 1 mM $CaCl_2$, 1 mM $MgCl_2$, 0.32 M sucrose, adjusted to pH 7.2. Add 500 ml dH_2O to a 1 l glass bottle and add 10 solid NaOH pellets while stirring. When the pellets have dissolved add 3 g PIPES, 0.22 g $CaCl_2 \cdot 6H_2O$, 0.2 g $MgCl_2 \cdot 6H_2O$, and 0.58 g NaCl. Titrate to pH 7.2 while mixing, using 1 M NaOH solution. Add 109.44 g sucrose to this solution. Keep mixing until completely dissolved and fill up to 1 l with dH_2O.
3. 166 mM PIPES: 166 mM NaCl, 166 mM piperazine-*N*,*N′*-bis (2-ethanesulfonic acid), 16.6 mM $CaCl_2$, 16.6 mM $MgCl_2$, adjusted to pH 7.2. Prepare as indicated for 10 mM PIPES, but omitting the sucrose.
4. 1 M Ca^{2+} solution.
5. 2 M sucrose solution.
6. 5 mM E-64: dissolve 5 mg in 2920 μl DMSO.
7. 20 mM Leupeptin hydrochloride: dissolve 5 mg in 525 μl ddH_2O.
8. 3 mM Pepstatin A: dissolve 5 mg in 2425 μl 100% ethanol and incubate for 1 h at 60 °C.
9. 200 mM Phenylmethylsulfonyl fluoride (PMSF): dissolve 100 mg in 2850 μl 100% methanol.
10. 1000× Hoechst: Dissolve 100 mg Hoechst 33342 in 10 ml dH_2O (10 mg/ml stock). Protect tube from light and keep under agitation overnight until completely dissolved.
11. Equipment and consumables: 200 μl plastic gel loading pipette tip (Starlab) (*see* **Note 2**), 10 ml disposable syringe, hemocytometer (*see* **Note 3**), microcentrifuge, benchtop centrifuge, ultracentrifuge and ultracentrifugation tubes, phase contrast microscope, fluorescence microscope.

3 Methods

An overview of the workflow is shown in Fig. 1.

3.1 Preparing Cells

1. Use an exponentially growing *Leishmania* promastigote culture (*see* **Notes 4** and **5**) to set up a 200 ml culture starting with 1×10^6 cells/ml, then grow for ~24 h until there are 1×10^7 cells/ml.
2. Decant culture into four 50 ml Falcon centrifuge tubes and collect 2×10^9 cells by centrifugation at $800 \times g$ for 15 min at 4 °C.
3. For all following steps, keep samples at 4 °C and cool buffers on ice before adding to samples.
4. Discard supernatant and combine the four cell pellets by resuspending in a total of 20 ml PBS and centrifuge as above.
5. Discard the supernatant and resuspended the cells in 5 ml 10 mM PIPES.
6. Place 8 μl cell suspension on a microscope slide and add a small volume of 1000× Hoechst stock (*see* **Note 6**). Examine sample on a fluorescence microscope (Fig. 2b).

3.2 Deflagellation

1. Add 0.375 ml of 1 M Ca^{2+} solution (final conc. 0.075 M) and protease inhibitors (12.5 μl Leupeptin, 12.5 μl PMSF, 12.5 μl Pepstatin A, and 5 μl E-64) to the cell suspension.
2. Attach a 200 μl gel loading pipette tip to a 10 ml disposable syringe.
3. Deflagellate cells by repeatedly drawing the cell suspension through the gel loading tip into the syringe and pushing out again. Perform this a total of 100 times until flagella are sheared from the *Leishmania* cell bodies (*see* **Note 7**).
4. Make a 1:2 dilution of the sample by mixing 10 μl sample with 10 μl 10 mM PIPES and then dilute again 1:25 (1:50 dilution of the sample). Add 10 μl of the 1:50 dilution of the sample onto a hemocytometer and quantify the number of flagella and cell bodies and the percentage of deflagellated cells in a 0.1 μl square with a phase contrast microscope (Fig. 2b).
5. If tagged cells are used, place 7 μl of the 1:2 sample dilution on a glass microscope slide, add a small volume of 1000× Hoechst (*see* **Note 6**) and examine sample on a fluorescence microscope to quantify the percentage of flagella retaining their membrane (Fig. 2b).

Table 1
Preparation of sucrose density gradient

Sucrose (%)	V [ml] 2 M sucrose	V [ml] ddH_2O	V [ml] 0.166 M PIPES pH 7.2
33	1.446	1.374	0.18
53	2.323	0.497	0.18
63	2.761	0.059	0.18

3.3 Separation of Flagella and Deflagellated Cell Bodies

Flagella and cell bodies are separated through density gradient centrifugation, using a modified version of the protocol in [9].

1. Prepare one 9 ml sucrose-bed containing three layers of 10 mM PIPES with 33% (upper), 53% (middle) and 63% (bottom) (w/v) sucrose: Mix the ingredients listed in Table 1 for each sucrose concentration. Place the 63% sucrose solution in a 15 ml Falcon tube, then carefully layer the 53% and the 33% sucrose solutions on top.
2. Carefully place the sample (from Subheading 3.2 above) on top of the sucrose-bed. Take care not to mix the layers.
3. Centrifuge at 800 × *g* for 15 min at 4 °C.
4. Prepare another 33% sucrose layer (as specified in Table 1) and pipette in a 15 ml Falcon tube.
5. Collect the top layer of the first sucrose-bed (~4.5 ml, flagella fraction) and place it on top of the 33% sucrose layer (from **step 4** above).
6. Discard the other sucrose layers, which contain a mixture of flagella and cell bodies (*see* **Note 8**).
7. Resuspend the pellet in the 63% sucrose layer in 10 ml 10 mM PIPES (contains the deflagellated cell bodies (*see* **Note 9**)) and keep on ice.
8. Centrifuge both the second sucrose-bed with the flagella fraction and the resuspended pellet (cell body fraction) at 800 × *g* for 10 min at 4 °C.
9. Discard the supernatant from the cell body fraction and add 20 μl 10 mM PIPES to the pellet. With remnants from the supernatant the final volume should be ~40 μl.
10. Transfer 36.5 μl of this fraction to a 0.5 ml Eppendorf tube and keep on ice.
11. Transfer the top layer of the flagella fraction to a 3.5 ml ultracentrifugation tube.
12. Discard the remainder of the second sucrose bed.
13. Centrifuge the flagella fraction at 100,000 × *g* for 1 h at 4 °C.

14. Discard the supernatant and resuspend the pellet containing the isolated flagella in 10 mM PIPES, adding PIPES in small volumes so that the final volume is exactly 36.5 μl.
15. Remove 0.5 μl from the flagella fraction and dilute with 10 mM PIPES (first 1:40 and then 1:25, to a final dilution of 1:1000). Use the 1:000 dilution to determine the yield and purity (*see* **Note 10**) by counting on a hemocytometer and if a tagged cell line was used, use the 1:40 dilution to determine the proportion of flagella with retained membrane using a fluorescence microscope (Fig. 2b).
16. Remove 0.5 μl from the final cell body fraction and analyze as for the flagella fraction (**step 15** above; Fig. 2b).
17. The isolated flagella and cell bodies can then be used for protein mass spectrometry, further biochemical fractionation (Fig. 2c) (*see* **Note 11**) or light and transmission electron microscopy (*see* **Note 12**).

4 Notes

1. PIPES buffer is used to prepare samples compatible with glutaraldehyde fixation for transmission electron microscopy analysis. An alternative buffer that works for the deflagellation protocol (but is not compatible with glutaraldehyde fixation because it contains Tris) is STC isotonic buffer (0.32 M sucrose containing 0.03 M Tris pH 7.2, 0.001 M $CaCl_2$). The addition of Ca^{2+} to the deflagellation buffer precludes resuspending samples in PBS as we noted a phosphate precipitation.
2. Plastic gel loading tips are used instead of syringe needles for safety reasons to avoid the possibility of needlestick injuries. The tips used in this protocol had an inner diameter of ~0.35 mm, which corresponds to a 23 gauge needle.
3. For counting of live *Leishmania*, we recommend using disposable hemocytometers such as "C-Chip" Digital Bio, Neubauer Improved DMC-N01 for safety reasons.
4. The density and health of the *Leishmania* culture at the start before homogenization are crucial to ensure a high yield.
5. This protocol can be used with *Leishmania* wild-type promastigotes or with a cell line that expresses fluorescently tagged proteins marking subcellular structures of interest. Expression of the small myristoylated protein 1 (SMP1 [29]; LmxM.20.1310) fused to a fluorescent protein at the C-terminus (e.g., SMP1::GFP) allows monitoring of the presence of the flagellar membrane throughout the isolation procedure. Tagged cell lines can be generated by transgene expression from an episome [30], using CRISPR-Cas9 tagging [15] or Fusion PCR tagging [31].

6. To achieve this, use a P10 pipette with tip and set pipette to 1 μl. Pipette Hoechst 1000× stock solution in and out. Using the same pipette tip, pipette 8 μl cell suspension on the microscope slide up and down.
7. The number of passages is optimized to yield a sample where >99% of all cells are deflagellated.
8. Attempts to purify this layer further to increase the flagellar yield resulted in flagella without attached membrane.
9. The sucrose bed exhibits different gradient properties when using PIPES or a Tris-based buffer (STC). While a clear a pellet is visible in the 63% layer of the PIPES sucrose-bed, this is not obvious for Tris sucrose-beds. Therefore, when using STC (*see* **Note 1**), take both the 53% and 63% layer and dilute to 15 ml with STC to recover cell bodies from the Tris sucrose-bed.
10. This protocol is optimized for high purity of isolated flagella. Expect a yield of ca. 2×10^8 flagella (about 10% of the starting material).
11. For protein analysis (e.g., mass spectrometry or Western blots) supplement cell body and flagellar fractions with 4 μl prediluted protease inhibitor cocktail (1 μl Leupeptin (1:10 dilution of stock), 1 μl PMSF (1:10 dilution of stock), 1 μl Pepstatin A (1:10 dilution of stock) and 1 μl E-64 (1:25 dilution of stock)). Samples can then be subjected to further fractionation (e.g., separation into detergent-soluble and insoluble components by extraction with 1% octylglucoside [28]). Samples should be resuspended in suitable sample buffer (e.g., Laemmli buffer) and these samples can be stored at −80 °C.
12. For transmission electron microscopy, collect cell fractions by centrifugation (flagellar fraction: 30 min at 18,500 × *g*; cell body fraction: 15 min, 800 × *g*) and fix by overlaying pellets with 500 μl 10 mM PIPES containing 2.5% (v/v) glutaraldehyde overnight at 4 °C. Prepare samples for transmission electron microscopy using the chemical fixation protocol described in [32].

Funding Statement

T.B. was supported by a Medical Research Council PhD studentship (15/16_MSD_836338) and an Erasmus grant, F.D. was supported by an Erasmus grant, R.W. is a Sir Henry Dale Fellow, supported by Wellcome Trust grant 211,075/Z/18/Z, and E.G. is a Royal Society University Research Fellow.

References

1. Hilgendorf KI, Johnson CT, Jackson PK (2016) The primary cilium as a cellular receiver: organizing ciliary GPCR signaling. Curr Opin Cell Biol 39:84–92. https://doi.org/10.1016/j.ceb.2016.02.008
2. Ostrowski LE, Blackburn K, Radde KM, Moyer MB, Schlatzer DM, Moseley A, Boucher RC (2002) A proteomic analysis of human cilia: identification of novel components. Mol Cell Proteomics 1(6):451–465
3. Pazour GJ, Agrin N, Leszyk J, Witman GB (2005) Proteomic analysis of a eukaryotic cilium. J Cell Biol 170(1):103–113. https://doi.org/10.1083/jcb.200504008
4. Ishikawa H, Thompson J, Yates JR 3rd, Marshall WF (2012) Proteomic analysis of mammalian primary cilia. Curr Biol 22(5):414–419. https://doi.org/10.1016/j.cub.2012.01.031
5. Amaral A, Castillo J, Estanyol JM, Ballesca JL, Ramalho-Santos J, Oliva R (2013) Human sperm tail proteome suggests new endogenous metabolic pathways. Mol Cell Proteomics 12 (2):330–342. https://doi.org/10.1074/mcp.M112.020552
6. Broadhead R, Dawe HR, Farr H, Griffiths S, Hart SR, Portman N, Shaw MK, Ginger ML, Gaskell SJ, McKean PG, Gull K (2006) Flagellar motility is required for the viability of the bloodstream trypanosome. Nature 440 (7081):224–227. https://doi.org/10.1038/nature04541. nature04541 [pii]
7. Subota I, Julkowska D, Vincensini L, Reeg N, Buisson J, Blisnick T, Huet D, Perrot S, Santi-Rocca J, Duchateau M, Hourdel V, Rousselle JC, Cayet N, Namane A, Chamot-Rooke J, Bastin P (2014) Proteomic analysis of intact flagella of procyclic *Trypanosoma brucei* cells identifies novel flagellar proteins with unique sub-localization and dynamics. Mol Cell Proteomics 13(7):1769–1786. https://doi.org/10.1074/mcp.M113.033357
8. Dupe A, Dumas C, Papadopoulou B (2015) Differential subcellular localization of *Leishmania* Alba-domain proteins throughout the parasite development. PLoS One 10(9): e0137243. https://doi.org/10.1371/journal.pone.0137243
9. Oberholzer M, Langousis G, Nguyen HT, Saada EA, Shimogawa MM, Jonsson ZO, Nguyen SM, Wohlschlegel JA, Hill KL (2011) Independent analysis of the flagellum surface and matrix proteomes provides insight into flagellum signaling in mammalian-infectious *Trypanosoma brucei*. Mol Cell Proteomics 10(10): M111 010538. https://doi.org/10.1074/mcp.M111.010538. M111.010538 [pii]
10. van Dam TJ, Wheway G, Slaats GG, Huynen MA, Giles RH (2013) The SYSCILIA gold standard (SCGSv1) of known ciliary components and its applications within a systems biology consortium. Cilia 2(1):7. https://doi.org/10.1186/2046-2530-2-7
11. Lindemann CB, Lesich KA (2010) Flagellar and ciliary beating: the proven and the possible. J Cell Sci 123(Pt 4):519–528. https://doi.org/10.1242/jcs.051326
12. Satir P, Heuser T, Sale WS (2014) A structural basis for how motile cilia beat. Bioscience 64 (12):1073–1083. https://doi.org/10.1093/biosci/biu180
13. Ishikawa T (2015) Cryo-electron tomography of motile cilia and flagella. Cilia 4(1):3. https://doi.org/10.1186/s13630-014-0012-7
14. Lin J, Nicastro D (2018) Asymmetric distribution and spatial switching of dynein activity generates ciliary motility. Science 360(6387). https://doi.org/10.1126/science.aar1968
15. Beneke T, Madden R, Makin L, Valli J, Sunter J, Gluenz E (2017) A CRISPR Cas9 high-throughput genome editing toolkit for kinetoplastids. R Soc Open Sci 4(5):170095. https://doi.org/10.1098/rsos.170095
16. Landfear SM, Tran KD, Sanchez MA (2015) Flagellar membrane proteins in kinetoplastid parasites. IUBMB Life 67(9):668–676. https://doi.org/10.1002/iub.1411
17. Saada EA, Kabututu ZP, Lopez M, Shimogawa MM, Langousis G, Oberholzer M, Riestra A, Jonsson ZO, Wohlschlegel JA, Hill KL (2014) Insect stage-specific receptor adenylate cyclases are localized to distinct subdomains of the *Trypanosoma brucei* flagellar membrane. Eukaryot Cell 13(8):1064–1076. https://doi.org/10.1128/EC.00019-14
18. Child FM (1959) The characterization of the cilia of Tetrahymena pyriformis. Exp Cell Res 18:258–267
19. Watson MR, Hopkins JM (1962) Isolated cilia from Tetrahymena pyriformis. Exp Cell Res 28:280–295
20. Rosenbaum JL, Carlson K (1969) Cilia regeneration in *Tetrahymena* and its inhibition by colchicine. J Cell Biol 40(2):415–425
21. Craige B, Brown JM, Witman GB (2013) Isolation of *Chlamydomonas* flagella. Curr Protoc Cell Biol 3(41):41–49. https://doi.org/10.1002/0471143030.cb0341s59
22. Pereira NM, de Souza W, Machado RD, de Castro FT (1977) Isolation and properties of

flagella of trypanosomatids. J Protozool 24 (4):511–514

23. Segura EL, Vazquez C, Bronzina A, Campos JM, Cerisola JA, Cappa SM (1977) Antigens of the subcellular fractions of *Trypanosoma cruzi*. II. Flagellar and membrane fraction. J Protozool 24(4):540–543

24. Piras MM, De Rodriguez OO, Piras R (1981) *Trypanosoma cruzi*: antigenic composition of axonemes and flagellar membranes of epimastigotes cultured in vitro. Exp Parasitol 51 (1):59–73

25. da Cunha e Silva NL, Hasson-Voloch A, de Souza W (1989) Isolation and characterization of a highly purified flagellar membrane fraction from trypanosomatids. Mol Biochem Parasitol 37(1):129–136

26. Ismach R, Cianci CM, Caulfield JP, Langer PJ, Hein A, McMahon-Pratt D (1989) Flagellar membrane and paraxial rod proteins of *Leishmania*: characterization employing monoclonal antibodies. J Protozool 36(6):617–624

27. Warburg A, Tesh RB, McMahon-Pratt D (1989) Studies on the attachment of *Leishmania* flagella to sand fly midgut epithelium. J Protozool 36(6):613–617

28. Beneke T, Demay F, Hookway E, Ashman N, Jeffery H, Smith J, Valli J, Becvar T, Myskova T, Lestinova T, Shafiq S, Sadlova J, Volf P, Wheeler RJ, Gluenz E (2018) Genetic dissection of a *Leishmania* flagellar proteome demonstrates requirement for directional motility in sand fly infections. bioRxiv:476994. https://doi.org/10.1101/476994

29. Tull D, Vince JE, Callaghan JM, Naderer T, Spurck T, McFadden GI, Currie G, Ferguson K, Bacic A, McConville MJ (2004) SMP-1, a member of a new family of small myristoylated proteins in kinetoplastid parasites, is targeted to the flagellum membrane in *Leishmania*. Mol Biol Cell 15(11):4775–4786. https://doi.org/10.1091/mbc.E04-06-0457

30. Tetaud E, Lecuix I, Sheldrake T, Baltz T, Fairlamb AH (2002) A new expression vector for *Crithidia fasciculata* and *Leishmania*. Mol Biochem Parasitol 120(2):195–204

31. Dean S, Sunter J, Wheeler RJ, Hodkinson I, Gluenz E, Gull K (2015) A toolkit enabling efficient, scalable and reproducible gene tagging in trypanosomatids. Open Biol 5 (1):140197. https://doi.org/10.1098/rsob.140197

32. Hoog JL, Gluenz E, Vaughan S, Gull K (2010) Ultrastructural investigation methods for *Trypanosoma brucei*. Methods Cell Biol 96:175–196. https://doi.org/10.1016/S0091-679X(10)96008-1

Chapter 30

Gel-Based Methods for the Investigation of Signal Transduction Pathways in *Trypanosoma brucei*

Balázs Szöőr and Mathieu Cayla

Abstract

In the cell, reversible phosphorylation, controlled by protein phosphatases and protein kinases, initiates and regulates various signaling-dependent processes such as enzyme–substrate interactions, the cell cycle, differentiation, and immune responses. In addition to these processes, in unicellular parasites like *Trypanosoma brucei*, the causative agent of African sleeping sickness, additional signaling pathways have evolved to enable the survival of parasites in the changing environment of the vector and mammalian host. In this chapter, we describe two in vitro kinase assays and the use of the phosphoprotein chelator Phos-tag and show that these three polyacrylamide gel-based assays can be used for rapid target validation and detection of changes in phosphorylation.

Key words Signal transduction, Protein kinases, Protein phosphatases, Phospho substrate, Kinase assays, SDS-PAGE, Phos-tag

1 Introduction

Investigations of signal transduction pathways can be challenging in the trypanosome field due to the early divergence of these organisms from other eukaryotic lineages that may have resulted in the evolution of unique mechanisms and components. One of the main regulatory mechanisms of signaling events is the regulation of the phosphorylation states of the components involved. Two families of antagonistic enzymes are responsible for such regulation, that is, protein kinases that transfer the γ-phosphate of ATP molecules on the substrate acceptor residues and protein phosphatases that are responsible for the dephosphorylation of these proteins. Based on their analysis of the human phosphoproteome, in which 50,000 distinct phosphopeptides were detected, Sharma et al. [1] have revealed that at least 75% of the proteome is phosphorylated. In kinetoplastids, recent phosphoproteomic studies identified

Balázs Szöőr and Mathieu Cayla contributed equally to this work.

Paul A. M. Michels et al. (eds.), *Trypanosomatids: Methods and Protocols*, Methods in Molecular Biology, vol. 2116,
https://doi.org/10.1007/978-1-0716-0294-2_30, © The Author(s) 2020

thousands of phosphosites [2–4], suggesting important roles for kinases and phosphatases regulating various signaling networks in these parasites.

Several high-throughput quantitative methods have been developed and are being used to study changes in phosphorylation (reviewed in [5]). However, there are cases when low cost, rapid, semiquantitative methods can be useful as the first step to identify a phosphosubstrate or the phosphorylation state of a target protein or to manually validate hits obtained by high-throughput technologies. Unfortunately, various phospho stains and commercial antibodies against phosphorylated S/T/Y residues of many signaling molecules cannot always be used on trypanosome cell lysates, for example, because of high background signal and low reproducibility.

Understanding the mode of regulation of kinases and phosphatases, as well as identifying their substrates, is therefore essential to unravel signaling pathways in trypanosomes. We here present a series of methods that can be easily implemented in any laboratory and used to determine the activity of protein kinases and phosphatases.

Kinases are often expressed at low level to facilitate the regulation of these important enzymes, rendering their purification from a physiologically relevant system, such as the parasite itself, potentially challenging. Commonly, bacterial systems are used to express proteins at a high level. However, the main weakness of these expression systems appears when researchers need an active enzyme because often *Escherichia coli* (and other prokaryote expression systems) cannot be used to produce active kinase, for example, due to the lack of eukaryotic posttranscriptional modifications. To overcome this limitation, we describe the use of an insect expression system to produce active trypanosome enzyme and, in combination with site-directed mutagenesis, to generate mutated versions of the kinase.

We also describe two in vitro kinase assays to identify a generic substrate that could be used for a structure/function analysis of different mutant versions of the kinase expressed. In the first instance, we recommend to use the "Cold" in vitro kinase assay with a modified ATP containing a substitution of the terminal oxygen of the γ-phosphate with a sulfur, based on the approach developed by Allen et al. [6]. This modified γ-phosphate is transferred to the substrate, and after an alkylation step, the modified substrate can be detected by a western blot probed with a commercially available antibody recognizing thiophosphate. If a stronger signal is required, we also describe an alternative approach that uses classical radioactive ATP, labeled on the γ-phosphate by the ^{32}P isotope. This method is also based on the migration of the phosphorylated substrates on SDS-PAGE and their transfer onto PVDF membrane. The activity for this "Hot" kinase assay is detected on

X-ray sensitive film and the excised bands corresponding to the substrates quantified by a scintillation counter. The advantages of these two kinase assays are that they are both based on the use of western blots that allow the detection of any other proteins of interest with corresponding antibodies, even when expressed at low level.

As a last gel-based method and as the first step to analyze changes in phosphorylation in *Trypanosoma brucei* cell lysates, we also describe Mn^{2+}-Phos-tag SDS-PAGE [7]. This method avoids the use of radioactive or chemical labels and is based on the Phos-tag molecule (1,3-bis[bis(pyridin-2-ylmethyl)amino]propan-2-olato dizinc(II) complex). This acts as a chelator in the presence of two divalent metal ions (preferably Mn^{2+} and Zn^{2+}) and binds specifically the phosphate monoester group regardless of the amino acid sequence context, such that it is equally potent in the detection of phosphorylation of Ser/Thr/Tyr. The other advantage of the method is that it uses conditions almost identical to standard SDS-PAGE conditions and can be combined with western blotting to investigate protein phosphorylation following electrophoresis. When Phos-tag (and Mn^{2+}) is added to the separating gel, it binds to the phosphoproteins and slows their migration with respect to unbound nonphosphorylated proteins, enabling separation of phosphorylated and nonphosphorylated molecules. Phosphoprotein isotypes can be also detected as multiple bands, with differential migration in the same lane, when Phos-tag SDS-PAGE is followed by western blotting and antibodies are used to detect the target protein.

2 Materials

2.1 PCR/Mutagenesis

- M13 Forward primer (-40) (TGTAAAACGACGGCCAGT).
- M13 Reverse primer (CAGGAAACAGCTATGACC).
- Site-directed mutagenesis Forward and Reverse primers.
- Taq DNA polymerase kit, NEB.
- Phusion DNA polymerase kit, Invitrogen.
- Gene of interest cloned in the desired intermediate plasmid backbone.
- pFastBac™.
- 200 μL PCR tubes.
- dNTPs 10 mM.
- DMSO.
- DpnI restriction enzyme.
- Nucleases-free water.

- Agarose gel at desired percentage, containing the DNA specific dye of your choice (e.g., ethidium bromide, SYBR Safe).
- Appropriate DNA ladder.
- TAE 10× buffer (use at 1×): 400 mM Tris-base, 200 mM acetic acid, 10 mM EDTA, solution adjusted at pH 7.6.
- Thermocycler (e.g., TProfessional Basic gradient PCR Thermocycler).
- Power supply.

2.2 Bacterial Transformation/Culture

- Your purified pFastBac™ construct (200 pg/μL in TE buffer: 10 mM Tris–HCl, pH 8, 1 mM EDTA).
- Positive expression control (i.e., pFastBac™1-Gus, used as a control for transposition).
- MAX Efficiency® E. coli DH10Bac™ chemically competent cells.
- *E. coli* XL1-Blue competent cells.
- LB agar plates containing 50 μg/mL kanamycin, 7 μg/mL gentamicin, 10 μg/mL tetracycline, 100 μg/mL Bluo-gal, and 40 μg/mL IPTG to select for DH10Bac™ transformants.
- LB agar plates containing 50 μg/mL ampicillin.
- LB liquid medium (using same antibiotic concentration as for the plates when required).
- Super Optimal broth with Catabolite repression (SOC) Medium, Invitrogen.
- 42 °C water bath.
- 37 °C shaking and nonshaking incubator.

2.3 Insect Cell Culture/Infection/Pulldown

- Sf9 cells.
- Sf-900 II serum-free medium (SFM) supplemented with 50 units/mL penicillin and 50 μg/mL streptomycin (final concentration).
- Grace's Medium.
- Cellfectin® Reagent.
- Purified bacmid.
- 0.2 μm filter (low protein binding).
- Fetal bovine serum.
- Radioimmunoprecipitation assay (RIPA) lysis buffer: 25 mM Tris–HCl, pH 7–8, 150 mM NaCl, 0.1% SDS, 0.5% sodium deoxycholate, 1% Triton X-100, protease inhibitor cocktail.
- Dynabeads™ Protein G–coupled magnetic beads, Invitrogen.
- Purification magnet.

- Elution buffer: 100 μL 25 mM Tris–HCl, pH 7.4 and 10% glycerol.
- 15 and 50 mL Falcon tubes.
- Eppendorf tubes.
- Centrifuges (benchtop mini centrifuge for 1.5 mL tubes and centrifuge suitable for 15 and 50 mL tubes).
- Vortex.
- 200 and 500 mL glass bottles (Autoclaved).
- 6-well culture plates.
- 27 °C humidified incubator.
- 27 °C shaking incubator.

2.4 Kinase Assay

- MOPS kinase buffer 1×: 50 mM MOPS (3-(*N*-morpholino) propanesulfonic acid) adjusted at pH 7.5, 100 mM NaCl, 10 mM $MgCl_2$, 10 mM $MnCl_2$.
- 50 mM PNBM (*p*-nitrobenzyl mesylate) in DMSO [6].
- 10 mM (ATP)-γ-S in distilled water (ddH_2O) [6].
- 250 μCi of 1 mCi [γ-^{32}P]-ATP (3000 Ci/mmol).
- Dephosphorylated MBP (myelin basic protein).
- Histone H1.
- Histone cores H2A, H2B, H3, H4.
- Dephosphorylated casein.
- ß-Casein.
- Recombinant *Mus musculus* caspase 9 (Casp9, first 200 amino acids).
- X-ray film developer.
- X-ray film.
- Scintillation counter.
- Scintillation vials.

2.5 Phos-Tag Assay

2.5.1 Sample Preparation

- *Trypanosoma brucei* cell lines: pleomorphic *Trypanosoma brucei* EATRO 1125 AnTat1.1 90:13 (TETR T7POL NEO HYG) [8] or double marker 29-13 procyclic form [9] trypanosomes, cultured in vitro in HMI-9 [10] medium at 37 °C under 5% CO_2 or in SDM-79 [11] medium at 27 °C, respectively.
- PBS (phosphate-buffered saline): 137 mM NaCl, 3 mM KCl, 16 mM Na_2HPO_4, 3 mM KH_2PO_4, pH 7.6.
- 50 mL Falcon tubes.
- Centrifuge capable of centrifuging 50 mL Falcon tubes at 1500 × *g*.

- Tabletop centrifuge capable of centrifuging 1.5 mL Eppendorf tubes and reaching 6200 × *g*.
- 1.5 mL Eppendorf tubes.
- Laemmli 6× sample buffer: 62.5 mM Tris–HCl, pH 6.8, 2% SDS, 10% glycerol, bromophenol blue, add β-mercaptoethanol (5%) immediately prior to use (50 μL in 1 mL).

2.6 SDS-PAGE and Western Blot

2.6.1 General

- Laemmli 6× sample buffer.
- Appropriate prestained and unstained protein ladders.
- ddH_2O.
- Transfer buffer 10×: 250 mM Tris–HCl, 1.92 M glycine (1×: 25 mM Tris–HCl, 192 mM glycine + 20% methanol).
- Methanol.
- Odyssey® Blocking buffer, Li-COR.
- TBS (Tris-buffered saline): 50 mM Tris–HCl, pH 7.5, 150 mM NaCl.
- Whatman 3MM Chr Chromatography Paper (GE Healthcare).
- Secondary antibodies conjugated to fluorescent dyes (i.e., secondary antibody: IRDye® 800CW Goat anti-Mouse IgG (H + L) (Li-COR Biosciences product n°: 926-32210, in 1:7000 dilution), anti-rabbit red IRDye® 680RD Goat anti-Mouse IgG (H + L) (Li-COR Biosciences product n°: 925-68070, in 1:7000 dilution)).
- Polyvinylidene difluoride membrane (PVDF, Immobilon-P, Millipore).
- SYPRO Ruby stain.
- SYPRO fixing solution: 7% acetic acid, 50% methanol.
- SYPRO destaining solution: 7% acetic acid, 10% methanol.
- Ponceau S stain: 0.4% Ponceau S and 3% trichloroacetic acid.
- Microwave oven.
- Typhoon scanner, GE Healthcare (or any other fluorescent/UV gel imager system).
- Li-COR Odyssey® imager system (or any other fluorescent western blot imager system).
- Power supply.
- Protein gel electrophoresis chamber system.
- Mini Trans-Blot apparatus (Bio-Rad).
- Icepack.
- Rocking table.

2.6.2 Kinase Assays

- NuPAGE® Bis-Tris polyacrylamide gradient gels 4–12% (ThermoFischer Scientific).
- NuPAGE® MES 20× running buffer (ThermoFischer Scientific).
- TBS 0.1% Tween: TBS + 0.1% Tween.
- The primary antibodies αBB2 (1:5, [12]); αGST (1:1000); αThioP (1:1000, Anti-Thiophosphate ester clone 51-8, Abcam).

2.6.3 Phos-Tag Aassay

- 5 mM Phos-tag™ Acrylamide AAL-107 aqueous solution 0.3 mL manufactured by Wako Nard Institute and distributed by Alpha Laboratories.
- 10 mM $MnCl_2$ stock solution.
- Separating gel buffer: 1.5 M Tris–HCl, pH 8.8, 0.4% SDS.
- Stacking gel buffer: 0.5 M Tris–HCl, pH 6.8, 0.4% SDS.
- 30% w/v acrylamide/bisacrylamide ratio 37.5:1.
- 10% ammonium persulfate (APS).
- *N′*,*N*,*N*,*N′*-Tetramethylethylene-diamine (TEMED).
- Bio-Rad PROTEAN II apparatus (glass plates, combs, casting stand, clamps).
- Running buffer 10× (use 1×): 1.92 M glycine 0.25 M Tris–HCl, pH 8.3.
- TBS 0.05% Tween: TBS + 0.05% Tween.
- Li-COR Block 50% Odyssey® block (Li-COR Biosciences) in TBS.

  Primary antibodies: anti-rabbit *Tb*PGKC (Tb927.1.700, 47 kDa, 1:75,000 dilution), anti-rabbit *Tb*PEX14 (Tb927.10.240, 39.9 kDa, 1:10,000 dilution), anti-rabbit *Tb*PIP39 (Tb927.9.6090, 39 kDa, 1:750 dilution), anti-mouse *Tb*TAT (Tb927.1.2340, 49.7 kDa, 1:5000 dilution).

Pretransfer treatment

- Appropriate containers.
- ddH_2O.
- 2 mM EDTA.

3 Methods

3.1 Site-Directed Mutagenesis

- The principle of this method is to introduce point mutations inside the gene of interest. To do so, two complementary primers are designed, integrating the point mutation in the middle of their sequences. For the design of those primers, we advise to use the QuickChange primer design tool from Agilent (https://www.agilent.com/store/primerDesignProgram.jsp), which is a user-friendly interface that gives good results.

– The PCR-based reaction could be done from the final plasmid but would require full sequencing to ensure that no other mutations have been introduced. Therefore, we would advise to perform the reaction on an intermediate plasmid before the final cloning as this would only require validation sequencing of the mutated gene of interest.

3.1.1 PCR and DpnI Digestion

1. The PCR-based reaction is performed under the following conditions (*see* **Note 1**):

5× HF buffer (GC rich)	4 μL
DNA (50 ng)	*x* μL
Primer Fwd (10 μM)	1 μL
Primer Rev (10 μM)	1 μL
dNTP (10 mM)	0.4 μL
DMSO (3% final)	0.6 μL
H_2O (up to 20 μL)	*y* μL
Phusion DNA polymerase	0.2 μL

98 °C	2 min	
98 °C 60 °C 72 °C	10 s 30 s 10 min	18 cycles
72 °C	10 min	

2. After the PCR reaction, add 20 units of DpnI to the 20 μL PCR reaction and incubate at 37 °C for 1 h to digest the parental (i.e., nonmutated) methylated DNA (*see* **Note 2**).

3.1.2 Bacterial Transformation

1. Gently thaw the *E. coli* XL1 Blue cells on ice. For each sample reaction to be transformed, aliquot 100 μL of the competent cells into an Eppendorf tube.
2. Swirl the contents of the tube gently. Incubate the cells on ice for 10 min, swirling gently every 2 min.
3. Transfer 5 μL of the DpnI-treated PCR reaction product from each sample reaction into separate aliquots of competent cells.

4. Swirl the transformation reactions gently to mix and incubate the reactions on ice for 30 min.
5. Heat-pulse the tubes in a 42 °C water bath for 45 s.
6. Incubate the tubes on ice for 2 min.
7. Add 0.5 mL of LB broth or SOC medium to each tube, then incubate the tubes at 37 °C for at least 1 h, with shaking at 225–250 rpm.
8. Centrifuge the culture, discard the supernatant, resuspend the pellet in 100 μL of LB, and plate all of each transformation reaction on agar plates, containing the appropriate antibiotic for selection of the plasmid vector.
9. Leave the plates in a 37 °C incubator overnight.
10. On the next morning, select colonies and grow them for at least 5 h in LB medium containing the appropriate drug selection.
11. Extract the plasmid DNA with the protocol of your choice.
12. The desired mutation and the integrity of the rest of the gene should be assessed by sequencing.

3.2 SF9 Insect Cells Expression System

- The expression of protein kinases and phosphatases in insect cells requires several steps, including the generation of the bacmid that will allow the infection of the insect cells. After the first step of infection has been performed, the virus needs to be amplified to obtain a sufficient titer for the subsequent infection, necessary for protein expression. The last step of the process consists of cell lysis and the pulldown of the target protein using the method of choice. Here, we describe the purification of proteins tagged with the combination of a TY1-epitope tag and YFP tag, to allow rapid screening of infected cells and the production and effective purification of expressed protein using the anti-TY1 BB2 antibody and magnetic Protein G-coupled Dynabeads.
- A comprehensive and extended protocol, including troubleshooting, of the insect cell expression system can be found at: http://tools.thermofisher.com/content/sfs/manuals/bactobac_man.pdf. Therefore, we only briefly describe the different steps.

3.2.1 Transformation

1. Proceed to the transformation of the DH10Bac™ cells as described earlier, using 100 ng of the pFastBac™ constructs.

2. After the heat-shock and the addition of LB or SOC medium, allow the cells to grow for 4 h at 37 °C, with shaking at 225–250 rpm.
3. For each pFastBac™ transformation, prepare tenfold serial dilutions of the cells (10^{-1}, 10^{-2}, 10^{-3}) with LB or SOC medium. Plate 100 μL of each dilution on a LB agar plate containing the three selective antibiotics, Bluo-gal, and IPTG.
4. Incubate the plates for 48 h at 37 °C.
5. Pick ten white colonies and re-streak them on fresh LB agar plates containing the three selective antibiotics, Bluo-gal and IPTG. Incubate the plates overnight at 37 °C.
6. The colonies for which the white phenotype is confirmed are then inoculated in liquid culture containing 50 μg/mL kanamycin, 7 μg/mL gentamicin, and 10 μg/mL tetracycline, followed by overnight culture at 37 °C.
7. Recombinant bacmid DNA is then isolated using the method of your choice, and the successful transposition of the gene of interest to the bacmid is assessed by PCR using the M13 Forward (-40) and M13 Reverse primers and Taq DNA polymerase, with the following conditions:

10× PCR Buffer (appropriate for enzyme)	2 μL
Recombinant bacmid DNA (100 ng)	*x* μL
Primer Fwd (Stock 10 μM)	1 μL
Primer Rev (Stock 10 μM)	1 μL
dNTP (10 mM)	0.4 μL
$MgCl_2$ (if required)	*y* μL
H_2O (up to 20 μL)	*z* μL
Taq DNA polymerase	0.2 μL

94 °C	3 min	
94 °C 55 °C 72 °C	45 s 45 s 5 min	25–35 cycles
72 °C	10 min	

8. Load 5–10 μL from the reaction mixture on an agarose gel, and if transposition has occurred, a band should be visible at ~2300 bp + the size of your insert (*see* **Note 3**). If the transposition failed, a band corresponding to the bacmid alone will be visible at ~300 bp.

3.2.2 Transfecting Insect Cells

1. In a 6-well culture plate, seed 9×10^5 Sf9 cells per well in 2 mL of growth medium containing antibiotics (e.g., Sf-900 II SFM containing 50 units/mL penicillin and 50 μg/mL streptomycin final concentration (*see* **Note 4**)). Allow the cells to attach at 27 °C for at least 1 h.
2. During this time, for each transfection, prepare the DNA:lipid complexes as follows:
   - Dilute 1 μg of purified bacmid DNA (do not exceed a volume of 10 μL) in 100 μL of unsupplemented Grace's Medium in an Eppendorf tube.
   - In a second Eppendorf tube, mix 6 μL of Cellfectin® Reagent with 100 μL of unsupplemented Grace's Medium.
   - Then, combine the two tubes (total volume is ~210 μL), mix gently, and incubate for 15–45 min at room temperature.
3. Wash the cells once with 2 mL of unsupplemented Grace's Medium and remove the wash medium.
4. Add 0.8 mL of unsupplemented Grace's Medium to each tube containing the DNA:lipid complexes, mix gently, and add the DNA:lipid complexes dropwise to each well containing cells.
5. Incubate in a 27 °C incubator for 5 h.
6. Remove the DNA:lipid complexes and add 2 mL of complete Sf-900 II SFM (containing antibiotics) to the cells.
7. Incubate in a 27 °C humidified incubator for 72 h or until signs of late viral infection are visible (*see* **Note 5**) (Fig. 1a).
8. Once signs of late stage infection (e.g., at 72 h post transfection) are observed, collect the medium containing virus from each well and centrifuge the tubes at 500 × *g* for 5 min to remove cells and large cell debris.
9. Filter the supernatant through a 0.2 μm filter (low protein binding) and add 2% of fetal bovine serum, to protect virus from digestion by proteases.
10. Store this P1 viral stock at +4 °C, protected from light.
11. Optional: determine the titer of your viral stock by performing a Viral Plaque Assay. You should expect a viral titer around 10^6–10^7 plaque forming units (pfu)/mL.

3.2.3 Amplifying Baculoviral Stock

1. Prepare a 20 mL Sf9 cell suspension at 2×10^6 cells/mL (>97% viability (*see* **Note 6**)) in an autoclaved 200-mL glass bottle (*see* **Note 7**).
2. Add the appropriate volume of P1 viral stock to the suspension culture to obtain a multiplicity of infection (MOI) of 0.1 (*see* **Note 8**).

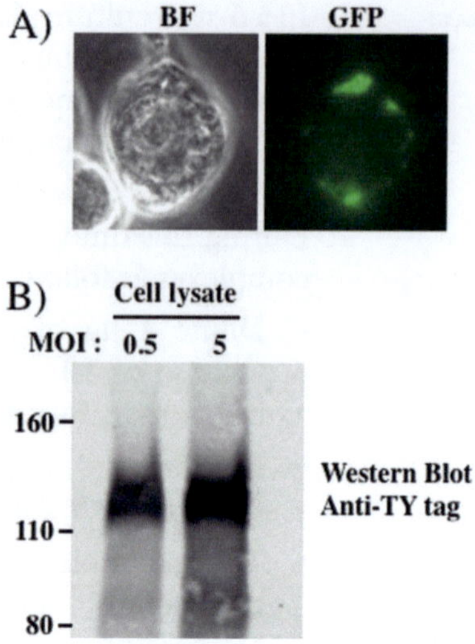

Fig. 1 Test of expression of a trypanosome protein kinase. (**a**) Infected insect cells can be quickly screened for TY1-YFP tagged target protein expression by mounting 10 μL of the insect cell culture, after 72 h of incubation, between a slide and coverslip and observing the GFP fluorescence under a fluorescence microscope. (**b**) Western blot of a crude insect cell lysate infected with a MOI of 0.5 or 5, where the TY1-YFP tagged target protein expression is revealed using an antibody raised against the TY1-tag

3. Incubate the cells for 48 h in a 27 °C incubator, with shaking at 120 rpm (*see* **Note 9**).
4. At 48–72 h post infection, collect the medium containing the virus from each bottle and transfer the medium to sterile Falcon tubes. Centrifuge the tubes at 500 × *g* for 5 min to remove cells and large debris.
5. Transfer the supernatant to fresh Falcon tubes. This is the P2 viral stock. Store at +4 °C, protected from light. For long-term storage, you may store an aliquot of the P2 stock at −80 °C, protected from light (*see* **Note 10**).
6. Optional: determine the titer of your P2 viral stock by performing a Viral Plaque Assay. You should expect a virus titer around 10^7–10^8 pfu/mL.

3.2.4 Expression and Purification of the Recombinant Protein

1. Prepare a 100 mL Sf9 cell suspension at 2.10^6 cells/mL (>97% viability) in an autoclaved 500 mL cylindrical glass bottle.
2. Add the P2 baculoviral stock to each well at the desired MOI (*see* **Note 11**) (Fig. 1b).
3. Incubate the cells in a 27 °C incubator, with shaking at 120 rpm (*see* **Note 9**).

4. Harvest the cells (for nonsecreted proteins) at the appropriate time (e.g., 24, 48, 72, 96 h post infection; this will need to be determined empirically, but a good starting point will be between 48 and 72 h).
5. Centrifuge the cells for 10 min at 500 × *g*.
6. Remove the supernatant and rinse the cells once with serum-free medium.
7. Lyse the cells with 15 mL of RIPA lysis buffer. Incubate on ice for 30 min.
8. Sonicate the samples to shear the DNA with the sonicator five times for 10 s ON followed by 20 s OFF at 5 Amp.
9. Clear the lysate by centrifugation for 15 min at 15,000 × *g* and 4 °C.
10. Keep the supernatant and discard the pellet (*see* **Note 12**).
11. For the pulldown of TY1-tagged protein, add the appropriate amount of αBB2 antibody (depending on the titer of the antibody) (*see* **Note 13**).
12. Incubate on a rotating wheel for 2 h at 4 °C.
13. Add 70 μL Protein G Dynabeads preequilibrated in lysis buffer.
14. Incubate for 1 h at 4 °C on a rotating wheel.
15. Pull down using a magnetic field and wash three times with 500 μL lysis buffer (for each wash, incubate on ice for 2 min).
16. Wash once with 500 μL of Elution buffer.
17. Native elution can be performed, with the beads, outside the magnetic field with 100 μL of Elution buffer.
18. Aliquot samples and freeze at −80 °C.
19. The pulldown quality is assessed by migration of the samples after SDS-PAGE:
    - Boil samples for 5 min in the presence of 1× Laemmli buffer.
    - Separate the proteins by SDS-PAGE.
    - Reveal the resolved proteins using SYPRO Ruby staining according to manufacturer's instructions. The relative quantity between different mutants can be assessed by this method, permitting determination of the correct dilutions for the future enzymatic assays (Fig. 2a).
    - Alternatively, proteins can be transferred onto PVDF membrane and the proteins detected by western blotting using appropriate antibodies (Fig. 2b).

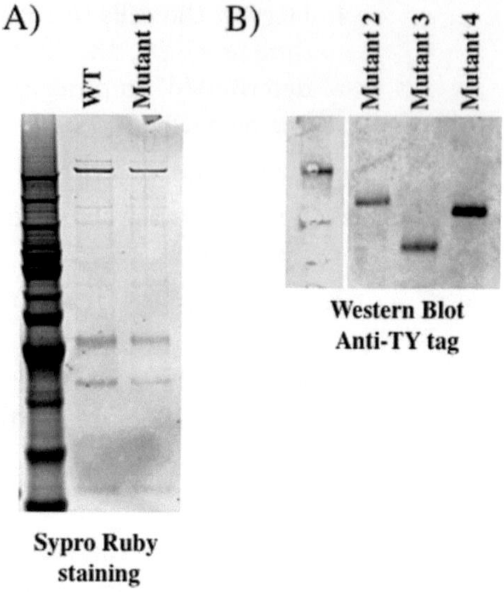

Fig. 2 Analysis of the quality of the pulldown from insect cells of the tagged protein kinase shown in Fig. 1, either as a wild-type or mutated protein. (**a**) Gel stained by SYPRO Ruby revealing the high quality of the purification of the wild-type and mutant 1 protein. (**b**) Alternatively, protein purification can be revealed by western blot here using an antibody detecting the TY1-tag incorporated into each expressed protein

3.3 Kinase Assays

3.3.1 "Cold" Kinase Assay

1. Prepare the "kinase mix" with the appropriate amount of MOPS kinase buffer 1× (*see* Subheading 2.4) and 5% of the purified kinase (including magnetic beads).
2. In a separate tube, prepare the "substrate mix" with 250 μM of (ATP)-γ-S, 200 μM ATP and the appropriate amount of substrate (*see* **Note 14**).
3. Start the kinase assay with mixing both the "kinase mix" and the "substrate mix" (*see* **Note 15**) and incubate for 30 min at 37 °C (*see* **Note 16**).
4. Stop the phosphotransferase reaction by incubating for 10 min at 95 °C.
5. Incubate the reaction with 5 mM (final concentration) PNBM for 2 h at 20 °C to initiate the alkylation reaction as described in Allen et al. [6].
6. The reaction is then stopped with 5 μL of Laemmli 6× loading buffer.

3.3.2 "Hot" Kinase Assay

If a more sensitive assay is required, we recommend to use the "hot" kinase assay, based on the presence of radioactive ATP, with the gamma phosphate group having a ^{32}P isotope.

1. As previously described, prepare the "kinase mix" with the appropriate amount of MOPS kinase buffer 1× (*see* Subheading 2.4) and 5% of the purified kinase (including magnetic beads).
2. In a separate tube, prepare the "substrate mix" with 1 mCi [γ-^{32}P]-ATP (3000 Ci/mmol), 200 μM ATP, and the appropriate amount of substrate.
3. Start the kinase assay with mixing both the "kinase mix" and the "substrate mix" (*see* **Note 15**) and incubate 30 min at 37 °C (*see* **Note 16**).
4. Stop the reaction with 5 μL of Laemmli 6× loading buffer.

3.3.3 SDS-PAGE and Transfer Onto PVDF Membrane

1. Boil the protein samples for 5 min in 1× Laemmli loading buffer.
2. Load the samples on a NuPAGE® gel 4–12% Bis-Tris and separate them by SDS-PAGE for 10 min at 100 V, followed by ~90 min at 120 V or until the desired protein separation is achieved.
3. Transfer the proteins onto PVDF membranes by the method of choice. We obtain good and reproducible results using wet transfer in 1× transfer buffer +20% methanol, for 2 h at 100 V (*see* **Note 17**).
4. Assess the quality of the separation and transfer by Ponceau S staining. Incubate the PVDF membrane for 5 min with 15 mL of Ponceau S, wash several times with ddH_2O or until the background staining remains stable and the protein bands become visible.
5. Images of the membrane can be captured at this point.

3.3.4 Phosphotransferase Activity Measurement

"Hot" kinase assay

1. ^{32}P incorporation is monitored by exposing an X-ray sensitive film to the membrane (*see* **Note 18**) at −80 °C.
2. After exposure, the bands corresponding to the substrates can be excised from the PVDF membrane and placed into individual scintillation vials.
3. Cherenkov radiation (as count per minute (cpm)) is quantified by a scintillation counter using the ^{32}P program, with three readings being taken for each sample (*see* **Note 19**).
4. If protein loading assessments require more sensitive methods than simple Ponceau S staining, a western blot analysis can be performed as described below for the "cold" kinase assay using appropriate antibodies, before excision of the bands from the membrane (Fig. 3).

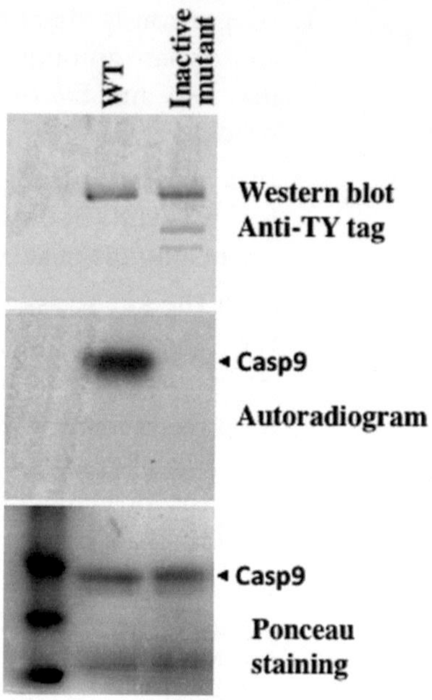

Fig. 3 "Hot" kinase assay of wild-type and an inactive mutant of the kinase expressed in Fig. 1, purified from insect cells and reacted against the Mus musculus Casp9 as a generic substrate. The loading of the kinase was revealed by western blot using the anti-TY1-tag antibody. The loading of the Casp9 was revealed by Ponceau S staining and the phosphotransferase activity of the kinase revealed by 5 h exposure of *X*-ray sensitive film (autoradiogram)

"Cold" kinase assay

1. Following Ponceau S staining, the membrane is blocked for 45 min at room temperature with Li-COR Odyssey® Blocking buffer (*see* **Note 20**).
2. Incubate the membrane with primary antibodies for 1–3 h at room temperature or overnight at 4 °C with agitation in 50% TBS-T and 50% Odyssey® Blocking buffer (*see* **Note 20**).
3. Use the following antibody dilutions: αBB2 (1:5, detecting the TY1-tag); αGST (1:1000); αThioP (1:1000, for the detection of the transferred thiophosphate).
4. Wash three times for 10 min with TBS-T at room temperature.
5. Incubate the membrane with secondary antibodies conjugated to a fluorescent dye diluted 1:5000 in 50% Li-COR Odyssey® Blocking buffer (*see* **Note 20**) and 50% TBS-T for 1 h at room temperature.
6. Wash three times for 10 min with TBS-T at room temperature.
7. Scan the membrane with a Li-COR Odyssey® imager system (*see* **Note 21**).

3.4 Phos-Tag Assay of Phosphorylated Proteins

3.4.1 Sample Prep

1. Harvest 2.5×10^7 cells in a 50 mL Falcon tube for 10 min at $1500 \times g$.
2. Pour off most of the supernatant from the cell pellet and resuspend in 500 μL of PBS.
3. Transfer all the resuspended cells to a labeled Eppendorf tube and spin down at $6200 \times g$ for 5 min in a benchtop centrifuge.
4. Remove all the supernatant carefully and add 62.5 μL Laemmli 6× buffer and pipette up and down several times until the sample is less viscous.
5. Boil the sample for 5 min in a heating block, and either load the samples on SDS-PAGE gels or freeze them and store at −20 °C.
6. Load $2–4 \times 10^6$ of cells in Laemmli 6× buffer per lane for SDS-PAGE.

3.4.2 SDS PAGE Using Mini Protean Gel Equipment (Bio-Rad)

Gel preparation

1. Wash and clean the glass plates (with ddH_2O and 70% ethanol) and assemble the glass plate sandwich (*see* **Note 22**).
2. Mix together the solutions (*except TEMED*) required for the separating (Table 1) and stacking (Table 2) gels in sterile tubes. For a single 0.75-mm thick protein gel, prepare 4 mL separating solution and 1.5 mL stacking solution. Supplement the separating gel mix with 10 mM $MnCl_2$ and the Phos-tag gel mix with 10 mM $MnCl_2$ and 5 mM Phos-tag solutions (Fig. 4, Table 1) (*see* **Notes 23–25**).
3. Add TEMED to the separating solution, swirl the mixture and pipette the solution between the gap between the plates, leaving sufficient space for the stacking gel (the length of the teeth of the comb plus 1 cm). Retain the leftover stacking gel mix in the tube, to monitor polymerization.
4. Prior to polymerization, overlay the gel carefully with a layer of 70% ethanol (this prevents oxygen from inhibiting polymerization and also creates an even surface).
5. After polymerization is complete (this depending on the volume of APS and TEMED added), pour off the 70% ethanol.
6. Add TEMED to the stacking solution. Pipette the stacking gel solution directly onto the surface of the polymerized resolving gel, to reach the edge of the glass sandwich. Keep the remainder of the stacking gel mix in the tube, to monitor polymerization.
7. Insert a clean comb carefully to avoid trapping air bubbles (first lower one side, then the other into the stacking gel solution). Leave the gel to set at room temperature.

Table 1
Solutions used for a 10% 0.75-mm thick normal and Phos-tag (supplemented with 10 μM Phos-tag compound) resolving gels

	Normal gel	Phos-tag gel
H_2O	2.06 mL	2.05 mL
PhosTag reagent (5 mM)	0	10 μL
$MnCl_2$ (10 mM)	20 μL	20 μL
Lower gel buffer	1.25 mL	1.25 mL
Acrylamide	1.67 mL	1.67 mL
10% APS	33 μL	33 μL
TEMED	5 μL	5 μL

Table 2
Solutions used for one 0.75 mm stacking gel

	1 gel
H_2O	1.5 mL
Lower gel buffer	0.375 mL
Acrylamide	0.625 mL
10% APS	12.5 μL
TEMED	4 μL

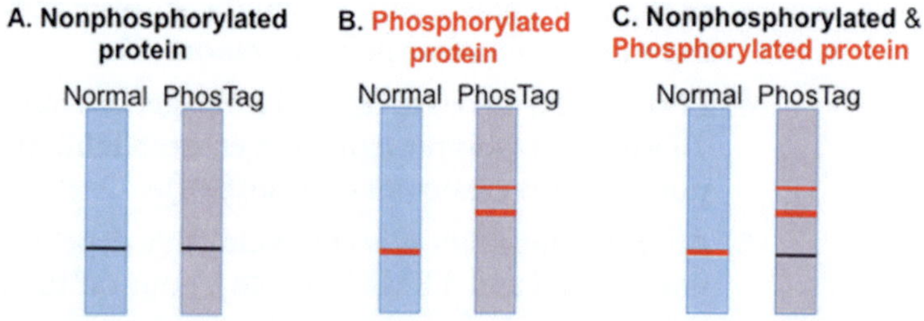

Fig. 4 (**a**) Nonphosphorylated "Protein X" (black band on schematic figure) migrates as a single band both on normal and PhosTag gel. (**b**) On a normal SDS gel, distinct phosphoprotein isotypes with different positions or numbers of phosphorylation migrate as a single band, but on PhosTag gel, they can also be separated depending upon the degree of phosphorylation. The thick red band denotes "Protein X" phosphorylated on a single residue, while the thin red band corresponds to a diphosphorylated "Protein X". (**c**) The mix of nonphosphorylated "Protein X" and phosphoprotein isotypes with different positions or numbers of phosphorylation migrate as a single band, but on a PhosTag gel, they can also be separated depending upon the degree of phosphorylation. Fastest migration: nonphosphorylated (black band), followed by uniphosphorylated (thick red band) and diphosphorylated "Protein X"

8. After the gel has polymerized, remove the comb and wash the wells with ddH_2O to remove any nonpolymerized acrylamide solution. The assembled gel sandwiches can be stored flat, wrapped in wet tissue in the fridge for few days.

Assembling, loading, and running the gel

1. Assemble the gel sandwiches in the electrophoresis apparatus (two gels can be run per tank; if only one gel is being run, a plastic buffer dam should be used to separate the upper and lower buffer in the tank).
2. Add Tris-glycine electrophoresis buffer to the top and bottom reservoirs.
3. Load up to 20 μL of sample to the wells of a 10-well gel (*see* **Note 26**).
4. Load 5–7.5 μL of appropriate protein marker to one lane of the gel (*see* **Note 27**). This allows estimation of resolved protein sizes and can be used to monitor the efficacy of transfer from the gel to the membrane after visualization by staining with Ponceau S stain. The use of prestained protein markers is not recommended with on Phos-tag gels, however these can be used on "normal" gels used as controls.
5. Run the gel at 100 V for 1.5–2.5 h or until the blue dye from the sample buffer reaches the very bottom of the gel (*see* **Note 28**).
6. Remove the glass plates from the electrophoresis apparatus and carefully take apart the glass–gel sandwich. Never use metal tools in this process; if needed, use the plastic wedge included with the Mini Protean II system.

Gel treatment before western blotting

1. After SDS-PAGE separation, rinse the gel in ddH_2O for 10 min, on a rocking platform, at room temperature.
2. Discard the ddH_2O and soak the gel in 2 mM EDTA for at least 20 min on a rocking platform at room temperature to chelate free Mn^{2+}. Omitting this step will reduce the efficiency of the protein transfer.
3. Discard the 2 mM EDTA solution and wash the gel with transfer buffer for 60 min on a rocking platform, at room temperature.
4. After this, the gel is ready for transfer.

Western blot

1. Cut four Whatman filter papers and a PVDF membrane into 8.5 × 5 cm pieces for a Bio-Rad minigel (use tweezers to handle these components). Use pencil to mark the membranes (*see* **Note 29**).

2. PVDF membranes should be activated for 60 s by submerging them in methanol. Soak the four Whatman papers, a PVDF membrane, and two sponges in transfer buffer before use. Always keep the PVDF membrane and Whatman papers wet throughout the process.
3. Assemble the gel sandwich for transfer in the order as follows (*see* **Note 30**):
   - The gel sandwich is prepared by placing the provided cassette in a small tray containing blotting buffer with the black side facing down. On top of the black side of the cassette, the other components were assembled in the following order: one of the fiber pads (provided with the Mini Trans-Blot apparatus (Bio-Rad)), two pieces of filter paper, the gel, the membrane, the other two pieces of filter paper, and the other fiber pad. To make sure that no bubbles are trapped between the different layers a 10-mL pipette is rolled on top of the assembled gel sandwich applying gentle pressure. The cassette was closed and placed in the apparatus, with the black side facing the black side (negative side) of the blotting device.
4. Fill the transfer tank with transfer buffer for 1 h at 80 V or overnight at 15 V. Avoid the buffer warming up during transfer using icepacks in the transfer tank and by placing the tank apparatus into wet ice in a large container.
5. After the transfer, disassemble the apparatus. Remove the PVDF membrane from the sandwich and place it in a small plastic tray.
6. Mark the PVDF membrane with pencil and stain the western blot with Ponceau S (to assist staining, place on a platform shaker for 5 min) to ensure the efficacy of transfer and to demonstrate even sample loading. Wash out the unspecific Ponceau staining with ddH_2O and take an image of the stained blot stained.
7. Wash off the Ponceau S solution with ddH_2O (by placing the blot on a platform shaker for 5 min and then by washing 3×).
8. Add 50% Li-COR block solution to the membrane in 1× TBS (note: different blocking solutions can be used depending the antibody used). Cover the tray and incubate the membrane with the blocking solution at room temperature for at least 45 min (or overnight in the cold room) on an orbital shaker.

Detection

1. Pour off the blocking solution (there is no need to wash if the primary antibody is diluted in the same blocking solution). Add primary antibody diluted in the blocking solution (*see* **Note 31**).

2. Incubate for a minimum of 1 h at room temperature (or overnight in the cold room) on an orbital shaker.
3. Wash the membrane 3× with TBS Tween (0.05% Tween)—each time add enough solution to cover the membrane, place it on a platform shaker for 10 min, then pour off the wash solution.
4. Add secondary antibody diluted in blocking solution.
5. Incubate for a minimum of 1 h at room temperature (or overnight in the cold room) on an orbital shaker.
6. Wash the membrane 3× with TBS Tween—each time add enough solution to cover the membrane, place it on a platform shaker for 10 min, pour off the solution.
7. The membrane is now ready to be scanned on the Li-COR/Odysseys® scanner.
8. The membrane can be washed in TBS Tween and dried by touching a paper towel for storage in cling film at −20 °C.

4 Notes

1. It is recommended to use a proofreading polymerase, such as Phusion DNA polymerase, to avoid mutations occurring at undesired position in the gene and/or the backbone plasmid.
2. Before bacterial transformation, the PCR reaction should be analyzed on an agarose gel by loading 5 μL of the reaction. A band at the expected size of the plasmid should be observed. If no band is observed, we would advise to repeat the PCR reaction with modified conditions. If a band is observed, proceed to the transformation of XL1 Blue bacteria.
3. The sizes indicated are the ones observed if you choose to use the pFastBac™1 plasmid. For other plasmids, you should refer to the manual with the link provided earlier.
4. We recommend the use of SF900 II for the culture of the insect SF9 cells, as this does not contain serum (SF9 cells have been adapted to culture without serum). This facilitates the subsequent steps of infection and protein purification. We also recommend to use this medium supplemented with 50 units/mL penicillin and 50 μg/mL streptomycin (final concentration) to avoid contamination.
5. The early infection stage is represented by growth arrest, followed by an increase in the cell and nucleus diameter, a granular appearance and a detachment of the cells from the plate. The very late stage of infection is characterized by cell lysis and a disappearance of the cell monolayer.

6. To assess the viability of the cells, dilute 5 μL of Trypan blue (stock 4%, final concentration 0.4%) with 45 μL of the cell culture. Pipette 10 μL of the mixture on a hemocytometer and count the cells under a microscope. The white/transparent cells are healthy cells, and the blue/dark cells are damaged or dead cells.
7. In our lab, we have found that the use of cylindrical glass bottles is most convenient for the culture of insect cells as they are inexpensive, cap sealed, and reusable and can be sterilized by autoclave. However, it is essential to thoroughly clean and rinse the bottles before autoclaving, in order to remove any trace of detergent, which is lethal for the insect cells.
8. To calculate the inoculum required, you can use the following formula:

$$\text{Volume required (mL)} = (\text{MOI (pfu/cell)} \times \text{number of cells}) / \text{titre of viral stock (pfu/mL)}.$$

9. If you are using glass bottles as recommended, remember to slightly loosen the cap to allow gas exchange.
10. As previously mentioned, the viral stock can be sterilized with a low binding 0.2 μm filter, which may also increase the pfu/mL.
11. Different MOI can be tested, for example, 1, 2, 5, 10, 20, and the most suitable will need to be determined empirically for the protein of interest. However, a good starting point would be a MOI of 2.
12. Optional: protein samples can be resolved by SDS-PAGE and transferred onto PVDF membrane to analyze the protein expression using appropriate antibodies by western blot (pellets/flow throughs/washes can also be analyzed to see whether the protein is lost in the insoluble fraction or during the different purification steps).
13. If you choose to use other tags, conditions will have to be empirically tested with the appropriate antibody or methodology.
14. If the substrates of the kinase of interest are unknown, identifying a generic substrate will be essential and a good starting point would be to test the following molecules:
    (a) 10 μg dephosphorylated MBP.
    (b) 40 μg histone H1.
    (c) 1 μg histone cores H2A, H2B, H3, H4.
    (d) 20 μg dephosphorylated casein.
    (e) 1 μg ß-casein.
    (f) 1 μg of the recombinant Mus musculus caspase 9 (Casp9, first 200 amino acids).

15. Make sure that the final volume does not exceed 25 μL, to be able to load the entire reaction into the gel.
16. The optimal temperature and time should be adjusted for each individual protein kinase.
17. During the transfer procedure, it is important to maintain the temperature of the transfer buffer below 15 °C to avoid changes in the pH of the solution. To do so, simply place your transfer tank in an ice bucket during the transfer.
18. We highly recommend sealing the membrane in a transparent plastic envelope, before exposure to the X-ray films at −80 °C. This prevents any liquid contacting the film, which can create background signal.
19. When measuring the ^{32}P isotope by its Cherenkov radiation, it is not necessary to add any scintillation liquid into the vial before measurement to obtain a reliable and reproducible signal.
20. Other blocking buffers could be used but will require appropriate optimization before preforming the kinase assay.
21. Other fluorescent gel imagers could be used.
22. In our assays, to study the phosphorylation state of target proteins, we mixed the Phos-tag reagent in Bis-Tris acrylamide gels at an appropriate concentration, instead of buying the premixed Phos-tag precast acrylamide gels from the provider. This allowed us to screen various Phos-tag compound concentrations and various % acrylamide gels to identify the best resolution/separation of the target proteins.
23. A nonsupplemented "normal" gel (no Phos-tag reagent added) with identical % of acrylamide to the Phos-tag gel must be run in parallel in the same electrophoresis apparatus. The "normal" gel will be used as a control for the unaltered mobility of your target protein.
24. We have used various concentrations of Phos-tag (30, 40, 60, and 80 μM) and achieved various results (Fig. 5), depending on the target protein. According to our experiments, an increased concentration of Phos-tag reagent in the separating gel can provide better resolution and resolve two bands, which might appear as a single band at lower concentration (*see* Fig. 5: PEX14, 40 μM vs. 30 μM). We would recommend <40 μM Phos-tag as a starting concentration and, depending on the outcome, titrate the compound further to increase resolution.
25. High Phos-tag concentrations can negatively affect SDS-PAGE resolution and lead to distorted bands.
26. A recombinant version of the target protein produced in a prokaryote expression system should be loaded on the Phos-

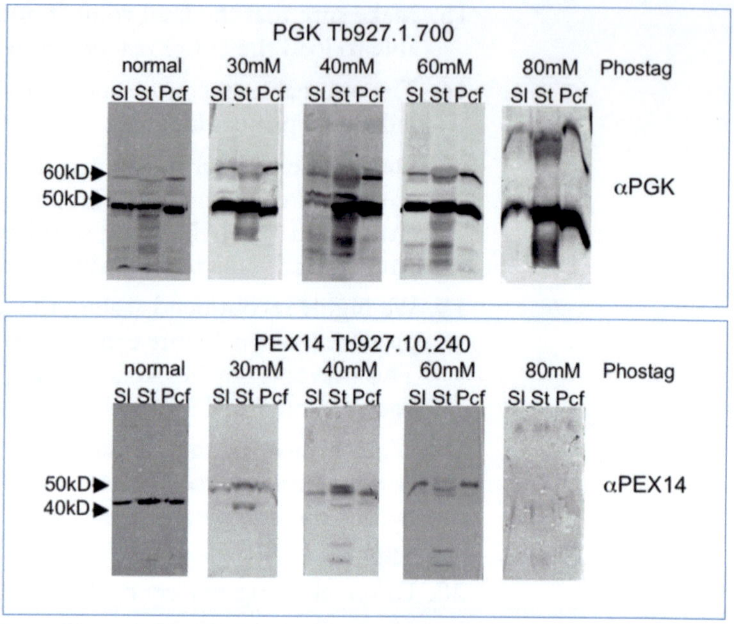

Fig. 5 Effect of increasing Phos-tag concentration on the migration of phosphoproteins. We used the Phos-tag SDS-PAGE method followed by western blotting to investigate how the phosphorylation of TbPGK and TbPEX14 changes in three different lifeforms (slender (sl), stumpy (st), and procyclic (pcf) forms) of *Trypanosoma brucei*. Trypanosome lysates equivalent to 2×10^6 cells were separated on 8% polyacrylamide gels and the Phos-tag gels were supplemented with 30–40–60–80 μM Phos-tag. No changes were detected in the TbPGK band pattern, but in the case of TbPEX14, the middle lane (st) and, possibly, the last lane (pcf) have more bands detected compared with the "normal" gel's band pattern. This suggests TbPEX14 is likely di or triphosphorylated in "st" and possible monophosphorylated in "pcf" The same protein is nonphosphorylated in "sl." The increasing concentration of Phos-tag has improved the separation of the target phosphoproteins (60 μM vs. 40 μM vs. 30 μM), but the highest concentration (80 μM) led to distorted bands

tag gel (and the "normal" gel, also) providing a negative control, revealing the migration of a nonphosphorylated version of the target protein.

27. Protein markers should be avoided (especially prestained markers, which can distort protein bands) because the protein separation on Phos-tag SDS-PAGE does not depend solely on molecular weight.

28. In our experiments, we found that for the best resolution, the gels need to be run very slowly at low voltage (100 V or lower).

29. After the SDS-PAGE separation, we used western blots probed with the appropriate antibodies for the detection of target proteins with altered mobility (phosphorylation).

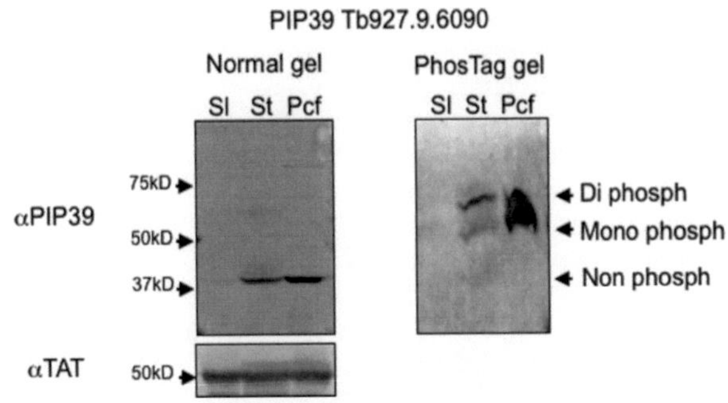

Fig. 6 TbPIP39 is differentially phosphorylated in slender, stumpy, and procyclic forms (*see* **Note 32**). *Trypanosoma brucei* lysates equivalent to 2×10^6 cells were separated on 8% polyacrylamide gels. The Phos-tag gel was supplemented with 40 μM Phos-tag compound

30. Wet overnight transfer provided better transfer of proteins from Phos-tag gels than the use of semidry apparatus.
31. For the success of this reasonably rapid and cost-effective method, it is important to have good antibodies. If these are not available, antibodies against tagged proteins can be used.
32. We used 8% 40 μM Phos-tag gel to investigate *Tb*PIP39 differential phosphorylation in slender, stumpy, and procyclic forms. According to the western blot probed with anti-*Tb*PIP39 antibody, we suggest that *Tb*PIP39 is phosphorylated on at least two residues in stumpy and procyclic forms. Analyzing the band pattern, we propose that the ratio of the phosphorylated residues differs in these two lifeforms (Fig. 6).

Acknowledgments

We thank Professor Keith Matthews, the University of Edinburgh, for advice and constructive comments on the manuscript.

B.Sz. and M.C. are funded by a Wellcome Trust Investigator award for Professor Keith Matthews (103740/Z14/Z).

References

1. Sharma K, D'Souza RC, Tyanova S et al (2014) Ultradeep human phosphoproteome reveals a distinct regulatory nature of Tyr and Ser/Thr-based signaling. Cell Rep 8(5):1583–1594
2. Domingo-Sananes MR, Szöőr B, Ferguson MA et al (2015) Molecular control of irreversible bistability during trypanosome developmental commitment. J Cell Biol 211 (2):455–468
3. Marchini FK, de Godoy LM, Rampazzo RC et al (2011) Profiling the Trypanosoma cruzi phosphoproteome. PLoS One 6(9):e25381
4. Nett IR, Martin DM, Miranda-Saavedra D et al (2009) The phosphoproteome of bloodstream form Trypanosoma brucei, causative agent of African sleeping sickness. Mol Cell Proteomics 8(7):1527–1538
5. Marchini FK, de Godoy LM, Batista M et al (2014) Towards the phosphoproteome of trypanosomatids. Subcell Biochem 74:351–378
6. Allen JJ, Li M, Brinkworth CS et al (2007) A semisynthetic epitope for kinase substrates. Nat Methods 4(6):511–516

7. Kinoshita-Kikuta E, Kinoshita E, Yamada A et al (2006) Enrichment of phosphorylated proteins from cell lysate using a novel phosphate-affinity chromatography at physiological pH. Proteomics 6(19):5088–5095
8. Engstler M, Boshart M (2004) Cold shock and regulation of surface protein trafficking convey sensitization to inducers of stage differentiation in Trypanosoma brucei. Genes Dev 18 (22):2798–2811
9. Wirtz E, Leal S, Ochatt C, Cross GA (1999) A tightly regulated inducible expression system for conditional gene knock-outs and dominant-negative genetics in Trypanosoma brucei. Mol Biochem Parasitol 99(1):89–101
10. Hirumi H, Hirumi K (1989) Continuous cultivation of Trypanosoma brucei blood stream forms in a medium containing a low concentration of serum protein without feeder cell layers. J Parasitol 75(6):985–989
11. Brun R, Schonenberger S (1979) Cultivation and in vitro cloning or procyclic culture forms of Trypanosoma brucei in a semi-defined medium. Short communication. Acta Trop 36 (3):289–292
12. Bastin P, Bagherzadeh Z, Matthews KR, Gull K (1996) A novel epitope tag system to study protein targeting and organelle biogenesis in Trypanosoma brucei. Mol Biochem Parasitol 77(2):235–239

Chapter 31

Methods to Investigate Signal Transduction Pathways in *Trypanosoma cruzi*: Cyclic Nucleotide Phosphodiesterases Assay Protocols

Alejandra C. Schoijet, Tamara Sternlieb, and Guillermo D. Alonso

Abstract

Intracellular levels of cyclic nucleotide second messengers are regulated predominantly by a large superfamily of phosphodiesterases (PDEs). Most of the different PDE variants play specific physiological functions; in fact, PDEs can associate with other proteins allowing them to be strategically anchored throughout the cell. In this regard, precise cellular expression and compartmentalization of these enzymes produce the specific control of cyclic adenosine monophosphate (cAMP) and cyclic guanosine monophosphate (cGMP) gradients in cells and enable their integration with other signaling pathways.

In trypanosomatids, some PDEs are essential for their survival and play fundamental roles in the adaptation of these parasites to different environmental stresses, as well as in the differentiation between their different life cycle forms. Given that these enzymes not only are similar to human PDEs but also have differential biochemical properties, and due to the great knowledge of drugs that target human PDEs, trypanosomatid PDEs could be postulated as important therapeutic targets through the repositioning of drugs.

In this chapter, we describe a simple and sensitive radioisotope-based method to measure cyclic 3′,5-′-nucleotide phosphodiesterase using [^{3}H]cAMP.

Key words Cyclic adenosine monophosphate (cAMP), Phosphodiesterase (PDE), Protein kinase A (PKA), Chagas disease, Therapeutic target, Drug discovery, Drug repositioning

1 Introduction

Cyclic adenosine monophosphate (cAMP) levels in most eukaryotes increase by stimulation of the activity of adenylyl cyclases (ACs), which use ATP as a substrate. However, cyclic nucleotide phosphodiesterases (PDEs) catalyze the hydrolysis of the phosphodiester bond in cAMP to give 5′-AMP, thereby decreasing the intracellular pool of this second messenger.

One of the principal cAMP effectors is the cAMP-dependent protein kinase (PKA), a serine/threonine kinase whose activity is dependent on the cAMP levels within the cell. In *Trypanosoma*

Paul A. M. Michels et al. (eds.), *Trypanosomatids: Methods and Protocols*, Methods in Molecular Biology, vol. 2116, https://doi.org/10.1007/978-1-0716-0294-2_31, © Springer Science+Business Media, LLC, part of Springer Nature 2020

cruzi, both catalytic and regulatory subunits (TcPKAc and TcPKAr, respectively) localized to the plasma membrane and the flagellar region with their catalytic sites at the cytoplasmic side of the membrane [1–3]. TcPKA has been implicated as a regulator of stage differentiation in *T. cruzi*, and it was shown that PKA enzymatic activity is essential for parasite survival [4].

Phosphodiesterases have been grouped into three classes based on their different catalytic domains. Class I PDEs are found in all eukaryotes and are the only form of PDEs in higher eukaryotes. These are the only enzymes that are capable of efficiently hydrolyzing cyclic nucleotides. In mammals, class I PDEs comprise 11 families, transcribed from 21 genes that in turn generate nearly 100 different isoforms. All members share a similar structure, but each one is functionally unique. The extensive number of isoforms arising from multiple transcription start sites and alternative splicing, along with tissue- or cell-specific expression and intracellular localization, results in individualized signaling roles [5]. All class I PDEs contain three functional domains: a C-terminal domain, a conserved catalytic core, and a regulatory N-terminal domain [6–8]. The C-terminal domain is similar in all PDE families, while the N-terminal domain shows high diversity, and the differences in this part are crucial for the regulation and subcellular localization of different PDEs. Within this domain, there are regions that are essential for ligand binding, oligomerization, kinase recognition, and phosphorylation which regulate PDE function. Class II PDEs are found in certain prokaryotes (e.g., *Vibrio fischeri*), in fungi (e.g., *Saccharomyces, Candida*), and in many early-branching eukaryotes (e.g., *Dictyostelium discoideum*). These PDEs also catalyze the hydrolysis of phosphodiester bonds, but they do not show the same substrate selectivity as the class I enzymes [9]. Class III PDEs are restricted to bacteria [10].

The genome of kinetoplastids encodes four different class I PDEs (PDE-A to PDE-D) in contrast to the human genome and does not contain members of the other PDE classes [11]. Our laboratory has focused on the study of the cAMP signal transduction pathway in *T. cruzi*, the causative agent of Chagas disease, which represents a major cause of cardiomyopathy. It affects around eight million people worldwide, most of them in Latin America [12]. Previously, we have described three cAMP-specific PDEs in *T. cruzi*: TcrPDEB2, which was the first PDE cloned and biochemically characterized in this parasite and was found to localize in the plasma membrane and in the flagellum, an essential organelle for the attachment, motility, and viability of the parasite [13]. In addition to TcrPDEB2, there is a closely related gene tandemly arranged with it that encodes TcrPDEB1, which is also a cAMP-specific phosphodiesterase [14]. In *T. brucei*, simultaneous RNAi against both TbrPDEB1 and TbrPDEB2 completely prevents infection and eliminates ongoing infections [15]. TcrPDEA1 has the singularity of being resistant to the typical PDE inhibitors of mammalian cells, has a high cAMP Km value (~200 μM) and possesses a cytosolic localization [16]. TcrPDEC2 is a cAMP-specific PDE and is distinguished by the presence of a FYVE domain close to its N-terminus, which is known to specifically recognize phosphatidylinositol 3-phosphate (PI3P) and recruit many proteins to PI3P-enriched membranes. TcrPDEC2 is localized in the contractile vacuole complex and participates in osmoregulation in *T. cruzi*, an essential mechanism in this parasite [17, 18]. In addition to TcrPDEC2, another allele was found, named TcrPDEC1, that is able to hydrolyze both cAMP and cGMP [19]. Finally, TcrPDED and its orthologous genes in other kinetoplastids are the least studied PDEs, and TcrPDED's function remains unclear (Fig. 1 and Table 1).

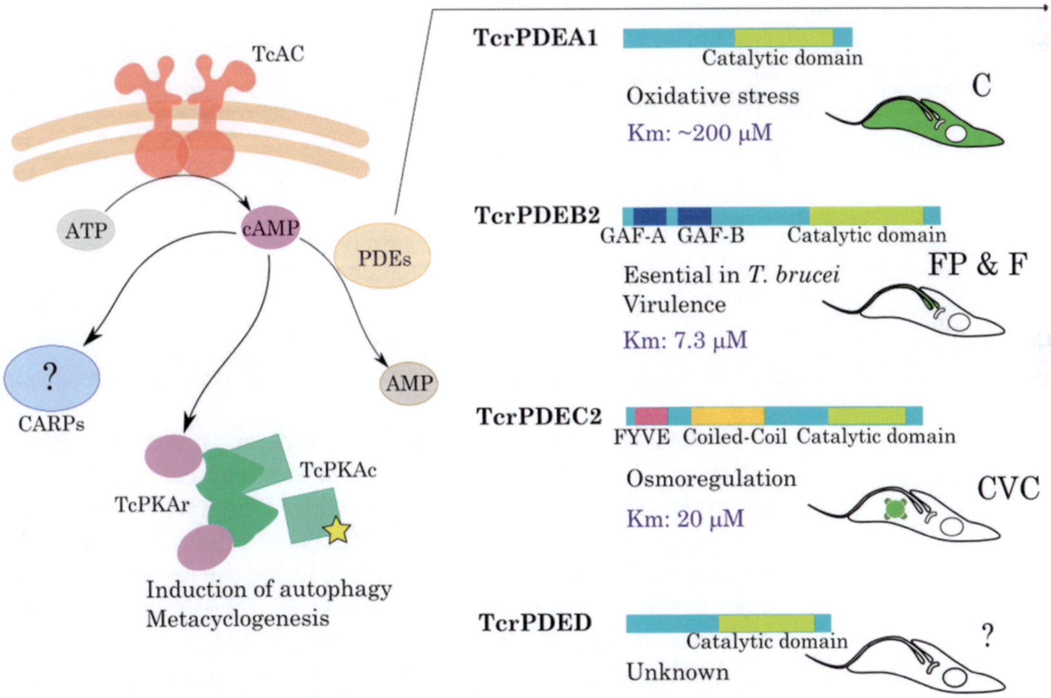

Fig. 1 Schematic representation of the signaling pathways mediated by cyclic nucleotides in *Trypanosoma cruzi*, highlighting the regulatory role of phosphodiesterases (PDEs). cAMP is a common second messenger with several important roles in trypanosomatids. In *T. cruzi*, a dimeric adenylyl cyclase (TcAC) uses ATP as substrate to produce cAMP. Downstream to cAMP, PDEs hydrolyze cAMP to 5′AMP. There are four different PDEs in *T. cruzi* (TcrPDEA1, TcrPDEB2, TcrPDEC2, and TcrPDED). TcrPDEA1 localizes to the cytosol (*C*); TcrPDEB2 localizes to the flagellum (*F*) and the flagellar pocket (*FP*); TcrPDEC2 is characterized by the presence of a FYVE domain, which is a phosphoinositide-binding motif and localizes to the contractile vacuole complex (*CVC*); and the TcrPDED localization is not defined. The main effector of cAMP is the cAMP-dependent protein kinase A (TcPKA), which exists as a tetramer consisting of two catalytic subunits (TcPKAc) and two regulatory subunits (TcPKAr). Regarding other cAMP effectors, cAMP responsive proteins (CARPs) were identified recently in *T. brucei*, although the molecules on which they exert their function are still unknown

Table 1
Classification and characteristics of phosphodiesterases (PDEs) from *Trypanosoma cruzi*

Name	TcrPDEA1	TcrPDEB1/2	TcrPDEC1/2	TcrPDED
Domains	Catalytic (Ct)	GAF-A, GAF-B, catalytic (Ct)	FYVE, catalytic (middle)	Catalytic (Ct)
Km for cAMP	High (~200 μM)	Low (4–8 μM)	Intermediate (~20 μM)	Nondetermined
Specificity	cAMP	cAMP	cAMP/cGMP (TcrPDEC1) cAMP (TrcPDEC2)	Nondetermined
Not affected by	Ca^{2+}-calmodulin	Ca^{2+}-calmodulin	Ca^{2+}-calmodulin	Nondetermined
Inhibitors	Not inhibited by the typical mammalian PDE inhibitors	Dipyridamole	Rolipram, etazolate, dipyridamole, IBMX	Nondetermined
Localization	Cytosolic (TcrPDEA1)	Plasma membrane, concentrated in the flagellum	Spongiome, in the contractile vacuole complex (TcrPDEC2)	Nondetermined
Tips to take into account to measure catalytic activity	Reaction mix 2× for PDEs with high Km value. Use soluble fraction (S100)	Reaction mix 2× for PDEs with low Km value. Use microsomal membranes (P100)	Reaction mix 2× for PDEs with low Km value. Use microsomal membranes (P100)	Nondetermined

Taken together, several studies have demonstrated that PDEs are essential for parasite survival and play prominent roles in their life cycle. The fact that trypanosomatid PDEs have characteristic binding pockets that allow for a differential inhibition from their human orthologues [20–22] and considering the extensive knowledge in the field of human PDE inhibitors, these enzymes can be positioned as interesting therapeutic drug targets.

In this chapter, we describe a rapid, sensitive, and efficient radioenzymatic assay using [^{3}H]cAMP, useful to measure PDE activity in cytosolic and membrane fractions, thus contributing to unravel the functional roles of PDEs in trypanosomatids. In this protocol, the separation of the enzymatic reaction product ([^{3}H]5′-AMP) formed by the hydrolysis of the phosphodiester bond of [^{3}H]3′,5′-cAMP by the phosphodiesterase reaction is carried out by a second step consisting in fully converting the [^{3}H]5′-AMP to [^{3}H]adenosine by means of the nucleotidase activity found in king cobra snake venom. It is important to highlight that the reaction catalyzed by the king cobra snake venom transforms all the [^{3}H]5′-AMP to [^{3}H]adenosine. Finally, the [^{3}H]adenosine can be easily

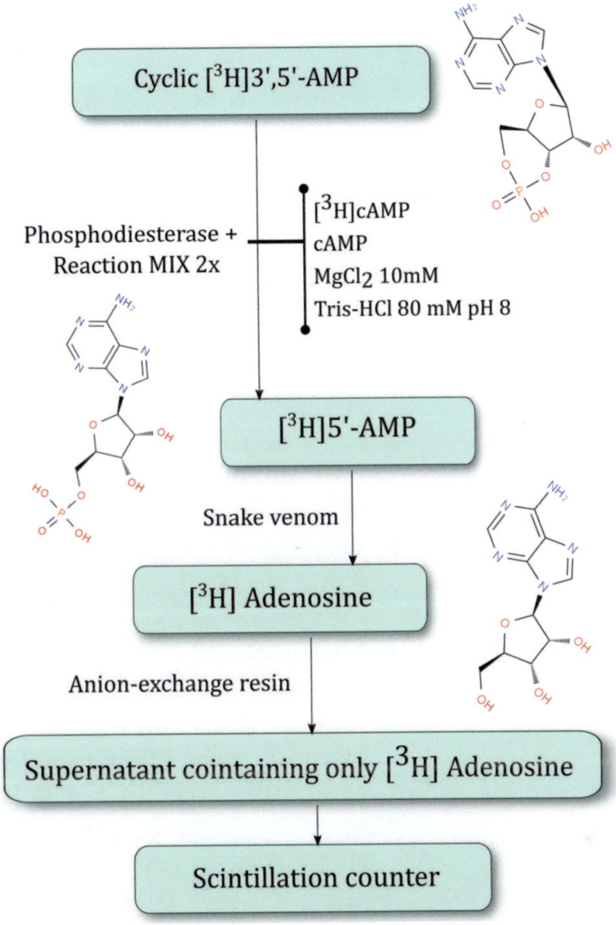

Fig. 2 Schematic representation of cyclic phosphodiesterase enzymatic assay

separated from the radioactive cyclic nucleotide substrate by retaining the [^{3}H]3′,5′-cAMP with an anion-exchange resin. The radioactive [^{3}H]adenosine remains in the supernatant and can be measured by liquid scintillation (Fig. 2).

In addition, we briefly describe how to apply this protocol to evaluate the possible activation of PDEs by Ca^{2+}-calmodulin (Ca^{2+}-CaM) and the ion dependence of trypanosomatid PDEs. Finally, suggestions are made on how to adapt this protocol to determine the sensitivity to specific PDE inhibitors, allowing a more precise PDE family identification and searching in turn for new compounds that could be used as trypanocidal drugs. Furthermore, these methods will enable readers to design themselves protocols to evaluate compounds with possible phosphodiesterase inhibitory properties.

2 Materials

Radiochemicals were purchased from PerkinElmer Life Sciences. Bacto-tryptose and liver infusion were from Difco. All other reagents were purchased from Sigma.

Prepare all solutions using ultrapure (milli-Q) water.

2.1 Parasite Culture and Extracts

1. LIT medium: 5 g/l liver infusion, 5 g/l bacto-tryptose, 68 mM NaCl, 5.3 mM KCl, 22 mM Na_2PO_4, 0.2% (w/v) glucose, 0.002% (w/v) hemin supplemented with 10% (v/v) newborn calf serum, 100,000 units/l penicillin, and 100 mg/l streptomycin.
2. Lysis buffer: 50 mM HEPES buffer, pH 7.3, containing 0.01 mg/ml leupeptin, 25 units/ml aprotinin, 0.5 mM phenylmethylsulfonyl fluoride, and 14 mM 2-mercaptoethanol.
3. Phosphate-buffered saline (PBS): 137 mM NaCl, 2.7 mM KCl, 8 mM Na_2HPO_4, and 2 mM KH_2PO_4, pH 7.4.

2.2 Phosphodiesterase Assay

1. Khan tubes, 12 × 75 mm.
2. Reaction mix 2× for PDEs with low Km value: 80 mM Tris–HCl, pH 8, 10 mM $MgCl_2$, 100 μM [^{3}H]cAMP (0.025 μCi/tube). *T. cruzi* PDEs measured with this mix: TcrPDEB1, TcrPDEB2, TcrPDEC1, and TcrPDEC2.
3. Reaction mix 2× for PDEs with high Km value: 80 mM Tris–HCl, pH 8, 10 mM $MgCl_2$, 400 μM [^{3}H]cAMP (0.05 μCi/tube). *T. cruzi* PDE measured with this mix: TcrPDEA1.
4. Prepare $MgCl_2$ as a 1-M solution and store at 4 °C.
5. Snake *(Ophiophagus hannah)* venom is obtained from Sigma Chemical Co., and the solution of use is prepared at 2 mg/ml in 10 mM Tris–HCl, pH 7.5–8. Lyophilized venom powder and the solution of use should be stored at −20 °C.
6. STOP solution: 50 mM EDTA and 5 mM adenosine. EDTA is used as a divalent ion chelator to stop the catalytic activity, and adenosine causes "product inhibition" where the reaction product competes with the substrate for free enzyme.
7. Anion-exchange resin: Bio-Rad AG® 1-X2 Anion-Exchange Resin, analytical grade, 200–400 mesh, chloride form (Bio-Rad Laboratories). To prepare the resin, add 33% of resin and 30% of ethanol (EtOH), and complete with distilled water. Store at 4 °C.

3 Methods

3.1 Trypanosoma cruzi Culture and Extracts Preparation

1. Culture *T. cruzi* epimastigote forms (CL Brener strain) at 28 °C for 7 days in LIT medium.
2. For *T. cruzi* extracts, from a culture at approximately 5×10^7 cells/ml, harvest 10^8 epimastigotes by centrifugation at $1500 \times g$ for 10 min, and wash two times with phosphate-buffered saline (PBS).
3. Resuspend pellets in lysis buffer, so that the cells are approximately 50 times concentrated (e.g., if you started from 2 ml of culture, you should resuspend the cells in approximately 40 μl of lysis buffer), and make six cycles of freezing in liquid N_2 and thawing at 4 °C in distilled water (*see* **Note 1**).
4. To obtain a cleared homogenate, centrifuge at $10{,}000 \times g$ for 10 min and discard the pellet containing the cellular debris.
5. If you want to separate the soluble fraction (S100) from microsomal membranes (P100), centrifuge the clarified extract (obtained at step 4) at $100{,}000 \times g$ for 1 h at 4 °C. Collect the supernatant (S100) and resuspend the pellet in lysis buffer, in approximately 50% of the volume of lysis buffer used in **step 3**.
6. In those cases where the studied protein turns out to be associated with membranes, it could be necessary to determine whether it is a peripheral or an integral membrane protein. To further evaluate the membrane protein type, take the P100 fraction and sequentially incubate it at 4 °C for 30 min with lysis buffer containing either 1 M NaCl (first fraction), 0.1% (w/v) sodium cholate (second fraction), 0.5% (w/v) sodium cholate (third fraction), or 8 M urea (fourth fraction). After each incubation, centrifuge for 40 min at $100{,}000 \times g$, recover the supernatant, and load it onto SDS-polyacrylamide gels. Peripheral proteins should be obtained in the first fraction, while integral proteins are released with more severe treatments and are obtained in the second, third, or fourth fraction according to the strength of the association with the membrane.
7. Store the remaining protein extracts at −70 °C or in liquid nitrogen (*see* **Note 2**).

3.2 Phosphodiesterase Assay

PDE activity is determined by a variation of the protocol described by Thompson and Appleman [23], with the modifications introduced by Londesborough [24].

1. Start the reaction by putting the Khan tubes in a rack set into a tray containing ice-cold water. Add the required volume of protein extract according to the μg of the enzymatic source previously determined. Complete to 50 μl by adding milli-Q water.

2. Initiate the reaction by adding 50 μl of the corresponding reaction mix 2× (for high or low Km as appropriate) (*see* **Notes 3–6**).
3. Gently vortex the samples and incubate the reaction for 10 min at 30 °C in a shaking water bath.
4. Stop the reaction by placing the tubes in a bath with boiling water for 1 min.
5. Place the tubes again in a tray containing ice-water and add 40 μl of snake venom solution (*see* **Note 7**).
6. Vortex thoroughly the tubes and incubate for 30 min at 30 °C in a water bath shaker. Since the snake venom contains 5-′-nucleotidase activity, it is added in excess, and the reaction is allowed to develop for 30 min. The result of this second enzymatic reaction is the full conversion of [^{3}H]5′-AMP (the specific product obtained as result of the PDE activity) to [^{3}H] adenosine.
7. Remove the tubes from the water bath and add 20 μl of the STOP solution.
8. Add 1 ml of the stirred resin slurry and allow the mixtures to equilibrate for 15 min at room temperature (*see* **Notes 8–10**).
9. Centrifuge the tubes at approximately 500 × *g* for 5 min at room temperature to form a resin pellet at the bottom of the tube (*see* **Note 11**).
10. Carefully pipette 0.4 ml of the supernatant, add 2 ml of scintillation liquid Ultima Gold™.
11. Measure the samples in the scintillation counter (*see* **Notes 12–13**).
12. For determination of Ca^{2+}-calmodulin dependence, use 0.05 or 0.5 units of calmodulin (from bovine brain) and 2.5 mM calcium, added previously to the reaction mix, along with the enzymatic source.
13. For determination of ion dependence, take into account not to include magnesium in the reaction mix. Additionally, to remove contaminating ions add 1 mM EDTA or 1 mM EGTA to chelate divalent ions or only Ca^{2+}, respectively. Once an ion-free condition has been obtained, add 5 mM Mg^{2+}, Mn^{2+}, or Ca^{2+} to identify possible ion dependencies (*see* **Note 14**).
14. For inhibition studies, add the concentration range of each compound according to the inhibitor used. The corresponding inhibitor is added previously to the mix, together with the enzymatic source. Take into account to include a control without inhibitor.

15. This assay can also be very useful for drug screening to evaluate trypanocidal activity of PDE inhibitors in vivo, using Vero cells in culture infected with *T. cruzi* Tulahuen strain expressing the *Escherichia coli* β-galactosidase gene (Tul-β-gal). The amount of β-galactosidase activity in a well is directly proportional to the number of parasites per well, and this activity can be easily and accurately quantitated in 96-well tissue culture plates with an enzyme-linked immunosorbent assay (ELISA) reader.

Additional equipment required

- Water bath shaker or incubator capable of uniformly heating tubes at 30 °C.
- Vortex.
- Scintillation counter.

4 Notes

1. Be careful about the possible opening of the Eppendorf tubes because of pressure changes due to the temperature changes during the freezing and thawing in the preparation of protein extracts. Eppendorf tubes with locked lids can be used for greater security.
2. To better preserve the protein source in extracts preparation, addition of 5–10% glycerol can help if the protein of interest is unstable.
3. [^{3}H]cAMP (Perkin Elmer, catalog number NET275250UC) comes in a vial as 250 μCi in 250 μl 1:1 ethanol-water (this is important because hydrogen-tritium exchange as occurs with water alone is prevented in this 1:1 mixture) and has an activity of 31.3 Ci/mmol. Therefore, the 0.05 μCi that is added for the high Km PDEs represents 1.6 pmol/0.025 μCi and for the low Km PDEs represents 0.8 pmol/0.025 μCi. It is worth to remark that this contribution is not significant in comparison with the 20,000 pmol in the 200 μM mix or the 100 pmol in the 50 μM mix.
4. Tritium is a very low-energy beta emitter. The major concern for individuals working with this isotope is the possibility of internal exposure. In this respect, care should be taken to prevent ingestion or contact with skin or clothing. Protective clothing, such as laboratory overalls and gloves, should be worn whenever radioactive tritium materials are handled.
5. Work should be carried out on a surface covered with absorbent material in order to contain any spillage. Working areas should be monitored regularly.

6. In the blank assay, the enzymatic source is replaced with the equivalent volume of lysis buffer or distilled water.
7. Use gloves to weigh snake venom. Do not breathe dust. Store at −20 °C.
8. When adding the resin, take into account to stir beforehand to obtain a homogenous mixture and avoid decanting.
9. At the end of the assay, distilled water can be added to the resin pellets. Vortex the tubes and store the suspension in a bottle with 20% EtOH.
10. To regenerate the anion-exchange resin, first wash it repeatedly with distilled water. Then the resin must be washed with a solution containing 0.1 N HCl and 1 M NaCl, at least twice. Check that the pH is close to 5. If necessary, the pH can be adjusted with a small amount of Tris base.
11. After adding stirred resin slurry, instead of centrifuging, the resin can be left to decant for a few min and the supernatant then directly taken.
12. To calculate the enzymatic activity (e.g., pmol/min), you must first calculate the pmoles of cold cAMP. Then a factor called *factor F* is calculated: (pmol of cold cAMP × 1.16 ml)/(0.4 × time of incubation × total cpm). Where 1.16 ml is the total assay volume per tube, 0.4 is the volume taken from the supernatant in the final step after adding the resin, and the total cpm is the measured reaction mix.

    F = pmol of cold cAMP × 1.16 ml/ 0.5 ml × time (min) × total cmp.

    Finally, you can calculate the enzymatic activity as follows:

    $$\begin{aligned}\text{Activity} &= \text{pmol of hydrolyzed cAMPc/ min}\\ &= F \times \text{average of counted cpm}\end{aligned}$$

    $$\text{Specific activity} = \text{A/mg of protein}$$

13. cGMP phosphodiesterase activity can be measured similarly using cold cGMP and [^{3}H]cGMP.
14. Magnesium chloride can come in its anhydrous or hydrated form. Take this into account when calculating the molecular weight. Also, remember to keep the bottle containing the solid drug tightly closed as it hydrates easily.

Acknowledgments

We are grateful to Dr. Rita Ulloa (INGEBI, Buenos Aires, Argentina) for helpful comments on the manuscript. This work was supported by the Consejo Nacional de Investigaciones Científicas y Técnicas (PIP 2013-00351); Departamento de Fisiología,

Biología Molecular y Celular, Facultad de Ciencias Exactas y Naturales, Universidad de Buenos Aires (UBACyT 2014-2017, Nro 00155BA); and Agencia Nacional de Promoción Científica y Tecnológica (PICT 2013–2015 and PICT 2015-0898). G.D.A. and A.C.S. are members of the Research Career of Consejo Nacional de Investigaciones Científicas y Técnicas, and T.S. is a fellow of the same institution.

References

1. Huang H, Werner C, Weiss LM et al (2002) Molecular cloning and expression of the catalytic subunit of protein kinase A from *Trypanosoma cruzi*. Int J Parasitol 32:1107–1115
2. Huang H, Weiss LM, Nagajyothi F et al (2006) Molecular cloning and characterization of the protein kinase A regulatory subunit of *Trypanosoma cruzi*. Mol Biochem Parasitol 149:242–245. https://doi.org/10.1016/j.molbiopara.2006.05.008
3. Bao Y, Weiss LM, Ma YF et al (2010) Protein kinase A catalytic subunit interacts and phosphorylates members of trans-sialidase superfamily in *Trypanosoma cruzi*. Microbes Infect 12:716–726. https://doi.org/10.1016/j.micinf.2010.04.014
4. Bao Y, Weiss LM, Braunstein VL, Huang H (2008) Role of protein kinase A in *Trypanosoma cruzi*. Infect Immun 76:4757–4763. https://doi.org/10.1128/IAI.00527-08
5. Kokkonen K, Kass DA (2017) Nanodomain regulation of cardiac cyclic nucleotide signaling by phosphodiesterases. Annu Rev Pharmacol Toxicol 57:455–479. https://doi.org/10.1146/annurev-pharmtox-010716-104756
6. Conti M, Beavo J (2007) Biochemistry and physiology of cyclic nucleotide phosphodiesterases: essential components in cyclic nucleotide signaling. Annu Rev Biochem 76:481–511. https://doi.org/10.1146/annurev.biochem.76.060305.150444
7. Thompson WJ (1991) Cyclic nucleotide phosphodiesterases: pharmacology, biochemistry and function. Pharmacol Ther 51:13–33
8. Bolger GB (1994) Molecular biology of the cyclic AMP-specific cyclic nucleotide phosphodiesterases: a diverse family of regulatory enzymes. Cell Signal 6:851–859
9. Bender AT, Beavo JA (2006) Cyclic nucleotide phosphodiesterases: molecular regulation to clinical use. Pharmacol Rev 58:488–520. https://doi.org/10.1124/pr.58.3.5
10. Gancedo JM (2013) Biological roles of cAMP: variations on a theme in the different kingdoms of life. Biol Rev Camb Philos Soc 88:645–668. https://doi.org/10.1111/brv.12020
11. Kunz S, Beavo JA, D'Angelo MA et al (2006) Cyclic nucleotide specific phosphodiesterases of the kinetoplastida: a unified nomenclature. Mol Biochem Parasitol 145:133–135. https://doi.org/10.1016/j.molbiopara.2005.09.018
12. WHO (2016) What is Chagas disease? WHO, Geneva
13. D'Angelo MA, Sanguineti S, Reece JM et al (2004) Identification, characterization and subcellular localization of TcPDE1, a novel cAMP-specific phosphodiesterase from *Trypanosoma cruzi*. Biochem J 378:63–72. https://doi.org/10.1042/BJ20031147
14. Díaz-Benjumea R, Laxman S, Hinds TR et al (2006) Characterization of a novel cAMP-binding, cAMP-specific cyclic nucleotide phosphodiesterase (TcrPDEB1) from *Trypanosoma cruzi*. Biochem J 399:305–314. https://doi.org/10.1042/BJ20060757
15. Oberholzer M, Marti G, Baresic M et al (2007) The *Trypanosoma brucei* cAMP phosphodiesterases TbrPDEB1 and TbrPDEB2: flagellar enzymes that are essential for parasite virulence. FASEB J 21:720–731. https://doi.org/10.1096/fj.06-6818com
16. Alonso GD, Schoijet AC, Torres HN, Flawiá MM (2007) TcrPDEA1, a cAMP-specific phosphodiesterase with atypical pharmacological properties from *Trypanosoma cruzi*. Mol Biochem Parasitol 152:72–79. https://doi.org/10.1016/j.molbiopara.2006.12.002
17. Alonso GD, Schoijet AC, Torres HN, Flawiá MM (2006) TcPDE4, a novel membrane-associated cAMP-specific phosphodiesterase from *Trypanosoma cruzi*. Mol Biochem Parasitol 145:40–49. https://doi.org/10.1016/j.molbiopara.2005.09.005
18. Schoijet AC, Miranda K, Medeiros LCS et al (2011) Defining the role of a FYVE domain in the localization and activity of a cAMP phosphodiesterase implicated in osmoregulation in *Trypanosoma cruzi*. Mol Microbiol 79:50–62.

https://doi.org/10.1111/j.1365-2958.2010.07429.x

19. Kunz S, Oberholzer M, Seebeck T (2005) A FYVE-containing unusual cyclic nucleotide phosphodiesterase from *Trypanosoma cruzi*. FEBS J 272:6412–6422. https://doi.org/10.1111/j.1742-4658.2005.05039.x
20. Jansen C, Wang H, Kooistra AJ et al (2013) Discovery of novel *Trypanosoma brucei* phosphodiesterase B1 inhibitors by virtual screening against the unliganded TbrPDEB1 crystal structure. J Med Chem 56:2087–2096. https://doi.org/10.1021/jm3017877
21. Wang H, Yan Z, Geng J et al (2007) Crystal structure of the *Leishmania major* phosphodiesterase LmjPDEB1 and insight into the design of the parasite-selective inhibitors. Mol Microbiol 66:1029–1038. https://doi.org/10.1111/j.1365-2958.2007.05976.x
22. Wang H, Kunz S, Chen G et al (2012) Biological and structural characterization of *Trypanosoma cruzi* phosphodiesterase C and implications for design of parasite selective inhibitors. J Biol Chem 287:11788–11797. https://doi.org/10.1074/jbc.M111.326777
23. Thompson WJ, Appleman MM (1971) Multiple cyclic nucleotide phosphodiesterase activities from rat brain. Biochemistry 10:311–316
24. Londesborough J (1976) Quantitative estimation of 3′5′ cyclic AMP phosphodiesterase using anion exchange resin in a batch process. Anal Biochem 71:623–628

Chapter 32

Methods for the Investigation of *Trypanosoma cruzi* Amastigote Proliferation in Mammalian Host Cells

Peter C. Dumoulin and Barbara A. Burleigh

Abstract

In its mammalian host, the kinetoplastid protozoan parasite, *Trypanosoma cruzi,* is obliged to establish intracellular residence in order to replicate. This parasite can infect and replicate within a diverse array of cell and tissue types across many mammalian host species. The establishment of quantitative assays to assess the replicative capacity of intracellular *T. cruzi* amastigotes under different conditions is a critical facet to understanding this host–pathogen interaction. Several complementary methods are outlined here. Their strengths and deficiencies in quantifying intracellular amastigote growth and death are discussed. We describe three assays to assess growth/replication. (1) A high throughput multiplexed plate-based assay that quantifies both host cell and parasite abundance. This method allows for the rapid and simultaneous screening of many conditions (e.g., small molecule inhibitors, the impact of host gene knockdown or of altered environmental parameters). (2) Simple fluorescence microscopy-based enumeration of amastigotes within host cells and (3) flow cytometry-based quantification of amastigote proliferation following isolation from host cells. Each approach has advantages but none of these can assess lethal outcomes in a quantitative manner. For this, we describe a clonal outgrowth assay that identifies the proportion of parasites that succumb to a defined exposure. Even using these assays, it can be challenging to differentiate between direct (targeting the parasite) and/or indirect (targeting the host) effects of a given treatment on amastigote growth. Therefore, we also outline a method of purification of intracellular amastigotes that allows for downstream biochemical and metabolic investigations specifically on the isolated amastigote.

Key words *Trypanosoma cruzi*, Amastigote, Proliferation, Cell cycle, Trypanocidal, Trypanostatic, Chagas disease

1 Introduction

Infection with the protozoan parasite *Trypanosoma cruzi* can result in debilitating cardiomyopathies and mega organ syndromes, the hallmarks of chronic Chagas disease [1]. These clinical pathologies are linked with the continued presence of the parasite, which only replicates intracellularly in the mammalian host [2, 3]. The ability of *T. cruzi* to persist for decades demonstrates an intimate relationship with its host. This interaction is of direct clinical relevance as there is no well-tolerated trypanocidal treatment with clear clinical

Paul A. M. Michels et al. (eds.), *Trypanosomatids: Methods and Protocols*, Methods in Molecular Biology, vol. 2116,
https://doi.org/10.1007/978-1-0716-0294-2_32,

benefits for the treatment of chronic disease [4, 5]. Additionally, many basic questions remain regarding the potential for metabolic flexibility and redundancies in the parasite that allow for its wide tissue tropism and, potentially, its escape from drug treatment. The recent observation that amastigotes have a highly plastic doubling time and dynamic cell cycle is indicative of an ability of the parasite to sense and respond to its environment to ensure productive replication in mammalian host cells [6]. Yet the mechanisms by which this is achieved and the specific elements being detected within the host are unknown and areas of ongoing research. This proliferative flexibility is especially important when prioritizing lead compounds as either trypanocidal or trypanostatic and in establishing metabolic dependencies of intracellular amastigotes that may be exploitable as therapeutic targets.

In this chapter, we outline several complementary methods for investigating intracellular *T. cruzi* amastigote growth and survival. Due to inherent limitations of scalability and/or readout for each assay, more than one assay is required to fully support conclusions about amastigote growth. Furthermore, the heterogeneity within a population of amastigotes cannot be adequately measured using a single technique. It is also important to note that for each technique, it is necessary to optimize assay parameters for different parasite strain–host cell combinations. Key points that should be considered are indicated. Here, we outline protocols that have been optimized for *T. cruzi* Tulahuén-LacZ ("Tula β-gal") clone C4 [7] infection of primary neonatal human dermal fibroblasts (NHDF).

1.1 Multiplexed Plate Assay to Measure Intracellular Parasite and Host Cell Abundance

The use of transgenic *T. cruzi* parasites for high throughput screening (e.g., detection based on *Escherichia coli* beta-galactosidase expressing transgenic lines) has facilitated the search for compounds with growth inhibitory properties [8–12]. The multiplexed plate-based assay outlined here (Subheading 3.2) measures relative amastigote and host cell abundance in single wells across a 384-well plate and is readily scalable for high throughput screening. This method is advantageous when many conditions need to be compared simultaneously, such as in an siRNA screen [13] or for screening of small molecules and IC_{50} determinations. Since host cell abundance is measured in each well, along with parasite load, treatments that impair host cell growth or viability and secondarily alter parasite load can be identified as toxic and triaged. The major limitation of this readout is that a reduction in parasite levels can be the result of either amastigote growth suppression or elimination (death) and, depending on when the perturbation is applied, a function of altered invasion properties. Automated high throughput imaging-based methodologies also exist [9, 14, 15], with inherent limits of detection (>1 parasite per cell) and consequently also do not allow for absolute determination of parasite growth suppression versus elimination.

1.2 Fluorescence Microscopy

Simple manual fluorescent microscopy using DNA stains to visualize both host cells and parasites (Subheading 3.3) can be used to complement high throughput approaches to distinguish between amastigote growth suppression or parasite elimination [6]. This technique is one of the most frequently used methods to measure amastigote growth in the *T. cruzi* literature. However, unless the inoculating dose of trypomastigotes is carefully titrated to minimize multiple invasion events, it is difficult to draw conclusions regarding amastigote growth. The second potential confounder is the division of infected host cells, where parasites are distributed between two daughter host cells, leading to artificial reduction in the measured number of amastigotes per cell. Therefore, any treatment or comparison that alters these processes can artificially skew interpretation of simple parasite counts by microscopy. For instance, the doubling time of different host cells can alter the number of amastigotes per cell without changing amastigote proliferation. In addition, the enumeration of amastigotes by microscopy does not assess their viability or current replicative state or their cell cycle, variables that can be important for understanding the impacts of any treatment.

1.3 Proliferation and Cell Cycle Quantification by Flow Cytometry

To complement a microscopic approach, we outline a flow-based method that can simultaneously measure the number of divisions an individual amastigote has undergone and the current state of its cell cycle (Subheading 3.4). As each amastigote divides, a stain (e.g., carboxyfluorescein succinimidyl ester, CFSE) is diluted and the number of divisions can be enumerated based on relative fluorescence intensity. Simultaneously, quantification of DNA content (e.g., DAPI) at the time of isolation allows for determination of cell cycle states. Therefore, the detection of CFSE identifies the extent to which parasites have divided. Since flow cytometry relies on relative fluorescence, several important controls are required to ensure proper interpretation of any dye-based proliferation measurement. First, undivided amastigotes must be collected (e.g., 18 h post infection (hpi)) for each experiment to set a relative 100%, and the fluorescent signal of unstained amastigotes must be known to identify the dynamic range. Without these metrics, the detection of proliferation dyes in a parasite has no relevance. Similarly, detection of these stains by microscopy cannot provide a quantitative measurement of amastigote proliferation.

1.4 Clonal Outgrowth to Measure Trypanocidal Activity

While direct measurement of proliferation and cell cycle by flow cytometry is informative with regard to amastigote growth suppression, the method only allows for detection of intact amastigotes. If a treatment kills a fraction of the parasite population, these events will go undetected. To distinguish lethal outcomes, a reciprocal assay that uses the extent of clonal outgrowth as a metric can be employed. The principles of this technique are adapted from published work and are not unique to *T. cruzi* [16]. The multiwell plate assay described (Subheading 3.5) was optimized, so that one parasite (intracellular amastigote), or fewer on average, is initially present in a given experimental well such that any detectable growth is the result of propagation of a clone. Treatments that result in a significant reduction in clonal outgrowth (i.e., the number of wells that become positive for parasite growth over time) as compared with mock-treated controls will be identified as having trypanocidal activity. Furthermore, this method is useful for determining the LD_{50} of cidal compounds [6]. The use of nonclonal (multiply infected) outgrowth measures provides a simpler and faster alternative but can only measure two outcomes; if no parasites survive a treatment or >1 parasites survive. The importance of this distinction is evident with benznidazole exposure where a range of concentrations exert growth suppressive effects, and as drug concentration is increased, these outcomes shift to a predominantly trypanocidal consequences that could not be detected without use of clonal outgrowth [6].

1.5 Purification of Intracellular Amastigotes

Since amastigote replication is intracellular, it is often difficult to separate direct versus indirect mechanisms of action for unknown compounds or treatments. Therefore, we also outline a methodology for the isolation and purification of intracellular amastigotes using a PD-10 column (Subheading 3.6). This technique allows for the separation of intracellular amastigotes from nonlysed host cells and host contaminants. These amastigotes are viable and can be used in downstream applications such as Seahorse metabolic flux analysis [17], ^{13}C metabolic tracing [18], and OMICS-based profiling [19]. We find that this method generally is more rapid and has lower levels of amastigote loss than anion-exchange chromatography methods [20], but PD-10 columns cannot separate trypomastigotes from amastigotes as anion-exchange chromatography can. While the purification of intracellular amastigotes is an important tool, these amastigotes do not divide under any conditions tested to date and therefore amastigote growth comparisons still require the use of host cells.

2 Materials

1. Rhesus Monkey Kidney Epithelial Cells, cell line LLC-MK_2 (ATCC, CCL-7).
2. Human Dermal Fibroblasts (e.g., cell line NHDF-Neo Lonza CC-2509).
3. *T. cruzi* Tulahuén-β-galactosidase clone C4 (ATCC, PRA-330) or other β-gal expressing clones.

4. Dulbecco's modified Eagle medium (DMEM) with or without phenol-red: 25 mM glucose, 2 mM L-glutamine, 100 U/mL penicillin-streptomycin, variable % FBS (D10 = 10% FBS, D2 = 2% FBS).
5. Humidified CO_2 incubator at 37 °C.
6. 75-cm^2 tissue culture flasks with vent cap (T-75).
7. Trypsin-EDTA (0.5%).
8. Phosphate Buffer Saline (PBS): without calcium or magnesium.
9. Centrifuge capable of 2060 × *g* with 15–50 mL tubes.
10. Centrifuge capable of 4000 × *g* using 1.5 mL tubes.
11. CellTiter-Fluor (CTF) from Promega.
12. Beta-Glo (βglo) from Promega.
13. Plate reader capable of fluorescence and luminescence in 384/96-well formats (e.g., EnVision Multimode Plate Reader from PerkinElmer).
14. 384-well clear flat-bottom black-walled polystyrene tissue culture treated microplates (e.g., Corning 3701).
15. BackSeal 96/384 black adhesive seal for microplates (PerkinElmer).
16. Hemocytometer.
17. Stainless steel vacuum manifold for microplates (e.g., Drummond scientific 3-000-101 for 384-well plates).
18. Multichannel pipette with volume capabilities from 10 to 60 μL.
19. 16% Paraformaldehyde stock solution.
20. Glass coverslips, 12 mm diameter.
21. Forceps.
22. ProLong Antifade Mounting solution (ThermoFisher Scientific).
23. Triton X-100.
24. DAPI (4′,6-diamidino-2-phenylindole).
25. Fluorescence microscope.
26. Flow cytometer with 405 nm laser and 488 nm laser.
27. DMSO (anhydrous).
28. CFSE (e.g., CellTrace CFSE Cell Proliferation Kit, ThermoFisher C34570).
29. 28 G blunt needles, 19 mm length (e.g., Harvard Apparatus 72-5485).
30. 1 mL syringe (e.g., BD Luer-Lok 309,628).
31. 1.5 mL microcentrifuge tubes.

3 Methods

3.1 Preparation of T. cruzi Trypomastigotes for Use in In Vitro Infections

1. Parasites are maintained in LLC-MK_2 (ATCC, CCL-7) cells (*see* **Note 1**). Confluent 75-cm^2 flasks are infected with 1×10^7 (high), 2×10^6 (medium), or 1×10^6 (low) trypomastigotes per flask weekly in D2 (*see* **Note 2**).
2. Collect the supernatant from parasite maintenance cultures and spin at $300 \times g$ for 5 min.
3. Collect the supernatant containing trypomastigotes in a new tube.
4. Spin the supernatant at $\geq 2060 \times g$ for 10 min to pellet trypomastigotes and any extracellular amastigotes. Do not remove the supernatant. Place the tube in a 5% CO_2 incubator at 37 °C.
5. Allow trypomastigotes to "swim" from the pellet for ≥2 h while in a 5% CO_2 incubator at 37 °C.
6. Collect the supernatant and place in a new tube.
7. Spin the supernatant at $\geq 2060 \times g$ for 10 min to pellet trypomastigotes. Remove the supernatant and resuspend the pellet in complete D2.
8. Spin the cell suspension again at $\geq 2060 \times g$ for 10 min to pellet trypomastigotes. Remove the supernatant and resuspend the pellet in complete D2 (*see* **Note 3**).
9. Count trypomastigotes on a hemocytometer and dilute to the desired concentration for the assay (*see* **Note 4**).

3.2 Multiplexed Assay to Measure Intracellular Parasite and Host Cell Abundance

1. Grow human dermal fibroblasts near confluence in 75-cm^2 flasks in D10 medium. Trypsinize and count cells using a hemocytometer (*see* **Note 5**).
2. Dilute fibroblasts to 5×10^4 per mL in D10. Using a multichannel pipette, add 30 μL per well of cells that corresponds to 1.5×10^3 cells per well in a 384-well plate (*see* **Note 6**). Allow cells to adhere to the plate overnight in a 5% CO_2 incubator at 37 °C.
3. Collect purified trypomastigotes (*see* Subheading 3.1).
4. Count trypomastigotes using a hemocytometer and dilute to 1.875×10^5 parasites per mL (*see* **Note 7**). Add 10 μL of diluted trypomastigotes per well (1.875×10^3 trypomastigotes per well, corresponding to an MOI of 1.25). Maintain uninfected wells for each condition to be tested.
5. Two hours following addition of trypomastigotes (2 hpi), remove growth medium from each well using a vacuum manifold and wash two times with PBS (30 μL per well) (*see* **Note 8**). Subsequently, add 30 μL per well complete D2 without phenol-red (*see* **Note 9**). Place plate back in a 5% CO_2 incubator at 37 °C.

6. At 18 hpi (*see* **Note 10**), add the treatment of interest. For example, 10 μL of a 4× compound can be added (final volume per well of 40 μL resulting in 1× of compound). Place plate back in a 5% CO_2 incubator at 37 °C.
7. At 66 hpi (*see* **Note 7**), place the 384-well plate at room temperature for at least 30 min (*see* **Note 11**).
8. Remove medium from each well using the vacuum manifold. Add 10 μL/well CTF and spin the plate briefly to ensure liquid is not on the side of any well. Incubate the plate at room temperature for 10 min and measure relative fluorescence units (RFU) (*see* **Note 12** and Fig. 1).
9. Add 10 μL/well βglo and spin the plate briefly to ensure liquid is not on the side of any well. Incubate the plate at room temperature for at least 30 min and measure luminescence (*see* **Note 13**). Use the uninfected wells in a given treatment condition to subtract luminescence values derived from the host cell and not the parasite (*see* **Note 14** and Fig. 1).

3.3 Enumeration of Amastigote Growth by Microscopy

1. Grow human dermal fibroblasts near confluence in 75-cm^2 flasks in D10 medium. Trypsinize and count cells using a hemocytometer.
2. Dilute fibroblasts to 8 × 10^4 cells per mL in D10.
3. Using a sterile pipette with vacuum or sterile tweezers, place one 12 mm diameter glass coverslip (sterile) per well in a 24-well cell culture plate.

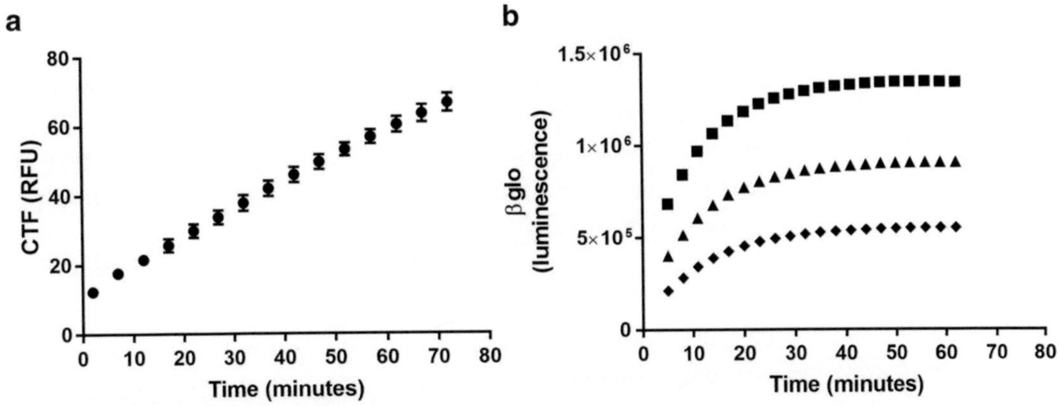

Fig. 1 CellTiter-Fluor (CTF) fluorescence and Beta-Glo (βglo) luminescence over time. (**a**) Cells were seeded and allowed to adhere for 24 h. Growth medium was removed and 10 μL/well CTF added ($n = 6$). Fluorescence was read sequentially at the indicated time points (*x*-axis), and relative fluorescence (RFU) values are shown (filled circles, mean and SD shown). (**b**) 10 μL of purified extracellular trypomastigotes were plated corresponding to 5 × 10^4 (squares), 2.5 × 10^4 (triangles), or 1.25 × 10^4 (diamonds), and 10 μL βglo was immediately added. Luminescence was read over time ($n = 6$ per condition)

4. Add 500 μL/well diluted fibroblasts in D10 (from **step 2**) (*see* **Note 15**).
5. Allow cells to adhere to the plate overnight in a 5% CO_2 incubator at 37 °C.
6. Collect purified trypomastigotes (*see* Subheading 3.1).
7. Count trypomastigotes using a hemocytometer and dilute to 1.6×10^5 trypomastigotes per mL in D2 (*see* **Note 7**). Remove growth medium from the fibroblast culture and add 500 μL/well of the trypomastigotes dilution (MOI 2). Place the plate in a 5% CO_2 incubator at 37 °C.
8. After 2 h, remove the trypomastigotes, wash each well two times with PBS. Add 500 μL/well D2, and place the plate in a 5% CO_2 incubator at 37 °C.
9. At 18 hpi, collect at least one coverslip using tweezers and place in a new 24 well plate (*see* **Note 16**). Place the plate with the remaining coverslips in a 5% CO_2 incubator at 37 °C until **step 11**.
10. Add 400 μL fixative (1% PFA/PBS) per well and place at 4 °C until staining (*see* **Note 17**).
11. At the desired time points post infection, collect coverslips in the same manner as **steps 9** and **10**.
12. Coverslips can be stained directly in 24-well plates used for fixation. Remove fixation solution and wash two times with PBS.
13. Add DAPI staining solution (0.1% Triton X-100 with 1 ug/mL DAPI) at room temperature.
14. Incubate at room temperature for 5 min.
15. Wash coverslips four times with PBS.
16. Place a single drop ~5 μL of ProLong mounting solution on a clean glass slide.
17. Pick up a single coverslip with forceps. Remove excess PBS by blotting around the edges of the coverslip with a kimwipe, careful not to disturb the cells.
18. Place coverslip cell side down on the ProLong solution (on slide from **step 16**).
19. Allow mounting solution to cure for ~24 h at room temperature in the dark.
20. Seal coverslips along their edges with nail polish for long-term storage.

3.4 Flow Cytometry-Based Detection of Amastigote Proliferation

1. Grow human dermal fibroblasts near confluence in 75-cm^2 flasks in D10 medium. Trypsinize and count cells using a hemocytometer (*see* **Note 5**).
2. Dilute fibroblasts to 2×10^5 per 3 mL in D10. Add 3 mL per well of a six-well plate. Allow cells to adhere to the plate overnight in a 5% CO_2 incubator at 37 °C.
3. Collect purified trypomastigotes (*see* Subheading 3.1).
4. Spin collected trypomastigotes at $\geq 2060 \times g$ for 10 min at room temperature. Resuspend trypomastigotes from the pellet in PBS.
5. Count trypomastigotes using a hemocytometer and dilute to 1×10^7 trypomastigotes per mL in PBS (2× staining concentration).
6. Add DMSO (*see* **Note 18**) to lyophilized CFSE for a stock concentration of 5 mM.
7. Add 1 μL of the 5 mM CFSE stock per 5 mL PBS (2× staining concentration) (*see* **Note 19**).
8. Add an equal volume of 2× stain (**step 7**) to 2× trypomastigotes (**step 5**) quickly to ensure homogeneity of the stain.
9. Incubate at 37 °C for 15 min.
10. Add ½ volume of warm D2 and mix by pipetting.
11. Immediately spin trypomastigotes at $\geq 2060 \times g$ for 10 min at room temperature. Resuspend trypomastigotes in D2 to wash and spin at $\geq 2060 \times g$ for 10 min at room temperature.
12. Resuspend the pellet (*see* **Note 20**) in D2 and count trypomastigotes using a hemocytometer. Dilute to the desired concentration (*see* **Note 21**).
13. Add CFSE stained trypomastigotes to fibroblasts in six-well plates. Two hours following addition of trypomastigotes (2 hpi), remove growth medium from each well, wash two times with PBS and replace with 3 mL/well D2.
14. At 18 hpi (*see* **Note 10**), the desired treatment can be initiated. Also at 18 hpi, one or two wells are collected, and amastigotes are isolated (*see* **steps 15–21**) (*see* **Note 22**).
15. At the desired time point for amastigote collection, wash each well with PBS and trypsinize host cells with 500 μL trypsin/well.
16. Quench the trypsinization with 500 μL/well D2 and transfer the cell suspension to a 1.5 mL tube. Spin cell suspension at $300 \times g$ for 5 min.
17. Remove the supernatant and resuspend the pellet in 500 μL PBS without calcium or magnesium (*see* **Note 23**).

18. Lyse host cells by passing the cell suspension twenty times through a 28 G needle (*see* **Note 24**).
19. Add paraformaldehyde to a final concentration of 1% and fix on ice for 20 min.
20. Following fixation, spin lysate for 10 min at 4000 × *g*.
21. Resuspend the pellet in 500 μL PBS and store at 4 °C until DAPI staining on the day of acquisition (**steps 22–24**).
22. On the day of acquisition, prepare a staining solution of PBS/Triton X-100 (0.1% v:v) with 10 ng/mL DAPI (4′,6-diamidino-2-phenylindole).
23. Spin lysate for 10 min at 4000 × *g* and resuspend the pellet in 200 μL staining solution (from **step 22**).
24. Place tubes on ice for ≥20 min and run on a flow cytometer (*see* **Note 25** and Fig. 2).

3.5 Quantification of Lethal Versus Static Effects on Amastigotes Through Clonal Outgrowth

1. Grow human dermal fibroblasts near confluence in 75-cm^2 flasks in D10 medium. Trypsinize and count cells using a hemocytometer (*see* **Note 5**).
2. Dilute fibroblasts to 5×10^4 cells per mL in D10 for seeding to a 384-well plate (add 30 μL/well) or 1×10^5 for a 96-well plate (add 100 μL/well). Allow cells to adhere to the plate overnight in a 5% CO_2 incubator at 37 °C. All subsequent steps pertain to 384-well plates with detection by luminescence (*see* **Note 26**).
3. Collect purified trypomastigotes (*see* Subheading 3.1).
4. Count trypomastigotes using a hemocytometer and dilute to 2.5×10^3 trypomastigotes per mL in D2. Add 10 μL of diluted trypomastigotes per well. The inoculating dose of trypomastigotes must be empirically determined (*see* **Note 27**).
5. Two hours following addition of trypomastigotes (2 hpi), remove growth medium from each well using a vacuum manifold and wash two times with PBS (30 μL per well) (*see* **Note 8**). Subsequently, add 30 μL per well complete D2 without phenol-red (*see* **Note 9**). Place plate back in a 5% CO_2 incubator at 37 °C.
6. At 18 hpi (*see* **Note 10**), initiate the treatment of interest.
7. After a predetermined exposure time (e.g., 24 h), remove growth medium from each well using a vacuum manifold and wash two times with PBS (30 μL per well). Subsequently, add 60 μL per well complete D2 without phenol-red. Place plate back in a 5% CO_2 incubator at 37 °C.
8. Allow parasites to grow for 14 days post infection (*see* **Note 28**).

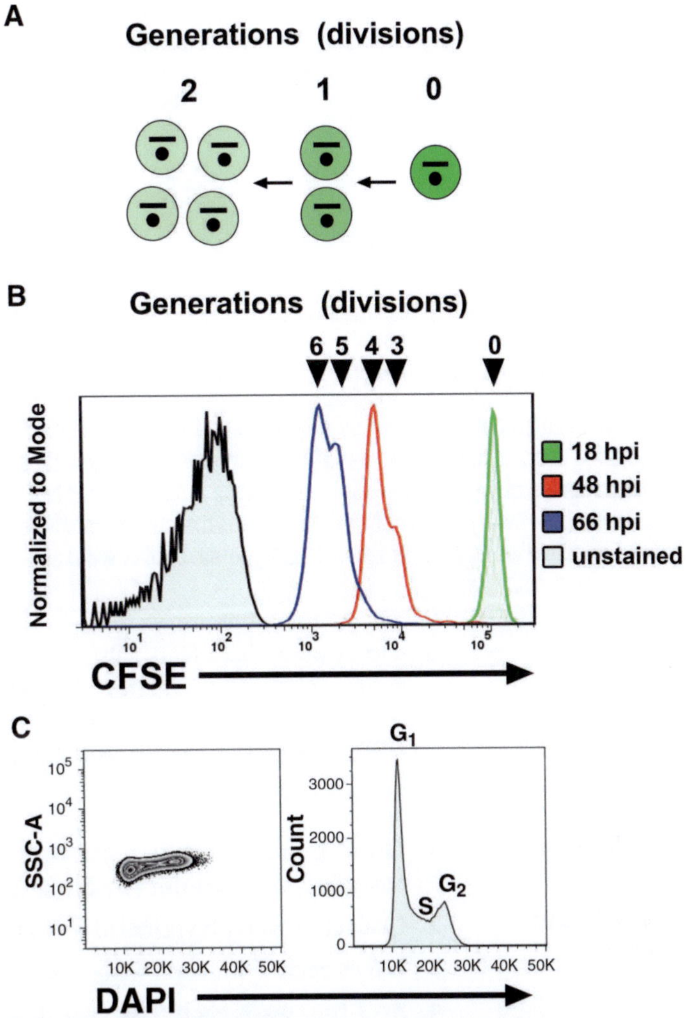

Fig. 2 Simultaneous measurement of amastigote proliferation and cell cycle by flow cytometry. (**a**) Cartoon depiction of amastigote proliferation and dilution of CFSE dye as parasites move from a nondividing state (18 hpi) through sequential rounds of division (right to left). (**b**) Histograms of relative CFSE fluorescence associated with intracellular *Trypanosoma cruzi* amastigotes isolated at indicated time points post infection. Unstained amastigotes are also plotted to demonstrate the dynamic range of CFSE. (**c**) Contour (left) and histogram (right) of DNA content of isolated amastigotes stained with DAPI

9. Remove medium from each well using the vacuum manifold (*see* **Note 29**).
10. Add 10 μL/well βglo and spin the plate briefly to ensure that liquid is not on the side of any well.
11. Read plate immediately and repeatedly for 30 min (*see* **Note 30**).

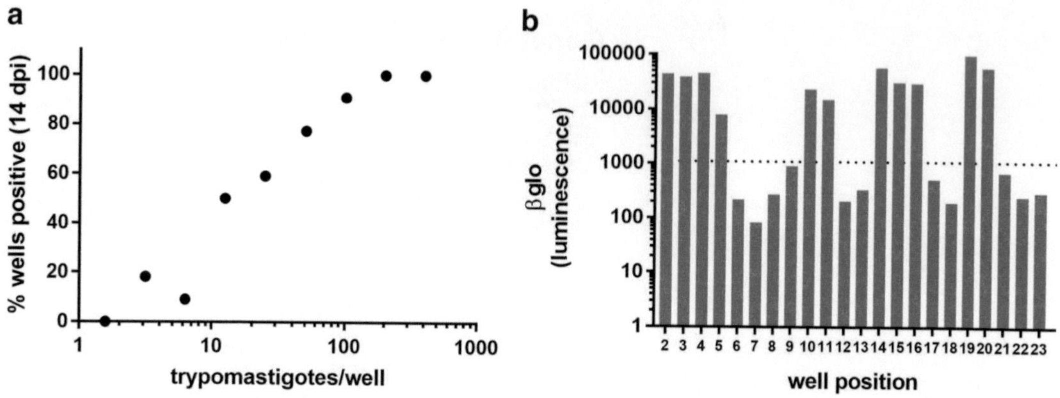

Fig. 3 Detection of clonal outgrowth by luminescence. (A) Plot of the relationship between the number of trypomastigotes used to initiate infection of NHDF (trypomastigotes/well) and the percentage of wells ($n = 22$) positive for parasites at 14 dpi using luminescence as a readout (*see* **Note 27**). (**b**) Luminescence signal from individual wells (384-well plate) is shown along with the cutoff (horizontal line) for discrimination of parasite positive and negative wells. An average of 12.5 trypomastigotes were added per well for 2 h. Plate was read at 14 dpi

12. Determine the mean signal from uninfected wells at a time point when the reaction has stabilized (*see* **Note 30** and Fig. 1). Set a discriminating value of 3× uninfected wells to differentiate between positive and negative clonal outgrowth (*see* Fig. 3).

3.6 PD-10 Column Purification of Intracellular T. cruzi *Amastigotes*

1. Grow human dermal fibroblasts near confluence in 75-cm^2 flasks in D10 medium (*see* **Note 5**).
2. Collect purified trypomastigotes (*see* Subheading 3.1).
3. Infect each T-75 flask with 5×10^6 trypomastigotes.
4. At 2 hpi, wash each flask two times with PBS and add 10 mL D2 per flask.
5. Between 48 and 66 hpi (*see* **Note 31**), remove D2 growth medium and wash cells one time with PBS.
6. Remove PBS and add 0.5 mL trypsin per flask and monitor for cell detachment.
7. Add 5 mL D2 to stop trypsinization and collect in a 15 mL tube.
8. Spin cell suspension at $300 \times g$ for 5 min and resuspend the pellet in 0.5 mL PBS. Move the cell suspension to a 1.5-mL microfuge tube.
9. Lyse host cells by passing the cell suspension twenty times through a 28 G needle (*see* **Note 24**).
10. Prepare PD-10 columns by removing the cap on the top of the column and pouring off the storage liquid.

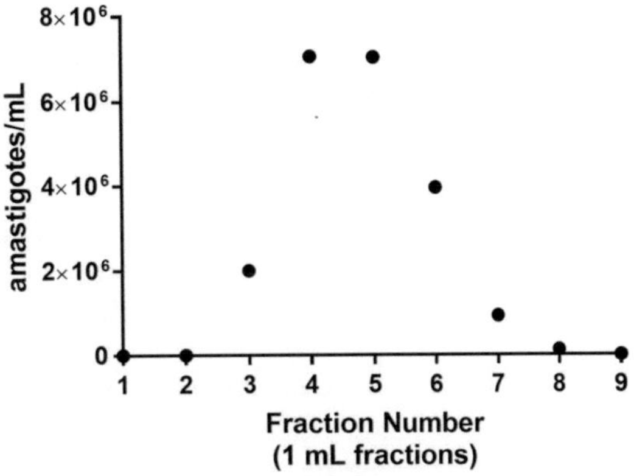

Fig. 4 Purification of intracellular *Trypanosoma cruzi* amastigotes. Host cells were lysed by syringe passage at 66 hpi, and lysate was applied to equilibrated PD-10 column. Fractions were collected immediately following addition of amastigotes to the column, and the number of amastigotes per fraction was counted following elution

11. Place the column so it is vertical and secure with a waste collection container underneath.
12. Remove the end of the column using scissors and fill the top of the column with PBS (equilibrium buffer). Allow the PBS to enter the column by gravity flow and drip into the waste container. Repeat until ~25 mL of PBS has passed through the column (*see* **Note 32**).
13. Dilute the lysate from **step 9** with PBS to a final volume of 2.5 mL.
14. Apply the lysate from **step 13** to one pre-equilibrated (**steps 10–12**) and allow the lysate to enter the column.
15. Apply PBS to the top of the column and collect 1 mL fractions (*see* Fig. 4).
16. Take 10 μL per fraction, and using a light microscope, look for the presence of amastigotes.
17. Pool fractions with amastigotes and spin at 4000 × *g* for 10 min.
18. Resuspend the resulting pellet in the desired buffer for downstream applications (*see* **Note 33**).

4 Notes

1. Uninfected confluent monolayers of LLC-MK$_2$ cells are trypsinized and split at a 1:20 ratio weekly and grown in D10 prior to infection. Allow growth for ~6 days in D10 prior to infection at which time the monolayer should be confluent. An

advantage of using LLC-MK_2 as host cells for maintenance of *T. cruzi* in vitro is that once a confluent monolayer is formed, it remains adherent after infection, allowing for daily harvesting of emerging trypomastigotes.

2. The intracellular *T. cruzi* maintenance strategy is as follows: T-75 flasks with confluent LLC-MK_2 cells are infected with between 1×10^7 and 1×10^6 *T. cruzi* trypomastigotes in D2 (harvested from the previous week's infection, or from a thawed previously frozen stock) on a Wednesday. The medium is changed to fresh D2 48 h later. Extracellular trypomastigotes are visible the following Monday, and subsequently, the medium is changed daily. Depending on the initial infecting dose, extracellular trypomastigotes can be harvested for the next 6–7 days before the cultures are no longer viable. Extracellular amastigotes will also be present in the supernatant with increasing numbers as the cultures age. Harvesting and preparing trypomastigotes for infections is described in Subheading 3.1.
3. Washing the purified trypomastigotes is important to remove soluble factors (e.g., cytokines) that may be present in the supernatant of the maintenance cultures.
4. The appropriate multiplicity of infection is determined by the parasite/host cell combination used, time of infection, time of detection, and specific technique to be used. The principles behind these determinations for each assay are discussed in their respective notes.
5. This specific protocol uses nonimmortalized human dermal fibroblasts. However, the principles of this assay allow for use with any host cell type, including immortalized or differentiated cells.
6. All wells of the 384-well plate should have liquid even if they will not be used for detection. Empty wells will interfere with the proper use of the vacuum manifold. Use of black-walled plates allows for the detection of fluorescence followed by luminescence. Clear bottom plates allow for visualization of cells during the experiment but require a black back seal prior to reading plates for fluorescence. This basic protocol can be adapted to a 96-well plate format, but reagent volumes and seeding densities should be optimized. This protocol is also compatible for use with automated liquid handling devices.
7. This protocol uses the parasite Tulahuén-β-gal clone C4 (ATCC, PRA-330) and nonimmortalized human dermal fibroblasts (Lonza CC-2509). The multiplicity of infection, time for invasion, and subsequent plate reading have all been optimized to (a) allow for maximum growth of amastigotes without conversion to trypomastigotes and (b) ensure that detection is

within the linear range of the reagents. It is *essential* that these parameters are empirically determined for every host cell–parasite strain combination to ensure proper interpretation of results.

8. Proper use of the vacuum manifold requires ensuring (a) that all wells in a given row to be used have liquid, (b) that the manifold does not touch the monolayer, and (c) that the force of the vacuum is appropriate to remove liquid but leave cells unperturbed (*see* **Note 6**).
9. Phenol-red in the medium has the potential to interference with downstream fluorescence measurements; use medium without phenol-red.
10. Since trypomastigotes are allowed to invade for 2 h and we initiate treatments at 18 hpi (trypomastigotes have invaded host cells, converted to the replicative amastigote stage but have not begun to divide—again the timing of these events should be empirically determined for each new parasite strain tested), we can ask questions regarding amastigote growth without differences in parasite invasion and/or differentiation into amastigotes confounding the interpretation of results.
11. The 384-well plate will cool once it is removed from the 37 °C incubator. Cooling is not uniform and will proceed from the edges inward. The rate of each reaction is temperature dependent, and plates are read at room temperature; therefore, if plates are not precooled to room temperature, the signals detected will be impacted by uneven temperature as the plate is read.
12. CellTiter-Fluor has an excitation efficiency maximum of ~360 nm and an emission efficiency maximum of ~490 nm. Some instruments may not detect at the emission maximum but may still be able to detect in a range near 490 nm. The CTF generated fluorescence increases with time in a linear fashion (*see* Fig. 1).
13. The βglo reaction and the derived luminescence do not proceed in a linear fashion (unlike fluorescence generated using CTF). The reaction must be allowed to reach equilibrium before proper comparisons can be made because the reaction in wells with greater parasite numbers initially proceeds more rapidly than wells with fewer parasites (*see* Fig. 1). The process generally takes >30 min, but the precise timing should be empirically determined using a titration of parasites.
14. Luminescence will occur simultaneously across all wells of the plate unlike fluorescence (detection of RFU requires excitation of individual wells one at a time). As a result, luminescence from adjacent wells can impact wells of interest as the plate is sequentially read. Use of physical barriers to block out light

from adjacent wells and/or mathematical adjustments can account for this well cross-talk.

Mammalian host cells have a low level of endogenous enzymatic activity that is detectable by the βglo reaction. Subtracting values from uninfected wells allows for determination of parasite-derived signal because in infected wells, the total luminescence signal is a sum of both parasite and host cell enzymatic activity. For assays such as antiparasitic compound titrations, we do not recommend normalizing βglo values (i.e., setting maximal values to 100 and minimum values to 0). However, normalization of data may be necessary in certain comparisons, such as determining IC_{50} shifts. Important: A decrease in βglo luminescence relative to a control does not necessarily indicate parasite death and can only be interpreted as an absence of growth.

15. Slowly pipette cells into the well, taking care to evenly distribute cells. Some cell lines may require special treatments such as addition of collagen to the coverslips to allow for proper attached.
16. By 18 hpi, the internalized trypomastigotes have completed their differentiation into amastigotes but have yet to undergo the first division. Therefore, any host cell that contains more than one amastigote at 18 hpi has been invaded by more than one trypomastigote. When the parasite growth assay is visual (i.e., by microscopy), multiple invasion events should be avoided by optimizing the multiplicity of infection, or growth data will be confounded. Always be aware of which side of the coverslip has adherent cells.
17. Coverslips can be left at 4 °C in fixative until all time points have been collected. Subsequently, all samples can be stained simultaneously.
18. Use anhydrous DMSO.
19. The final staining concentrations of CFSE or a similar dye should be empirically determined with the following considerations taken into account. First the staining concentration should not impact the proliferative capacity of the amastigotes. Staining concentrations should be titrated and can be compared with unstained controls by microscopy (*see* Subheading 3.3). Use of unnecessary high staining concentrations that impact proliferation can lead to dubious conclusions with regard to proliferation or proliferative capacity of intracellular amastigotes. In general, we find that optimal staining concentrations relative to cell number are much lower than those typically used for mammalian cells. The second consideration for staining concentration is the signal over unstaining amastigotes. The fluorescence intensity of a given amastigote will be

the sum of native fluorescence of the parasite and CFSE. Therefore, it is important to determine the difference in fluorescence between stained (undivided) and unstained parasites because this separation will determine the number of generations that can be measured before fluorescence values are indistinguishable from native fluorescence (*see* Fig. 2).

20. If the staining is successful, the pellet should now be a pale green that is distinguishable by eye.
21. Typically, we use a multiplicity of infection of 5–10 for Tulahuén-β-gal CFSE stained trypomastigotes.
22. Collection of amastigotes at 18 hpi is an *essential* step in properly quantifying amastigote proliferation and must be done for each experiment. Without this determination, subsequent fluorescence intensity will not be able to inform the number of divisions an amastigote has undergone.
23. Lysis of host cells by syringe passage is more efficient in PBS than medium.
24. For safety, DO NOT use a sharp tip needle. Blunt tip needles are readily available and can be reused. Count host cells using a hemocytometer before and after syringe lysis. After lysis, amastigotes should be present and appear similar in shape to watermelon seeds. If host cells are still present following lysis, additional syringe passages can be applied.
25. DO NOT wash samples after addition of staining solution, run directly on a suitable cytometer. To detect DAPI and CFSE, a cytometer must have the adequate lasers for excitation (e.g., 405 nM DAPI and 488 nM CFSE) and filters for detection of emission. Dyes with similar chemistry to CFSE or DAPI are available with alternative excitation and emission properties. Analysis can be performed using software such as FlowJo and proliferation models can be generated using the 18 hpi fluorescence intensity as the undivided value (*see* Fig. 2). In general, we find that CFSE stain after a single round of division is ~47% of the prior generation, and coefficients of variation of CFSE peaks slightly increase with each generation. Using a model (log scale for CFSE), the average number of generations from the culture can be determined along with the standard deviation of this measurement [21]. This calculation is important because as cells divide they contribute more events and therefore must be normalized. Models for cell cycle can also be fit using a linear scale for relative DAPI fluorescence. As in other systems, amastigotes in the G_2 phase of their cell cycle will be larger than G_1 parasites (*see* Fig. 2).
26. Infections can be carried out in 96-well plates, and visual inspection can be used to monitor for parasite outgrowth. This method is particularly laborious. However, it has been

used to validate and optimize detection by luminescence (*see* Fig. 3), especially since treatments such as benznidazole have growth suppressive effects that last even after drug exposure [6]. Visual identification of parasites can be performed on successive days, while detection by luminescence is an end point assay.

27. To differentiate between lethal or inhibitory effects of a given treatment, we adapted the principle of clonal outgrowth. In these assays, parasites are diluted, so that the eventual parasite outgrowth is likely the product of a single clone. In this system, the number of wells that have detectable parasite outgrowth is the measured parameter and approximates the number of surviving clones following a treatment. Since not all trypomastigotes invade the host cells present, it is necessary to deliver >1 parasites to individual wells to achieve infection in ~50% of wells. The number of trypomastigotes needed to be added to each well must be empirically predetermined by performing a titration where outgrowth is measured (*see* Fig. 3a). Our assay is optimized so that on average ~50% of wells under control conditions will have detectable parasitemia at 14 dpi when NHDF are exposed to on average 12.5–25 trypomastigotes per well for 2 h (*see* Fig. 3b). Titration of trypomastigotes is an important control to optimize the infection protocol, so that outgrowth is predominantly the result of single clones. In our hands, the number of parasite positive wells in the control conditions can vary from 40% to 60% of infected wells, and therefore, it is essential to have a control for normalization in each assay. Since multiple trypomastigotes are required per well to achieve ~50% well outgrowth, it is possible that multiple invasion events can occur at low frequency.

28. The use of 14 dpi was determined to be a time point at which (a) infected wells with outgrowth are readily detectable and (b) no difference in sensitivity was observed when compared with visual detection of parasites (*see* **Note 26**). Plates read at >14 dpi showed similar results.

29. The manifold should not remove the entire liquid contents of the well. If clear bottom 384-well plates are used, trypomastigotes should still be present in positive wells. Detection using βglo will be a combination of signal from remaining uninfected host cells (minimal, *see* **Note 10**), extracellular trypomastigotes and intracellular amastigotes.

30. To ensure that luminescence is stable (*see* Fig. 1), it is important to measure luminescence over time. If the reaction substrate is depleted, the luminescence signal will eventually fall to background and generate a false negative. We have not observed this phenomenon using this protocol, but care should be taken to ensure lack of signal in positive wells is not a function of time during plate reading.

31. If amastigotes are collected at time points, <66 hpi higher MOIs can be used.
32. The white filter on top of the packed portion of the column can be removed to increase flow rate or in conditions with a large amount of cell debris after lysis. In general, one to two 75-cm^2 flasks are used per column. If desired, the purification process can be repeated with a new column to further purify amastigotes.
33. Soluble host proteins elute in similar fractions to the amastigotes. Spins at 4000 × *g* can wash amastigotes and remove soluble host proteins. Purity should be independently assessed for alternative host cell types and with consideration to the specific downstream application.

References

1. Bern C (2015) Chagas' disease. N Engl J Med 373:456–466. https://doi.org/10.1056/NEJMra1410150
2. Zhang L, Tarleton RL (1999) Parasite persistence correlates with disease severity and localization in chronic Chagas' disease. J Infect Dis 180:480–486. https://doi.org/10.1086/314889
3. Tarleton RL, Zhang L, Downs MO (1997) "Autoimmune rejection" of neonatal heart transplants in experimental Chagas disease is a parasite-specific response to infected host tissue. Proc Natl Acad Sci U S A 94:3932–3937
4. Morillo CA, Marin-Neto JA, Avezum A, Sosa-Estani S, Rassi A, Rosas F, Villena E, Quiroz R, Bonilla R, Britto C, Guhl F, Velazquez E, Bonilla L, Meeks B, Rao-Melacini P, Pogue J, Mattos A, Lazdins J, Rassi A, Connolly SJ, Yusuf S, Investigators BENEFIT (2015) Randomized trial of benznidazole for chronic Chagas' cardiomyopathy. N Engl J Med 373:1295–1306. https://doi.org/10.1056/NEJMoa1507574
5. Murcia L, Carrilero B, Muñoz MJ, Iborra MA, Segovia M (2010) Usefulness of PCR for monitoring benznidazole response in patients with chronic Chagas' disease: a prospective study in a non-disease-endemic country. J Antimicrob Chemother 65:1759–1764. https://doi.org/10.1093/jac/dkq201
6. Dumoulin PC, Burleigh BA (2018) Stress-induced proliferation and cell cycle plasticity of intracellular *Trypanosoma cruzi* amastigotes. mBio 9. https://doi.org/10.1128/mBio.00673-18
7. Buckner FS, Verlinde CL, La Flamme AC, Van Voorhis WC (1996) Efficient technique for screening drugs for activity against *Trypanosoma cruzi* using parasites expressing beta-galactosidase. Antimicrob Agents Chemother 40:2592–2597
8. Romanha AJ, de CSL, Soeiro M de NC, Lannes-Vieira J, Ribeiro I, Talvani A, Bourdin B, Blum B, Olivieri B, Zani C, Spadafora C, Chiari E, Chatelain E, Chaves G, Calzada JE, Bustamante JM, Freitas-Junior LH, Romero LI, Bahia MT, Lotrowska M, Soares M, Andrade SG, Armstrong T, Degrave W, Andrade Z de A (2010) *In vitro* and *in vivo* experimental models for drug screening and development for Chagas disease. Mem Inst Oswaldo Cruz 105:233–238
9. Peña I, Pilar Manzano M, Cantizani J, Kessler A, Alonso-Padilla J, Bardera AI, Alvarez E, Colmenarejo G, Cotillo I, Roquero I, de Dios-Anton F, Barroso V, Rodriguez A, Gray DW, Navarro M, Kumar V, Sherstnev A, Drewry DH, Brown JR, Fiandor JM, Julio Martin J (2015) New compound sets identified from high throughput phenotypic screening against three kinetoplastid parasites: an open resource. Sci Rep 5:8771. https://doi.org/10.1038/srep08771
10. Khare S, Nagle AS, Biggart A, Lai YH, Liang F, Davis LC, Barnes SW, Mathison CJN, Myburgh E, Gao M-Y, Gillespie JR, Liu X, Tan JL, Stinson M, Rivera IC, Ballard J, Yeh V, Groessl T, Federe G, Koh HXY, Venable JD, Bursulaya B, Shapiro M, Mishra PK, Spraggon G, Brock A, Mottram JC, Buckner FS, Rao SPS, Wen BG, Walker JR, Tuntland T, Molteni V, Glynne RJ, Supek F (2016) Proteasome inhibition for treatment of leishmaniasis, Chagas disease and sleeping sickness. Nature

537:229–233. https://doi.org/10.1038/nature19339

11. Diaz-Gonzalez R, Kuhlmann FM, Galan-Rodriguez C, Madeira da Silva L, Saldivia M, Karver CE, Rodriguez A, Beverley SM, Navarro M, Pollastri MP (2011) The susceptibility of trypanosomatid pathogens to PI3/m-TOR kinase inhibitors affords a new opportunity for drug repurposing. PLoS Negl Trop Dis 5:e1297. https://doi.org/10.1371/journal.pntd.0001297
12. Bettiol E, Samanovic M, Murkin AS, Raper J, Buckner F, Rodriguez A (2009) Identification of three classes of heteroaromatic compounds with activity against intracellular *Trypanosoma cruzi* by chemical library screening. PLoS Negl Trop Dis 3:e384. https://doi.org/10.1371/journal.pntd.0000384
13. Caradonna KL, Engel JC, Jacobi D, Lee C-H, Burleigh BA (2013) Host metabolism regulates intracellular growth of *Trypanosoma cruzi*. Cell Host Microbe 13:108–117. https://doi.org/10.1016/j.chom.2012.11.011
14. Alonso-Padilla J, Cotillo I, Presa JL, Cantizani J, Peña I, Bardera AI, Martín JJ, Rodriguez A (2015) Automated high-content assay for compounds selectively toxic to *Trypanosoma cruzi* in a myoblastic cell line. PLoS Negl Trop Dis 9:e0003493. https://doi.org/10.1371/journal.pntd.0003493
15. Sykes ML, Avery VM (2015) Development and application of a sensitive, phenotypic, high-throughput image-based assay to identify compound activity against *Trypanosoma cruzi* amastigotes. Int J Parasitol Drugs Drug Resist 5:215–228. https://doi.org/10.1016/j.ijpddr.2015.10.001
16. Young RD, Rathod PK (1993) Clonal viability measurements on *Plasmodium falciparum* to assess *in vitro* schizonticidal activity of leupeptin, chloroquine, and 5-fluoroorotate. Antimicrob Agents Chemother 37:1102–1107
17. Shah-Simpson S, Pereira CFA, Dumoulin PC, Caradonna KL, Burleigh BA (2016) Bioenergetic profiling of *Trypanosoma cruzi* life stages using Seahorse extracellular flux technology. Mol Biochem Parasitol 208:91–95. https://doi.org/10.1016/j.molbiopara.2016.07.001
18. Shah-Simpson S, Lentini G, Dumoulin PC, Burleigh BA (2017) Modulation of host central carbon metabolism and *in situ* glucose uptake by intracellular *Trypanosoma cruzi* amastigotes. PLoS Pathog 13:e1006747. https://doi.org/10.1371/journal.ppat.1006747
19. Gazos-Lopes F, Martin JL, Dumoulin PC, Burleigh BA (2017) Host triacylglycerols shape the lipidome of intracellular trypanosomes and modulate their growth. PLoS Pathog 13:e1006800. https://doi.org/10.1371/journal.ppat.1006800
20. Marques A, Marques A, Nakayasu E, Almeida I (2011) Purification of extracellular and intracellular amastigotes of *Trypanosoma cruzi* from mammalian host-infected cells. Protoc Exch. https://doi.org/10.1038/protex.2011.265
21. Roederer M (2011) Interpretation of cellular proliferation data: avoid the panglossian. Cytom Part J Int Soc Anal Cytol 79:95–101. https://doi.org/10.1002/cyto.a.21010

Chapter 33

Isolation of Extracellular Vesicles from *Leishmania* spp.

Andrea Vucetic, Alonso Da Silva Lira Filho, George Dong, and Martin Olivier

Abstract

Exosomes, a class of extracellular vesicles, are released by eukaryotes, bacteria, and archaea, as evident from both in vitro and in vivo studies. These nano-sized double-membraned vesicles play an important role in cell-to-cell communication, dysregulation of the immune system, and pathogenesis in a number of diseases, including leishmaniasis. *Leishmania* is a genus of obligate intracellular parasites, which infect host macrophages, are transmitted through the bite of a sandfly, and are shown to secrete exosomes with immunomodulatory activities. Given the importance of these vesicles in *Leishmania* spp. virulence, it is necessary to perform appropriate isolation and characterization in order to further study their relevance in the parasite's infectious life cycle. In this chapter, we describe four methods for the isolation of extracellular vesicles derived from *Leishmania* species including ultracentrifugation, polyethylene glycol-based precipitation, size-exclusion chromatography, and sucrose-gradient fractionation. Further, we describe the preparation of isolated samples for characterization by nanoparticle tracking analysis, transmission electron microscopy, and proteomic profiling.

Key words Extracellular vesicles, Exosomes, Leishmania, Ultracentrifugation, ExtraPEG, Size exclusion chromatography, Sucrose gradient, Micro BCA, Nanoparticle tracking analysis, Transmission electron microscopy, Trichloroacetic acid protein precipitation

1 Introduction

Exosomes are a class of extracellular vesicles (EVs) that are ubiquitous among eukaryotes and have been implicated in numerous diseases, leishmaniasis included. It has been recently shown that *Leishmania* exosomes are both constitutively enriched with virulence factors, such as GP63, that are capable of immune modulation of host macrophages and released in the sandfly midgut [1]. Exosomes are 40–120 nm in diameter, possess a specific density of 1.13–1.19 g/mL, and are characterized by physical properties that allow for their purification from a liquid culture of *Leishmania* [2]. This purification or isolation can be conducted by high-speed ultracentrifugation, size exclusion chromatography, and polyethylene glycol-based methods (ExtraPEG) [2–5].

Paul A. M. Michels et al. (eds.), *Trypanosomatids: Methods and Protocols*, Methods in Molecular Biology, vol. 2116, https://doi.org/10.1007/978-1-0716-0294-2_33, © Springer Science+Business Media, LLC, part of Springer Nature 2020

The method selected should align with the scientific question and the intended downstream experimental applications [6]. Following their separation, it is important to perform a number of analyses to characterize the exosomes, for which the International Society for Extracellular Vesicles (ISEV) recently released an updated set of guidelines required for the study of EVs in order to improve the reproducibility and reliability of experimental data in the field [7]. However, our protocols will focus on the preparation of EV samples for downstream characterization analysis. To determine the morphology and size of EVs, nanoparticle tracking analysis (NTA) and transmission electron microscopy (TEM) are used [8, 9]. NTA is performed using the commercially available platforms NanoSight and ZetaView, while TEM is performed on samples that have been negatively stained [10–12]. EV density is characterized using a sucrose gradient, which can also be used to further purify exosomes [2]. Proteomic analysis is performed using liquid chromatography–mass spectrometry (LC-MS/MS), and the resulting protein hits are identified using a database of *Leishmania* proteins [13, 14]. Our lab has shown that the release of *Leishmania* exosomes is greatly increased upon a temperature shift to 37 °C, and we use this property to increase exosome production before purification, leading to a higher yield [14].

2 Materials

Prepare all solutions using ultrapure (double-distilled) water to attain a sensitivity of 18 MΩ cm at 25 °C and analytical grade reagents. Pass all buffers through a 0.22-μm filter if the final use of the EVs will require sterility. Prepare and store all reagents at 4 °C.

2.1 Parasite Culture, Cleaning of Parasite Conditioned Medium

1. Parasite culture medium: Schneider's *Drosophila* Medium (SDM) supplemented with 10% heat-inactivated fetal bovine serum (FBS), 5 μg/mL hemin, 100 U/mL penicillin, and 100 μg/mL streptomycin.
2. Phosphate-buffered saline (PBS): 155.17 mM NaCl, 1.54 mM KH_2PO_4, 2.71 mM Na_2HPO_4, pH 7.4.
3. RPMI 1640, 1× medium without phenol red.
4. 50 mL conical centrifuge tubes.
5. High-speed centrifuge: e.g., Beckman Allegra 6R Refrigerated Centrifuge (Beckman Coulter Life Sciences, Indianapolis, IN, USA).

2.2 Ultracentrifugation

1. Exosome buffer: 137 mM NaCl, 20 mM HEPES, pH 7.5. Add approximately 100 mL water to a 1-L graduated cylinder. Weigh 8 g sodium chloride and 4.77 g HEPES and transfer to the cylinder. Add water to a volume of 900 mL. Mix and adjust pH with HCl (*see* **Note 1**). Make up volume to 1 L with water.
2. Ultracentrifuge: e.g., Beckman Optima™ XPN-90 (Beckman Coulter Life Sciences, Indianapolis, IN, USA).
3. Ultracentrifuge rotor: Beckman Coulter SW 32.1 Ti swinging-bucket (Beckman Coulter Life Sciences, Indianapolis, IN, USA).
4. Ultracentrifuge tubes: open-top thin wall polypropylene tube (16 × 102 mm) (Beckman Coulter, Brea, CA, USA) (*see* **Note 2**).
5. Precision balance with minimum readability of 0.01 g: e.g., Mettler Toledo ML3002T (Mettler Toledo Canada, Mississauga, ON, Canada).

2.3 Polyethylene Glycol-Based Method (ExtraPEG)

1. ExtraPEG stock solution (2×) (16%): Dissolve 16 g of polyethylene glycol (Sigma, 81260) and 5.84 g of NaCl in water for a final volume of 100 mL.
2. Refrigerated tabletop centrifuge: e.g., Eppendorf 5424 R (Eppendorf Canada, Mississauga, ON, Canada).
3. 1.5 mL microcentrifuge tubes.
4. Exosome buffer: 137 mM NaCl, 20 mM HEPES, pH 7.5. Add approximately 100 mL water to a 1-L graduated cylinder. Weigh 8 g sodium chloride and 4.77 g HEPES and transfer to the cylinder. Add water to a volume of 900 mL. Mix and adjust pH with HCl (*see* **Note 1**). Make up volume to 1 L with water.

2.4 Size-Exclusion Chromatography

1. Equilibration and run-through buffer stock: 200 mM ammonium acetate, pH 6.5. Add approximately 100 mL water to a 1-L graduated cylinder. Weigh 15.42 g ammonium acetate and transfer to the cylinder. Add water to a volume of 900 mL. Mix and adjust pH with HCl (*see* **Note 1**). Make up volume to 1 L with water.
2. Column preservation solution stock: 0.02% sodium azide. Add approximately 90 mL water to a 100-mL graduated cylinder. Weigh 0.02 g sodium azide and transfer to the cylinder. Make up volume to 100 mL with water.
3. Phosphate-buffered saline (PBS): 155.17 mM NaCl, 1.54 mM KH_2PO_4, 2.71 mM Na_2HPO_4, pH 7.4.
4. Pierce™ Disposable 10 mL polypropylene columns (Thermo-Scientific, Rockford, IL, USA).

5. Sepharose™ CL-4B (GE Healthcare, Uppsala, Sweden).
6. 50 mL conical centrifuge tubes.
7. 1.5 mL microcentrifuge tubes.

2.5 Sucrose-Gradient Purification

1. Exosome buffer: 137 mM NaCl, 20 mM HEPES, pH 7.5. Add approximately 100 mL water to a 1-L graduated cylinder. Weigh 8 g sodium chloride and 4.77 g HEPES and transfer to the cylinder. Add water to a volume of 900 mL. Mix and adjust pH with HCl (*see* **Note 1**). Make up volume to 1 L with water.
2. 2 M sucrose solution: Add 684.6 g of sucrose in 600 mL of Exosome buffer and continue to stir until completely dissolved. Make up volume to 1 L with water. Smaller volumes of solution can be made, keeping in mind the ratio of sucrose to the volume of buffer (*see* **Note 3**).
3. Ultracentrifuge: e.g., Beckman Optima™ XPN-90 (Beckman Coulter Life Sciences, Indianapolis, IN, USA).
4. Ultracentrifuge rotor: Beckman Coulter SW 32.1 Ti swinging-bucket and Type 90 Ti fixed-angle (Beckman Coulter Life Sciences, Indianapolis, IN, USA).
5. Ultracentrifuge tubes: open-top thin wall polypropylene tube (16 × 102 mm) (Beckman Coulter, Brea, CA, USA) and polycarbonate bottles with cap (10.4 mL) (16 × 76 mm) (code 355603, Beckman Coulter, Brea, CA, USA) (*see* **Note 2**).
6. Precision balance with minimum readability of 0.01 g: e.g., Mettler Toledo ML3002T (Mettler Toledo Canada, Mississauga, ON, Canada).

2.6 Micro BCA Protein Assay

1. Exosome buffer: 137 mM NaCl, 20 mM HEPES, pH 7.5. Add approximately 100 mL water to a 1-L graduated cylinder. Weigh 8 g sodium chloride and 4.77 g HEPES and transfer to the cylinder. Add water to a volume of 900 mL. Mix and adjust pH with HCl (*see* **Note 1**). Make up volume to 1 L with water.
2. Micro BCA™ Protein Assay Kit, catalog number 23235 (ThermoFisher Scientific, Rockford, IL, USA).
3. 96-well plate.
4. Sealing tape for 96-well plates (ThermoFisher Scientific, Waltham, MA, USA).
5. Plate reader with plate shaker (e.g., ASYS UVM 340 Microplate Reader, Biochrom Ltd., Cambourne, Cambridge, UK).

2.7 Nanoparticle Tracking Analysis

1. Exosome buffer: 137 mM NaCl, 20 mM HEPES, pH 7.5. Add approximately 100 mL water to a 1-L graduated cylinder. Weigh 8 g sodium chloride and 4.77 g HEPES and transfer to the cylinder. Add water to a volume of 900 mL. Mix and adjust pH with HCl (*see* **Note 1**). Make up volume to 1 L with water.
2. NTA device: e.g., Nanosight NS500 (Malvern Panalytical, Malvern, Worcestershire, UK).
3. 1.5 mL microcentrifuge tubes.

2.8 Negative Staining for TEM

1. Copper grids for TEM with carbon/Formvar film: e.g., Carbon Films on 200 Mesh Grids Copper (Agar Scientific Ltd., Stansted, Essex, UK).
2. Grid tweezers: e.g., PELCO® Pro Reverse (self-closing) Tweezers (Ted Pella Inc., Redding, CA, USA).
3. 2.0% glutaraldehyde in 0.1 M sodium cacodylate buffer, pH 7.4. Add 0.8 mL EM-grade 25% glutaraldehyde aqueous solution (Millipore Sigma, Burlington, MA, USA) and 0.214 g of sodium cacodylate trihydrate (Millipore Sigma, Burlington, MA, USA) to a 10-mL graduated cylinder. Mix and adjust pH with HCl. Make up volume to 10 mL with water. Store up to 6 months at −20 °C or up to 1 week at 4 °C after thawing.
4. 1.0% uranyl acetate.
5. Grid holder: e.g., PELCO® TEM Grid Storage Box (Ted Pella Inc., Redding, CA, USA).

2.9 Trichloroacetic Acid (TCA) Protein Precipitation

1. 10× TE Buffer: 1 M Tris–HCl (pH 8.0), 0.5 M EDTA. Add 1 mL Tris–HCl and 0.8 mL EDTA to a 10-mL graduated cylinder. Add water to a volume of 10 mL.
2. 0.3% sodium deoxycholate (NaDoc). Add approximately 90 mL water to a 100 mL graduated cylinder. Weigh 0.3 g of NaDoc and transfer to the cylinder. Make up volume to 100 mL with water.
3. 72% TCA. Add approximately 40 mL water to a 100 mL graduated cylinder. Weigh 72 g of TCA and transfer to the cylinder. Make up volume to 100 mL with water.
4. 90% acetone. Add 1 mL of water to 9 mL of 100% acetone in a 10-mL graduated cylinder.
5. Refrigerated tabletop centrifuge: e.g., Eppendorf 5424 R (Eppendorf Canada, Mississauga, ON, Canada).
6. 1.5 mL microcentrifuge tubes.

3 Methods

3.1 Cell Culture, Cleaning of Parasite Conditioned Medium

1. Culture parasites in SDM until they reach stationary phase (about 7–8 days following the last passage). Determine the density of *Leishmania* cells in the culture (*see* **Notes 4** and **5**).
2. Transfer parasite culture into 50 mL tubes. Centrifuge at 300 × *g* at room temperature (RT; 25 °C) for 5 min (*see* **Note 6**). Discard the medium into waste containers.
3. Lightly resuspend the pellet by agitating the bottom of the tube and top up volume to 50 mL with PBS. Centrifuge at 300 × *g* at RT for 5 min. Pour off the PBS into waste containers. Gently resuspend the pellet as described and repeat the washing process with PBS once more (*see* **Note 7**).
4. Resuspend the *Leishmania* pellet in 10 mL of RPMI 1640, 1× at a concentration of approximately 1–4 × 10^8 parasites/mL.
5. Place tubes in a horizontal position and incubate for 4 h at 37 °C with low agitation (40–60 rpm) (*see* **Note 8**).
6. Centrifuge tubes at 1000 × *g* (avg) at RT for 5 min and quickly transfer the supernatant containing *Leishmania*-derived EVs using a serological pipette into clean centrifuge tubes. Repeat this step once more (*see* **Note 9**).

3.2 Ultra-centrifugation

1. Pass the supernatant from the second centrifugation through a 0.45-μm syringe filter, followed by a 0.22-μm syringe filter, using 20 mL syringes (*see* **Note 10**).
2. Transfer filtered supernatant to ultracentrifuge tubes.
3. Load the filled ultracentrifuge tubes into the SW 32.1 Ti buckets.
4. Carefully weigh and then balance the tubes in the buckets (*see* **Note 11**).
5. Match the bucket caps with the numbered buckets. Tightly close the caps by aligning the pins on each side of the cap with the guide slots in the bucket and then twisting clockwise one-quarter turn.
6. Holding the tabs of the bucket caps, lower the buckets into the corresponding numbered openings on the rotor body (*see* **Note 12**).
7. Centrifuge at 100,000 × *g* at 4 °C for 70 min.
8. Carefully aspirate the supernatant from each tube (*see* **Note 13**).
9. Pool all pellets together into one tube and complete volume with Exosome buffer.
10. Repeat **steps 4–6**.

11. Centrifuge at 100,000 × *g* at 4 °C for 70 min.
12. With extra caution, carefully aspirate supernatant from the tube. Leave approximately 200–300 μL of volume.
13. Resuspend pellet in Exosome buffer and aliquot the sample.
14. Store samples at −80 °C.

3.3 Polyethylene Glycol-Based Method (ExtraPEG)

1. Follow steps described in Subheadings 3.1 and 3.2, **step 1**.
2. Add equal volumes of ExtraPEG Stock Solution (2×) (16%) and conditioned medium to acquire a final concentration of 8% PEG (*see* **Note 14**) [5].
3. Incubate solution at 4 °C overnight. Keep tubes upright. Do not agitate or rotate during incubation time.
4. The following day, centrifuge tubes at 3000 × *g* at 4 °C for 30 min (or up to 1 h to increase yield). Vesicles will be precipitated as pellet.
5. Gently aspirate supernatant, making sure to leave some volume behind to avoid accidental aspiration of the pellet.
6. Spin down residual solution at 3000 × *g* at 4 °C for 30 min.
7. Aspirate the supernatant. Do not disturb pellet.
8. Resuspend the pellet in 50–500 μL of Exosome buffer.

3.4 Size-Exclusion Chromatography

1. Equilibrate the column, resin slurry, and buffers to RT (*see* **Note 15**).
2. Position the empty 10-mL column upright in a clamp or column rack and cut the bottom tip with scissors. Put the bottom cap in place.
3. Prepare a 100 mL solution of 100 mM ammonium acetate by diluting the 200 mM ammonium acetate stock with water. Soak the porous filter disc in a small volume of this solution.
4. Use the reverse end of a Pasteur pipette or 1000 μL pipette tip to push the disc evenly to the bottom of the column, ensuring that the filter disc lays flat.
5. Homogenize the bottle of resin slurry by stirring or swirling the bottle. Pour approximately 15 mL of the slurry into a 50-mL tube (*see* **Note 16**).
6. Pour the resin slurry from the conical tube slowly into the column. Wait at least 30 min to allow the resin to settle in the column.
7. Remove the bottom cap and allow the liquid to flow through, permitting the beads to pack into the column.
8. Continue to pour the beads while the liquid drains from the bottom of the column until the level of the resin bed reaches approximately 1.5 cm below the opening of the column (*see* **Note 17**).

9. Equilibrate the packed column by slowly adding 100 mM ammonium acetate on top of the resin bed, ensuring that the surface area is consistently covered evenly (*see* **Notes 18** and **19**). Continue to wash the column with a total of 100 mL of buffer, adding it slowly each time with a 1000 μL pipettor (*see* **Note 20**).
10. Dilute 1 mL of supernatant from the last centrifugation step in Subheading 3.1 in 1 mL of 200 mM ammonium acetate (*see* **Note 21**).
11. Once the layer of buffer reaches a height of approximately 1–2 mm above the surface of the packed resin bed, load the diluted supernatant (2 mL) to the top of the column.
12. Elute the column with the same buffer, collecting fractions of volume 500 μL to 1 mL, depending on the approach, in appropriately labeled microcentrifuge tubes (*see* **Notes 22** and **23**). Store fractions at −80 °C.
13. Dilute 5 mL of 0.02% sodium azide with an equal volume of 200 mM ammonium acetate. Following collection of the final fraction, add approximately 5 mL of diluted sodium azide to the top of the packed resin bed and allow to run throughout the column (*see* **Note 24**).
14. Cap the bottom of the column, add 1–2 mL of the ammonium acetate buffer to the surface of the resin bed to prevent drying, and then cap the top of the column.
15. Store the packed column upright and capped at both the top and bottom ends at 4 °C (*see* **Notes 25** and **26**).

3.5 Sucrose-Gradient Purification

1. Follow steps described in Subheadings 3.1 and 3.2, **step 1**.
2. Using the 2-M sucrose stock solution, create 1.5 M, 1 M, and 0.5 M dilutions using Exosome buffer.
3. Create a sucrose gradient in each polycarbonate bottle in the following order: Bottom → Top (2, 1.5, 1, 0.5 M). Each layer of sucrose in the gradient should have a volume of 2 mL. Position the ultracentrifuge bottle at a 45° angle and slowly pour the different dilutions with a 1000-μL pipettor, making sure not to disrupt the layers.
4. Carefully place the extracted sample on top of the upper-most sucrose layer, making sure not to disturb the gradient.
5. Carefully weigh and then balance the bottles (*see* **Note 11**).
6. Load the filled bottles symmetrically in the rotor (*see* **Note 27**).
7. Centrifuge bottles at 110,000 × *g* at 4 °C for 90 min.
8. Number ten open-top thin wall polypropylene ultracentrifuge tubes (1–10).

9. After centrifugation, collect ten fractions of 1 mL and place each fraction into the corresponding labeled ultracentrifuge tube in the order of removal.
10. Wash each fraction with Exosome buffer, following the steps outlined in Subheading 3.2, **steps 2–14**.
11. Exosomes are typically found in fractions 4, 5, and 6, corresponding to concentrations of 0.8–1.2 M of sucrose and densities of 1.10–1.15 g/mL (*see* **Note 28**).
12. Resuspend the pellet in Exosome buffer and aliquot the sample.
13. Store samples at −80 °C.

3.6 Micro BCA Protein Assay

1. Prepare protein standards according to the following table using one bovine serum albumin (BSA) standard ampule and Exosome buffer:

Protein standard	Volume of exosome buffer (mL)	Volume and source of BSA	Final BSA concentration (μg/mL)
A	4.5	0.5 mL of stock	200
B	8.0	2.0 mL of A	40
C	4.0	4.0 mL of B	20
D	4.0	4.0 mL of C	10
E	4.0	4.0 mL of D	5
F	4.0	4.0 mL of E	2.5
G	4.8	3.2 mL of F	1.0
H	4.0	4.0 mL of G	0.5
I	8.0	0 mL	0 = BLANK

2. Prepare the working reagent using 25 parts reagent MA, 24 parts reagent MB, and 1 part reagent MC, which is represented by the following formulas (*see* **Notes 29** and **30**):

$$\text{Total volume} = (\text{of standards} + \text{of samples}) \times 100\ \mu\text{L} \times 2 \times 1.2$$

$$\text{Volume of MA} = \frac{\text{Total volume}}{2}$$

$$\text{Volume of MB} = \frac{\text{Total volume}}{50} \times 24$$

$$\text{Volume of MC} = \frac{\text{Total volume}}{50}$$

3. Dilute samples by 1:20 in Exosome buffer to achieve a final volume of 240 μL per sample (*see* **Note 31**).
4. Pipette 100 μL of each standard into duplicate wells in descending order of protein concentration, followed by the samples and Exosome buffer blank.
5. Pipette 100 μL of working reagent into each well, mixing gently by pipette or on a plate shaker for 30 s (*see* **Note 32**).
6. Cover plate using sealing tape or plate lid and incubate at 37 °C for 2 h (*see* **Note 33**).
7. Cool plate to RT for approximately 15–30 min.
8. Measure absorbance at 562 nm using a plate reader.
9. Create a standard curve by plotting the average blank-corrected 562 nm reading of each BSA standard versus its known protein concentration, then use this curve to calculate the protein concentration of the desired sample, making sure to multiply by the correct dilution factor (*see* **Note 34**).

3.7 Nanoparticle Tracking Analysis

1. Dilute samples to a protein concentration of 2 μg/mL, based on Micro BCA results, using Exosome buffer to achieve a total volume of 1000 μL in a microcentrifuge tube (*see* **Note 35**).
2. Prepare the NanoSight machine with a liquid waste container and a 15-mL tube of distilled water placed in one of the openings in the metal platform of the NanoSight.
3. Place the thin plastic tube used for flushing in another container filled with distilled water.
4. Open the NanoSight software and prime the fluidics of the NanoSight.
5. Turn on the camera and set the SOP with the following settings:

   SETTEMP 37.

   CAMERASETTINGMSG.

   REPEATSTART.

   PUMPADV.

   DELAY 5.

   CAPTURE 30.

   DELAY 1.

   REPEAT 2.

   TEMPERATURECONTROLOFF.

   PROCESSSINGLESETTING.

   EXPORTRESULTS.

6. Insert the loading tube into the 15 mL tube with distilled water and select "load" in the hardware control screen.
7. Vortex the diluted sample, and place microcentrifuge tube in the other opening of the metal platform.
8. Wipe the loading tube with a Kimwipe and insert into the sample (*see* **Note 36**) and then select "load."
9. Name the file appropriately in the SOP tab.
10. Once the sample is loaded, adjust the camera level, so that there are particles visible, but background is low, and then adjust the focus (*see* **Note 37**). Select "advance" to verify the focus with different portions of the sample.
11. Once the camera is set, select "run."
12. Once all the videos are captured and analysis begins, you may remove the sample after confirming the processing settings. Connect the loading tube to the waste container and select "flush" in the hardware control screen.
13. Once analysis is complete, select the files that are to be generated and export the results (Fig. 1) (*see* **Note 38**).
14. Repeat **steps 6–13** for each following sample (*see* **Note 39**).
15. Once finished, flush an additional time to fully clean the system.

3.8 Negative Staining for TEM

1. Spread parafilm on a tabletop (*see* **Note 40**).
2. Place a drop of glutaraldehyde, three drops of ultrapure (double-distilled) water, and uranyl acetate, arranging the five drops in a row as depicted:

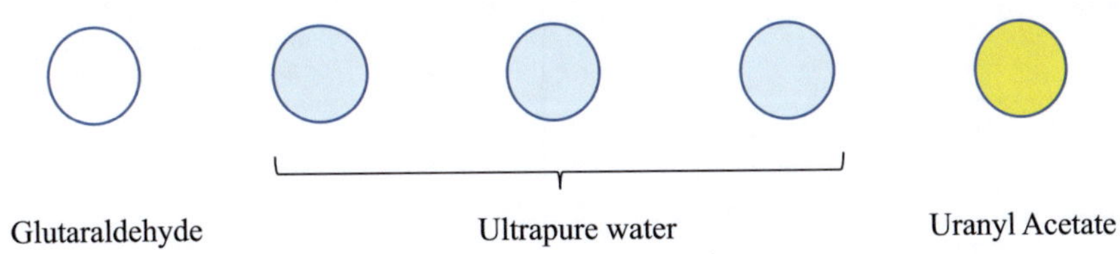

3. Using grid tweezers, gently pick up a grid and place a droplet of sample onto the carbon-side of the grid (black) for 1 min. Gently touch the edge of the grid to a Kimwipe to remove excess sample (*see* **Note 41**).
4. Place the grid carbon-side down onto the droplet of glutaraldehyde for 1 min.
5. Wash three times by placing the grid carbon-side down onto the three successive water droplets for 1 min each.

NANOSIGHT WT9_2_18 2018 2018-02-15 13-25-12

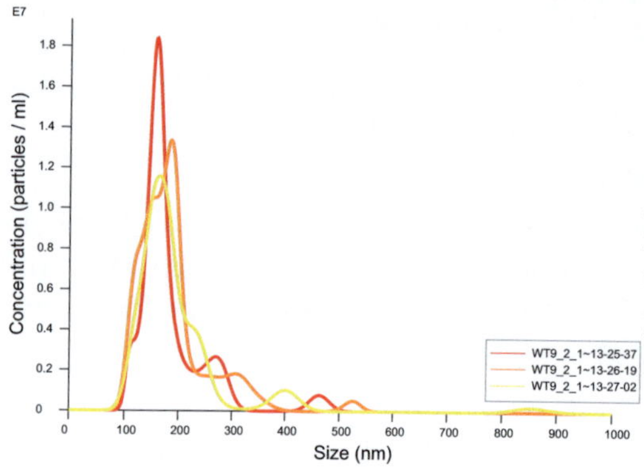

FTLA Concentration / Size graph for Experiment:
WT9_2_18 2018 2018-02-15 13-25-12

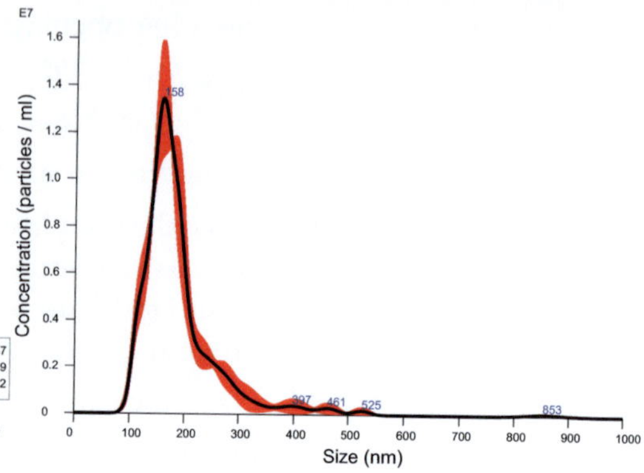

Averaged FTLA Concentration / Size for Experiment:
WT9_2_18 2018 2018-02-15 13-25-12
Error bars indicate + / -1 standard error of the mean

Included Files

WT9_2_18 2018 2018-02-15 13-25-37
WT9_2_18 2018 2018-02-15 13-26-19
WT9_2_18 2018 2018-02-15 13-27-02

Details

NTA Version:	NTA 3.1 Build 3.1.46
Script Used:	3 videos 30sec NO TEMP CONTROL with analy~
Time Captured:	13:25:12 15/02/2018
Operator:	George
Pre-treatment:	
Sample Name:	WT exo
Diluent:	1/50
Remarks:	camera level 15 FOCUS 360

Capture Settings

Camera Type:	EMCCD
Camera Level:	Manual settings used
Slider Shutter:	1205
Slider Gain:	437
FPS	14.9
Number of Frames:	445
Temperature:	37.0 °C
Viscosity:	(Water) 0.7 cP
Dilution factor:	Dilution not recorded

Analysis Settings

Detect Threshold:	5
Blur Size:	Auto
Max Jump Distance:	Auto: 13.9 - 14.6 pix

Results

Stats: Merged Data

Mean:	190.8 nm
Mode:	157.9 nm
SD:	83.2 nm
D10:	124.7 nm
D50:	169.4 nm
D90:	271.6 nm

Stats: Mean +/- Standard Error

Mean:	190.9 +/- 3.8 nm
Mode:	168.2 +/- 8.2 nm
SD:	81.7 +/- 12.0 nm
D10:	125.5 +/- 2.9 nm
D50:	170.0 +/- 3.3 nm
D90:	271.5 +/- 7.7 nm
Concentration:	1.21e+009 +/- 6.38e+007 particles/ml
	61.3 +/- 3.2 particles/frame
	70.2 +/- 2.6 centres/frame

Fig. 1 Typical graphical figure representing estimated particle size (nm) distribution of sample containing exosomes generated by NanoSight analysis. (Left) Representation of three separate video analyses performed by the software. (Right) Representation of combined average of the three video analyses. Error bars in red indicate ± 1 standard error of the mean. A relatively pure sample should have at most two large peaks in the size range pertaining to exosomes ($<$200 nm)

NANOSIGHT WT9_2_18 2018 2018-02-15 13-25-12

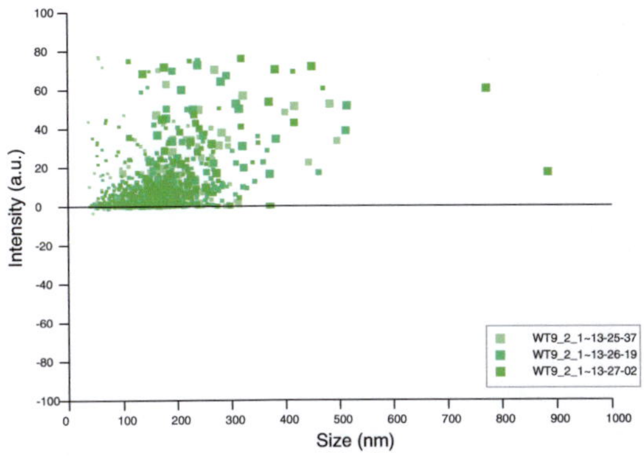

Intensity / Size graph for Experiment:
WT9_2_18 2018 2018-02-15 13-25-12

Script Used: (Full Text):

3 videos 30sec NO TEMP CONTROL with analysis.txt

Fig. 1 (continued)

6. Place the grid onto the uranyl acetate droplet for exactly 1 min (*see* **Note 42**). Dry the grid by touching the edge to a Kimwipe and place carbon-side up for at least 30 min, then store the grids in a grid holder.
7. Repeat **steps 2–6** for each following sample.
8. View each grid using a transmission electron microscope (e.g., FEI Tecnai 12 BioTwin 120 kV TEM) (Fig. 2).

3.9 TCA Protein Precipitation

1. Dilute 1–5 μg of total protein based on Micro BCA results to achieve a final volume of 100–500 μL of Exosome buffer.
2. Add 100 μL of 10× TE buffer.
3. Add 100 μL of 0.3% NaDoc.
4. Add 100 μL of 72% TCA.
5. Incubate on ice for 1 h.
6. Centrifuge at 18,400 × *g* at 4 °C for 20 min.
7. Aspirate supernatant using a 200 μL pipette.
8. Resuspend pellet in 90% acetone at RT, using the same volume as the starting volume of sample.
9. Wrap samples in plastic wrap and incubate at −20 °C overnight.
10. Centrifuge at 18,400 × *g* at 4 °C for 20 min.
11. Aspirate supernatant using a 200 μL pipette.

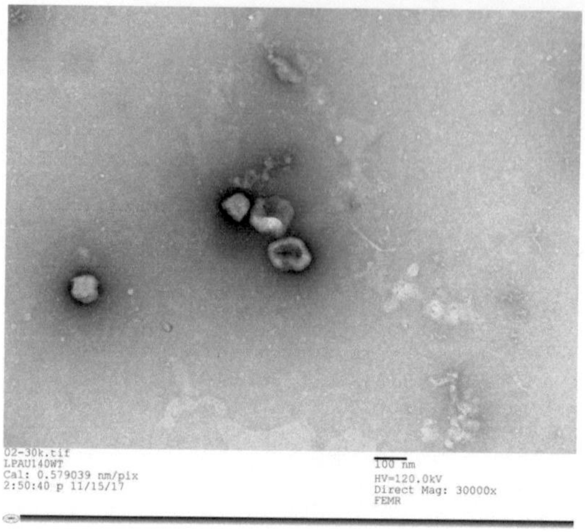

Fig. 2 Typical electron micrograph of exosomes at 30,000× magnification. Characteristic double membrane layer is visible. The cup-shaped morphology is due to shrinking during negative staining and should be regarded as an artifact

12. Air dry samples for 15 min or until microcentrifuge tubes are completely dry.
13. Store samples at −80 °C.

4 Notes

1. If the gap between the starting pH and the required pH is large, small quantities of concentrated HCl (12 N) can be used at the beginning. Afterwards, HCl of lower ionic strength (1 N) is recommended to achieve the required pH for the reagent.
2. All tubes should be prewashed with a mild detergent solution, rinsed with double-distilled water and left to air-dry. It is also advisable to autoclave tubes upside down in a tube rack at 121 °C and 15 psi for 20 min prior to utilization. Note that the number of heat sterilizations can alter the life of the tube. Alternatively, cold sterilization methods can be used, which can include soaking the tubes in a solution of ethanol (70%) or hydrogen peroxide (10%) for a minimum of 10 min. For procedures and experiments where endotoxin-free conditions are critical, such as in vitro immune assays, heat sterilization is preferable.
3. If sterility is necessary, pass the solution through a 0.22 μm membrane filter. Heat sterilization methods are not advisable, as hot temperatures can lead to the charring of sugars such as sucrose.

4. Stationary phase parasite-derived EVs are used in order to mimic EVs that are secreted by infective forms when in contact with the host. Logarithmic phase parasites may be used as an alternate approach, depending on the question and desired outcome.
5. In order to acquire an adequate amount of isolated EVs for nanoparticle tracking analysis, TEM, proteomics, and other assays/experiments, it is necessary to use a sufficient volume of parasites (i.e., 1 L of *Leishmania* culture at a concentration of $1–4 \times 10^7$ parasites/mL will yield approximately 300 μg of exosomes).
6. The lengths of time required for centrifugation at a given gravitational force (g-force) provided in this protocol are based on the *k* factor calculated for fully filled 50 mL conical tubes spun with the rotor of a standard high-speed centrifuge (e.g., Beckman Coulter GH-3.8 swinging-bucket stainless steel rotor for use in Allegra 6 series centrifuges). If the protocol will be modified for tubes or volumes of different size, it is important to recalculate the centrifugation time corresponding to the appropriate *k* factor. To note, the *k* factor represents the relative efficiency of a given centrifuge rotor at maximum rotation speed to pellet a desired component. Thus, the *k* factor allows for one to estimate the run time required for sedimentation of a material at a desired g-force.
7. FBS contains an abundance of extracellular proteins such as albumin, along with a large number of EVs derived from the serum, both of which can be co-sedimented during ultracentrifugation leading to bovine contamination of the isolated preparation. Thus, it is important to remove the FBS from the culture by washing with PBS.
8. Incubation at 37 °C with low agitation stimulates a marked environmental temperature shift during transmission from the sandfly vector (ambient temperature, 25–26 °C) to the mammalian host (37 °C). This temperature shift induces an increase in EVs released into the media from *Leishmania* within 4 h.
9. Centrifugation in this step will pellet the parasites and other debris, allowing for isolation and collection of the supernatant that contains the EVs.
10. After the supernatant is collected and filtered, it is highly recommended that the purification of the EVs is performed immediately. If absolutely necessary, it is also possible to store the supernatant at −80 °C, but this may lead to some degradation of the EVs, resulting in a lower yield preparation of poorer quality.

11. When balancing the tubes, buckets, and caps, it is very important to leave 0 to minimal difference (±0.01 g) between the matched pairs that will be symmetrically arranged in the rotor (1–4, 2–5, 3–6). This is necessary because failing to do so can lead to permanent damage of the ultracentrifuge machine and even potentially severe damage to other structures surrounding the equipment.
12. It is advisable to leave a small volume remaining at the bottom of the tube after aspirating the supernatant.
13. Whether they are loaded or empty, all six bucket assemblies must be attached to the rotor prior to spinning. If fewer than six tubes are being run in the ultracentrifuge, they must be arranged symmetrically in the rotor, so that opposing tubes are filled with the same weight of liquid.
14. For better purity and TEM image quality of vesicles, it is advisable to reprecipitate vesicles in a lower concentration PEG solution (e.g., 5%) or to wash the resuspended pellet with Exosome buffer and then ultracentrifuge at 100,000 × *g* at 4 °C for 70 min.
15. The column, resin slurry, and buffer should all have the same temperature prior to use. Introducing the equilibration and run-through buffer at RT to a packed column from a cold room at 4 °C can lead to air bubbles in the packed bed, which can ultimately result in poorer separation.
16. The volume of resin slurry required to obtain the desired settled resin-bed volume is based on the percentage of ethanol used to store the slurry. Thus, 20 mL of slurry in 50% ethanol will result in a 10 mL packed bed, while approximately 12 mL of slurry in 20% ethanol is required to achieve the same packed bed volume.
17. A gap of approximately 1.5 cm below the opening of the column and the top of the resin bed is necessary to have sufficient room for a layer of ammonium acetate buffer to prevent the resin bed from becoming dry or a layer of sodium azide for storage. A gap is also necessary in order to be able to appropriately cap the top of the column for storage.
18. It is highly recommended that all solutions and buffers used for size-exclusion chromatography are degassed in order to prevent air bubbles from forming in the resin bed, which can reduce performance by preventing contact with the resin and impeding flow. Filtering buffers under vacuum will allow for the solution to become degassed.
19. If there are air bubbles within the resin bed that persist, it is necessary to remove them prior to running the sample through the column. First ensure that the equilibration buffer is

covering the resin bed with approximately 1–2 cm of solution. The entire bottom-capped column can then be placed in a centrifuge tube and centrifuged for 10 min at 1000 × g at RT. This centrifugation step should be sufficient to remove all of the air that has been entrapped. Alternatively, with the bottom of the column capped, the resin matrix can be stirred gently with a clean weighing spatula or a 1000 μL pipette tip, focusing on areas containing the most air bubbles. After the resin bed has been disrupted, wait for about 5–10 min prior to buffer equilibration to allow for the resin to settle again.

20. It is very important to ensure that the resin does not become dry at any point. Do not allow for the level of buffer to fall below the top of the packed resin bed in the column.
21. Given that the column has been equilibrated with 100 mM ammonium acetate, every sample or solution added to the column going forward should be formulated with this concentration of buffer.
22. Prior to isolating EVs from precious experimental samples, it is highly recommended to optimize the column with less valuable samples (i.e., supernatant obtained from wild type culture). During optimization, it is suggested that 50–70 fractions are collection by column elution, followed by NTA of the fractions in a sequential manner. This will allow one to determine the initial volume of waste eluate, along with the number of fractions necessary to collect the EVs when working with experimental samples.
23. Following collection of the fractions, it is necessary to screen the samples by NTA to locate and quantify the isolated EVs. Extracellular vesicles should elute in the earlier fractions, whereas other soluble contaminants such as proteins, ribonucleoproteins, and some lipoproteins will elute in the later fractions [7].
24. Buffer containing sodium azide is added to the column prior to storage in order to prevent microbial growth in the resin supports composed of a base matrix of agarose, a carbohydrate. To ensure that the sodium azide buffer has dispersed throughout the resin, allow for approximately 3–4 mL of liquid to pass through as waste, and then cap the bottom of the column.
25. Upon subsequent use of the prepacked column, remember to remove the top cap of the column prior to the bottom cap, in order to prevent the entrance of large air bubbles into the resin bed. When both ends of the column are open, always cap the bottom before the top, for the same reason.
26. Prior to every new use of the size exclusion column to isolate EVs, it is necessary to re-equilibrate the column resin with 50–100 mL of ammonium acetate buffer.

27. If there are less than eight buckets being run in the ultracentrifuge, they must be arranged symmetrically in the rotor, so that opposing buckets are filled with the same weight of liquid.
28. Depending on the preciseness of the pipetting technique performed during the layering of the sucrose density gradient, it is possible to have a shift in the fractions where the exosomes will be located.
29. The ThermoFisher™ user guide suggests using a total well volume of 300 μL, but 200 μL of total volume is sufficient to generate a robust signal. Thus, total volume calculations are performed to achieve a volume of 100 μL of working reagent per well, and then multiplied by a factor of 1.2 to account for pipetting errors.
30. Once all three reagents are mixed properly, the working reagent should turn into a light green color.
31. The sample is diluted by a factor of 20 to conserve isolated material. However, if the pellet is not visible after the final round of ultracentrifugation and/or the final volume of Exosome buffer used to resuspend the pellet is greater than 300 μL, it may be necessary to reduce the dilution factor.
32. When mixing with the micropipette, do not push the plunger to the first stopping point until the final mix and make sure to never depress the plunger past this point of first resistance. This is to avoid the creation of bubbles in the well.
33. If the signal is weak, the plate can be left covered and protected from light overnight at RT, and then remeasured the following day.
34. Although standard curves calculated using a linear function are often sufficient, using a second order polynomial function can generate a more accurate curve.
35. It is recommended that a total volume of 1000 μL is used for analysis by NanoSight, but this can be reduced to 500 μL as long as the sample is loaded to 70% instead of 100%.
36. It is important to make sure that the plastic tubing is fully submerged in the sample but does not touch the bottom of the microcentrifuge tube. This is necessary to prevent the tube from sticking to the bottom or generating air bubbles in the sample.
37. When loading the sample, it is sufficient to load to 70%. If using a total sample volume of 500 μL, this is necessary to avoid the generation of air bubbles.
38. If particles passing the camera appear to slant, it is likely that air bubbles have entered the system and are interfering with the camera. If the problem worsens or other camera issues arise, it

will be necessary to open the machine and clean the camera before continuing analysis. The fluidics must also be reprimed at this stage.

39. If the sample is too dilute ($<4.0 \times 10^8$ particles/mL) or too concentrated ($>2.5 \times 10^9$ particles/mL), it is necessary to prepare the sample again and run a new analysis.
40. It is important to not wear nitrile rubber gloves or other typical laboratory gloves while performing the negative stain in order to avoid the creation of static that can interfere with the process.
41. If samples are suspended in PBS, this can interfere with the negative staining and result in artifacts when viewing the sample grid under the TEM.
42. It is imperative to stain the sample for exactly 1 min with uranyl acetate. To ensure this, grasp the edge of the grid with the tweezers at least 10 s in advance and remove the grid from the droplet at an angle to reduce the amount of uranyl acetate clinging to the grid.

Acknowledgments

Work performed in the M.O.'s laboratory is supported by grants from the Canadian Institutes of Health Research, and Natural Sciences and Engineering Research Council (NSERC). A.V., A.S. L.F., and G.D. are studentship recipients from NSERC, Science without Borders, and Fonds de Recherche du Québec Santé, respectively. We thank Professor Ana Claudia Trocoli Torrecilhas for generously helping with the size exclusion chromatography set-up and protocol.

References

1. Atayde VD, Aslan H, Townsend S et al (2015) Exosome secretion by the parasitic protozoan leishmania within the sand fly midgut. Cell Rep 13(5):957–967. https://doi.org/10.1016/j.celrep.2015.09.058
2. Raposo G, Nijman HW, Stoorvogel W et al (1996) B lymphocytes secrete antigen-presenting vesicles. J Exp Med 183 (3):1161–1172
3. Ogawa Y, Kanai-Azuma M, Akimoto Y et al (2008) Exosome-like vesicles with dipeptidyl peptidase IV in human saliva. Biol Pharm Bull 31(6):1059–1062. https://doi.org/10.1248/bpb.31.1059
4. Trocoli Torrecilhas AC, Tonelli RR, Pavanelli WR et al (2009) *Trypanosoma cruzi*: parasite shed vesicles increase heart parasitism and generate an intense inflammatory response. Microbes Infect 11(1):29–39. https://doi.org/10.1016/j.micinf.2008.10.003
5. Rider MA, Hurwitz SN, Meckes DG Jr (2016) ExtraPEG: a polyethylene glycol-based method for enrichment of extracellular vesicles. Sci Rep 6:23978. https://doi.org/10.1038/srep23978. https://www.nature.com/articles/srep23978#supplementary-information
6. Witwer KW, Soekmadji C, Hill AF et al (2017) Updating the MISEV minimal requirements for extracellular vesicle studies: building bridges to reproducibility. J Extracell Vesicles 6(1):1396823–1396823. https://doi.org/10.1080/20013078.2017.1396823

7. Théry C, Witwer KW, Aikawa E et al (2018) Minimal information for studies of extracellular vesicles 2018 (MISEV2018): a position statement of the International Society for Extracellular Vesicles and update of the MISEV2014 guidelines. J Extracell Vesicles 7(1):1535750. https://doi.org/10.1080/20013078.2018.1535750
8. Dragovic RA, Gardiner C, Brooks AS et al (2011) Sizing and phenotyping of cellular vesicles using nanoparticle tracking analysis. Nanomed Nanotechnol Biol Med 7 (6):780–788. https://doi.org/10.1016/j.nano.2011.04.003
9. Linares R, Tan S, Gounou C et al (2017) Imaging and quantification of extracellular vesicles by transmission electron microscopy. Methods Mol Biol (Clifton, NJ) 1545:43–54. https://doi.org/10.1007/978-1-4939-6728-5_4
10. Carr B, Warren J (2012) Company profile: NanoSight: delivering practical solutions for biological nanotechnology. Nanomedicine (Lond) 7(8):1129–1132. https://doi.org/10.2217/nnm.12.43
11. Mehdiani A, Maier A, Pinto A et al (2015) An innovative method for exosome quantification and size measurement. J Vis Exp 95:50974–50974. https://doi.org/10.3791/50974
12. Brenner S, Horne RW (1959) A negative staining method for high resolution electron microscopy of viruses. Biochim Biophys Acta 34:103–110
13. Silverman JM, Chan SK, Robinson DP et al (2008) Proteomic analysis of the secretome of Leishmania donovani. Genome Biol 9(2):R35. https://doi.org/10.1186/gb-2008-9-2-r35
14. Hassani K, Antoniak E, Jardim A et al (2011) Temperature-induced protein secretion by Leishmania mexicana modulates macrophage signalling and function. PLoS One 6(5): e18724. https://doi.org/10.1371/journal.pone.0018724

Part V

Biochemistry

Chapter 34

2D Gel Electrophoresis Analysis of *Leishmania* Proteomes

Christina Naula and Richard Burchmore

Abstract

2D gel electrophoresis enables resolution of intact proteins in complex mixtures and is thus useful for comparative proteomic analysis, particularly of posttranslationally modified proteoforms that might not be distinguished by shotgun proteomic analysis of peptides. 2D gel electrophoresis is a multistep procedure that can require sample-specific optimization. We present a comprehensive protocol that is effective for 2D electrophoretic analysis of proteins from *Leishmania* promastigotes and may also be employed for *Leishmania* amastigotes and for trypanosomes.

Key words *Leishmania*, 2D gel electrophoresis, Proteomics, Isoelectric focusing

1 Introduction

Electrophoresis for the separation of proteins is ubiquitous in biochemistry, and the original publication reporting sodium dodecyl sulfate polyacrylamide gel electrophoresis (SDS-PAGE) for the separation of reduced proteins by apparent molecular weight is one of the most highly cited papers [1]. Combined with antibody-based detection of the separated proteins, SDS-PAGE forms the basis of the western blot.

Two-dimensional gel electrophoresis (2DE) aims to improve the separation of proteins in complex mixtures, through sequential orthogonal electrophoretic separation. The archetypal 2DE method [2] employs separation of proteins according to their native charge, by isoelectric focusing, followed by reduction of the proteins and separation according to apparent molecular weight, by SDS-PAGE. Developed in the 1970s, 2DE experienced a renaissance in the 1990s as the favored protein separation method for proteomic analyses. Technical advances increased the reproducibility and resolution of 2DE, such that several thousand proteoforms could be resolved in a single gel, and their expression compared between different gels. Multiplexing approaches, such

Paul A. M. Michels et al. (eds.), *Trypanosomatids: Methods and Protocols*, Methods in Molecular Biology, vol. 2116, https://doi.org/10.1007/978-1-0716-0294-2_34,

as difference gel electrophoresis [3], established 2DE as the proteomics analogue of microarray analyses for RNA expression studies.

Shotgun proteomics [4], involving separation of peptides rather than proteins by chromatography rather than electrophoresis, has now largely replaced 2DE as the standard separation technology in proteomics labs, principally because liquid chromatography–mass spectrometry (LC-MS) is highly automatable, while 2D gels are labor intensive and have limited throughput. 2DE is also challenged by the dynamic range that is characteristic of proteomes and by proteins with extreme charge or hydrophobicity. Nevertheless, 2DE retains some important advantages over shotgun LC-MS, in particular, because it separates intact proteins and can thus resolve proteoforms with different posttranslational modifications [5]. The visual output from 2DE facilitates relative quantitation and comparison of proteomes, without recourse to complex software. 2DE also requires limited equipment, much of which is ubiquitous in biochemistry laboratories, and it is thus accessible to researchers without sufficient resource to undertake shotgun proteomic analyses.

There are four major steps involved in 2DE. Firstly, proteins must be extracted from biological material into a solvent system that is compatible with isoelectric focusing. It is critical to avoid protein modification or degradation. Secondly, isoelectric focusing is performed. This is best achieved using a commercial system involving immobilized pH gradient (IPG) gels. Thirdly, SDS polyacrylamide gel electrophoresis is performed as the second dimension separation. This can be achieved using a standard minigel system, although greater resolution can be obtained with larger format gels, which can be combined with longer IPG gel strips. Finally, the 2D gel is visualized using a protein stain, or the gel may be used to generate a 2D western blot.

Typically, this process is aimed at producing a 2D map, in which individual protein species can be annotated. Often, 2D maps from related samples will be compared, with the aim of detecting differences in protein expression that correlate with a phenotype of interest; with this approach, reproducibility is critical. Protein spots of interest can be excised from the gel and subjected to mass spectrometry analysis, and because 2D gel spots are typically composed mostly of a single protein species, confident identification can generally be achieved using a relatively inexpensive mass spectrometer, such as a MALDI-ToF or ion trap.

While the second dimension is in 2DE is quite robust, isoelectric focusing requires careful sample preparation for success. Only proteins that are solubilized will feature on the resulting 2D map, but the inclusion of ionic reagents, such as SDS, which is commonly used to solubilize proteins for SDS-PAGE, in sample buffer is not compatible with isoelectric focusing. The conventional protocols for protein solubilization for isoelectric focusing utilize a chaotrope (usually urea), a reducing agent (usually DTT), nonionic detergents (often CHAPS), and carrier ampholytes to promote establishment of a stable pH gradient. This cocktail effectively solubilizes the majority of proteins, so that they can be efficiently focused by p*I*. Not all classes of protein are readily soluble under these conditions, and these proteins will be underrepresented in the 2D map. In particular, hydrophobic proteins such as integral membrane proteins are difficult to solubilize; since many membrane proteins are also low abundance, they are often considered unsuitable for 2D electrophoresis. However, there are a number of modified detergent systems that may improve the solubility of membrane proteins [5]. Proteins that associate with nucleic acid, lipid, or polysaccharide may also be problematic, and it may be helpful to treat samples with nuclease and/or to precipitate proteins from lysis buffer for resuspension in appropriate sample buffer. The simplest approach (described herein) is to disrupt cells in the presence of urea and CHAPs, then add DTT, ampholytes, and bromophenol blue to complete the standard sample buffer. The sample is mixed, centrifuged to remove particulates, and loaded onto the IPG strip. This approach is a recommended starting point for projects that aim to generate a complete proteomic map.

The method described here was optimized for *Leishmania* promastigotes and works well for all species we have tested, including *L. mexicana*, *L. infantum*, and *L. major*. It also works well for procyclic *Trypanosoma brucei*. It has been used for bloodstream form trypanosomes, obtained ex vivo from infected rats, and for *L. mexicana* amastigotes, obtained through axenic culture, though the resolution of the resulting 2D gels is poorer than that obtained with procyclic forms. This may due to the greater protease activity expressed in mammalian-infective stages and may be ameliorated by the inclusion of protease inhibitors, although we have not systematically addressed this. Approximately 0.5–1 mg of protein may be obtained from 1×10^8 cells. This will be sufficient for several 2D gels. If possible, 1×10^9 cells should be used as starting material.

2 Materials

All reagents should be of good quality and purity (*see* **Note 1**):

1. Phosphate-buffered saline (PBS): 137 mM NaCl, 2.7 mM KCl, 4.3 mM Na_2HPO_4, 1.47 mM KH_2PO_4; adjust to a final pH of 7.4.
2. Cell lysis buffer: 6 M urea, 2 M thiourea, 4% CHAPS, 25 mM Tris base; do not adjust pH.
3. IPG strip rehydration buffer: 6 M urea, 2 M thiourea, 4% CHAPS, 0.5% IPG buffer, 65 mM DTT, trace bromophenol blue; do not adjust pH.

4. SDS-PAGE gel running buffer: 25 mM Tris, 192 mM glycine, 0.1% (w/v) SDS, pH 8.8.
5. IPG strip equilibration buffer stock solution: 100 mM Tris–HCl, pH 8.8, 6 M urea, 30% (v/v) glycerol (87% [v/v]), 2% (w/v) SDS. This stock solution can be stored at room temperature. Stable for 6 months. Immediately prior to use, add 0.5% DTT or 4.5% iodoacetamide for equilibration solution 1 or 2, respectively.
6. Gel fixation solution: 30% (v/v) methanol, 7.5% (v/v) acetic acid.
7. Coomassie stock: 5% (w/v) Coomassie Brilliant Blue G-250 in water. Shake before use.
8. Colloidal Coomassie dye stock: 10% (w/v) ammonium sulfate, 1% (v/v) phosphoric acid, 2% (v/v) Colloidal Coomassie dye stock, in dH_2O. Shake before use.
9. Colloidal Coomassie stain: 80% (v/v) Colloidal Coomassie dye stock, 20% (v/v) methanol. Prepare fresh for each use.
10. IPG strips: Purchase from commercial source, store frozen in sealed packaging until use. Purchase together with appropriate IPG buffer or carrier ampholytes. Various pH ranges are available.

3 Methods

3.1 Protein Extraction From Leishmania Promastigotes for 2D Gel Electrophoresis

Goal: To prepare proteins in an appropriate buffer and concentration for isoelectric focusing.

3.1.1 Wash Cells

Goal: To remove soluble macromolecules and salts without lysing the cells.

1. Wash cells two times in ice cold PBS. Collect cells from each wash by centrifugation and decanting supernatant. Centrifuge cells at low speed (below 1000 × *g*) to avoid lysis.
2. After decanting the second wash, return pellets to the centrifuge for a brief spin, then remove as much as possible of the remaining supernatant with a micropipette (*see* **Note 2**). Cell pellets may be snap frozen at this point and can be stored at −20 °C for several months. We have not systematically assessed long-term stability of proteins under longer storage conditions.

3.1.2 Lyse Cells

Goal: To solubilize proteins efficiently while limiting protein modification.

1. Resuspend cell pellet in ice cold lysis buffer. Lysis buffer (1 ml) is appropriate for 1×10^9 promastigotes, which should be rapidly resuspended by vigorous pipetting in a microcentrifuge tube.
2. Immediately lyse the cells by up to ten brief (1–2 s) cycles of probe sonication (MSE soniprep or similar), with 1 min cooling on ice between each sonication. *Avoid foaming and heating* (*see* **Note 3**).
3. Incubate for 10 min at room temperature, with gentle mixing.
4. Centrifuge for 10 min at 13,000 × *g* (benchtop microfuge) to remove insoluble material, and transfer supernatant to a fresh microcentrifuge tube.

3.1.3 Protein Precipitation

Goal: Precipitate solubilized proteins to remove lipids, salts, polysaccharides, and so on, which may cause subsequent issues with isoelectric focusing.

1. Add 4× sample volume of cold (−20 °C) acetone to protein. Vortex tube and incubate for >1 h at −20 °C. Centrifuge at 4 °C for 10 min at 13,000 × *g* (benchtop microfuge).
2. Decant supernatant and wash pellet twice with cold 80% acetone, disrupting the pellet and recentrifuging with each wash. Centrifuge, decant supernatant, centrifuge briefly, and remove residual supernatant with pipette.
3. Air dry pellet ~5 min at room temperature. *Do not overdry.* Resuspension is more difficult if the pellet is first allowed to dry completely (*see* **Note 4**).
4. Resuspend in a small volume of lysis buffer. This volume should be sufficiently small that the final protein content will be >5 mg/ml. Typically, 1×10^9 promastigotes will yield between 5 and 10 mg of total protein.
5. After thorough resuspension, centrifuge for 10 min at 13,000 × *g* (benchtop microfuge) to remove insoluble material, and transfer supernatant to a fresh microcentrifuge tube.
6. Insoluble material may be reserved for analysis by 1D SDS-PAGE—this pellet is likely enriched for hydrophobic and structural proteins.

3.1.4 Determine and Adjust Protein Content

Goal: To adjust protein content to a working concentration of 5 mg/ml.

1. Determine protein content of aliquots of each sample, using a commercial protein assay kit, such as 2D Quant kit (GE Healthcare) or Bradford assay (Bio-Rad). Add lysis buffer

to give a final protein content of 5 mg/ml. Use lysis buffer also to prepare protein assay standards, as components such as urea and CHAPS may interfere with the protein assay readings.

2. Samples can be stored at −20 °C prior to 2D electrophoresis.

3.2 Isoelectric Focussing (IEF)

Goal: Separate proteins by isoelectric focusing, according to their native pI.

3.2.1 Load Protein Sample Into IPG Gel Strip

Goal: To introduce proteins to the IPG gel matrix.

1. Identify the recommended volume and protein load for the IPG strips you will use (see manufacturer's instructions).
2. Pipette the required volume of protein sample into a microcentrifuge tube.
3. Add the required volume of rehydration buffer to obtain the final volume recommended for rehydration of the IPG strip. The rehydration buffer should contain the appropriate IPG buffer or carrier ampholyte mixture for the pH range of the IPG strip used (*see* **Note 5**).
4. Thoroughly mix each sample and incubate for ~1 h at room temperature.
5. Centrifuge for 3 min at full speed in a microcentrifuge to collect aggregates that might interfere with focusing or precipitate on the IPG strip.
6. Load supernatant into the IPG strip holder, distributing along the bed of the strip holder. Avoid bubbles.
7. Remove the IPG strip from the protective package and, handling with forceps and gloves, peel away the plastic cover. Do not touch the gel. Hold the strip by the gel-free plastic backing at either end.
8. Lay the IPG strip (more rigid than the plastic cover) into the IPG strip holder, so that the dehydrated IPG gel (opaque, sticky, was in contact with plastic cover) faces down and is in contact with the sample solution. Avoid bubbles under the strip. Overlay the strip with mineral oil, sufficient to cover the entire strip and limit evaporation.
9. Place the IPG strips, in holders with samples prepared as described above, on the electrode bed of the isoelectric focusing unit, so that the acid end of the strip (marked on the plastic backing) is oriented toward the anode.

3.2.2 Isoelectric Focusing of Protein Mixture

Goal: To apply a voltage potential that is sufficient to move proteins within the IPG gel until they achieve their isoelectric point.

1. Allow rehydration loading to proceed for a minimum of 10 h, but this is conveniently done as the first step of the focusing protocol. Depending on the isoelectric focusing system

available, this can permit temperature control, a small voltage to help maintain protein solubility and an automatic start to the focusing program.

2. A typical IEF protocol (for a 7-cm IPG strip) comprises the following:
   (a) 10–15 h at 30 V (rehydration step).
   (b) 2 h at 300 V.
   (c) 2 h at 600 V.
   (d) 2 h at 1000 V.
   (e) 2 h at 5000 V.
3. For longer IPG strips, the final isoelectric focusing voltage can be up to 8000 V, maintained for up to 8 h.
4. The increasing voltage is best applied stepwise or increased as a gradient (depending on the isoelectric focusing system available).
5. The rate at which high voltages are attained will depend upon the conductivity of the sample(s), and the final high voltage may not be attained at all if the ionic strength of the sample is too high. If this situation occurs, it may be beneficial to increase focusing time and/or to extend the period during which voltage is ramping to the focussing voltage. However, problems attaining high voltage reflect excess ions in the sample, and it is desirable to reduce conductivity to improve focusing efficiency. This is most readily achieved by precipitation of the sample prior to isoelectric focusing.
6. Normally, temperature is maintained throughout IEF at 20 °C and current limited at 50 μA/IPG strip, to prevent heating if sample conductivity is an issue.
7. If the isoelectric focusing equipment is able to display accumulated volt/hours for the entire IEF separation, it can be useful to record this for comparison between different samples. Approximately ten accumulated kVh would be anticipated for a 7-cm IPG strip.
8. At the end of the protocol, strips should be immediately processed for the second dimension. If there will be a short delay (less than 1 h), 1000 V can be applied to maintain focusing until ready. If there will be a longer delay, strips can be removed and stored at −20 °C.

3.3 SDS-PAGE

Goal: To separate proteins according to their molecular weight.

3.3.1 IPG Strip Equilibration

Goal: To add SDS to proteins in the IPG strip, as a prerequisite to SDS-PAGE.

1. Remove focused IPG strips from IPG strip holders (or from −20 °C storage) with forceps, and transfer to a suitable tube, with the plastic backing side in contact with the tube wall. Do not touch the gel. Hold the strip by the gel-free plastic backing at either end. *Note the state of the rehydrated IPG strip at this point; uneven swelling may indicate problems with focusing.*
2. Add equilibration buffer, completed with 100 mg DTT/10 ml, and rock gently, so that the strip is well covered with equilibration buffer.
3. Incubate, with gentle mixing (by hand or on a rocker platform), ensuring that the IPG strip remains submerged in equilibration buffer.
4. After 15 min, pour off the first equilibration buffer and replace with equilibration buffer completed with 250 mg iodoacetamide/10 ml and equilibrate for 15 min.
5. Incubate, with gentle mixing (by hand or on a rocker platform), ensuring that the IPG strip remains submerged in equilibration buffer (*see* **Note 6**).

3.3.2 SDS-PAGE Gel Preparation

1. Ensure that preparations for gel assembly are complete prior to commencing IPG strip equilibration, as extended equilibration times may lead to a loss of focusing resolution.
2. Second dimension gels may be prepared using standard recipes but should be cast without stacking gels or well-forming combs. The gel can be overlaid with ~1 ml water-saturated butanol prior to polymerization, to ensure a flat surface at the top of the gel. Alternatively, precast gels may be purchased.
3. Position equilibrated strips onto the top of the SDS gel, so that there is complete contact between gel and strip. By convention, the acidic end of the strip is oriented toward the left hand side of the gel.
4. Fix the IPG strip in place by the addition of molten 0.5% low melting temperature agarose in SDS-PAGE running buffer with bromophenol blue. Avoid bubbles or air gaps at the interface between the IPG strip and the gel as these can hinder protein transfer.

3.3.3 SDS-PAGE Electrophoresis

1. Perform electrophoresis at constant power, as recommended by the gel apparatus manufacturer, until the bromophenol blue dye front reaches the base of the gel (or until the dye front has just run off the gel). We have observed that gels run at higher power are better resolved.

3.3.4 Colloidal Coomassie Blue staining (See **Note 7**)

Perform these steps with gentle agitation on a rocker or orbital platform.

1. Fix gel(s) 1–2 h in 40% ethanol, 10% acetic acid.
2. Wash gel(s) 10 min in distilled H_2O. Repeat.
3. Stain gel(s) in freshly prepared colloidal dye solution for up to 1 week. *Overnight may be sufficient, but sensitivity may improve by extending staining for several days.*
4. Rinse gel(s) in several changes of distilled H_2O.

4 Notes

1. The purity of some reagents is critical for high resolution isoelectric focusing. In particular, urea and thiourea should be of good quality and from a fresh source. CHAPS should be of the highest purity available.
2. Salt is a major issue in 2D electrophoresis as conductivity in the sample limits the isoelectric focusing voltage potential that can be achieved. It is therefore helpful to remove as much of the PBS as possible after the final cell washing step, and prior to cell lysis or freezing.
3. Urea can spontaneously degrade to form cyanate ions, which attack and modify proteins. Always use high quality urea, freshly prepared. Avoid heating urea, especially protein samples in urea-containing buffers.
4. Resuspension of acetone-precipitated protein pellets may take some time and may require approaches such as sonication, vigorous vortexing, repeated pipetting, stirring, or grinding. Freeze-thaw cycling may help if all else fails but avoid heating (*see* **Note 2**). Resuspension is more difficult if the pellet is first allowed to dry completely.
5. The length of IPG strip that is employed is an important consideration. The smallest format (7 cm) is appropriate for most pilot studies since it can be combined with a standard (lab-made) minigel for the second dimension step. This is quicker and more economical. Larger format IPG strips have a higher protein load capacity and focusing resolution. However, they require larger format SDS-PAGE gels for the second dimension, and these take longer (typically o/n) to run in larger, more costly, and less ubiquitous apparatus.
6. Prior to SDS-PAGE, focused proteins must be equilibrated with SDS, so that all proteins are saturated with SDS. This equilibration normally takes place in two steps, firstly in the presence of DTT (to maintain proteins in a fully reduced state) and secondly in the presence of iodoacetamide (to alkylate thiol

groups and prevent reoxidation of cysteine residues). Two equilibration steps of 15 min each is sufficient. Longer equilibration will permit focused proteins to diffuse within the IPG strip (the IPG strip is a low percentage polyacrylamide, and the proteins are not fixed).

7. Proteins can be visualized by a variety of methods. Coomassie staining is the most straightforward approach and is appropriate when maximum sensitivity is not critical. Colloidal Coomassie stains can detect ~100 ng/protein spot. Fluorescent stains are rather more sensitive (SYRPO Ruby™, ~10 ng/protein spot) and also have a much broader dynamic range. This can be critical for quantitative approaches.

   Silver staining is still the most sensitive stain for protein gels (~1 ng/protein spot) but has a poor dynamic range, significant variability in results and is not compatible with subsequent mass spectrometry unless the protocol is modified, at a cost to sensitivity.

References

1. Laemmli UK (1970) Cleavage of structural proteins during the assembly of the head of bacteriophage T4. Nature 227(5259):680–685
2. O'Farrell PH (1975) High resolution two-dimensional electrophoresis of proteins. J Biol Chem 250(10):4007–4021
3. Alban A, David SO, Bjorkesten L, Andersson C, Sloge E, Lewis S et al (2003) A novel experimental design for comparative two-dimensional gel analysis: two-dimensional difference gel electrophoresis incorporating a pooled internal standard. Proteomics 3(1):36–44
4. Washburn MP, Wolters D, Yates JR III (2001) Large-scale analysis of the yeast proteome by multidimensional protein identification technology 14. Nat Biotechnol 19(3):242–247
5. Rabilloud T, Chevallet M, Luche S, Lelong C (2010) Two-dimensional gel electrophoresis in proteomics: past, present and future. J Proteome 73(11):2064–2077

Chapter 35

Analysis of the Physiological and Metabolic State of *Leishmania* Using Heavy Water Labeling

Joachim Kloehn and Malcolm J. McConville

Abstract

This protocol describes the use of heavy water (^2H_2O) labeling to determine the growth rate and metabolic state of *Leishmania* parasites in culture and in infected animals. In vitro labeling studies are undertaken by cultivating defined parasite developmental stages in standard medium supplemented with 5% ^2H_2O, resulting in the incorporation of deuterium (^2H) into a range of metabolic precursors used in macromolecule (DNA, RNA, protein, lipid, and glycan) synthesis. The rate of turnover of different parasite macromolecules can subsequently be determined by analysis of deuterium enrichment in the different constituents of these macromolecules by gas chromatography–mass spectrometry (GC-MS). To measure the growth rate and physiological state of parasite stages in lesion tissue, infected mice were provided with 9% ^2H_2O in their drinking water for various periods of time and ^2H-enrichment in the macromolecular constituents of isolated lesion-derived parasite stages determined by GC-MS. This protocol provides quantitative information on key cellular processes, such as replication (DNA turnover), transcription (RNA turnover), translation (protein turnover), membrane biogenesis (lipid turnover), and central carbon metabolism (glycan turnover) that define the growth state and phenome of different parasite stages in vitro and in vivo. This approach can be used to assess the impact of host immune responses on parasite growth and physiology (using different *Leishmania* strains/species, mouse lines), characterize different parasite populations during chronic and acute infections, and assess parasite responses to drug treatments. It is also broadly applicable to other microbial pathogens.

Key words Heavy water labeling, Parasite growth, Virulence, Microbial heterogeneity

1 Introduction

Trypanosomatid parasites belonging to the genus *Trypanosoma* (*T. brucei*, *T. cruzi*) and *Leishmania* transition between a number of different developmental stages during their complex digenetic life cycles in their respective insect vectors and mammalian hosts [1]. These developmental programs allow these parasites to exploit different nutrient conditions in different hosts and host niches and to adapt to host microbicidal responses and other environmental stresses (i.e., temperature, pH) [2]. Parasite differentiation often involves well-characterized changes in cell morphology and

Paul A. M. Michels et al. (eds.), *Trypanosomatids: Methods and Protocols*, Methods in Molecular Biology, vol. 2116, https://doi.org/10.1007/978-1-0716-0294-2_35,

ultrastructure, as well as the expression of surface antigens. However, much less is known about the extent to which the growth rate, metabolism, and macromolecule biosynthesis vary between and within different developmental stages. In particular, very little is known about the physiological state of mammalian infective stages that target different tissue niches in the mammalian host [3]. This information is critical for understanding how these parasites adapt to different tissue niches within the animal host; how they can switch from causing long-term persistent (chronic) infections to causing acute and, in some cases, life-threatening infections; and their ability to persist after drug treatment [4].

In this chapter, we describe a new method for measuring the growth and physiological state of *Leishmania* parasites in vitro and in vivo. *Leishmania* grow as flagellated promastigotes in the digestive tract of the sand fly vector, transitioning between several developmental states as they migrate from the midgut to the foregut, prior to transmission to the mammalian host. The best characterized of these developmental stages are the rapidly dividing procyclic and nondividing metacyclic promastigotes that play important roles in the initial establishment of infection in the sand fly midgut and subsequent transmission and infection of the mammalian host, respectively [5, 6]. Comparable promastigote stages are thought to occur in culture during log and stationary phase growth, respectively. Following infection of the mammalian host, metacyclic promastigotes target macrophages and other phagocytic cells and differentiate to nonmotile amastigotes in the mature phagolysosome compartment. Amastigotes proliferate within the phagolysosomes of macrophages and are the cause of both long-term chronic (asymptomatic) infections and acute infections. Depending on the *Leishmania* species involved, acute infections are characterized by the formation of large granulomatous inflammatory lesions in the skin, often at the site of the sand fly bite (cutaneous leishmaniasis), at the facial tissue (mucocutaneous disease), or in the spleen and liver (visceral disease). Recent studies suggest that amastigote differentiation and adaptation to the lesion microenvironment is associated with major changes in the growth rate and metabolic state of these stages [7–9]. While amastigotes are obligate intracellular parasites in vivo, culture conditions for axenic growth of these developmental stages have been developed for *Leishmania* species/strains [10, 11]. Axenic amastigotes have similar morphology to lesion-derived amastigotes, although differences in the transcriptome, physiology, and metabolism of these stages have been observed [8, 12], highlighting the need to assess amastigote physiology in vivo. Moreover, recent studies have suggested that distinct populations of *Leishmania* amastigotes, differing in their growth rate, may occur in vivo [13].

Heavy water (^2H_2O) is increasingly being used to measure a wide variety of metabolic processes in cells, tissues, and live animals [14–17]. Many enzyme reactions involve the addition of water or exchange of protons that lead to the incorporation of deuterium (^2H) into a wide range of metabolites (sugars, amino acids, fatty acids, etc.) in the presence of ^2H_2O. Incubation of cells in the presence of low levels of ^2H_2O (usually less than 10% (v/v)) can thus lead to the incorporation of ^2H-labeled metabolic precursors into the major cellular building blocks of cells (DNA, RNA, proteins, lipids, carbohydrates) with the level of enrichment providing a direct read-out of synthesis and turnover [14]. Compared with other stable isotope-labeling protocols (using, for example, ^{13}C-glucose), ^2H_2O is relatively inexpensive, easy to administer over long time periods (from hours to days and months), and accessible to all tissues [18]. It is particularly useful for measuring the growth rate (i.e., DNA turnover) or other cellular parameters in slow growing or metabolically quiescent cells or tissues [19].

In this protocol, we describe the use of ^2H_2O-labeling to measure the growth rate and physiological state of cultured *Leishmania* promastigotes and lesion-derived amastigotes [20]. In brief, the protocol involves cultivating parasite stages in standard medium containing 5% ^2H_2O or labeling *Leishmania*-infected mice with ^2H_2O (to give ~5% ^2H_2O body water levels). Following harvest or isolation from lesions, parasites are differentially extracted to enrich for different classes of macromolecules (DNA, RNA, protein, lipids, carbohydrates). The level of deuterium enrichment in core constituents (i.e., deoxyribose, ribose, amino acids, fatty acids, and sugars) is quantitated after depolymerization and derivatization by gas chromatography–mass spectrometry (GC-MS). The rate of turnover of macromolecular constituents is subsequently determined by comparing the level of ^2H-enrichment in key monomers at defined time points, with maximum ^2H-enrichment determined empirically following long-term (equilibrium) labeling. This method has a number of advantages over other approaches that have been used to measure *Leishmania* growth and macromolecular synthesis in vivo, such as the use of transgenic lines expressing luciferase or fluorescent reporter proteins [21–24]. In particular, the ^2H-labeling method is quantitative, does not require the generation of transgenic parasite lines (with concomitant possible loss of virulence during prolonged culture), provides a measure of global macromolecule turnover (not just expression of a single protein), and can be used to measure growth/metabolic dynamics at any stage of infection in different animal models (by judicious selection of labeling start/end points). While not described here, this method can also be extended to measure parasite heterogeneity in different tissues using imaging mass spectrometry [25].

2 Materials

2.1 Parasite Cultivation In Vitro, ^2H_2O Labeling, and Harvest

1. Laminar flow hood for cell culture.
2. Refrigerated centrifuge for 15 ml conical tubes.
3. Refrigerated centrifuge for microfuge tubes.
4. −80 °C freezer.
5. Light microscope.
6. pH-meter.
7. Neubauer hemocytometer.
8. Thermometer.
9. Sealed 25 ml tissue culture flask.
10. Small plastic/styrofoam container.
11. Pipettor/pipettes and pipette tips.
12. 15 ml conical tubes.
13. 1.5 ml safe lock microfuge tubes.
14. 0.22 μm pore-sized filter.
15. RPMI 1640 medium.
16. Heat inactivated FCS (hiFCS).
17. Sodium chloride (NaCl).
18. Heavy water, deuterium oxide 99.96% (^2H_2O, e.g., Cambridge stable isotope laboratories DLM-6). Use ^2H_2O to prepare a ^2H_2O-saline solution: weigh out 0.45 g NaCl in a 50-ml conical tube, add 50 ml pure ^2H_2O (99.96%), vortex until dissolved, and filter sterilize by filtering through a 0.22-μm pore-sized filter.
19. Ultrapure water (deionized, 18 Ω, sterile filtered).
20. Dry ice.
21. Ice bath.
22. Ethanol.
23. Phosphate buffered saline (PBS).

2.2 The Infection, In Vivo ^2H_2O Labeling, Parasite Harvest, and Purification

All materials as under Subheading 2.1. Additionally, the following materials are used:

1. 1, 5, and 10 ml disposable syringes.
2. 25, 27 G needles.
3. 15 and 50 ml conical tubes.
4. Sterilized tweezers, scalpels, and scissors.
5. Materials required for laboratory mouse husbandry (housing, bedding, food, water, enrichment).

6. 10 cm ø petri dish.
7. Cell strainer.
8. Filter system (e.g., Whatman plastic filter holders, WHA420400).
9. Filter membrane, 5 μm pore size (e.g., Merck, SMWP04700).
10. Magnesium chloride ($MgCl_2$).
11. Deoxyribonuclease I (DNase I, e.g., Sigma-Aldrich, 11284932001).

2.3 Chloroform/Methanol/Water Extraction

1. Chemical fume hood (work under the fume hood when handling solvents or fuming acids).
2. Refrigerated microfuge centrifuge.
3. Vortex mixer.
4. −80 °C freezer.
5. 1.5 ml safe lock microfuge tubes.
6. Pipette/pipette tips.
7. Ice bath.
8. Chloroform (high purity grade).
9. Methanol (high purity grade).
10. Ultrapure water (deionized, 18 Ω, sterile filtered).

2.4 Macromolecule Hydrolysis and Derivatization

2.4.1 DNA and RNA Hydrolysis and Derivatization

1. Chemical fume hood (work under the fume hood when handling solvents or fuming acids).
2. Nitrogen evaporator manifold with heating block.
3. Scientific oven (suitable for 90 °C heating).
4. Sample shaker at 37 °C.
5. Centrifuge holding below mentioned glass tubes.
6. Vortex mixer.
7. pH-meter.
8. 50 ml conical tubes.
9. Pipette/pipette tips.
10. 1.5 ml safe lock microfuge tubes.
11. Conical glass tubes with Teflon-lined lids (e.g., Corning, CL S995025, CL S9999132).
12. Hamilton syringe (e.g., Sigma-Aldrich, 20737).
13. 2 ml glass vials, lids, and inserts suitable for mass spectrometry (e.g., Agilent).
14. Ultrapure water (deionized, 18 Ω, sterile filtered).
15. Sodium acetate.

16. Glacial acetic acid.
17. Zinc sulphate.
18. Potato acid phosphatase (Calbiochem, 524529).
19. S1 nuclease (Sigma-Aldrich, N5661).
20. 5× DNA/RNA hydrolysis buffer: Add sodium acetate (3.08 g) and zinc sulfate (21.5 mg) to 100 ml ultrapure water and adjust the pH to 5.0 using glacial acetic acid.
21. Saturated saline solution (to prepare, add >7 g sodium chloride (NaCl) in 20 ml ultrapure water in a 50-ml conical tube vortex, spin at 500 × *g* for 1 min, and take saturated saline solution from supernatant).
22. Hexane (high purity grade).
23. Ethyl acetate (high purity grade).
24. Pyridine (high purity grade).
25. Hydrochloric acid (HCl) (concentrated, 32%).
26. Pentafluorobenzyl hydroxylamine hydrochloride (PFBHA-HCl, e.g., Sigma-Aldrich, 19448).
27. Bis(trimethylsilyl)trifluoroacetamide + 1% trimethylchlorosilane (BSTFA + 1% TMCS, e.g., ThermoFisher Scientific, TS 38831).

2.4.2 Protein Hydrolysis and Derivatization

1. Chemical fume hood.
2. Scientific oven (suitable for 110 °C heating).
3. Heatable nitrogen flow evaporator.
4. Conical glass tubes with Teflon-lined lids (e.g., Corning, CL S995025, CL S9999132).
5. 2 ml glass vials, lids, and inserts suitable for mass spectrometry (e.g., Agilent).
6. Pipette/pipette tips.
7. Methanol (high purity grade).
8. HCl (concentrated, 32%).
9. Pyridine (high purity grade).
10. (*N*-Methyl-*N*-(tert-butyldimethylsilyl)trifluoroacetamide, +1% tertbutylimetheylchlorosilane) (MTBSTFA + 1% TBDMCS, e.g., Sigma-Aldrich, 375934).

2.4.3 Mannogen (Oligosaccharide) Hydrolysis and Derivatization

1. Chemical fume hood.
2. Heatable nitrogen flow evaporator.
3. Scientific oven suitable for heating to 100 °C.
4. Glass vials, lids, and inserts suitable for mass spectrometry (e.g., Agilent).

5. Conical glass tubes with Teflon-lined lids (e.g., Corning, CL S995025, CL S9999132).
6. Pipette/pipette tips.
7. Pyridine (high purity grade).
8. Methoxyamine hydrochloride (MeOx-HCl, e.g., Sigma-Aldrich, 226904).
9. BSTFA + 1% TMCS (e.g., ThermoFisher Scientific, TS 38831).
10. Trifluoroacetic acid (TFA, e.g., Sigma-Aldrich, 302031).
11. Methanol (high purity grade).

2.4.4 Lipid Hydrolysis and Derivatization

1. Chemical fume hood.
2. Centrifugal evaporator (ideally with solvent trap).
3. 2 ml glass vials, lids, and 250 μl inserts suitable for mass spectrometry (e.g., Agilent).
4. 1.5 ml safe lock microfuge tubes.
5. 3-(trifluoromethyl)phenyltrimethylammonium hydroxide (*m*TFPTAH, e.g., TCI, T0961).
6. Chloroform (high purity grade).
7. Methanol (high purity grade).

2.5 GC-MS Measurement and Data Analysis

1. GC-MS instrument with an autosampler and suitable for chemical ionization (CI) analysis (e.g., Agilent HP 6890 GC system and an Agilent HP 5973 MSD (Agilent Technologies).
2. DB5 capillary column (J&W Scientific, 30 m, 250 μm inner diameter, 0.25 μm film thickness) with a 10-m inert duraguard).
3. Split/splitless inlet liner with glass wool (deactivated).
4. CI ion source.
5. Methane (high purity as reagent gas).
6. Helium (high purity as carrier gas).
7. Methanol (high purity grade).
8. Hexane (high purity grade).
9. Software for data analysis (e.g., Agilent Chemstation, Agilent MassHunter, Microsoft Excel, DExSI [26]).

3 Methods

3.1 Parasite Cultivation In Vitro, ^2H_2O Labeling, and Harvest

1. Culture *Leishmania mexicana* promastigotes in 9.5 ml RPMI 1640 medium, pH 7.4 supplemented with 10% (v/v) heat-inactivated fetal calf serum (hiFCS) in sealed tissue culture flasks at 27 °C. Subculture the cells regularly (usually twice

weekly) by adding 100 μl culture medium containing promastigotes in late log/early stationary phase to 9.4 ml fresh medium (*see* **Note 1**).

2. For in vitro labeling, add 0.5 ml ^2H_2O-saline solution directly to culture flasks containing 9.5 ml culture medium and parasites at selected stages of growth (final concentration 5% ^2H_2O (v/v)). Incubate cultures under standard conditions and in individual culture flasks. Harvest flasks at defined time points to measure labeling dynamics (e.g., after 2, 4, 8, 24, 48 h of labeling). Include a flask in which water-saline, rather than ^2H_2O-saline is added (unlabeled control), as well as a flask in which parasites were labeled to steady-state (maximum labeling control). The latter control is generated by adding ^2H_2O-saline to the flask at the same time as the culture inoculum (one drop of a log phase culture) and incubation in the presence of 5% ^2H_2O for at least 72 h. (*see* **Notes 2** and **3**).
3. To quench the metabolism at the time of harvest, prepare a dry ice/ethanol slurry (dry ice pellets in a small 3–5 cm deep ethanol bath). Insert a clean thermometer into the culture flask and immerse the culture flask in the dry ice/ethanol bath. Gently shake the flask to facilitate rapid, even cooling of the cell solution. When the thermometer reaches approximately 10 °C, remove the thermometer and transfer the culture flask to the ice bath (*see* **Note 4**).
4. Use a pipettor to transfer the chilled cell solution to a prechilled conical tube and spin the culture at 1500 × *g* for 10 min at 4 °C. Resuspended the cell pellet in 1 ml ice-cold PBS and transfer to prechilled microfuge tubes.
5. Take an aliquot and dilute 1:10 or 1:100 in PBS. Pipette 10 μl on a Neubauer hemocytometer and determine number of parasites using a standard light microscope.
6. Centrifuge 3×10^7 parasites at 15,000 × *g* for 3 min at 4 °C and wash the pellet three times with ice-cold PBS (in each case, parasite suspension is centrifuged 15,000 × *g*, 1 min, 4 °C, and PBS removed by aspiration). After the final wash, the cell pellets can be stored at −80 °C.

3.2 Infection, In Vivo ^2H_2O Labeling, Parasite Harvest, and Purification

1. Allow mice to adapt to your facility prior to use. BALB/c mice (all female) are commonly used as the preferred animal model as the lesion type generally mimics the lesion morphology seen in susceptible humans. For example, infection with *L. major* or *L. mexicana* generally leads to the formation of localized cutaneous lesions, while infection with *L. donovani* or *L. infantum* leads to visceral (liver, spleen) infections. While the procedure described below focuses on *L. mexicana*-induced cutaneous lesions in BALB/c mice, the same procedure is applicable to

visceral lesions. Animal handling and welfare differ between institutions. Be sure to follow the guidelines of your facility. All procedures involving animals should be carried out by trained personnel.

2. Remove hair on the back flank of the mice to expose a small circle (~1 cm in diameter) of bare skin.
3. Suspend *L. mexicana* stationary phase promastigotes (10^6) in 50 μl PBS and carefully inject subcutaneously into the skin using a 1-ml syringe equipped with a 27-G needle (*see* **Note 5**).
4. Monitor the well-being of the animals and development of the infection regularly (>2 times per week). Cutaneous lesions initially manifest as a swelling at the site of injection but can rapidly ulcerate with risk of secondary infections.
5. Initiate the ^2H_2O-labeling at any stage during the infection. To determine the maximal ^2H-molar enrichment in analytes of interest, initiate labeling shortly after the infection and continue the labelling for several weeks until the termination of the experiment.
6. To initiate in vivo ^2H_2O-labeling, inject a ^2H_2O-saline solution intraperitoneally (32 μl/g body weight) using a 1-ml syringe equipped with a 27-G needle. Provide mice subsequently with 9% ^2H_2O (v/v) in their drinking water for the rest of the labeling period (*see* **Note 6**).
7. Continue to monitor the well-being of the animal and the progression of the infection closely.
8. Harvest the infected tissue (murine skin lesion) at any stage during the infection. At the desired end point of the experiment, mice are culled humanely according to the guidelines of your institution. Carefully remove hair from the site of infection using sharp scissors or a scalpel. Gently excise the infected tissue using tweezers, sharp scissors, and a scalpel and place the lesion in a conical tube filled with 10 ml ice-cold PBS. Lesions can progress to up to 1 cm in diameter and can harbor as many as 10^9 parasites.
9. Pour the lesion and PBS into a wire-grid cell strainer that is propped over a glass petri dish. Use a syringe plunger (5 ml syringe) to press the lesion tissue through the strainer, and collect the disintegrated tissue in the petri dish.
10. Lyse host cells by passing the cell suspension through a 5-ml syringe equipped with a 25-G needle (×10), followed by a 27-G syringe needle (×5).
11. Transfer the lysate to a 15-ml conical tube and remove large host cell debris by low-speed centrifugation (60 × *g*, 5 min at room temperature (RT)).

12. Pour the supernatant into a new 10-ml syringe equipped with a 5-μm pore size filter and discard the pellet. Filter the cell suspension into a 15-ml conical tube and wash the filter membrane with an additional 5-ml PBS.
13. Harvest parasites in the filtrate by centrifugation (1500 × *g*, 10 min, RT) and resuspend the pellet in 10 ml PBS containing 5 mM $MgCl_2$ and DNase I (0.1 mg/ml)—incubate for 1 h at 33 °C (*see* **Note 7**).
14. After 1 h, insert a clean thermometer into the cell suspension and immerse the 15 ml conical tube in the dry ice/ethanol bath. Gently shake the flask to facilitate rapid and even cooling of the cell solution. When the thermometer reaches approximately 10 °C, remove the thermometer and place the culture flask on ice.
15. Harvest and wash the parasites as described in Subheading 3.1 **item 6** and store pellets at −80 °C prior to extraction.

Figure 1 provides a schematic summary of the key steps from infection and ^2H_2O labeling to the harvest of parasites and the analysis of macromolecule building blocks by GC-MS.

3.3 Macromolecule Extraction

1. Place freshly prepared or frozen cell pellets (from −80 °C freezer) on ice for 5 min before addition of 50 μl chloroform, and vigorously vortex the mixing. Place the tube on ice for 1 min after 30 s of vortexing (repeat this four times).
2. Add a further 200 μl methanol/water (3:1 v/v) to generate a single phase and vortex mix the suspension vigorously. Place the tube on ice for 1 min after 30 s of vortexing (repeat this four times).
3. Spin the solution at 25,000 × *g*, 5 min at 4 °C.
4. Transfer the supernatant to a new microfuge tube containing 100 μl ultrapure water and keep chilled in an ice bath. After vortex mixing (1 min), centrifuge the supernatant-water mixture at 25,000 × *g*, 5 min at 4 °C. Transfer the upper, methanol/water-enriched polar phase to a new clean microfuge tube and store at −80 °C (continue with Subheading 3.4.3).
5. Store the organic, chloroform-enriched apolar phase (50 μl) at −80 °C (continue with Subheading 3.4.4).
6. Suspend the delipidated cell pellet in 80 μl ultrapure water by vigorously pipetting up-and-down. Transfer 40 μl of the suspension to a new tube. One tube will be used for analysis of deuterium incorporation into the deoxyribose/ribose moieties of DNA/RNA, while the other will be used for analysis of proteinogenic amino acids. Store both tubes at −80 °C (continue with Subheadings 3.4.1 and 3.4.2).

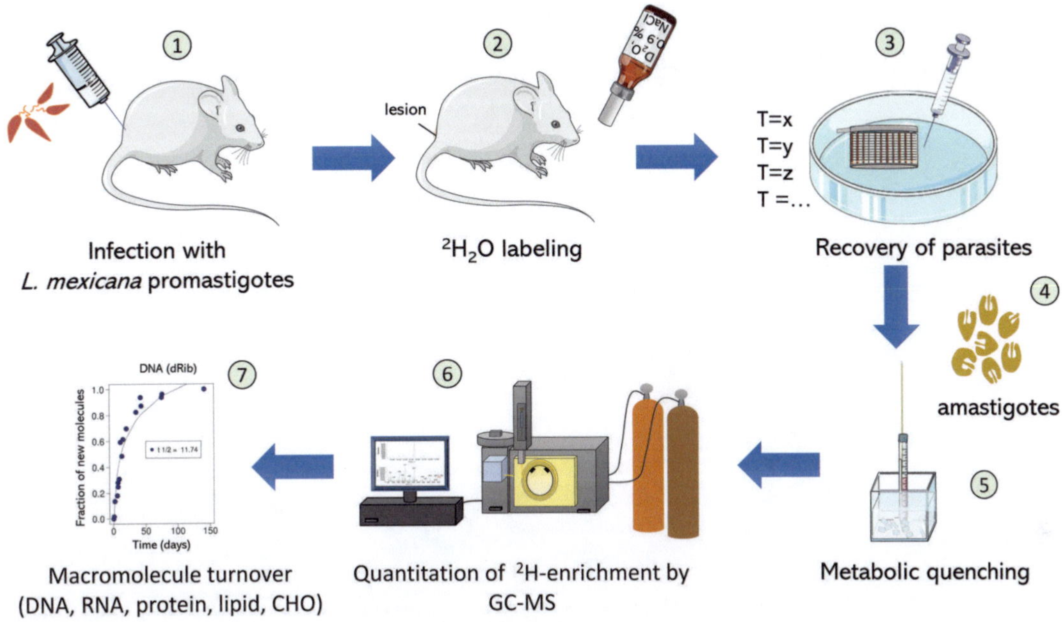

Fig. 1 Overview of the ^2H_2O labeling approach used to measure *Leishmania* growth and macromolecular turnover in infected animals. A mouse is infected with 10^6 stationary phase promastigotes (1). Following the formation of a skin lesion, the mouse is labeled through an initial bolus with 32 μl ^2H_2O per gram of body weight as 0.9% NaCl solution and consecutive feeding with 9% ^2H_2O in the drinking water (2). After the intended time of labeling (*Tx*, *Ty*, *Tz*, ...), the mouse is humanely euthanized, and parasites are released from the infected tissue by passage through a cell strainer and syringing with a narrow bore needle (3). To further minimize contamination with host cell material, purified parasites can be treated with nuclease to digest extracellular DNA and RNA (4). Parasites are rapidly chilled to quench metabolism and harvested (5). Macromolecules are extracted, hydrolyzed, and derivatized for analysis by gas chromatography–mass spectrometry (6). ^{2}H-enrichments in different macromolecule constituents are used to determine the half-life of parasite DNA, RNA, protein, lipids, oligosaccharides (7)

3.4 Macromolecule Hydrolysis and Derivatization

Figure 2 provides a summary of the differential extraction procedure and macromolecule/lipid depolymerization procedures used. Figure 3 provides a summary of the derivatization procedures used (together with structures and molecular weights of key metabolites) for analysis of macromolecule constituents by GC-MS.

3.4.1 DNA and RNA Hydrolysis and Derivatization

1. Prepare the 5× DNA/RNA hydrolysis buffer as described above and in [18].
2. Transfer 38 ml of 5× DNA/RNA hydrolysis buffer to a 50-ml conical tube.
3. Resuspend entire vial of potato acid phosphatase in 1 ml ultrapure ice-cold water and keep on ice while preparing enzyme cocktail.
4. Resuspend 2.5 μl of S1 nuclease in 2 ml 5× DNA/RNA hydrolysis buffer.

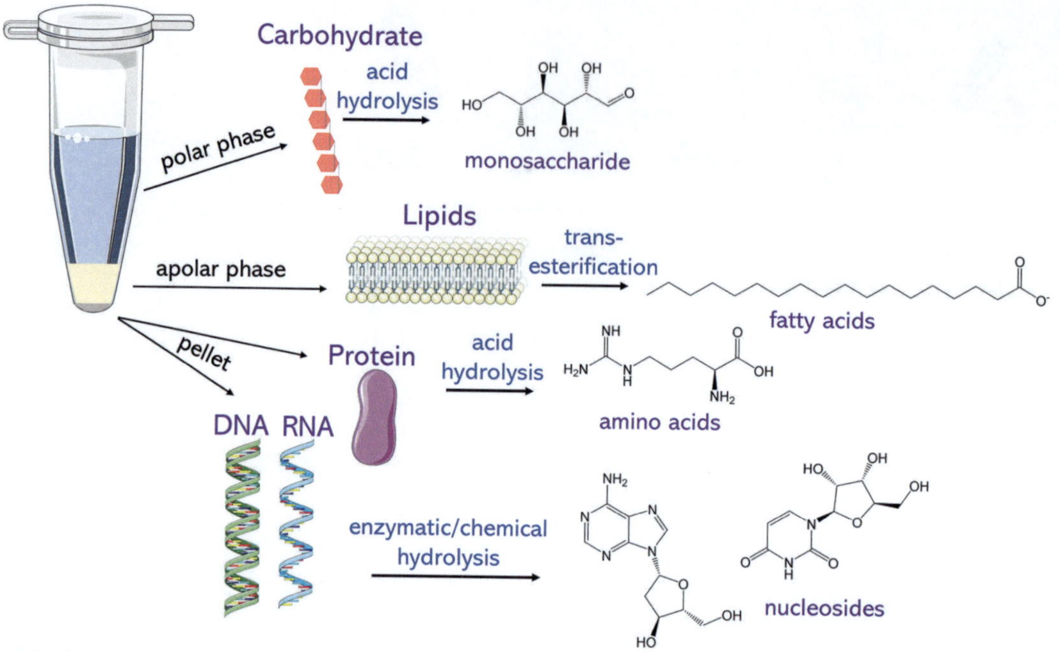

Fig. 2 Schematic overview of differential extraction protocol used to extract parasite macromolecules for analysis. Cultured or lesion-derived parasite stages are initially extracted in chloroform:methanol:water to extract lipids and water-soluble metabolites, including mannogen, the major carbohydrate reverse material of *Leishmania* [29]. After phase separation, lipids and water-soluble metabolites are recovered in the apolar and polar fractions, respectively, and the constituent fatty acid methyl esters and sugars are analyzed by GC-MS. The delipidated pellet is split into two fractions and subjected to S1 nuclease/phosphatase digestion and strong acid hydrolysis, respectively. After derivatization, the released deoxyribose/ribose and amino acids are also analyzed by GC-MS

5. Transfer 1 ml of acid phosphatase solution and 1 ml of the diluted S1 nuclease solution to the 38 ml of 5× DNA/RNA hydrolysis buffer (enzyme cocktail).
6. Aliquot the enzyme cocktail mix into 1.5 ml microfuge tubes (as 520 μl or 1 ml aliquots) and store at −80 °C for up to 12 months.
7. Thaw sample tubes containing delipidated parasite cell pellets (40 μl) and add 160 μl ultrapure water.
8. Add 50 μl enzyme cocktail and incubate the samples for >8 h at 37 °C with vigorous shaking (*see* **Note 8**).
9. For derivatization of the released purine deoxyribose, transfer phosphatase/S1 nuclease-treated samples (250 μl) to a 5-ml screw-capped glass vial with a V-bottom.
10. Add 1.84 ml 0.01 M HCl (pH 2) and 20 μl of pentafluoro-benzyl hydroxylamine hydrochloride (25 mg/ml in ultrapure water). Vortex briefly and incubate at 90 °C in an oven or heating block for 3 h (*see* **Note 9**).

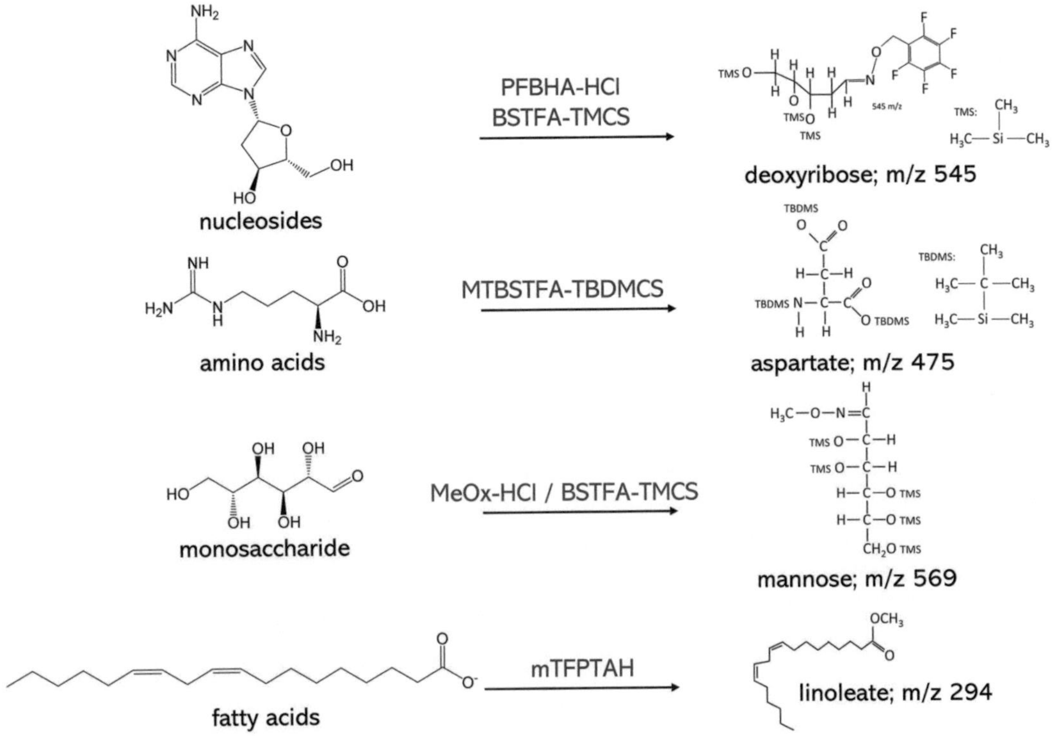

Fig. 3 Schematic overview of the different derivatization protocols used to analyze pentose sugars, amino acids, neutral hexoses, and fatty acids. Prior to GC-MS analysis, released DNA- and RNA-derived pentoses are oximated using pentafluorobenzyl hydroxylamine hydrochloride (PFBHA-HCl), followed by silylation using bis (trimethylsilyl) trifluoroacetamide + 1% trimethylchlorosilane (BSTFA-TMCS). Released proteinogenic amino acids are derivatized using *N*-methyl-*N*-(tert-butyldimethylsilyl)trifluoroacetamide, +1% tertbutylimetheyl-chlorosilane (MTBSTFA-TBDMCS). Mannogen derived mannose is oximated using methoxyamine hydrochloride (MeOx-HCl) and silylated using BSTFA-TMCS. Lipids are transesterified and converted to fatty acid methyl esters using 3-(trifluoromethyl)phenyltrimethylammonium hydroxide (mTFPTAH)

11. Allow the sample to cool to RT on the bench. Add 2 ml of saturated saline solution.
12. Add 1 ml of ethyl acetate/hexane (1:1 v/v) and vortex vigorously for 1 min.
13. Centrifuge at 500 × *g*, 5 min at RT.
14. Carefully remove 800 μl of the upper phase and transfer to a new/clean glass tube.
15. Add a further 1 ml of ethyl acetate to the 5 ml glass vial, and vortex mix for 1 min.
16. Spin the tube at 500 × *g* for 5 min at RT and transfer 800 μl of the upper phase to the tube containing the upper phase collected in **step 14**.

17. Place the tubes containing the pooled organic phases in a heating block with a nitrogen manifold and dry samples under a gentle stream of nitrogen at 40 °C (the nitrogen evaporator should be placed under a hood to avoid inhalation of solvent fumes).
18. Resuspend the dried sample in 30 μl pyridine and 30 μl BSTFA + 1% TMCS. Vortex vigorously and incubate the sample at 90 °C for 30 min (*see* **Note 10**).
19. Allow the sample to cool to RT and transfer the sample into GC-MS glass vial inserts using a gas-tight Hamilton syringe.
20. Incubate the samples for 30 min at RT gently rocking prior to analysis by GC-MS (*see* **Note 11**).

3.4.2 Protein Hydrolysis and Derivatization

1. Transfer the second delipidated cell pellet (40 μl) to a 2.5-ml screw-cap (Teflon-lined) glass vial.
2. Add 60 μl of concentrated (32%) hydrochloric acid (6 M final concentration).
3. Incubate the tube at 110 °C in a heating block or oven for 2 h.
4. Allow the samples to cool to RT on the bench and dry under a gentle stream of nitrogen at 40 °C. The nitrogen manifold and heating block should be placed inside a well-ventilated fume hood to avoid inhalation of acid fumes.
5. Add 80 μl methanol and dry under nitrogen to remove residual water.
6. Add 40 μl pyridine and 40 μl BSTFA + 1% TBDMCS (*see* **Note 12**).
7. Vortex vigorously and incubate the sample at 60 °C for 30 min.
8. Allow the samples to cool to RT and transfer samples to GC-MS glass vial inserts using a gas-tight Hamilton syringe.
9. Incubate the samples for 30 min at RT with gentle shaking prior to analysis by GC-MS (*see* **Note 13**).

3.4.3 Mannogen Hydrolysis and Derivatization

1. Thaw methanol/water polar phase parasite extracts (300 μl) on ice and transfer to a 2.5-ml screw-capped (Teflon-lined) glass tube with a V-bottom.
2. Dry the samples under a gentle stream of nitrogen at 40 °C and place tubes in a fume hood for addition of acid.
3. Add 80 μl of 2 M trifluoroacetic acid (TFA), vortex vigorously, and incubate in an oven or heating block at 100 °C for 3 h.
4. Allow the samples to cool to RT and dry under a stream of nitrogen at 40 °C.
5. Add 60 μl methanol and dry under nitrogen to remove any residual water/acid.

6. Add 40 μl of MeOx in pyridine (20 mg/ml), vortex vigorously, and incubate the sample at 90 °C for 30 min.
7. Allow the samples to cool to RT and add 40 μl of BSTFA + 1% TMCS.
8. Transfer the samples to GC-MS glass vial inserts using a gas-tight Hamilton syringe.
9. Incubate the samples for 30 min at RT with gentle rocking prior to analysis by GC-MS.

3.4.4 Lipid Hydrolysis and Derivatization

1. Thaw chloroform (apolar) phase parasite extracts and transfer to GC-MS glass vial inserts, which have been placed in a microfuge tube.
2. Dry the sample in a SpeedVac centrifugal vacuum evaporator at ambient temperature.
3. Transfer the glass vial inserts into GC-MS glass vials (suitable for loading on autosampler).
4. Add 60 μl chloroform/methanol (3:1 v/v) containing 3% (v/v) of *m*TFPTAH.
5. Incubate the samples gently rocking for 30 min at RT prior to analysis by GC-MS (*see* **Note 14**). Note that lipid transesterification and derivatization occurs by pyrolysis following injection into the GC-MS inlet.

Figure 4 shows the GC-MS total ion chromatogram of mannogen-derived mannose and lipid-derived fatty acids and their ion spectra.

3.5 GC-MS Measurement and Data Analysis

1. Utilize a GC-MS instrument equipped with an autosampler and chemical ionization mass detector in positive chemical ionization (PCI) mode with methane as reagent gas.
2. Set the injector insert and GC-MS transfer line temperatures to 250 °C and the ion source temperature to 300 °C.
3. Set the flow rate of the carrier gas to 1 ml/min, determine the optimal flow rate of the reagent gas using the autotune function.
4. Set the oven temperature gradient to 70 °C (1 min); 70–295 °C at 12.5 °C/min; 295–320 °C at 25 °C/min; 320 °C for 2 min (*see* **Note 15**).
5. Set the injection volume to 1–2 μl.
6. Program the injection needle to be washed extensively between samples to avoid carry-over (e.g., three washes with methanol, followed by three washes with hexane).
7. Set the instrument to PCI using methane as reagent gas.

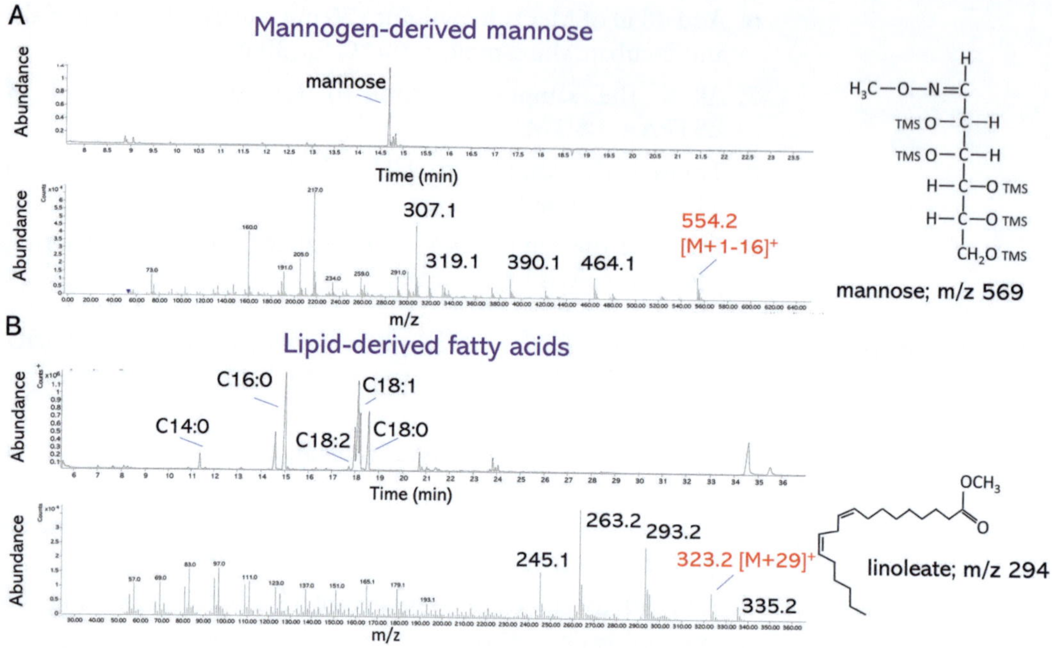

Fig. 4 Representative GC chromatograms and mass spectra of hexose sugars and fatty acids released from *Leishmania* mannogen and total lipids, respectively. All samples are analyzed by GC-PCI-MS. Mannogen is comprised entirely of mannose and is the major glycan component of the polar organic fraction [29]. The major fatty acids in *L. mexicana* promastigotes are C16:0 (palmitate), C18:0 (stearate), C18:1 (oleate), and C18:2 (linoleate). The ion spectra of mannose and linoleate are shown. The relevant molecular ions used to quantitate ^{2}H-enrichment are shown in red

8. Analyze samples in scan mode (50–700 m/z) and identify metabolites based on the GC-retention time and comparison with the mass spectra of authentic standards.
9. Selected ion monitoring (SIM) can be used for more accurate quantitation of M0/M1 mass isotopologues of specific analytes. The M0/M1 $[M + 1\text{–}16]^+$ mass isotopologues for DNA/RNA-derived pentose sugars are deoxyribose (m/z 530, 531) and ribose (m/z 618, 619), and for mannogen-derived, mannose (m/z 554, 555). M0/M1 mass isotopologues ($[MH]^{+}$) for protein-derived amino acids are alanine (m/z 318, 319), aspartate (m/z 475, 476), and glutamate (m/z 489, 490). M0 mass isotopologues for $[M + 29]^+$ fatty acid methyl ester are stearate (m/z 298), oleate (m/z 296), and linoleate (m/z 294). A representative ion chromatogram of deoxyribose and ribose peaks and corresponding mass spectrum for deoxyribose are shown in Fig. 5a, b. Ion chromatograms of deoxyribose M0 and M1 $[M + 1\text{–}16]^+$ ions before and after labeling of promastigotes with ^2H_2O in Fig. 5c, d.
10. Choose dwell times, so that more than eight data points are collected across a peak.

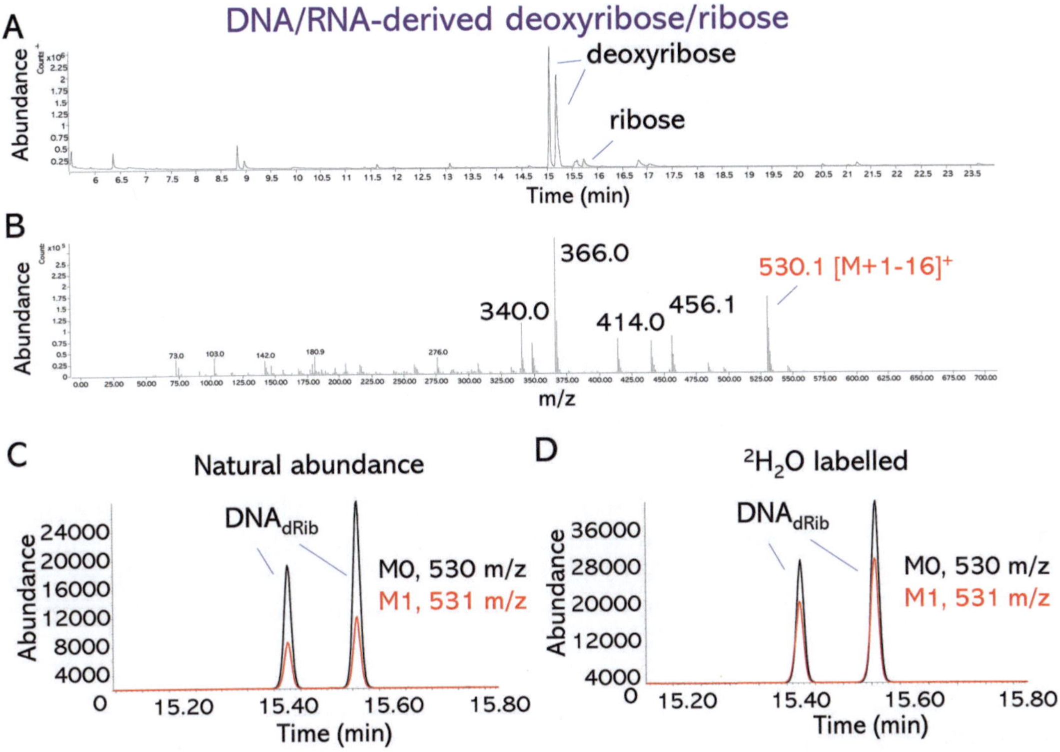

Fig. 5 Analysis of deoxyribose/ribose using GC-PCI-MS. After enzymatic depolymerization and dephosphorylation of extracted nucleic acids, nucleosides are oximated using PFBHA-HCl and silylated using BSTFA +1% TMCS. The base residue is lost during the derivatization and resulting derivatized sugar is analyzed by GC-MS in PCI mode. (**a**) Representative total ion chromatogram of derivatized deoxyribose and ribose. Deoxyribose runs as two identical peaks corresponding to their *cis/trans* isomers. (**b**) Representative positive ion mass spectrum of derivatized deoxyribose. The major ion at m/z 530 (red) corresponds to the molecular ion of the PFBHA/TMS derivative minus one of the TMS methyl groups. This abundant fragment contains all of the backbone carbons and hydrogens from the pentose sugar. (**c**, **d**) ^{2}H-enrichment in deoxyribose is determined by quantitating levels of the M0 and M1 mass isotopologues. Selected ion monitoring (SIM) is used to quantitate the levels of the deoxyribose M0 (m/z 530) and M1 (m/z 531) ions in DNA extracts from unlabeled (**c**) and ^2H_2O-labeled (**d**) *L. mexicana* lesion-derived amastigotes. Unlabeled samples contain a significant M1 mass isotopologue due primarily to natural abundance of ^{13}C in the environment. This value is invariant (M1/(M0 + M1) = 0.2728) and is subtracted from the M1 abundance observed in labeled samples. In the presence of ^2H_2O (5%, v/v), the abundance of the M1 relative to the M0 increases due to incorporation of ^{2}H into deoxyribose of newly formed DNA strands. The increase in M1/(M0 + M1) ratio over time can be used to calculate the rate of DNA turnover and parasite growth

11. Determine the abundance/area under the peak for each ion using GC-MS software. Data can also be exported and analyzed using software such as DExSI that also calculates natural abundance and isotopologue enrichment [26].
12. Calculate the excess molar enrichment in the M1 isotopologue (EM1, %) using the following formulae ("sample" refers to a sample labeled with ^2H_2O, while "unlab" refers to a sample of unlabeled cells, in absence of ^2H_2O:

$$\text{EMI}, \% = \left(\left[\frac{\text{M1 abundance}_{\text{sample}}}{(\text{M0} + \text{M1 abundance}_{\text{sample}})}\right] - \left[\frac{\text{M1 abundance}_{\text{unlab}}}{(\text{M0} + \text{M1 abundance}_{\text{unlab}})}\right]\right) \times 100$$

13. Determine the fraction of new molecules (new cells in the case of DNA labeling) relative to the maximal enrichment observed in fully turned over cells after prolonged labeling using the formula below:

$$\text{Fraction of new molecules/cells}, f = \frac{\text{EM1}_{\text{sample cells}}}{\text{EM1}_{\text{fully turned over cells}}}$$

14. Determine the half-life ($t_{½}$) by plotting data points on a log time (days) scale, fitting a straight line to the data points and solving the equation $y = mx + c$ for $y = 0.5$. The $t_{½}$ is given by exp. (log (days)).

Figure 5 show the total GC-MS ion chromatogram of nucleic acid-derived pentoses (deoxyribose/ribose), the mass spectrum of the PFBHA/TMS derivative of DNA-derived deoxyribose, and selected ion chromatograms of the M0/M1 ions of deoxyribose from unlabeled and labeled lesion-derived amastigotes.

4 Notes

1. The virulence of *Leishmania* promastigotes in BALB/c mice often decreases with continuous cultivation in rich medium. Parasite lines should therefore be regularly passaged through BALB/c mice and not subcultured more than 20 times in medium. Cryopreserved parasite stocks can be used as long as they have not been subcultured more than 20 times. The extent to which different species/strains lose virulence in culture varies considerably and needs to be tested empirically in each case.
2. High concentrations of ^2H_2O can lead to reduced growth and eventual toxicity as high levels of deuterium incorporation into some metabolites can alter enzyme efficiency (the deuterium isotope affect [18]). We have found that growth of *L. mexciana* is unaffected by concentrations of ^2H_2O up to 12%. However, growth was reduced at higher concentrations (>20%), similar to that reported for animal cells [27]. Administration of <15% (v/v) to animals is considered safe and has no effect on the animal or the progeny, while higher concentrations may lead to sterility, neurological symptoms, liver hyperplasia, and anemia [27].
3. The maximal molar enrichment of the M1 mass isotopologue of individual metabolites varies depending on the concentration of heavy water used and the number of enzymatic steps that lead to proton exchange within that metabolite under the

specific growth conditions used. For example, the ^{2}H-molar enrichment in sugar phosphates increases under glucose-limiting conditions as the de novo synthesis of sugar phosphates by gluconeogenesis results in additional incorporation of deuterium into the carbon backbone over and above that achieved by isomerization and epimerization reactions that occur during the interconversion of glucose 6-phosphate with other sugar phosphates. Hence, the maximal molar ^{2}H-enrichment of the M1 mass isotopologue must be determined empirically for each metabolite.

4. The precise temperature at which the 25-ml culture flask containing the cell suspension is transferred from the dry-ice-ethanol bath to the ice bath should be determined empirically. For a standard 25-ml culture flask containing 10 ml medium/parasite suspension, the flask is normally transferred when the temperature drops to ~10 °C (after a few seconds) as the temperature of the liquid continues to fall rapidly after transfer. It is important that the culture suspension does not freeze during this quenching steps as this can lead to cell lysis and loss of metabolites/macromolecules. We have found that this quenching procedure effectively halts central carbon metabolism and macromolecule/lipid biosynthesis and is highly reproducible. However, faster quenching procedures may be required if the investigator is interested in metabolites that have a very rapid turnover (e.g., ATP). The time between cold quenching and addition of chloroform (which inactivates most enzymes) should also be kept constant when processing samples.
5. Stationary phase promastigotes are used to infect mice. Stationary cultures are enriched in metacyclic promastigotes which are the transmission competent stages that accumulate in the foregut of the sand fly and are preadapted for life in the mammalian host. Log phase promastigote cultures are generally depleted of these stages and result in very poor, irreproducible, or delayed lesion development.
6. This protocol results in a level of ^{2}H-labeling of mouse body water of approximately 5% (v/v). However, the precise level of ^{2}H-enrichment can differ depending on the water content of the food, mouse strain, and so on. It is therefore advisable to regularly monitor ^{2}H-enrichment in body water using the protocol of Shah et al. [28]. In this simple protocol, mouse serum or urine samples (5 μl), together with equivalent samples from unlabeled mice which have been spiked with known amounts of ^2H_2O, are incubated with acetone (5 μl) and 5 M NaOH (2.5 μl; to facilitate exchange of ^2H_2O and acetone) in a tightly capped GC vial. A sample of the head-space volume is injected into the GC-MS for analysis of the M1/M0 ratios of acetone using selected ion monitoring (m/z 58–62) [28].

7. The parasites are purified from host cell material through differential centrifugation and filtration. Hence, the contamination with host cell material/debris is expected to be minimal. This should be confirmed by light microscopy (can be done during parasite cell counting). We additionally perform a DNase I treatment of intact parasites as negatively charged host-DNA may adhere to the positively charged surface of the parasites. We have previously shown that this treatment is efficient to remove any exogeneous/extracellular DNA from the parasite sample [20].
8. The differential extraction protocol described here can be used to analyze all major classes of macromolecules (DNA/RNA, protein, carbohydrate) and lipids. In particular, analyses of parasite (deoxy)ribose/ribose in DNA/RNA can be carried out utilizing the crude delipidated parasite extracts. We have found that this extraction gives high yield and very low background. However, other protocols, including the use of commercial kits for extracting DNA or RNA can also be used if the investigator is primarily interested in measuring parasite growth or RNA turnover [18].
9. In other protocols, the pentafluorobenzyl derivative of deoxyribose is commonly analyzed by negative chemical ionization [18]. While negative ion chemical ionization is highly sensitive, we have found that PCI is also suitable for these analyses, allowing all sample types to be analyzed using the same GC-MS program. The pentafluorobenzyl derivatization protocol was also selected for these analyses because it is robust and results in minimal background peaks. Following oximation with PFBHA-HCl, the analyte is recovered in the apolar phase during extraction, resulting in minimal contamination with salts and water which can interfere with the derivatization.
10. We have found that the BSTFA + 1% TMCS derivatization protocol for pentose and hexose sugars is rapid and robust. Other derivatization protocols, such as acetylation using acetic anhydride which generates a single derivative for each sugar can also be used [18].
11. We have found that this procedure is suitable for quantifying both RNA and DNA levels in delipidated cell extracts as both DNA-deoxyribose and RNA-ribose are released and quantitated in the same GC-MS run. The level of DNA-deoxyribose is directly related to cell equivalents and serves as the internal standard in these analyses. Most of the cellular RNA-ribose is associated with ribosomal RNA (rRNA), while mRNAs and tRNAs generally account for less than 20% of total RNA pool. In *Leishmania*, total RNA-ribose levels vary in different developmental stages. Levels are lowest in lesion-derived

amastigotes, 7–16 times higher in nondividing promastigotes and 10–20 times higher in rapidly dividing (log phase) promastigotes.

12. BSTFA + 1% TBDMCS is the most suitable derivatizing agent for amino acids. It is particularly insensitive to residual moisture and acid in the samples and enables more robust analysis compared with other derivatizing agents. All derivatization steps using this reagent should be undertaken in a well-ventilated fume hood.

13. Most proteinogenic amino acids are labeled with deuterium in the presence of ^2H_2O as a result of labeling of their corresponding keto-acids and subsequent transamination reactions. However, the level of labeling in individual amino acids differ greatly, depending on the activity of these pathways, as well as the rate of uptake of exogenous amino acids. In cultured *L. mexicana* promastigotes, the highest level of ^{2}H-enrichment occurs in the nonessential amino acids, alanine and glutamate, while very little or no enrichment is observed in valine and threonine, which are directly acquired from the medium. In contrast, intracellular amastigotes can acquire ^{2}H-labeled amino acids derived from the host cell. For example, protein-derived valine in lesion-derived amastigotes is well labeled due to the uptake of host valine, which is labeled via transamination reactions (unlike the parasite pool). Analysis of the labeling of amino acids thus provides insights into differences in host and parasite metabolism, as well as the rate of amino acid uptake by intracellular parasite stages. Regardless of the origin of labeling, the global rate of protein turnover in different parasite developmental stages can be inferred from deuterium incorporation into any of the protein-derived amino acids.

14. The *m*TFPTAH protocol results in the release and derivatization of all ester-linked fatty acids by reactive pyrolysis with high reproducibility. Alternative derivatization procedures can be used to also detect the glycerol moieties of membrane lipids. Quantitation of ^{2}H-enrichment in the glycerol backbone provides a robust measure of cellular lipid membrane turnover. In this protocol, samples are transesterified in 3 N methanolic HCl (250 μl) at 60 °C for 1 h. After removal of the acid under a stream of nitrogen, released glycerol is derivatized by suspending the samples in acetic anhydride:pyridine (50 μl:50 μl) at 60 °C for 30 min [16].

15. A single extended GC oven temperature gradient is provided in the protocol which is suitable for analyses of the different metabolite classes ((deoxy)ribose, amino acids, fatty acids). Shorter oven ramp gradients (from 25 to 12 min) can be used for the analysis of simple mixtures, such as purine

deoxyribose/ribose and released sugars from the mannogen carbohydrate reserve, in order to reduce analysis time and increase throughput.

Acknowledgments

This work was supported by the Australian National Health and Medical Research Council (NHMRC Project Grant APP1100000). M.J.M. is an NHMRC Principal Research Fellow.

References

1. Stuart K, Brun R, Croft S, Fairlamb A, Gürtler RE, McKerrow J, Reed S, Tarleton R (2008) Kinetoplastids: related protozoan pathogens, different diseases. J Clin Invest 118:1301–1310
2. Rojas F, Silvester E, Young J, Milne R, Tettey M, Houston DR, Walkinshaw MD, Pérez-Pi I, Auer M, Denton H, Smith TK, Thompson J, Matthews KR (2018) Oligopeptide signaling through TbGPR89 drives trypanosome quorum sensing. Cell 176 (1–2):306–317.e16
3. Tanowitz HB, Scherer PE, Mota MM, Figueiredo LM (2017) Adipose tissue: a safe haven for parasites? Trends Parasitol 33:276–284
4. Fairlamb AH, Gow NA, Matthews KR, Waters AP (2016) Drug resistance in eukaryotic microorganisms. Nat Microbiol 1:16092
5. Bates PA (1994) The developmental biology of Leishmania promastigotes. Exp Parasitol 79:215–218
6. Gossage SM, Rogers ME, Bates PA (2003) Two separate growth phases during the development of Leishmania in sand flies: implications for understanding the life cycle. Int J Parasitol 33:1027–1034
7. McConville MJ, Saunders EC, Kloehn J, Dagley MJ (2015) Leishmania carbon metabolism in the macrophage phagolysosome—feast or famine? F1000Res 4:938
8. Saunders EC, Ng WW, Kloehn J, Chambers JM, Ng M, McConville MJ (2014) Induction of a stringent metabolic response in intracellular stages of Leishmania mexicana leads to increased dependence on mitochondrial metabolism. PLoS Pathog 10:e1003888
9. Naderer T, Heng J, Saunders EC, Kloehn J, Rupasinghe TW, Brown TJ, McConville MJ (2015) Intracellular survival of leishmania major depends on uptake and degradation of extracellular matrix glycosaminoglycans by macrophages. PLoS Pathog 11:e1005136
10. Barak E, Amin-Spector S, Gerliak E, Goyard S, Holland N, Zilberstein D (2005) Differentiation of Leishmania donovani in host-free system: analysis of signal perception and response. Mol Biochem Parasitol 141:99–108
11. Bates PA, Robertson CD, Tetley L, Coombs GH (1992) Axenic cultivation and characterization of Leishmania mexicana amastigote-like forms. Parasitology 105(Pt 2):193–202
12. Fiebig M, Kelly S, Gluenz E (2015) Comparative life cycle transcriptomics revises Leishmania mexicana genome annotation and links a chromosome duplication with parasitism of vertebrates. PLoS Pathog 11:e1005186
13. Mandell MA, Beverley SM (2017) Continual renewal and replication of persistent Leishmania major parasites in concomitantly immune hosts. Proc Natl Acad Sci U S A 114: E801–E810
14. Hellerstein MK (2003) In vivo measurement of fluxes through metabolic pathways: the missing link in functional genomics and pharmaceutical research. Annu Rev Nutr 23:379–402
15. Berry D, Mader E, Lee TK, Woebken D, Wang Y, Zhu D, Palatinszky M, Schintlmeister A, Schmid MC, Hanson BT, Shterzer N, Mizrahi I, Rauch I, Decker T, Bocklitz T, Popp J, Gibson CM, Fowler PW, Huang WE, Wagner M (2015) Tracking heavy water (D_2O) incorporation for identifying and sorting active microbial cells. Proc Natl Acad Sci U S A 112:E194–E203
16. Foletta VC, Palmieri M, Kloehn J, Mason S, Previs SF, McConville MJ, Sieber OM, Bruce CR, Kowalski GM (2016) Analysis of mammalian cell proliferation and macromolecule synthesis using deuterated water and gas chromatography-mass spectrometry. Metabolites 6(4):E34

17. Goh B, Kim J, Seo S, Kim TY (2018) High-throughput measurement of lipid turnover rates using partial metabolic heavy water labeling. Anal Chem 90:6509–6518
18. Busch R, Neese RA, Awada M, Hayes GM, Hellerstein MK (2007) Measurement of cell proliferation by heavy water labeling. Nat Protoc 2:3045–3057
19. Neese RA, Misell LM, Turner S, Chu A, Kim J, Cesar D, Hoh R, Antelo F, Strawford A, McCune JM, Christiansen M, Hellerstein MK (2002) Measurement in vivo of proliferation rates of slow turnover cells by $2H_2O$ labeling of the deoxyribose moiety of DNA. Proc Natl Acad Sci U S A 99:15345–15350
20. Kloehn J, Saunders EC, O'Callaghan S, Dagley MJ, McConville MJ (2015) Characterization of metabolically quiescent Leishmania parasites in murine lesions using heavy water labeling. PLoS Pathog 11:e1004683
21. Lang T, Goyard S, Lebastard M, Milon G (2005) Bioluminescent Leishmania expressing luciferase for rapid and high throughput screening of drugs acting on amastigote-harbouring macrophages and for quantitative real-time monitoring of parasitism features in living mice. Cell Microbiol 7:383–392
22. Romero I, Téllez J, Suárez Y, Cardona M, Figueroa R, Zelazny A, Gore Saravia N (2010) Viability and burden of Leishmania in extralesional sites during human dermal leishmaniasis. PLoS Negl Trop Dis 4:pii: e819
23. Michel G, Ferrua B, Lang T, Maddugoda MP, Munro P, Pomares C, Lemichez E, Marty P (2011) Luciferase-expressing Leishmania infantum allows the monitoring of amastigote population size, in vivo, ex vivo and in vitro. PLoS Negl Trop Dis 5:e1323
24. Müller AJ, Aeschlimann S, Olekhnovitch R, Dacher M, Späth GF, Bousso P (2013) Photoconvertible pathogen labeling reveals nitric oxide control of Leishmania major infection in vivo via dampening of parasite metabolism. Cell Host Microbe 14:460–467
25. Prideaux B, Dartois V, Staab D, Weiner DM, Goh A, Via LE, Barry CE, Stoeckli M (2011) High-sensitivity MALDI-MRM-MS imaging of moxifloxacin distribution in tuberculosis-infected rabbit lungs and granulomatous lesions. Anal Chem 83:2112–2118
26. Dagley M, McConville M (2018) DExSI: a new tool for the rapid quantitation of 13C-labelled metabolites detected by GC-MS. Bioinformatics 34(11):1957–1958
27. Kushner DJ, Baker A, Dunstall TG (1999) Pharmacological uses and perspectives of heavy water and deuterated compounds. Can J Physiol Pharmacol 77:79–88
28. Shah V, Herath K, Previs SF, Hubbard BK, Roddy TP (2010) Headspace analyses of acetone: a rapid method for measuring the ^2H-labeling of water. Anal Biochem 404:235–237
29. Ralton JE, Naderer T, Piraino HL, Bashtannyk TA, Callaghan JM, McConville MJ (2003) Evidence that intracellular beta1-2 mannan is a virulence factor in Leishmania parasites. J Biol Chem 278:40757–40763

Chapter 36

A Scalable Purification Method for Mitochondria from *Trypanosoma brucei*

Moritz Niemann and André Schneider

Abstract

Due to its unique biology the mitochondrion of *Trypanosoma brucei* has attracted a lot of interest since many decades, making it arguably the best studied mitochondrion outside yeast and mammals. Here we describe a method allowing purification of mitochondria from procyclic trypanosomes that yields highly enriched and functional organelles. The method is based on isotonic lysis of cells by nitrogen cavitation, DNase I digestion, differential centrifugation and Nycodenz gradient centrifugation. The method is scalable and can be adapted to culture volumes a small as 100 mL or as large as 24 L.

Key words Trypanosomes, *Trypanosoma brucei*, Mitochondria, Subcellular fractionation, Nitrogen cavitation

1 Introduction

Mitochondria are a defining feature of eukaryotic cells. While their main function is oxidative phosphorylation, they are also the site of FeS-cluster biogenesis and play important roles in processes such as lipid synthesis, calcium homeostasis and apoptosis. Mitochondrial biology has attracted a lot of interest and has been studied in great detail [1]. However, most of these studies have been restricted to yeast and mammals, both of which belong to the eukaryotic supergroup of the Opisthokonts [2]. In contrast, we know very little about mitochondria of the remaining four supergroups with two exceptions.

One is plants (Archaeplastida supergroup) whose mitochondria have been studied quite extensively [3]. The other exception is the trypanosomatid parasites, which are members of the excavate supergroup, whose mitochondrion due to its many unique features has been studied since many years [4, 5]. Trypanosomes, unlike most other eukaryotes, have a single mitochondrion only with a single unit genome, termed kinetoplast DNA (kDNA). The kDNA is physically linked across the two mitochondrial membranes to the

Paul A. M. Michels et al. (eds.), *Trypanosomatids: Methods and Protocols*, Methods in Molecular Biology, vol. 2116, https://doi.org/10.1007/978-1-0716-0294-2_36, © Springer Science+Business Media, LLC, part of Springer Nature 2020

basal body of the flagellum by a structure termed tripartite attachment complex (TAC). As a consequence of its single unit nature, the kDNA replicates in coordination with the nuclear cell cycle and requires precise segregation mechanisms, which guarantee that each daughter organelle receives an intact and complete genome [6]. The kDNA consists of several dozen maxi circles (22 kb) that are identical in sequence and several thousands of minicircles (1 kb) which are heterogeneous in sequence. The two genetic elements of the kDNA are highly topologically interlocked forming a dense network. Sequence analysis of the maxicircles revealed that many of its genes are cryptogenes, whose primary transcripts have to be edited by multiple uridine insertions and or deletions to become functional mRNAs. In fact, it was in trypanosomes where RNA editing was first discovered, before the process was shown to be widespread among eukaryotes (reviewed in [7, 8]). Another unusual feature of the kDNA is that it does not encode any tRNA genes, indicating that the trypanosomal mitochondrion imports all of its tRNAs from the cytosol [9, 10].

More recently other aspects of mitochondrial biology in trypanosomes have also been studied. They include: FeS cluster biogenesis [11], the global metabolic changes of the mitochondrion during the *T. brucei* life cycle and the role the ATP synthase plays in this process [12, 13], the unusual mitochondrial protein import systems [14], the highly diverged trypanosomal MICOS complex that forms the cristae [15] and the structure of the highly unusual mitochondrial ribosomes [16].

The access to highly pure and functional mitochondria is of great benefit for all aspects of trypanosomal mitochondrial biology that are being studied. Here we present an isolation procedure for mitochondria of procyclic trypanosomes. It represents an updated and optimized version of a protocol that has been published in a previous volume of this series [17].

2 Materials

2.1 Cell Growth and Harvest

1. Procyclic *Trypanosoma brucei* cells (*see* **Note 1**).
2. Medium SDM-79 [18] containing 5–10% heat inactivated fetal bovine serum, depending on the cell line.
3. Centrifuge [e.g., Sorvall LYNX 6000 Superspeed centrifuge (Thermo Fisher Scientific, ref. No. 75006591) with appropriate fixed-angle rotor Fibrelite F9-6x1000 LEX (Thermo Fisher Scientific, ref. No. 096-061075) and fitting centrifugation bottles made from polypropylene copolymer (PPCO, Thermo Fisher Scientific, ref. No. 010-1491)].
4. Counting chambers (either reusable or disposable). Alternatively, an automated cell counting system can be used.

5. Generic paint brush (flat, 12 mm, hog bristle or synthetic).
6. 1× SBG: 20 mM sodium phosphate, pH 7.9, 20 mM glucose, 0.15 M NaCl. Prepare as 4× stock (*see* **Note 2**).

2.2 Breakage of Cells, DNase I Digestion, Low-Speed Centrifugation

1. 1× SoTE buffer: 20 mM Tris–HCl, pH 7.5, 0.6 M sorbitol, 2 mM EDTA, pH 7.5. Prepare as 2× stock solution.
2. Dounce homogenizer/tissue grinder, all-glass, 15 and 40 mL (e.g., Kimble Chase Life Science and Research Products ref. No. 885300-0015 and 885300-0040).
3. Cell disruption vessel for nitrogen cavitation [e.g., general purpose model 4635920 mL (600 mL capacity maximum, Parr instrument Company, Moline, Illinois, USA)]. For smaller scale preparations use general purpose model 463945 mL (capacity 30 mL maximum, Parr instrument Company, Moline, Illinois, USA).
4. Centrifuge [e.g., Sorvall LYNX 6000 Superspeed centrifuge as above with appropriate fixed-angle rotor (Thermo Fisher Scientific Fibrelite F21–8 × 50y, ref. No. 096-084275) and fitting centrifuge tubes made from PPCO (e.g., Nalgene round-bottom centrifuge tube, 50 mL capacity, lipped, open top, ref. No. 3110-9500)]. Alternatively, the same tubes fit with a generic SS-34 fixed-angle rotor (Thermo Fisher Scientific ref. No.28020TS) and complementary centrifuge (e.g., Sorvall RC 6 Plus, or RC 5B/RC 5B plus series).
5. Electronic pipette controller.
6. 1 M $MgCl_2$, 0.5 M EDTA, pH 7.5.
7. DNase I, grade II, from bovine pancreas.
8. Conical centrifuge tube, 50 mL capacity (e.g., Falcon, ref. No. 352070).
9. Swing-out centrifuge [e.g., SIGMA 3-16PK with rotor 11180 bucket 13194 and adaptor 18310 or Eppendorf 5810 R with rotor A-4-81, rectangular bucket 500 mL (ref. No. 5810730007) and adaptor for five conical tube 50 mL (ref. No. 5810723000)].

2.3 Density Gradient Centrifugation

1. Ultracentrifuge and rotors Beckman Coulter SW32 Ti or SW28. Use rotor SW41 Ti for smaller scale preparations.
2. Ultracentrifugation tubes for SW32 Ti or SW28 rotor (Ultra-Clear Tube, Beckman Coulter, capacity 38.5 mL, 25 × 89 mm, ref. No. 344058), or for SW41 rotor (Ultra-Clear Tube, Beckman Coulter, capacity 13.2 mL, 14 × 89 mm ref. No. 344059). Tubes can be washed and reused up to five times.
3. Nycodenz powder. Prepare 80% (w/v) Nycodenz stock solution in water (dissolves slowly). Use this 80% (w/v) Nycodenz stock solution and 2× SoTE stock solution (*see* Subheading

2.2, **step 1**) to produce Nycodenz gradient solutions 50%/28%/25%/21% and 18% (w/v) Nycodenz/1× SoTE.

4. Glass syringe Sanitex Eterna Matic (10 mL) with glass piston and clear glass barrel, metal Luer-lock center and long steel needle (1.4 × 100 mm).

2.4 Removal of Nycodenz and Storage

1. 1× SoTE, fixed-angle centrifuge and 50 mL-tubes (*see* Subheading 2.2, **step 4**).
2. Fatty acid-free BSA. Prepare 100 mg/mL stock solution.
3. BCA or Bradford protein assay kit.
4. Liquid nitrogen.

3 Methods

The single mitochondrion of *T. brucei* is a continuous network that extends through the entire cell. This structure cannot be purified as a whole entity, irrespectively of the cell lysis method used, the mitochondrial networks fragments into mitochondrial vesicles, which are subsequently separated from cellular debris, soluble components of the cytosol, flagella and other vesicles.

In short, the method works as follows: cells are resuspended in isotonic buffer and lysed by nitrogen-cavitation. After DNase digestion and low speed spins to remove intact cells, the organelles are purified using Nycodenz gradient centrifugation (for a schematic overview *see* Fig. 1a). Mitochondrial vesicles isolated with this method retain their membrane potential and in the presence of suitable substrates are competent to recapitulate mitochondrial processes in organello (*see* **Note 3**). Consequently, for functional biochemical assays or applications that require the presence of all four mitochondrial subcompartments (mitochondrial outer membrane, MOM; inter-membrane space, IMS; mitochondrial inner membrane, MIM and mitochondria matrix, MTX) the procedure is the method of choice (*see* **Note 4**). Moreover, the purification scheme grants access to precursor fractions that can be used to achieve further subcellular fractionation (*see* **Note 5**).

In the following we describe the mitochondrial isolation procedure for ca. 1×10^{11} cells corresponding to ca. 3 L culture volume of late log-phase cells (density of ca. 3.0–6.0 × 10^7 cells/mL, depending on the specific cell line). However, isolation of mitochondria from smaller culture volumes might be required for labeling experiments (e.g., with SILAC) [19], whereas upscaling might be necessary if very large amounts of mitochondria are needed (e. g. for structural studies of mitochondrial ribosomes using cryoEM, etc.) [16]. An advantage of the described method is that it is scalable and thus suitable for culture volumes ranging

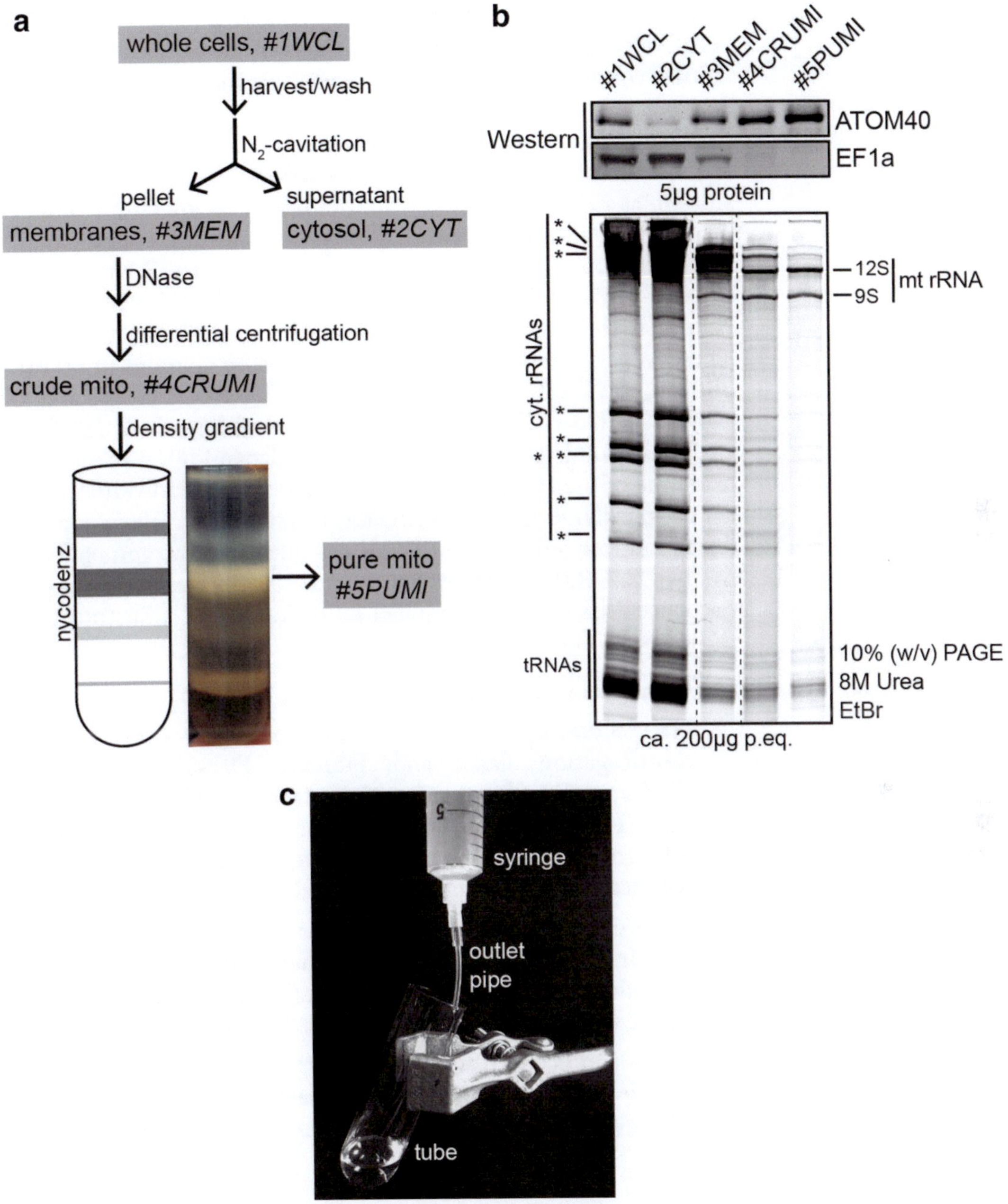

Fig. 1 (**a**) Overview of the purification procedure with schematic and picture of an optimal Nycodenz gradient enriched for mitochondrial vesicles (as detailed in *see* Subheading 3.5, **step 7**). Fractions underlaid in gray are used for quality control of the mitochondrial vesicle preparation as detailed in Subheading 4 (#1WCL, whole cell lysate; #2CYT, cytosol; #3MEM, membranes; #4CRUMI, crude mitochondria; #5PUMI, pure mitochondria). (**b**) Upper panel Equal amounts of protein from the five indicated fractions were subjected to Western blotting (5 µg protein per lane) and probed for the mitochondrial (mt) marker ATOM40 (atypical translocase of the MOM, 40 kDa) and the cytosolic protein EF1a (eukaryotic Elongation Factor 1 alpha); lower panel purified RNA of ca. 200 µg protein equivalents (p.eq.) of the indicated fractions separated by denaturing polyacrylamide gel electrophoresis (PAGE) containing 10% polyacrylamide and 8 M urea. RNAs were visualized by ethidium

from 0.1 up to 24 L (corresponding to 2×10^9 up to 1×10^{12} cells). Deviations of the protocol for very small and very large culture volumes are described in the text or the notes.

3.1 Cell Growth and Harvest

Procyclic stage *T. brucei* is grown in SDM-79 containing 5–10% (w/v) FCS (depending on the strain) in suspension culture at 27 °C shaking at 120 rpm using Erlenmeyer flasks. To guarantee optimal growth, the cultures should be diluted every day and scaled accordingly (*see* **Note 6**). Thus, to obtain 3 L of *T. brucei* 427, a preculture of ca. 3–5 mL late log-phase cells ($4–6 \times 10^7$ mL^{-1}) is needed. This culture is successively diluted 1:4 reaching a volume of 12 mL. These steps are repeated daily to reach culture volumes of 50 mL, 200 mL, 750 mL and finally ca. 3 L using Erlenmeyer flasks of 100 mL, 250 mL, 500 mL and 2.0 L volume, respectively (*see* **Note 7**). These numbers are approximate and depend upon the generation time of the strain used and need to be tested individually with the cells/cell lines under investigation (*see* **Note 8**). When comparing uninduced and induced RNAi cell lines, it is recommended to use two 1.5–2.0 L cultures (ca. 5×10^{10} cells each) and prepare mitochondrial vesicles in parallel following minor adjustments to the protocol (*see* **Note 9**).

1. Unless otherwise noted, all following steps are on ice.
2. Harvest cells by centrifugation in a fixed angle rotor [e.g., 1.0 L centrifugation flasks and Fibrelite F9-6x1000 LEX at 7100 rpm/11,000 × *g* (*see* **Note 10**) at 4 °C for 10 min (*see* **Note 11**)]. While the centrifugation is running determine the cell density using an appropriate aliquot with either a Coulter counter or a Neubauer chamber and a microscope.
3. Discard medium immediately after centrifugation (*see* **Note 12**). In case of large culture volumes, add the next round of cell culture to the same flasks on top of the pelleted cells and repeat **steps 2** and **3** until all cells are harvested.
4. Resuspend pellets using a paint brush and pool everything into a single centrifuge bottle using a small volume of prechilled 1× SBG. Add 1× SBG to the total volume of the centrifuge bottle.

Fig. 1 (continued) bromide staining (EtBr) depicting cytosolic rRNAs, tRNAs and mitochondrial rRNAs. An asterisk indicates the fragmented cytosolic rRNAs mostly visible in the fractions #1WCL and #2CYT (length 119–2251 nucleotides). Fraction #5PUMI is largely free of cytosolic contaminants and the only visible RNAs it contains are mt 9S and 12S rRNA and tRNAs. (**c**) Generation of Nycodenz step-gradients as described in **Note 26** by using a syringe connected to a small-diameter outlet pipe that allows for slow draining alongside the ultracentrifugation tube to achieve ideal phase separation

Repeat spin as above and discard wash buffer to remove remaining medium.

3.2 Breakage of Cells

1. Resuspend the cell pellet in 1× SoTE at 2×10^9 cells/mL with the help of a paint brush. Subsequently the suspension is homogenized thoroughly in a 40 mL glass Dounce homogenizer using the loose-fitting pestle (*see* **Note 13**). Transfer the cell suspension to a 100 mL plastic beaker that fits into the cavitation vessel and when necessary add 1× SoTE to reach the minimal volume of 60 mL (*see* **Note 14**).
2. Place cell suspension into the prechilled cavitation vessel sitting in an ice bath placed on top of a magnetic stirrer. Add magnetic stir bar and a protease inhibitor cocktail as specified by the manufacturer. Lock the vessel, close the outlet valve.
3. Slowly apply 60 bar pressure using nitrogen gas. Lock the inlet valve. Equilibrate nitrogen gas pressure between cells and the buffer by stirring slowly for 30 min (*see* **Note 15**).
4. Depressurize the cavitation vessel and collect the disrupted cells from the outlet valve in a large enough flask (e.g., 0.5 L Erlenmeyer) to accommodate all of the foamy suspension (*see* **Note 16**). Put on ice.
5. Examine the cell lysis efficiency microscopically (*see* **Note 17**).
6. To separate the particulate fraction containing the mitochondrial vesicles from the cytosolic fraction, spin out the lysate and including the foam on the top in a fixed-angle rotor (e.g., SS-34; 40 mL per tube; 16,000 rpm/30,600 × *g* for 10 min/4 °C). Prior to the harvesting spin collect excessive foam at the wall of the collection flask with additional 1× SoTE to minimize loss of material. Discard cytosolic fraction (*see* **Note 18**).

3.3 DNase I Digestion

1. Resuspend pellets in an equal volume of 1× SoTE using an electric pipettor and add 1× SoTE to a density of ca. 2×10^9 cell equivalents/mL. Homogenize suspension with a suitable glass Dounce homogenizer using the loose fitting pestle (*see* **Note 19**). Collect suspension in a suitable plastic beaker.
2. Adjust Mg^{2+}-concentration to 6 mM using 1 M $MgCl_2$ stock while stirring on ice.
3. Add DNase I to a final concentration of 0.1 mg/mL (*see* **Note 20**).
4. Cover beaker with parafilm, incubate 20 min on ice with a magnetic stirrer.
5. Stop the reaction by adding EDTA to 6 mM using a 0.5 M stock solution, stir for 1 min on ice (*see* **Note 21**).

3.4 Low-Speed Centrifugation

1. Spin DNase I-treated lysate in 50 mL Falcon tubes in a swing-out rotor for 20 min at 4 °C and at 555 × *g*/1700 rpm in the SIGMA 3-16PK swing-out centrifuge with rotor 11180, bucket 13194 and adapter 18310 to pellet the remaining intact cells and cellular debris. The mitochondrial vesicles will stay in the supernatant (*see* **Note 22**).
2. Collect supernatant in a beaker on ice. Pellets are very soft, do not decant, but use a 50 mL pipette for transferring the supernatant. Leave 1/10–1/4 of the supernatant in the tube. Resuspend and pool the soft pellets and dilute 1:2 with 1× SoTE and spin again as above (*see* **Note 23**).
3. Transfer second supernatant and pool with the first supernatant. The pellets after the reextraction should be much smaller (2–5 mL) and more clearly visible.
4. Harvest mitochondrial vesicles from the pooled supernatant in a fixed-angle rotor [e.g., SS-34 16,000 rpm/30,600 × *g* for 10 min at 4 °C (40 mL per tube)].
5. Decant supernatant. The pellets are now stable and will stay at the bottom (*see* **Note 24**).

3.5 Density Gradient Centrifugation

1. Calculate the number of gradient tubes needed. For a typical preparation (3 L-scale, 1 × 10^{11} cell equivalents), it is usually one 38.5 mL tube which fits into the SW32 Ti or the SW28 rotor (*see* **Note 25**).
2. During the nitrogen cavitation or the DNase I digestion prepare the Nycodenz step gradients and precool the ultracentrifuge, rotor and buckets. Pipet 8 mL ice-cold 28% (w/v) Nycodenz/1× SoTE into two 38.5 mL tubes (for the 3 L-scale one is used as a balance). Carefully overlay in a stepwise fashion with 8 mL of 25%/21% and 18% (w/v) of Nycodenz/1× SoTE (*see* **Note 26**).
3. Resuspend pellet(s) in 50% (w/v) Nycodenz/1× SoTE. Collect and pool in Dounce homogenizer and homogenize with the loose fitting pestle. Collect in a 50 mL Falcon tube (*see* **Note 27**).
4. Slowly underlay the gradients with the resulting suspension using the glass syringe with the long steel needle (e.g., Sanitex Eterna Matic 10 mL) (*see* **Note 28**).
5. Balance gradients with the 18% (w/v) Nycodenz/1× SoTE using fine balance (tolerance <10 mg).
6. Spin for 45 min at 27,000 rpm in SW32 Ti (=124,513 × *g*) or SW28 (=131,453 × *g*) at 4 °C (*see* **Note 29**).
7. Following centrifugation, the gradients show up to four bands of various densities corresponding to the interphases between the different Nycodenz layers (Fig. 1a). The four bands should

be microscopically examined. Typically, the second band from the top at the 25%/21% interphase is most enriched for the mitochondrial vesicles and ca. 3–5 mL of it (per gradient) should be collected from above with the glass syringe. Pool all collected mitochondrial vesicle fractions in a large beaker that accommodates a volume up to 640 mL (*see* **Note 30**).

3.6 Removal of Nycodenz and Storage

1. Dilute the pooled interphase(s) of the 25%/21% (and potentially the 21%/18%, *see* **Note 30**) Nycodenz layers at least 1:5 with 1× SoTE to allow for the sedimentation of the mitochondrial vesicles (*see* **Note 31**).
2. Mix well and distribute into fixed-angle centrifugation tubes to sediment vesicles (e.g., SS-34; 40 mL per tube; 16,000 rpm/ 30,600 × *g* for 10 min/4 °C).
3. Resuspend the pellets in as little 1× SoTE as possible, to reach a final concentration of ca. 2×10^{10} cell equivalents per 1 mL. Examine the vesicle suspension microscopically (e.g., magnification 500-1000×), the final fraction should contain mostly densely packed vesicles of homogeneous size, some flagella and possibly a few dead or alive whole cells might be visible as well (*see* **Note 32**).
4. Aliquot as desired and flash-freeze in liquid nitrogen and store at −80 °C. For functional assays that require the membrane potential, such as ATP-production assays [20–22] or protein import assays [23–25], add fatty acid free BSA to a final concentration of 10 mg/mL. Consider that BSA might interfere with certain downstream applications such as immunoblots or mass spectrometry.

4 Notes

Materials: Cell Growth and Harvest (See Subheading 2.1)

1. The protocol worked for all procyclic *T. brucei* cell lines we tested. We mainly have applied it to wild-type or transgenic 427 and 29–13 strains expressing tagged proteins or RNAi constructs.
2. The procedure is not carried out under sterile conditions. Accordingly, there is no need to sterilize the solutions described. For long-term storage, the solutions are kept at −20 °C, otherwise they are kept at 4 °C.

Methods

3. The mitochondrial vesicles were successfully employed for in-organellar ATP production assays [20–22] and in vitro protein import assays [23–25].
4. The mitochondrial vesicles originating from the purification protocol were used as starting material to isolate MOM and MIM vesicles and to characterize their proteome [26].

5. Among the subcellular fractions that were purified and characterized via proteomics is, for example, the "microsomal" or "crude ER" fraction. It was obtained by further processing of the "cytosolic fraction" (Subheading 3.2, **step 6**) using dilution and S100/P100 separation as described in [26, 27]. Furthermore, using a slightly altered ultracentrifugation approach employing a continuous 18–50% (w/v) Nycodenz gradient allows, in principle, for simultaneous isolation of a mitochondrial-enriched fraction and a fraction enriched for glycosomes [27].

Methods: Cell Growth and Harvest (See Subheading 3.1)

6. Daily dilutions and upscaling of the cultures are the best way to detect contaminations—should they occur—early and allow precise timing of the purification for optimal yield.
7. Keep the final volume at maximally 1.0 L in the 2.0 L Erlenmeyer flask, otherwise cell growth will slow down. (1.5 L cultures of WT 427 cells in a 2.0 L Erlenmeyer flask only tripled in 24 h instead of the quadruplication that was observed when lower volumes were used. Increasing the shaker speed to 140 rpm did not help).
8. The maximal cell densities of late-log *T. brucei* 427 and *T. brucei* 29–13 differ in our lab strains. Thus, we consider late-log phase for strain 427 to be acceptable up to 6×10^7 cells/mL, whereas for strain 29–13 the maximum is 4×10^7 cells/mL, even though the 29–13 strain is grown at the higher FCS concentration of 10% (w/v). In our experience a good indicator for the maximal acceptable late-log density is the presence of dividing cells. If many cells are visible that have a distorted morphology—thin at both ends with a bulge in the middle (reminiscent of a *Boa constrictor* that just swallowed a hog)—the culture is overgrown and should not be used.
9. Proceed with uninduced cells first through cell harvest (Subheading 3.1) and the nitrogen cavitation (Subheading 3.2) steps. While the uninduced cells incubate under pressurized nitrogen atmosphere (*see* Subheading 3.2, **step 3**), harvest and wash the induced cells (3.1) and prepare for the cavitation (*see* Subheading 3.2, **step 1**). Proceed with the uninduced cells through the lysis and sedimentation (*see* Subheading 3.2, **steps 4–6**) to separate the cytosolic fraction from the particulate fraction. Discard the supernatant (cytosolic fraction) and keep the mitochondria-containing pellet on ice. Meanwhile, subject the induced cells to nitrogen cavitation and fractionation (*see* Subheading 3.2, **steps 2–6**). Continue with the subsequent steps in parallel for uninduced and induced cells, starting with the DNase digestion (*see* Subheading 3.3).
10. Indicated *g* forces refer to the bottom of the tube.

11. Using the Fibrelite rotor with 1.0 L flasks is most convenient for larger culture volumes. Sorvall GS-3 or GSA work just as well, use them at 8000 rpm (10,800 and 10,440 × *g*, respectively) for 10 min. Older swing-out rotors such as Sorvall RC-3C plus/RC-3B plus (rotors H-4000A or H-6000A) reach ca. 7000 × *g* at top speed of ca. 5000 rpm, which is good enough to pellet ca. 90% of the cells within 20 min.
12. The pellets are firm enough to allow for careful decanting of the medium. However, since a subsequent wash step follows it is recommended to do so conservatively.

Methods: Breakage of Cells (See Subheading 3.2)

13. For smaller cell numbers, a smaller glass Dounce homogenizer (e.g., 15 mL) is more practical. Alternatively, the cell suspension can be homogenized by a passage through a syringe using a hypodermic needle 25G, 0.5 × 16 mm (orange).
14. A volume of at least 60 mL is required to prevent too much loss of the material during the cavitation step. In general, the cavitation is done at a density of 2×10^9 cells/mL. However, we have efficiently lysed cells at concentrations of $0.2\text{-}4 \times 10^9$ cells/mL. When processing large volumes of cell suspension, a bigger or even no beaker is used, the model 4635920 mL cell disruption vessel from Parr Instruments (*see* Subheading 2) can hold up to 600 mL volume (*see* Subheading 2). For less than 60 mL volume we recommend to use the smaller cavitation vessel (e.g., model 463945 mL, Parr Instruments), which works well for volumes in the range of 1 to 30 mL.
15. Although not experimentally verified, nitrogen gas equilibration between cells and buffer likely depends on the volume of the cell suspension. Thus, for larger volumes (>200 mL) of cell suspension the equilibration time and pressure were adjusted to 45–60 min and 70 bar, respectively.
16. Release the pressure slowly, yet fast enough to ensure steady flow of the foamy-white mixture; too abrupt discharge might lead to buildup of ice that clogs the outlet. Moreover, you may get soaked in cell suspension. If the pressure drops too slowly, cavitation becomes ineffective and the cells do not lyse.
17. Microscopic inspection will reveal vesicles of variable sizes, flagella, empty cell "ghosts" and living cells. Microscopic comparison of cell suspension before and after nitrogen cavitation allows to estimate the efficiency of cell lysis. If you want to monitor the purification by immunoblots or for their RNA content, collect an aliquot of the "whole cell lysate" sample (#1WCL, Fig. 1a). An example for both RNA and protein quality control is depicted in Fig. 1b.

18. A sample of the supernatant can be kept as "cytosol" (#2 CYT, Fig. 1a, b) for immunoblot and/or RNA analysis. This fraction consists of the crude cytosol and the microsomal vesicles, which can be further separated into "soluble cytosol" and "crude ER" fractions (*see* **Note 5**). For larger volumes, repeat **step 6** with the same 40 mL tubes, thus a second pellet is sedimented on top of the first one, until the whole lysate is processed.

Methods: DNase I Digestion (See Subheading 3.3)

19. Do not attempt to resuspend the white, hard material at the center of the pellet. It cannot readily be resuspended and represents contaminating material that should be left behind.
20. Mg^{2+} is needed for the activity of the DNase I. Without DNase I treatment the density gradient purification does not work since the mitochondrial vesicles are trapped in a viscous DNA solution. The effect of DNase I is often immediately visible as it decreases the viscosity of the suspension. For very large number of cell equivalents (in the range of 1×10^{12}), the volume can be reduced to $\leq$300 mL to economize DNase I usage. The volume then needs to be increased again before the low speed spins (*see* Subheading 3.4, **step 1**).
21. EDTA is added to inactivate DNase I and to prevent aggregation of vesicles in the presence of Mg^{2+}. A sample can be kept as "membranous fraction" (#3 MEM, Fig. 1a, b) for immunoblots and/or RNA analysis.

Methods: Low-Speed Centrifugation (See Subheading 3.4)

22. This is a critical step that needs to be optimized for each centrifuge and rotor pair separately. Low speeds are difficult to control when using older centrifuges and are often not accurate. Only marginal higher g-forces than 555 × g may result in pelleting of mitochondrial vesicles and thus a loss of the yield. This is why we changed from an old pair of Sorvall RC 5B/RC 5B plus centrifuges and a 10 min spin in the SS-34 fixed-angle rotor to the more reproducible swing-out rotor setup using 50 mL Falcon tubes and a 20 min spin in the SIGMA 3-16PK centrifuge in combination with the appropriate rotor, bucket, and adaptors as specified (*see* Subheading 3.4, **step 1**). Alternatively, the low speed spins can be carried out using the Eppendorf swing-out centrifuge 5810 R with rotor A-4-81, rectangular bucket 500 mL (ref. No. 5810730007) and adaptor for five conical 50 mL tubes (ref. No. 5810723000) for 20 min at 4 °C and precisely 555 × g/1660 rpm. Too dense suspensions do not work well for the low speed spins. Thus, for very large number of cell equivalents (in the range of 1×10^{12}) the concentration has to be adjusted with 1× SoTE to reach 2×10^9 cells/mL.

23. A very soft pellet should be visible, although it may look more like a phase separation between a dense and a less dense suspension. The denser phase can make up to 1/3 of the tube, which is why reextraction is essential. The supernatant should still be turbid. It is recommended to check the pellet and the supernatant fractions microscopically. The pellet should contain moving as well as dead cells and large debris, whereas in the supernatant much less of these contaminations should be seen (although it will be far from homogeneous). When in doubt, rather centrifuge at a lower speed to avoid losing the mitochondrial vesicles in this step. There is no need to extensively resuspend the pellets before the reextraction spin, since the mitochondrial vesicles that are potentially present in the pellet will resuspend very rapidly. Leave behind any hard debris visible at the bottom of the tube.
24. For very large number of cell equivalents (in the range of 1×10^{12}), it is preferable to spin consecutively the pellets on top of each other using the same tubes in order to minimize handling.

Methods: Density Gradient Centrifugation (See Subheading 3.5)

25. A single 38.5 mL tube of the SW32Ti/SW28 rotors can accommodate between 3.5×10^{10} and 1×10^{11} cell equivalents. If only one ultracentrifuge and rotor is available this becomes a limiting step for large preparations. You can process your samples in two subsequent runs but this will increase the time for the procedure accordingly. If two centrifuges and rotors are available 1×10^{12} cells can be processed simultaneously in parallel. For smaller preparations, use the SW41 rotor, whose 13.2 mL tubes can hold between 2×10^9 and 2×10^{10} cell equivalents/gradient. Prepare an even number of gradients (2, 4 or 6) to facilitate balancing.
26. The gradients can also be prepared the day before and stored at 4 °C. Using ice-cold Nycodenz/1× SoTE solutions helps to make the borders between the phases visible as they diffract the light slightly differently. For small preparations using the SW41 Ti rotor with 13.2 mL tubes use 3 mL each of the same Nycodenz/1× SoTE solutions. To prepare the step gradient tubes, let the solutions slowly drain along the inside of the tube wall. This can be done with a pipette. Alternatively, you can use the setup shown in Fig. 1c.
27. The volume of added 50% (w/v) Nycodenz/1× SoTE has to be large enough to reach a Nycodenz concentration of the total suspension that is greater than 28%; otherwise, the sample will not stay at the bottom of the gradient. A sample can be kept as "crude mitochondria" (#4 CRUMI, Fig. 1a, b) for Western blots and/or RNA analysis. As before, avoid

resuspending the white, hard pellets at the center (*see* **Note 19**).

28. Carefully check whether the suspension stays at the bottom of the tube. Should it float up, add more of the 50% (w/v) Nycodenz/1× SoTE to the suspension. To reduce the volume of the final sample you can also directly add a small amount of the 80% Nycodenz stock solution. If you want to avoid underlaying the gradients, you can pour the gradients "on top" of your suspension. However, also here you have to make sure that your sample is denser than the 28% (w/v) Nycodenz/1× SoTE solution.
29. The g-forces indicated refer to the bottom of the tube. For small preparations using the SW41 Ti rotor spin for 45 min at 27,000 rpm (=125,003 × *g*) at 4 °C.
30. A sketch and a picture of an ideal gradient are shown in Fig. 1a. Before starting with the collection of vesicles, remove the white floating layer of cell ghosts on top of the gradients with a piece of a paper towel. Microscopic investigation and evaluation reveals mainly flagella in the lowest, sharpest/most condensed band (50%/28% interphase). The least intense band at the 28%/25% interphase contains but a few larger vesicles, which are not very homogeneous. The intensities of the two top bands at the interphase of 25%/21% and 21%/18% Nycodenz can be quite variable between preparations. The former is usually the most prominent one and contains the most homogeneous fraction of mitochondrial vesicles and thus is collected as described (*see* Subheading 3.5, **step 7** and Fig. 1a). However, equal distribution of mitochondrial vesicles in both bands is common as well, especially when gradients are loaded with the upper limit of the suggested cell equivalents. Should that be the case, both bands should be collected. The band at the 28%/25% Nycodenz interphase should be discarded.

Methods: Removal of Nycodenz (See Subheading 3.6)

31. The removal of Nycodenz does not require extensive washes; however, at lower dilutions the pellets are fluffy and become detached easily. The 1:5 dilution in 1× SoTE is sufficient to obtain stable pellets, but the higher the dilution at this step, the better. For larger volumes repeat Subheading 3.6, **steps 1** and **2** until all vesicles are pelleted.
32. To determine the protein concentration of the mitochondrial vesicle preparation by, for example, BCA or Bradford assay retain 1–2 μL of the final fraction. A sample can be kept as "pure mitochondria" (#5 PUMI, Fig. 1a, b) for Western blots and/or RNA analysis. To assess the quality of the preparation, determine the concentration of the five samples (#1 WCL; #2

CYT; #3 MEM; #4 CRUMI; #5 PUMI, Fig. 1a, b) and separate equal amounts of protein (5–10 μg) of each fraction in a 12% (w/v) SDS-PAGE. Subsequent immunoblotting for mitochondrial marker proteins [26] as well as the cytosolic marker anti-EF1a (commercially available from Merck Millipore, clone CBP-KK1, #05–235) allows to determine the enrichment factor of mitochondrial vesicles compared to whole cells, which typically is about fivefold (Fig. 1b, *upper panel*). The yield of mitochondrial vesicles should be around 25 mg protein per 1×10^{11} cells but can be quite variable. Alternatively, the RNA content of the five fractions can be analyzed to assess the quality of the mitochondrial vesicle preparation (Fig. 1b, *lower panel*). RNA extracts [28] of the equivalent to 200 μg protein per fraction are separated in denaturing PAGE and visualized by ethidium bromide staining. The characteristic band pattern of the fragmented, cytosolic rRNAs (depicted by an ∗) should be reduced close to background, whereas only mt-rRNAs (9S + 12S) and mt-tRNAs should be visible in fraction #5PUMI (Fig. 1a, b, *lower panel*).

References

1. Friedman JR, Nunnari J (2014) Mitochondrial form and function. Nature 505:335–543
2. Burki F (2014) The eukaryotic tree of life from a global phylogenomic perspective. Cold Spring Harb Perspect Biol 6(5):a016147
3. Murcha MW, Wang Y, Narsai R, Whelan J (2013) The plant mitochondrial protein import apparatus – the differences make it interesting. Biochim Biophys Acta 1840:1233–1245
4. Schneider A (2001) Unique aspects of mitochondrial biogenesis in trypanosomatids. Int J Parasitol 31:1403–1415
5. Verner Z, Basu S, Benz C, Dixit S, Dobakova E, Faktorova D et al (2015) Malleable mitochondrion of *Trypanosoma brucei*. Int Rev Cell Mol Biol 315:73–151
6. Schneider A, Ochsenreiter T (2018) Failure is not an option – mitochondrial genome segregation in trypanosomes. J Cell Sci 131(18):pii: jcs221820
7. Siegel TN, Gunasekera K, Cross GA, Ochsenreiter T (2011) Gene expression in *Trypanosoma brucei*: lessons from high-throughput RNA sequencing. Trends Parasitol 27:434–441
8. Read LK, Lukes J, Hashimi H (2016) Trypanosome RNA editing: the complexity of getting U in and taking U out. Wiley Interdiscip Rev RNA 7:33–51
9. Schneider A (2011) Mitochondrial tRNA import and its consequences for mitochondrial translation. Annu Rev Biochem 80:1033–1053
10. Alfonzo JD, Söll D (2009) Mitochondrial tRNA import – the challenge to understand has just begun. Biol Chem 390:717–722
11. Lukes J, Basu S (2015) Fe/S protein biogenesis in trypanosomes – a review. Biochim Biophys Acta 1853:1481–1492
12. Schnaufer A, Domingo GJ, Stuart K (2002) Natural and induced dyskinetoplastic trypanosomatids: how to live without mitochondrial DNA. Int J Parasitol 32:1071–1084
13. Dean S, Gould MK, Dewar CE, Schnaufer AC (2013) Single point mutations in ATP synthase compensate for mitochondrial genome loss in trypanosomes. Proc Natl Acad Sci U S A 110:14741–14746
14. Harsman A, Schneider A (2017) Mitochondrial protein import in trypanosomes - Expect the unexpected. Traffic 18:96–109
15. Kaurov I, Vancova M, Schimanski B, Cadena LR, Heller J, Bily T et al (2018) The diverged trypanosome MICOS complex as a hub for mitochondrial cristae shaping and protein import. Curr Biol 28:3393–3407. e5
16. Ramrath DJF, Niemann M, Leibundgut M, Bieri P, Prange C, Horn EK et al (2018) Evolutionary shift toward protein-based

architecture in trypanosomal mitochondrial ribosomes. Science 362(6413):eaau7735

17. Schneider A, Charrière F, Pusnik M, Horn EK (2007) Isolation of mitochondria from procyclic *Trypanosoma brucei*. Methods Mol Biol 372:67–80
18. Brun R, Schönenberger M (1979) Cultivation an in vitro cloning of procyclic culture forms of *Trypansoma brucei* in a semi-defined medium. Acta Trop 36:289–292
19. Peikert CD, Mani J, Morgenstern M, Käser S, Knapp B, Wenger C et al (2017) Charting organellar importomes by quantitative mass spectrometry. Nat Commun 8:15272
20. Bochud-Allemann N, Schneider A (2002) Mitochondrial substrate level phosphorylation is essential for growth of procyclic *Trypanosoma brucei*. J Biol Chem 277:32849–32854
21. Allemann N, Schneider A (2000) ATP production in isolated mitochondria of procyclic *Trypanosoma brucei*. Mol Biochem Parasitol 111:87–94
22. Schneider A, Bouzaidi-Tiali N, Chanez A-L, Bulliard L (2007) ATP production in isolated mitochondria of procyclic *Trypanosoma brucei*. Methods Mol Biol 372:379–387
23. Hauser R, Pypaert M, Häusler T, Horn EK, Schneider A (1996) In vitro import of proteins into mitochondria of *Trypanosoma brucei* and *Leishmania tarentolae*. J Cell Sci 109:517–523
24. Mani J, Desy S, Niemann M, Chanfon A, Oeljeklaus S, Pusnik M et al (2015) Mitochondrial protein import receptors in kinetoplastids reveal convergent evolution over large phylogenetic distances. Nat Commun 6:6646
25. Pusnik M, Schmidt O, Perry AJ, Oeljeklaus S, Niemann M, Warscheid B et al (2015) Mitochondrial preprotein translocase of trypanosomatids has a bacterial origin. Curr Biol 21:1738–1743
26. Niemann M, Wiese S, Mani J, Chanfon A, Jackson C, Meisinger C et al (2013) Mitochondrial outer membrane proteome of *Trypanosoma brucei* reveals novel factors required to maintain mitochondrial morphology. Mol Cell Proteomics 12:515–528
27. Farine L, Niemann M, Schneider A, Butikofer P (2015) Phosphatidylethanolamine and phosphatidylcholine biosynthesis by the Kennedy pathway occurs at different sites in *Trypanosoma brucei*. Sci Rep 5:16787
28. Chomczyinski P, Sacchi N (1987) Single-step method of RNA isolation by acid guanidinium thiocyanate-phenol-chloroform extraction. Anal Biochem 162:156–159

Chapter 37

Isolation of Glycosomes from *Trypanosoma cruzi*

Héctor Acosta and Wilfredo Quiñones

Abstract

Glycosomes are peroxisome-related organelles of trypanosomatids in which the glycolytic and some other metabolic pathways are compartmentalized. We describe here two methods for the purification of glycosomes from *Trypanosoma cruzi* for preparative purposes, differential and isopycnic centrifugation. These are two techniques that allow the separation of different cellular compartments based on their different physicochemical characteristics. The first type of centrifugation is a rapid method that does not require large inputs and allows for fractions enriched in specific cell compartments to be obtained. The second type of centrifugation is a more elaborate method, but enables highly purified cellular compartments to be isolated. The success in obtaining these purified, intact organelles critically depends on using an appropriate method for controlled rupture of the cells.

Key words Differential centrifugation, Isopycnic centrifugation, Cellular compartments

1 Introduction

Separation of particles by centrifugation is one of the most powerful tools in cell biology. It is a technique to separate subcellular fractions according to differences in their sedimentation coefficient, that is, most often according to their mass differences [1] and thus can be used to separate cellular components (e.g., organelles, suborganellar vesicles, exosomes) from the cell cytosol into different fractions. The objective of this chapter is to describe in detail procedures for the isolation of glycosomes from cell homogenates obtained from cultures of *Trypanosoma cruzi*, with the purpose of isolating and characterizing soluble and/or membrane components of this organelle, as well as to use the organelles for functional studies such as uptake of proteins or metabolites, determination of topology of membrane proteins by protease protection or labeling of membrane proteins. The procedures described are for *T. cruzi*, but are also (with minor modifications) applicable to other kinetoplastids [2–5].

Paul A. M. Michels et al. (eds.), *Trypanosomatids: Methods and Protocols*, Methods in Molecular Biology, vol. 2116,
https://doi.org/10.1007/978-1-0716-0294-2_37,

Two types of centrifugation are most commonly used for the separation of the different cellular components. First, differential centrifugation (sometimes also called differential pelletization) is based mainly on the different physicochemical characteristics of the distinct cellular components that determine their sedimentation coefficient, such as density, shape, and size in the environment in which they are present. When these components are artificially subjected to a change in the force of gravity, produced by an increasing Relative Centrifugal Force (RCF), they will sediment at different rates (according to their sedimentation coefficient), with the larger and denser particles settling at the lowest centrifugal force. To pellet small and less dense organelles and particles, a higher RCF will be necessary [6]. Differential centrifugation was introduced for cellular research in the early 1940s by the renowned biologist and Nobel laureate Albert Claude [7]. This method is commonly used for subcellular fractionation in general and particularly to obtain enriched fractions of peroxisomes and glycosomes—the peroxisome-related organelles of trypanosomatids containing glycolytic and some other metabolic pathways [1, 8]. The procedure consists in centrifuging a cell homogenate, obtained by controlled rupture of the cells with silicon carbide, by stepwise increasing rates until the fraction enriched in glycosomes is obtained (Fig. 1). Differential centrifugation is a valuable purification method given its simplicity and low input requirements. However, it is based on differences in sedimentation rates of the components to be separated and therefore it is necessary that these differences are sufficiently large to obtain a good separation.

Since glycosomes have a similar sedimentation coefficient as some other organelles or vesicles derived from them, such as intact lysosomes and mitochondrial vesicles (this organelle is fragmented during the process to obtain the homogenate, because trypanosomatids have only a single, large ramified mitochondrion), it may be necessary to combine the procedure of differential centrifugation with a second centrifugation method, density gradient or isopycnic centrifugation, in order to increase the extent of purification of the organelle. This may be particularly critical for detailed characterization of specific glycosomal properties, like determining transporter activities, identification of the organelles' membrane proteins or studying the subcellular localization of metabolic pathway components. This additional isopycnic centrifugation is necessary to obtain a glycosomal fraction devoid of the mitochondrial vesicles and lysosomes, since these latter components are pelleted together with the glycosomes due to similar sedimentation coefficients (Fig. 1). However, if the purpose is merely the purification of some components from the glycosomes, the glycosome-enriched fraction obtained by differential centrifugation might be good enough as a starting point.

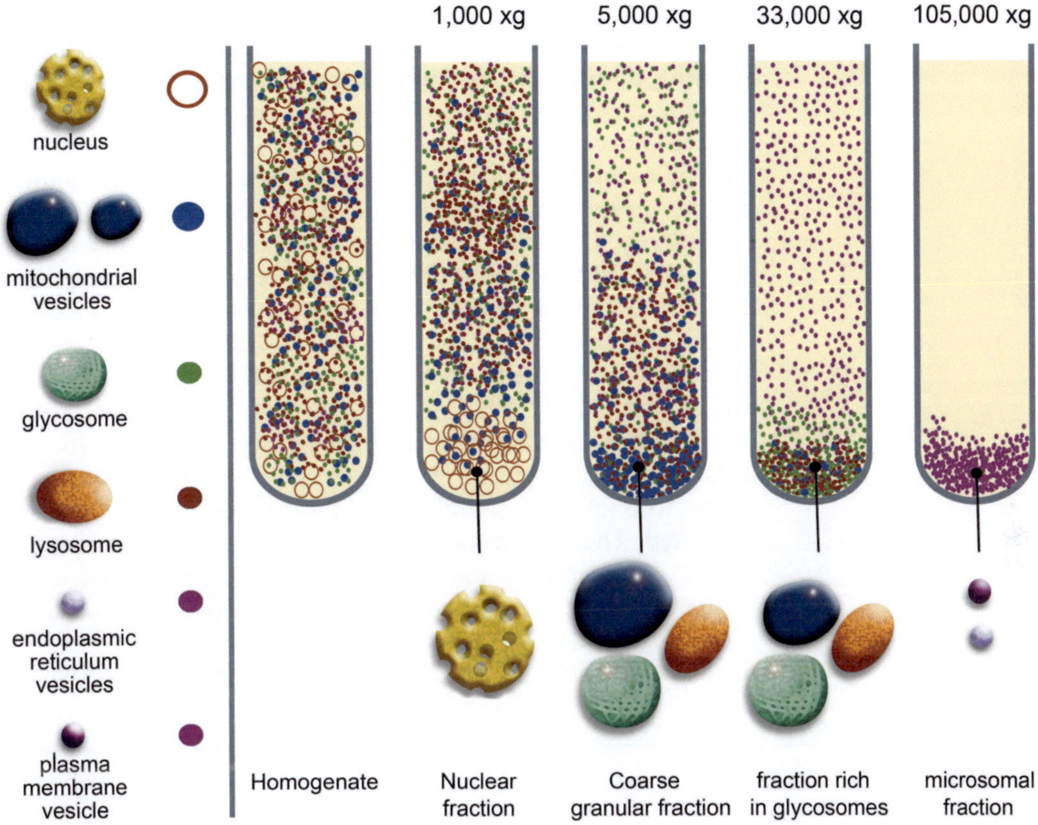

Fig. 1 Differential centrifugation. Particles of different densities or size will sediment at different rates with the largest and most dense particles sedimenting the fastest followed by less dense and smaller particles

Isopycnic-gradient centrifugation allows the separation of different cellular components according to their buoyancy coefficient [1, 9–11]. Isopycnic centrifugation refers to density gradient centrifugation methods in which macromolecular complexes or organelles end up in a position where their apparent density—or buoyant density—is equal to the local density of the gradient and no longer at a position in accordance with their sedimentation coefficients, as in zonal centrifugation. Organelles with different buoyant densities are distributed in bands that occupy different positions in the gradient. In this technique, the medium in which the samples are distributed can be sucrose, mannitol, glycerol, Ficoll 400 (a polymer of sucrose), Percoll (colloidal silica) or iodixanol (OptiPrep). The density range prepared with which these media can vary, and the medium to be chosen depends on the desired resolution in the separation of the components or the density of the component of interest. Purification of glycosomes with a high value of latency (indicator of the integrity of the organelles) has been achieved with different materials, usually by using linear sucrose gradients [8, 12–14]. This approach was first implemented to purify peroxisomes from rat liver [15] and later shown to be an effective methodology for purification of trypanosomatid glycosomes. However, recently it was reported that peroxisomes, including glycosomes contain channel-forming proteins in their surrounding membrane [16, 17]. The channels formed have an exclusion size that allows sucrose to cross the membrane and change the osmotic equilibrium of the organelle that may affect its integrity. This effect could thus change the distribution of the organelle in the density gradient or even result in the formation of the so-called ghost vesicles. Nonetheless, using sucrose gradients, we are able to obtain a homogeneous distribution of glycosomes with high yield and good latency from *Trypanosoma* and *Leishmania* species [18, 19].

In the protocols indicated in this chapter, methods for both differential centrifugation and isopycnic centrifugation using a linear sucrose gradient combined for purification of glycosomes are presented. The combination of differential centrifugation with isopycnic centrifugation methods allows glycosomes with a high degree of purity to be obtained. It is one of the most commonly used methods due to its low cost and that functional properties of the organelles and structure of its proteins are maintained [20, 21].

2 Materials

Prepare all solutions with ultrapure water and analytical grade reagents. Prepare and store all reagents at 5 °C (unless indicated otherwise).

2.1 Cell Culture

Trypanosoma cruzi epimastigotes (the multiplicative form of the parasite present in the midgut of the insect vector) are axenically grown in Liver Infusion Tryptose (LIT) medium [22] supplemented with hemin (20 μg/ml) and 5% heat-inactivated fetal bovine serum at 28 °C with strong aeration (*see* **Note 1**).

2.2 Materials and Standard Equipment

1. Micropipettes and micropipettes tips (20, 200, 1000, and 5000 μl).
2. Pipettes (2, 5, 10, and 25 ml).
3. Pasteur glass pipettes with cotton plugs.
4. Eppendorf tubes (1.5 and 1.8 ml).
5. Centrifuge tubes (polycarbonate thick-wall centrifuge tubes, 50 ml).
6. Slides and coverslips.
7. Stainless steel lab spoon spatula. Precooled at 5 °C.
8. Mortar and pestle. Precooled at 5 °C.

9. Optical microscope.
10. Analytical and precision balances.
11. Gradient maker.
12. Peristaltic pump, with tubing of tygon I.D. × O.D. 1/4 in. × 1/2 in.
13. Syringe needle of 22 G × 1¼ in. (for preparation of gradient).
14. Laboratory pipetting needle with blunt ends 16 G × 6 in. (for fractionation of the first gradient).
15. Steel needle gauge of 18 G × 1¼ in. (to collect glycosomes from the second gradient).
16. Refrigerated centrifuge for microcentrifuge tubes.
17. Superspeed centrifuge with fixed angle rotor.
18. Polyallomer oak ridge centrifuge bottles (250 ml).
19. Polypropylene flanged tubes (50 ml).
20. Ultracentrifuge with fixed angle and vertical rotor.
21. Ultracentrifuge tubes (polycarbonate thick-wall centrifuge tubes, 35 ml).
22. ULTRACRIMP Sealing Tool.
23. Glass tissue homogenizer with riding vessel of borosilicate glass and pestle. With stainless steel shaft. Precooled at 4 °C.
24. Spectrophotometer UV/VIS.
25. Quartz cuvette of 1 ml for UV/VIS spectrophotometry.
26. Magnetic stirrer and stirring bars.
27. pH meter.
28. Refractometer.

2.3 Reagents and Buffer Solutions for Cell Rupture and Gradient Centrifugation

1. *Cell washing buffer solution (Buffer A)*: 0.02 M Tris–HCl pH 7.2, 0.225 M sucrose, 0.020 M KCl, 0.010 M KH_2PO_4, 0.005 M $MgCl_2$, 0.005 M EDTA-Na_2. Add approximately 50 ml of water to a 250 ml beaker. Weigh 0.24 g of Tris base and transfer it to the beaker. Add 7.71 g sucrose, 0.15 g KCl, 0.14 g KH_2PO_4, 0.102 g $MgCl_2$ and 0.033 g EDTA-Na_2. Mix well using a magnetic stirring bar. Adjust the pH to 7.2 with HCl and make up to 100 ml with ultrapure water, using a graduated cylinder. Store at 5 °C (*see* **Note 2**).
2. *Cell rupture buffer solution (Buffer B)*: 0.025 M Tris–HCl, pH 7.6, 0.250 M sucrose, 0.025 M NaCl and 0.001 M EDTA-Na_2. Add approximately 50 ml of water to a 250 ml beaker. Weigh 0.3 g of Tris base and transfer it to the beaker. Add 8.557 g sucrose, 0.146 g NaCl and 0.033 g EDTA-Na_2. Mix well using a magnetic stirring bar. Adjust the pH to 7.6 with HCl and make up to 100 ml with ultrapure water, using a graduated cylinder. Store at 5 °C (*see* **Note 2**).

2.4 Solution of Sucrose for the Isopycnic Gradient

For the preparation of the isopycnic gradient, 15 ml of 0.3 M and 2.5 M sucrose solutions are used; both stock solutions are prepared in Buffer B (*see* **Note 3**).

1. *Solution of 0.05 M sucrose.* Dissolve 1.71 g of sucrose in 100 ml of Buffer B, mix well using a magnetic stirring bar (*see* **Note 4**).
2. *Solution of 2.5 M sucrose.* Dissolve 77.01 g of sucrose in 50 ml of Buffer B, in a glass beaker of 100 ml. Mix well using a magnetic stirring bar (*see* **Note 5**), and make up to 100 ml with ultrapure water, using a graduated cylinder (*see* **Note 4**).

2.5 Cocktail of Protease Inhibitors

For 200 ml of Buffer B, the following inhibitors are used: 1 mg leupeptin, 10 mg trypsin inhibitor, 31 mg benzamidine, 7.4 mg TLCK (Tosyl-L-lysyl-chloromethane hydrochloride), 10 μl antipain (2.4 mg/ml), 100 μl pepstatin (2 mg/ml), 100 μl E-64 (2 mg/ml), 10 μl chymostatin (7 mg/ml), 10 μl bestatin (7 mg/ml), and 100 μl PMSF (phenylmethylsulfonyl fluoride) (20 mg/ml dissolved in pure isopropanol or methanol) (*see* **Note 6**).

2.6 Silicon Carbide

Silicon Carbide powder ~200 Mesh. Store at 5 °C.

2.7 Marker Enzyme Assay Reagents

1. $NADP^+$ 12 mM stock solution prepared in ultrapure water and stored at −20 °C.
2. ATP 81 mM stock solution prepared in ultrapure water and stored at −20 °C.
3. Glucose 60 mM stock solution prepared in ultrapure water and stored at −20 °C.
4. Glucose-6-phosphate dehydrogenase (G6PDH), type VII, from baker's yeast (250 units). Store at −20 °C.
5. Phosphoenolpyruvate (PEP) 10.5 mM stock solution prepared in ultrapure water and stored at −20 °C.
6. ADP 94 mM stock solution prepared in ultrapure water and stored at −20 °C.
7. NADH 12 mM stock solution prepared in ultrapure water and stored at −20 °C.
8. Lactate dehydrogenase (LDH) from rabbit muscle (550 units/mg protein). Store at −20 °C.
9. α-Ketoglutarate 20 mM stock solution (*see* **Note 7**) prepared in ultrapure water and stored at −20 °C.
10. Ammonium acetate 100 mM stock solution prepared in ultrapure water and stored at −20 °C.
11. 1.5 M NaCl containing 1% Triton X-100 prepared in ultrapure water and stored at 4 °C.

12. Imidazole 0.1 M, supplemented with 3.6 mM EDTA, pH 7.8.
13. Tris–HCl 0.1 M, supplemented with 2 mM $MgCl_2$, pH 7.6.
14. Tris–HCl 0.1 M, supplemented with 2 mM $MgSO_4$, pH 7.6.
15. Hexokinase (HK) assay medium: 6 mM D-glucose, 4.8 mM ATP, 0.72 mM $NADP^+$, 2 U G6PDH in 0.1 M Tris–HCl, 2 mM $MgCl_2$, pH 7.6 [23] (*see* **Note 8**).
16. Pyruvate kinase (PK) assay medium: 0.4 mM PEP, 4 mM ADP, 0.24 mM NADH, 1 U LDH, in 20 mM Tris–HCl, 2 mM $MgSO_4$, pH 7.6 [24] (*see* **Note 8**).
17. Glutamate dehydrogenase (GDH) assay medium: 0.36 mM NADH, 7 mM α-ketoglutarate, 100 mM ammonium acetate, in 100 mM imidazole, 3.6 mM EDTA, pH 7.8 [24] (*see* **Note 8**).
18. Trichloroacetic acid (TCA).

3 Methods

Carry out the preparation of the gradient solutions and the gradient at room temperature, the rupture of the cells and the centrifugation steps at 4 °C, and the analyses of the fractions through activity assays of marker enzymes at 25 °C (standard condition).

3.1 Rupture of Parasites by Abrasion with Silicon Carbide

1. Parasites (from 1 l of culture) are harvested by centrifugation at 3000 × *g* for 15 min at 5 °C.
2. Wash the pellet twice with Buffer A (*see* **Note 9**) and once with Buffer B (*see* **Note 10**), centrifuging at 3000 × *g* for 15 min at 5 °C.
3. In a porcelain mortar (*see* **Note 11**), place an amount of cold silicon carbide (in a 1:1 (wet wt:wt) mixture of cells with silicon carbide (~200 mesh)), and put the pellet of parasites on the silicon carbide (*see* **Note 12**).
4. Mix the parasites with the silicon carbide using the pestle of the mortar (without applying any force); add Buffer B supplemented with the inhibitors cocktail (around 5 ml) (*see* **Note 13**).
5. After mixing the parasites with the silicon carbide, initiate the rupture of the cells by abrasion (*see* **Note 14**), macerating for 30 s in a homogeneous way (the procedure should be performed on ice), check the degree of rupture using the optical microscope (40×) (*see* **Note 15**). Repeat this step until approximately 90% of the parasites are broken (i.e., around one or two parasites visible per microscopic observation field).

6. Once 90% of the cells have been broken, add between 50 and 60 ml (per liter of parasite culture used) of Buffer B supplemented with the inhibitors cocktail, wash the wall of the mortar with this buffer in order to take off the material, mix with a spatula all content in the mortar (*see* **Note 16**), and leave the mixture for 5 min on ice.
7. Pour the suspension into a clean tube (*see* **Note 17**), to initiate the differential centrifugation steps.
8. Centrifuge the collected suspension at 300 × *g* for 3 min at 5 °C to remove the residual silicon carbide.
9. Collect the supernatant (*see* **Note 18**); it corresponds to the *cell homogenate*.

3.2 Preparation of an Enriched Fraction of Glycosomes by Differential Centrifugation

1. Centrifuge the cell homogenate at 1000 × *g* for 10 min at 4 °C. Separate the pellet (**P1**) (containing mainly nuclei and intact cells) from the supernatant (**S1**) (*see* **Note 19**); put **S1** into a new clean centrifuge tube for the next centrifugation step.
2. Centrifuge **S1** for 20 min at 5000 × *g* at 4 °C to separate a large granular fraction as a pellet (**P2**) from the supernatant (**S2**) (*see* **Note 20**); put **S2** into a new clean centrifuge tube for the next centrifugation step.
3. Centrifuge **S2** for 20 min at 33,000 × *g* at 4 °C to separate a fraction enriched in glycosomes (**P3**) from the supernatant (**S3**) (*see* **Note 21**).
4. Resuspend each of the pellet fractions (**P1**, **P2**, **P3**) separately in a volume of 5 ml of Buffer B supplemented with the inhibitors cocktail (*see* **Note 22**), in order to wash the fractions and eliminate remaining supernatant from the respective separation steps. Centrifuge all samples for 20 min at 33,000 × *g* at 4 °C. Discard the supernatants of this step. The pellets (**P1**, **P2**) will be resuspended in 5 ml of Buffer B supplemented with the inhibitors cocktail and used to determine the activities of marker enzymes.
5. Resuspend **P3** of **step 4**, in 1.5 ml of Buffer B containing the protease inhibitors cocktail and prepare the sample for the isopycnic centrifugation (*see* **Note 23**).

3.3 Preparation of Pure Glycosomes by Isopycnic Centrifugation

After having performed the differential centrifugation, the fraction enriched with glycosomes (**P3**) usually contains between 10% and 20% mitochondria-derived vesicles and 5% lysosomes, because their sedimentation coefficients are close to those of glycosomes. On some occasions, an improved degree of the purity is mandatory (for example for proteomics studies). In that case, further separation by isopycnic centrifugation is recommended, taking advantage of the difference in buoyant densities between the components.

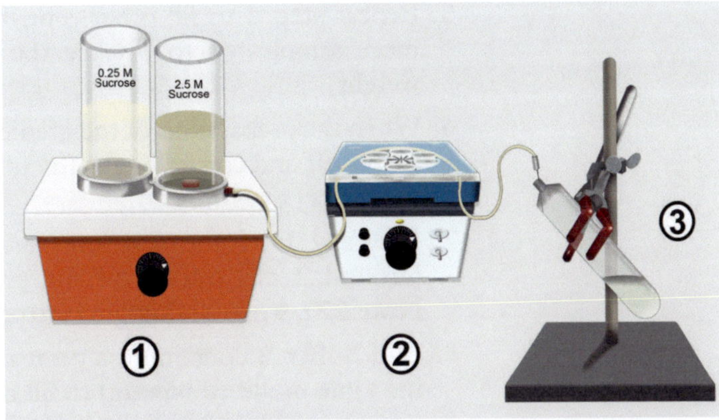

Fig. 2 Preparation of gradients for isopycnic-gradient centrifugation. (1) gradient maker, (2) peristaltic pump, (3) ultracentrifuge tube in which the gradient is formed

3.3.1 Making Gradients for Isopycnic Centrifugation

A linear and continuous gradient from 0.3 to 2.5 M sucrose will be prepared, with the highest concentration of sucrose at the base of the centrifuge tube.

1. Close the passage between the two chambers of the gradient maker. Add 15 ml of the 2.5 M sucrose solution in the chamber on the exit side of the gradient maker (with the magnetic stirring bar). Switch the magnetic stirrer on and add 15 ml of the 0.3 M sucrose solution in the other chamber (Fig. 2) (*see* **Note 24**).
2. Connect the gradient maker to a peristaltic pump and set a rate of 0.5 ml/min. Place a slightly inclined ultracentrifuge tube at the other end of the system (as indicated in Fig. 2). The centrifuge tube must be inclined 45° with respect to the surface of the bench. Add a needle (22 G × 1¼ in.) to the end of the peristaltic pump tubing and place it in the tube, near the top against the lower located side, in order to allow the solution to slide along the wall until the utmost layer of the gradient is formed. In this way, the solution will be gently added at the surface of the gradient being formed, thus avoiding the mixing of layers of different densities.
3. Allow approximately 0.5 ml of the 2.5 M sucrose solution to flow into the peristaltic pump tubing. Immediately open the passage between the two chambers containing the different sucrose solutions of the gradient maker. The solutions will be mixed in the chamber of the gradient maker nearest to the peristaltic pump (Fig. 2).
4. When the upper layer of the gradient reaches the tip of the needle, move the needle up until the solution will be finished and then take the needle out (*see* **Note 25**). Put the tube carefully right up.

5. Repeat **step 4** to fill other centrifuge tubes (for centrifuging more samples or to balance the rotor with tubes of equal weight).
6. When the preparation of the gradients is completed, switch the stirrer off and carefully take the ultracentrifuge tubes with the gradients (*see* **Note 26**).
7. Carefully load the fraction enriched in glycosomes (**P3**) (around 2 ml) on top of the gradient using a pipette (*see* **Note 27**), while avoiding to introduce any air bubbles.
8. Add Buffer B containing a protease inhibitors cocktail (using the same modified pipette) to fill the tube completely.
9. Seal the tube using a sealing tool (following recommendations of the manufacturer) and centrifuge at 170,000 × *g* for 2 h at 5 °C in a vertical rotor (*see* **Note 28**). If a swinging bucket rotor is used, the centrifugation time must be extended to 24 h.

3.3.2 Fractionating Gradients

In order to know the distribution of the glycosomes and the other components in the density gradient, it is necessary to fractionate and measure the activity of different markers in these fractions.

1. Rinse the pump tubing with distilled water and then dry it. Fill the fraction collector with 18 microcentrifuge tubes.
2. Cut the top of the ultracentrifuge tube, taking care not to disturb the gradient (*see* **Note 29**). Carefully insert a laboratory pipetting needle with blunt ends (16 G × 6 in.) into the ultracentrifuge tube, making sure that the needle rests at the bottom of the tube. The needle must be connected to the tubing of the peristaltic pump which is set at a speed of 1 ml/min (*see* **Note 30**) and the outlet of the tubing is placed at the first microcentrifuge tube. Set the size of the fractions at 2 min for a gradient volume of 35 ml. Consequently, 2 ml fractions of the gradient are collected from the bottom (dense fractions) to the top (light fractions).
3. After 35 min, verify that all sucrose has been discharged into the microcentrifuge tubes (there must be 18 fractions).

   When further improvement in the degree of purity of the glycosomal preparation obtained in this first isopycnic centrifugation is required, the procedure may be repeated as follows:
4. Pool the fractions with the highest activity of HK and the lowest activity of the other markers, PK and GDH (*see* Subheading 3.3.3), dilute this suspension four times with Buffer B containing a protease inhibitors cocktail and repeat all steps of Subheading 3.3.1 with previously prepared new gradients.

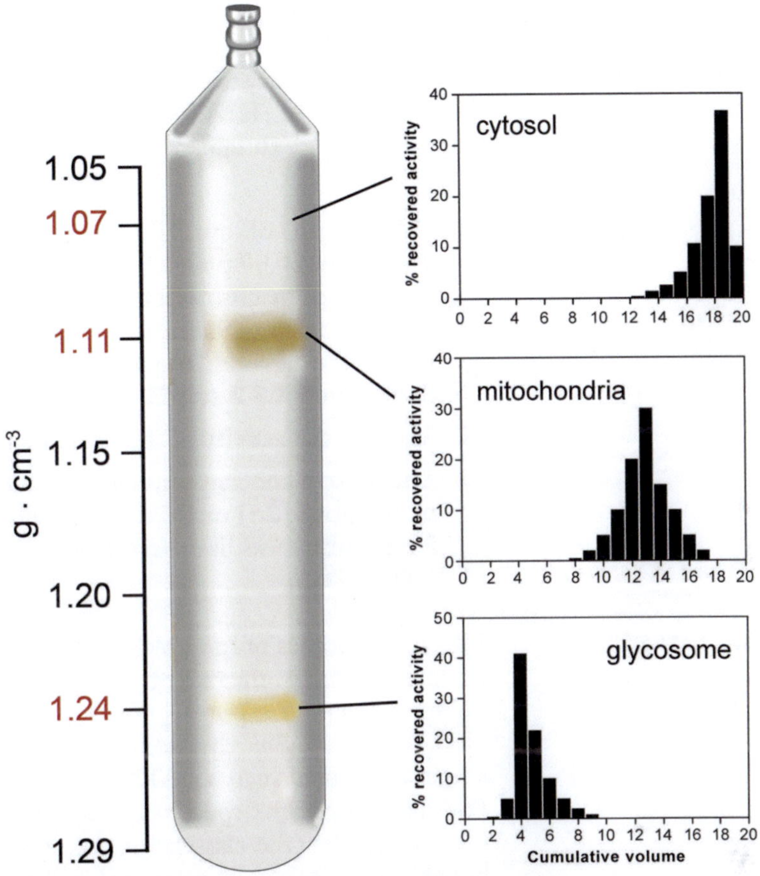

Fig. 3 Sucrose gradient where the zones corresponding to cytosol, mitochondrial vesicles and glycosomes are indicated as well as their buoyant densities and the distribution profiles of their marker enzymes. The enzyme activity profiles indicated were determined after isopycnic centrifugation of a glycosome-enriched (P3) fraction obtained by differential centrifugation of a *T. cruzi* homogenate

5. After the second round of ultracentrifugation, make a perforation in the lateral wall of the tube just below the lower band, with steel needle (18 G × 1¼ in.) connected to a syringe of 20 ml, puncture the wall and extract the band of the glycosomes. The organellar fractions are visible as brownish bands as shown in Fig. 3.
6. The density of the glycosomal and other subcellular components obtained in **step 2** can be determined by analysis of small samples of the respective gradient fractions using a refractometer. The concentrations and therefore also the densities of solutions like sucrose—and thus the subcellular structures equilibrated in them—are proportional to their refractive indices.

3.3.3 Location of Isolated Compartments Using Marker Enzymes

To determine the location of the compartments distributed along the first gradient, the activity of enzymes present in each compartment and characteristic of it ("marker enzymes") will be measured [e.g., hexokinase (HK) for glycosomes, pyruvate kinase (PK) for the cytosol, and glutamate dehydrogenase (GDH) for mitochondria (Fig. 3)].

1. Take a small volume (100 μl) of each fraction and add 10 μl of 1% Triton X-100 plus 1.5 M NaCl to solubilize the membrane and disrupt macromolecular interactions. At this point all fractions obtained in Subheading 3.2, that is, **P1**, **P2**, **P3**, and **S3**, must be evaluated, together with the fractions obtained in Subheading 3.3.2 **step 3**.
2. Measure the activity of the enzymes of interest.
3. The protein concentration is determined using the Lowry [25] or Bradford [26] methods, after elimination of possibly interfering substances like sucrose by precipitation of proteins, with 10% of TCA.

3.4 Determination of Intact Glycosomes: Latency

Intact membranes of the isolated glycosomes are in principle semipermeable, that is, they allow passage of most substrates and metabolites through pores formed by membrane proteins [17]. However, the glycosomal membrane is not permeable for larger molecules such as ATP, ADP, NAD(H), and NADP(H). For that reason, the specific activity of the enzyme representative of an organelle (the classical marker enzyme for glycosome being hexokinase) is generally measured in the presence and absence of a detergent that promotes rapid access of all substrates to the respective enzyme. This measure is usually expressed as a percentage of latency. Latency (%) is defined as [(activity of the enzyme in the presence of detergent *minus* enzyme activity in the absence of the detergent)/enzyme activity in the presence of the detergent × 100].

It is considered that the membrane of the purified glycosomes is largely intact when the value of the latency is close to 90%.

1. Solubilize 100 μl of purified glycosomes with 10 μl of 1% Triton X-100 plus 1.5 M NaCl.
2. Measure the hexokinase activity at 340 nm in a quartz cuvette of 1 ml for UV/VIS spectroscopy at 25 °C using the assay conditions mentioned in Subheading 2.7 **steps 15–17**. Start the reaction by adding a sample of the solubilized glycosome preparation (*see* **Note 31**), using a sample of between 2 and 10 μl.
3. Repeat the assay using the same volume of purified glycosomes employed in **step 2** in the absence of the detergent and NaCl.

4 Notes

1. Make sure that the volume of the flask is sufficient for correct aeration of the culture; a medium: empty space ratio of 1:2 is desirable.
2. The buffer should be stored at −20 °C when it will not be used on the day of preparation, in order to prevent contamination with bacteria, fungi or yeasts. At the moment when the buffer will be used it should be at room temperature to prevent a thermal shock to the trypanosomes.
3. When preparing the gradient stock solutions, be aware that these will be made in Buffer B that contains already 0.25 M of sucrose. Therefore, for solution A (2.5 M) 2.25 M of sucrose should be added and for solution B (0.3 M) 0.05 M of sucrose.
4. This solution should be made at the time when the gradient will be prepared.
5. Because of the high sucrose content, this solution should be prepared by incubation at 37–40 °C using a water bath, or by agitation at room temperature alternated with short periods (2 min) of incubation in the water bath, in order to promote complete dissolution of the sucrose.
6. The preparation of Buffer B supplemented with protease inhibitors should be done at least 1 day before the glycosome isolation procedure, except for the PMSF that should be added just before starting the procedure since the lifetime of this compound in the buffer is only 6 h.
7. Before use, the α-ketoglutarate stock solution must be neutralized by adding drops of 0.2 M NaOH while determining with a pH indicator when the solution reaches pH values in the basic range.
8. The reaction mix solution should be prepared for a 1 ml final volume, adding the components to the buffer and starting the reactions by addition of the sample.
9. The pellet of parasites must be resuspended carefully to avoid the forming of foam and premature mechanical rupture of the cells. For this purpose it is important to mix the cells several times with a small volume of buffer, until a homogeneous suspension is obtained, after which more buffer is added, but at least five times less than the initial culture volume.
10. For this wash step wash, the volume of buffer is at least 20 times less than that of the initial culture volume, and it is done in tubes of 50 ml volume, to have the parasites concentrated in a compact pellet that is put in the mortar.

11. The mortar and pestle should be previously cooled to approximately 5 °C to guarantee that, when the cells are ruptured, the procedure is done at this low temperature.
12. The pellet of parasites should be removed from the bottom of the tube with a spoon spatula precooled at 5 °C; make sure that the entire pellet is taken. Subsequently, use a small volume (approximately 2 ml) of Buffer B supplemented with the cocktail of inhibitors and a Pasteur pipette to wash the wall of the tubes to recover all the parasites. This parasite suspension is added to the mortar which contains the silicon carbide and the pellet of parasites.
13. The amount of buffer is critical; the consistency of the mixture should be viscous and homogeneous, not too liquid, in order to create the optimal environment for rupture of the cells. It should be taken into account that in a liquid mixture the contact between the silicon carbide and the cells is diminished preventing cell rupture, while a too viscous and less homogeneous suspension promotes an uncontrolled rupture of the cells.
14. Apply an homogeneous force while macerating the mixture over the entire surface of the mortar. Eventually the material adhered to the wall of the mortar must be taken off with the spatula.
15. To visualize the extent of cell rupture, take a small amount of the suspension, using a pipette tip, mix it with 5 μl of Buffer B supplemented with the inhibitor cocktail over a microscope slide and check it using the optical microscope (40×). Cells that have been broken will be visualized like dark spots moving randomly (Brownian movement); one will be able to distinguish these spots from the silicon carbide particles and unbroken cells.
16. Use of a sufficient volume of buffer guarantees that the material will be properly released from the silicon carbide and suspended, while the majority of the carbide will sediment at the bottom of the mortar.
17. Make sure to retrieve the entire content of the lysed cell suspension, while avoiding to collect silicon carbide. If the color of the sediment is black and homogeneous, do not add more buffer. In contrast, a different color indicates the presence of cell material trapped in the silicon carbide. To retrieve it, add 20 ml of Buffer B supplemented with the inhibitors cocktail and leave it on ice for 5 min. Subsequently, continue the extraction of the remaining material and mix it with the previously collected sample.

18. Be careful not to mix again the supernatant with the silicon carbide, since it does not form a tight pellet at the bottom of the tube.
19. Since the pellet of this step is not very compact, pay attention not to mix it with the supernatant. Take a small volume of the supernatant for determination of protein concentration and marker enzymes activity, and register the total volume of the fraction.
20. Take a small volume of the supernatant for protein concentration and marker enzymes activity determinations, and register the total volume of the fraction.
21. To perform a full subcellular fractionation and isolate also a microsomes-enriched fraction (comprising vesicles derived from the ER and plasma membrane), one may continue with an additional step of ultracentrifugation of **S3** at 105,000 × *g* for 90 min and 4 °C (*see* Fig. 1).
22. In this resuspension step avoid mechanical rupture of organelles in the sample, particularly of **P3** (glycosomes). Start using a small volume of buffer (1 ml) and a pipette of 1 ml, to avoid the formation of foam.
23. Use a glass tissue homogenizer to disrupt any aggregates in this sample. For this purpose, the suspension has to be placed in the vessel and put in contact with the pestle. Rotate the pestle a low speed (between 500 and 1000 rpm) for 1–2 min. This procedure is performed on ice, to avoid overheating of the sample.
24. Since the solutions in the chambers of the gradient maker have different densities, an empty test tube must be introduced in the chamber containing the 0.3 M sucrose to balance this difference. To avoid that the sucrose solution will enter the test tube, seal its extremity with Parafilm.
25. Before the sucrose solution of 0.3 M runs out, tilt slightly the gradient maker to allow that its entire content will be mixed in the chamber connected with the peristaltic pump.
26. The tube with the gradient must be withdrawn carefully to avoid disturbing the gradient. Do not shake the tube at any moment, and place it on ice until the sample will be loaded on it.
27. To load the sample use a pipette to which silicone tubing of around 5 cm is added. The end of the tubing must be in contact with the surface of the gradient at the moment of loading the sample; the sample is added slowly and the tip of the tubing must be withdrawn while the sample is being loaded.

28. Make sure that the tubes are completely full to guarantee their accurate balance in the ultracentrifuge. The machine's program must be set in the acceleration/deceleration mode with a slow speed at the start and end of the centrifugation, to prevent disturbance of the gradient.
29. The ultracentrifuge tube must be taken from the hole of the rotor with extremely care, to avoid disturbing the gradient and the distribution of the bands. Place the tube in a vertical position, using a rack to support it, and maintain the tube in position with a hand while cutting the tip from it with a knife.
30. Make sure that the speed of the peristaltic pump does not exceed the recommended value, since a higher speed could perturb the gradient and mix the bands.
31. The volume of the sample to be used should be chosen such that a measurable activity of the HK is obtained, while avoiding the rapidly exhaustion of substrates in the assay or that the HK activity exceeds the activity of the auxiliary assay enzyme glucose-6-phosphate dehydrogenase.

References

1. Fritsch A (1975) Preparative density gradient centrifugations. Beckman Instruments International S.A, Geneva
2. Opperdoes FR (1977) Particle-bound enzymes in the bloodstream form of *Trypanosoma brucei*. Eur J Biochem 76(1):21–28
3. Pabón MA, Cáceres AJ, Gualdrón M, Quiñones W, Avilán L, Concepción JL (2007) Purification and characterization of hexokinase from *Leishmania mexicana*. Parasitol Res 100 (4):803–810
4. Rivero LA, Concepción JL, Quintero-Troconis E, Quiñones W, Michels PA, Acosta H (2016) *Trypanosoma evansi* contains two auxiliary enzymes of glycolytic metabolism: phosphoenolpyruvate carboxykinase and pyruvate phosphate dikinase. Exp Parasitol 165:7–15. https://doi.org/10.1016/j.exppara.2016.03.003
5. Rondón-Mercado R, Acosta H, Cáceres AJ, Quiñones W, Concepción JL (2017) Subcellular localization of glycolytic enzymes and characterization of intermediary metabolism of *Trypanosoma rangeli*. Mol Biochem Parasitol 216:21–29. https://doi.org/10.1016/j.molbiopara.2017.06.007
6. Graham JM, Rickwood D (2001) Biological centrifugation. Springer, Berlin
7. Claude A (1946) Fractionation of mammalian liver cells by differential centrifugation: II. Experimental procedures and results. J Exp Med 84:61–89
8. Concepcion JL, Gonzalez-Pacanowska D, Urbina JA (1998) 3-Hydroxy-3-methyl-glutaryl-CoA reductase in *Trypanosoma (Schizotrypanum) cruzi*: subcellular localization and kinetic properties. Arch Biochem Biophys 352 (1):114–120
9. Fisher WD, Cline GB, Anderson NG (1964) Density gradient centrifugation in angle-head rotors. Anal Biochem 9:477–482
10. Price CA (1982) Centrifugation in density gradients, 1st edn. Academic, Cambridge, MA
11. Rødahl E (1998) Ultracentrifugation. In: Encyclopedia of immunology, 2nd edn. Elsevier, Amsterdam, pp 2446–2448
12. Opperdoes FR, Baudhuin P, Coppens I, De Roe C, Edwards SW, Weijers PJ, Misset O (1984) Purification, morphometric analysis, and characterization of the glycosomes (microbodies) of the protozoan hemoflagellate *Trypanosoma brucei*. J Cell Biol 98(4):1178–1184
13. Taylor MB, Gutteridge WE (1987) *Trypanosoma cruzi*: subcellular distribution of glycolytic and some related enzymes of epimastigotes. Exp Parasitol 63(1):84–97
14. Vertommen D, Van Roy J, Szikora JP, Rider MH, Michels PA, Opperdoes FR (2007) Differential expression of glycosomal and mitochondrial proteins in the two major life-cycle stages of *Trypanosoma brucei*. Mol Biochem Parasitol 158(2):189–201. https://doi.org/10.1016/j.molbiopara.2007.12.008.

15. Beaufay H, Jacques P, Baudhuin P, Sellinger OZ, Berthet J, de Duve C (1964) Tissue fractionation studies. 18. Resolution of mitochondrial fractions from rat liver into three distinct populations of cytoplasmic particles by means of density equilibrium in various gradients. Biochem J 92(1):184–205
16. Antonenkov VD, Hiltunen JK (2012) Transfer of metabolites across the peroxisomal membrane. Biochim Biophys Acta 1822 (9):1374–1386. https://doi.org/10.1016/j.bbadis.2011.12.011
17. Gualdron-López M, Vapola MH, Miinalainen IJ, Hiltunen JK, Michels PA, Antonenkov VD (2012) Channel-forming activities in the glycosomal fraction from the bloodstream form of *Trypanosoma brucei*. PLoS One 7(4):e34530. https://doi.org/10.1371/journal.pone.0034530
18. Quiñones W, Urbina JA, Dubourdieu M, Luis Concepción J (2004) The glycosome membrane of *Trypanosoma cruzi* epimastigotes: protein and lipid composition. Exp Parasitol 106 (3–4):135–149
19. Quiñones W, Cáceres AJ, Ruiz MT, Concepción JL (2015) Glycosomal membrane proteins and lipids from *Leishmania mexicana*. Comp Biochem Physiol B Biochem Mol Biol 182:27–36. https://doi.org/10.1016/j.cbpb.2014.11.012
20. Lee JC, Timasheff SN (1981) The stabilization of proteins by sucrose. J Biol Chem 256 (14):7193–7201
21. Aman RA, Wang CC (1986) An improved purification of glycosomes from the procyclic trypomastigotes of *Trypanosoma brucei*. Mol Biochem Parasitol 21(3):211–220
22. CAMARGO EP (1964) Growth and differentiation in *Trypanosoma cruzi*. I. Origin of metacyclic trypanosomes in liquid media. Rev Inst Med Trop Sao Paulo 6:93–100
23. Cáceres AJ, Portillo R, Acosta H, Rosales D, Quiñones W, Avilan L, Salazar L, Dubourdieu M, Michels PA, Concepción JL (2003) Molecular and biochemical characterization of hexokinase from *Trypanosoma cruzi*. Mol Biochem Parasitol 126(2):251–262
24. Bergmeyer HU (1983) Methods of enzymatic analysis. Academic, New York, NY
25. Lowry OH, Rosbrough NJ, Farr AL, Randall RJ (1951) Protein measurement with the Folin phenol reagent. J Biol Chem 193:265–275
26. Bradford MM (1976) A rapid and sensitive method for the quantitation of microgram quantities of protein utilizing the principle of protein-dye binding. Anal Biochem 72:248–254

Chapter 38

Sorting the Muck from the Brass: Analysis of Protein Complexes and Cell Lysates

Martin Zoltner, Ricardo Canavate del Pino, and Mark C. Field

Abstract

Reliable determination of protein complex composition or changes to protein levels in whole cells is challenging. Despite the multitude of methods now available for labeling, analysis, and the statistical processing of data, this large variety is of itself an issue: Which approach is most appropriate, where do you set cutoffs, and what is the most cost-effective strategy? One size does not fit all for such work, but some guidelines can help in terms of reducing cost, improving data quality, and ultimately advancing investigations. Here we describe two protocols and algorithms for facile sample preparation for mass spectrometric analysis, robust data processing, and considerations of how to interpret large proteomic datasets in a productive and robust manner.

Key words Proteomics, SDS-PAGE, Sample preparation, Data presentation, *Trypanosoma*, MaxQuant

1 Introduction

The ability to analyze changes to cellular protein levels, in response to stimuli or genetic modification and the composition of mixtures of proteins representing complexes, organelles, or extracts, has revolutionized biology, uncovering previously unknown mechanisms, components, and pathways [1]. Proteomics, which relies on mass spectrometry (MS) to identify peptides within mixtures, has evolved into a powerful tool, with modern instrumentation allowing detection of thousands of proteins within a single sample. This wealth of information does, however, have a robustness that is heavily dependent on the quality of the analysis and the manner in which the most salient data are extracted; failure to curate these data appropriately can, and likely will, devalue an otherwise high-quality and valuable dataset. Algorithms that analyze patterns within data, generating principal components for example, are powerful but frequently abstract data to the degree where the underlying biology can be cryptic, or is obscure. Furthermore,

Paul A. M. Michels et al. (eds.), *Trypanosomatids: Methods and Protocols*, Methods in Molecular Biology, vol. 2116,
https://doi.org/10.1007/978-1-0716-0294-2_38, © Springer Science+Business Media, LLC, part of Springer Nature 2020

Table 1
Possible contaminant proteins that are frequently observed in pull downs from *T. brucei*

Structural proteins
Tubulin, basal body component, paraflagellar rod proteins, BILBO1
Nucleic-acid interacting proteins
EF1alpha, EF2, Ran, Histone H2B, Histone H4, RNA-binding protein RBSR1, RNA helicases
Ribosomal proteins
40S and 60S ribosomal proteins
Enzymes
Glyceraldehyde 3-phosphate dehydrogenase (GAPDH), cysteine desulfurase, ATP-dependent phospho fructokinase, hexokinase, fructose-1,6-bisphosphatase, glycerol kinase. Other high-abundance glyco lytic enzymes are also frequent
Others
Ubiquitin, polyubiquitin, chaperonins (e.g., HSP60, HSP70, dynamin)

the riches within a list of proteins are frequently intermixed with the less valuable, and discrimination between high and low value identifications is frequently difficult (Table 1). While "where there's muck there's brass" is an old Yorkshire English adage, there is genuine hazard for the unwary.

For trypanosomatids, there are several advantages over many other organisms in context of proteomic analysis. There is little or no alternative splicing that generates more than one distinct protein per gene, the gene number is quite small (~8500 for *Trypanosoma brucei*) and the genomes of multiple species are now available and well annotated [2]. Culturing conditions for stable isotope labeling with amino acids in cell culture (SILAC) are well established [3], developmental transitions are now possible to model in vitro [4], and the power of modern MS instruments highly impressive, reliable and sensitive [5]. The advent of quantitative MS revolutionized the study and characterization of interactomes, allowing for identification of specific enrichment between interactors and therefore overcoming the requirement to purify protein complexes to, what is likely an arbitrary, homogeneity [6]. Importantly, the application of less stringent purification conditions facilitates capturing of weak and transient interactors. The recent development of intensity-based label-free quantification algorithms added a simpler, but powerful alternative to label-based methods [7]. To make full use of these approaches we have optimized protocols for isolation of complexes, preparation of samples for LC-MSMS and the analysis of the resulting data, to provide robust analytical pipelines within the means of most laboratories (Fig. 1). For information concerning the isolation for complexes from trypanosomes and the use of cryomilling, the reader is referred to an earlier article by us in this series [8].

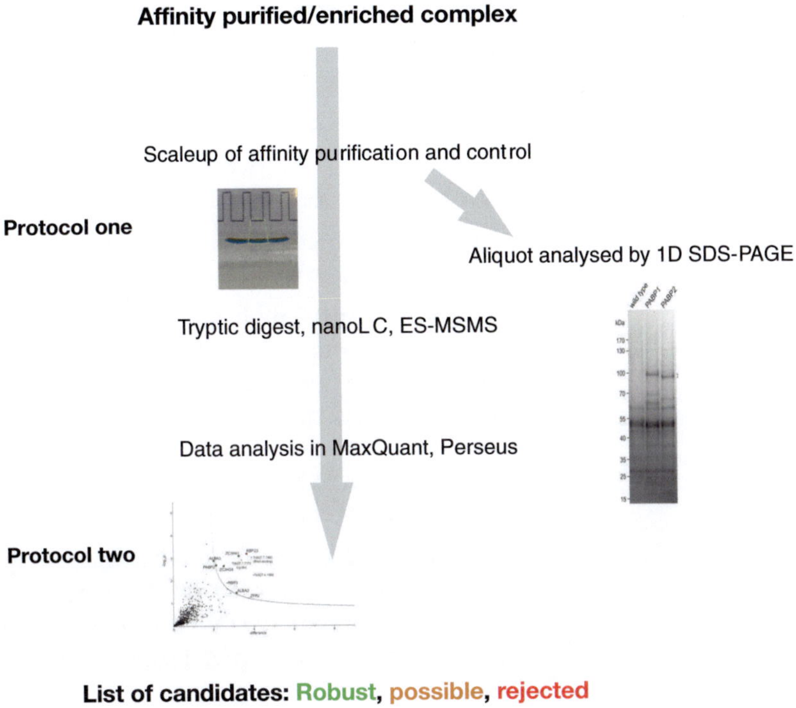

Fig. 1 Flowchart for analysis of protein mixtures using LC-MSMS. The protocols in this chapter require as a starting point one of a whole cell lysate, an isolated complex or a subcellular fraction. Protocol one describes a simple method for preparing samples for mass spectrometry as well as increasing the depth of analysis. Protocol two discusses analysis using MaxQuant software, and how to parse your data for likely artefacts and low-quality protein identifications

2 Materials

2.1 SDS–Polyacrylamide Gel

1. NuPAGE Sample Reducing Agent (10×) (Thermo Fisher Scientific).
2. Resolving gel buffer: 50 mM MOPS. 50 mM TRIS base. 3.5 mM SDS, 1.0 mM EDTA. Prepared using ultrapure (18 M ohm) water.
3. Precast NuPAGE 4–12% Bis-Tris polyacrylamide gel (Thermo Fisher Scientific).
4. Fixative: 40% ethanol, 10% acetic acid (v/v).

2.2 Data Processing and Analysis

1. MaxQuant and the Perseus framework, download https://maxquant.org.

3 Methods

3.1 SDS Polyacrylamide Gel Electrophoresis

1. Load the entire sample eluted from the nanobeads (supplemented with reducing agent if desired) into a single well of a Bis-Tris NuPAGE gel (*see* **Note 1**) and run at 100 V, 400 mA for 10 min or until the sample is 1–1.5 cm into the gel (Fig. 2).
2. Using a virgin scalpel, cut the entire band corresponding to your sample and transfer to a 15 ml Falcon tube.
3. Fill the Falcon tube with 5 ml fixative and incubate the gel slice for 10 minutes with rotation (*see* **Note 2**). Discard the fixative and repeat twice more (*see* **Note 3**), then transfer the slice into a 1.5 ml Protein LoBind tube (Eppendorf).

3.2 In-Gel Tryptic Digest and Mass Spectrometry

1. Subject gel slices to reductive alkylation and in-gel tryptic digest using routine procedures.
2. Analyze eluted peptides by liquid chromatography-tandem mass spectrometry (LC-MSMS) on an Ultimate3000 nano rapid separation LC system (Dionex) coupled to an LTQ Velos mass spectrometer (Thermo Fisher Scientific) or similar (*see* **Note 4**).

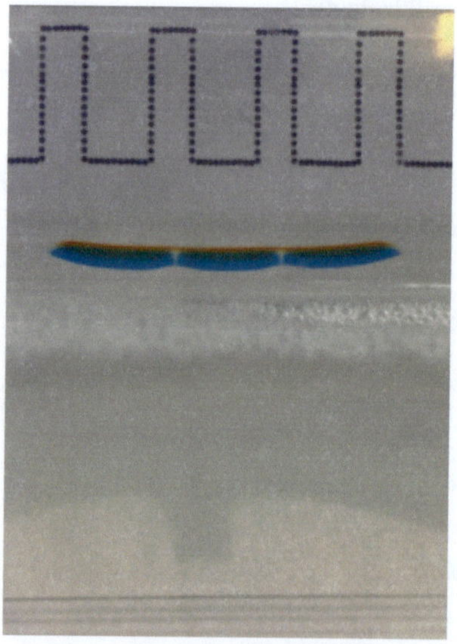

Fig. 2 Cutting gel slices. After running the sample 1.0–1.5 cm into the SDS–polyacrylamide gel (as judged by the migration of the bromophenol blue band) a slice is extracted. The dimensions are indicated by the dotted line and are compatible with standard tryptic digest procedures in 1.5 ml microfuge tube format

3.3 Data Processing and Label Free Quantification

Spectra are processed using the intensity-based label-free quantification (LFQ) method of MaxQuant [7, 9], which has been validated as a tool for affinity enrichment mass spectrometry [6].

1. Organize spectra (*.raw* files for Thermo Fisher Scientific mass spectrometers) into one folder, load these into MaxQuant and assign an experiment number to each in the tab "*Raw data.*"
2. Activate LFQ in the tab "*Group-specific parameters.*"
3. Add a search database (*.fasta* file) in the tab "*Global parameters*" (*see* **Note 5**) and enable "Match between runs" (*see* **Note 6**).
4. Select a "*Number of processors*" (bottom panel), defining the number of threads used for processing, and start the analysis. The progress is monitored in the tab "*Global parameters.*" Activating "Show all activities" will show a list of completed tasks.
5. Output files will be written to the same path as input files.

3.4 Data Analysis

The LFQ data are analyzed using the Perseus software [10].

1. Load the "proteingroups.txt" file, located in the folder/combined/txt of the input path, or using the Matrix/Generic Matrix Upload into *Perseus.*
2. Import LFQ intensities into the "*Main*" column and Fasta headers into the "*Text*" column.
3. Use "filter rows based on categorical columns" to eliminate hits to the contaminants and reverse database and proteins only identified by site (hits relying on modified peptides only).
4. Log2 transform LFQ intensities (using "*Basic/Transform*") and impute missing values from a normal distribution around the detection limit of the mass spectrometer (using "Imputation/Replace missing values from normal distribution") (*see* **Note 7**).
5. Group replicates using "Categorical annotation rows."
6. Perform a Student's *t*-test comparing the nontagged control sample group to the respective pull down with the tagged-protein group. Using "Processing/Tests/Two-sample *t*-test" will generate the additional columns "−log10 *t*-test *p* value," "*t*-test difference," "*t*-test *q*-value," and "*t*-test test statistic."
7. The −log10 *t*-test *p* value is plotted versus the *t*-test difference to generate a volcano plot. This can be done also in one step using Misc./Volcano plot, which generates a cutoff curve indicating which hits are significant (*see* **Note 8**). For an example *see* Fig. 3b, c.
8. Potential interactors are classified according to their position in the volcano plot.

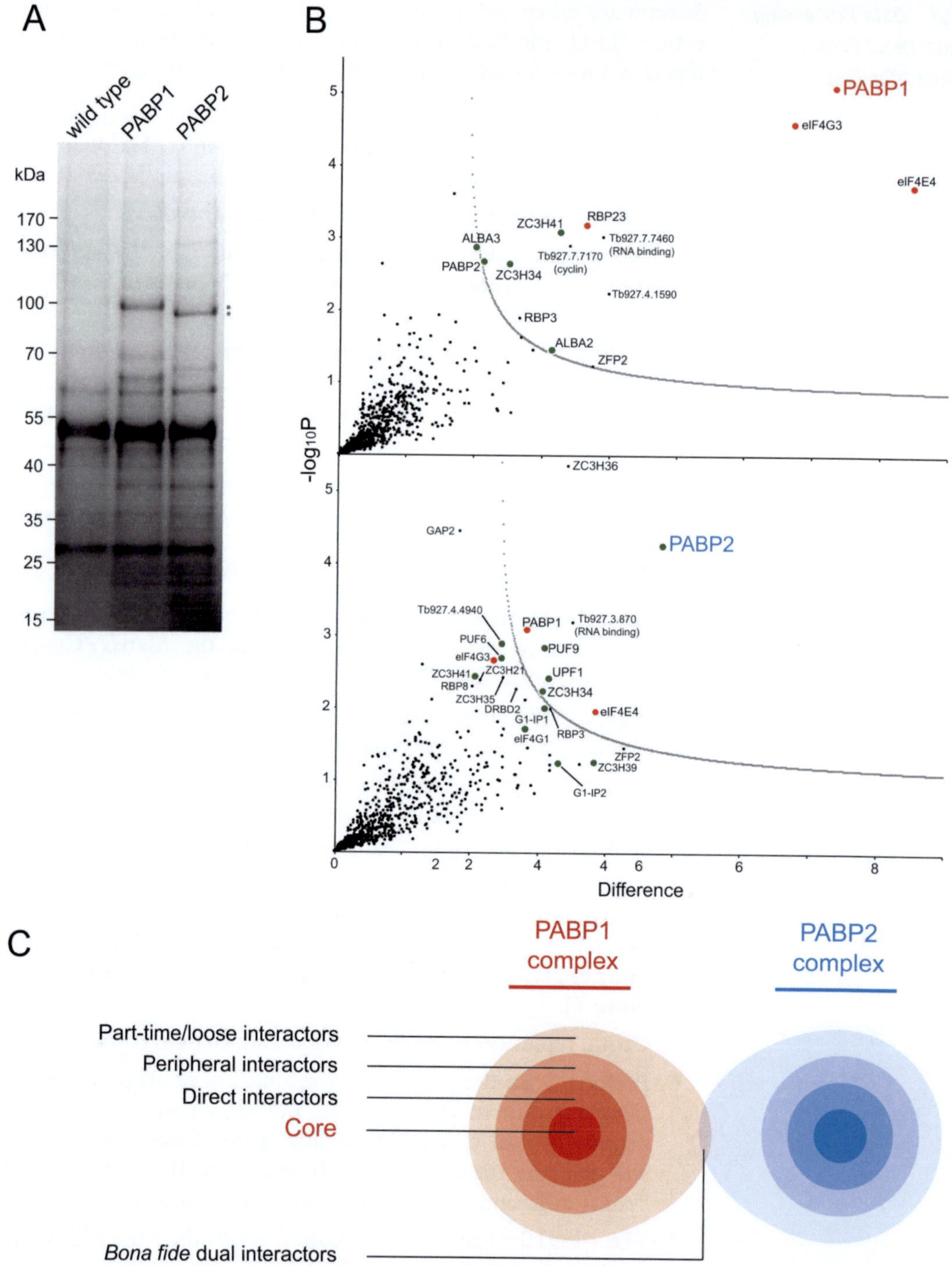

Fig. 3 Pull down of the two PolyA-binding proteins PABP1 and PABP2. Panel **a**: SDS-PAGE analysis of the elution from polyclonal anti-GFP nanobody beads, from *wild type* cells, cells expressing PABP1-eYFP and cells expressing PABP2-eYFP, respectively. The theoretical molecular weights of the bait proteins (95.6 kDa for PABP1-eYFP and 94.7 kDa PABP2-eYFP) are indicated by asterisks. Panel **b**: Volcano plots of pull downs for PABP1-eYFP and PABP2-eYFP, respectively, both analyzed in triplicate. Starvation stress granule localization

3.5 Validation

Even with a high number of replicates (we recommend at least three), false interactors can appear significantly enriched, which is likely due to nonspecific binding of contaminants to the complex during isolation and dependent on buffer conditions. On the other hand, some true interactors, which are only mildly enriched, can appear below the significance threshold cutoff and hence be discarded. The latter also depend on buffer conditions destabilizing individual interactions within the complex differentially. Moreover, substoichiometric and/or transient interactors can easily fall into this group. Ultimately, then, at least for a selection of key interactors, validation is essential. A reverse isolation, where the potential interactor serves as bait, is a straightforward way to improve confidence. Optionally, the analysis of this reverse isolation can be performed by western immunoblotting. Colocalization by immunofluorescence can deliver strong supporting evidence when the complex under investigation has a discrete localization within the cell.

An example is given in Fig. 3. A comparative interactome analysis of the two paralogs of poly(A) binding protein, PABP1 and PABP2, controlling mRNA stability and translation initiation in *Trypanosoma brucei*, revealed partly overlapping, but distinct, interactomes, consistent with roles in regulation of distinct sets of mRNAs [11]. Extensive localization studies after induction of stress granules (ribonucleoprotein assemblies regulating the fate of mRNAs in eukaryotes) were used to interpret the interactomes (indicated in Fig. 3b) and to put them into biological context. Additionally, a key interactor for each isoform was validated by reverse IP. PABP1 engages in strong associations with eIF4G3 and eIF4E4 and is largely excluded from stress granules. PABP2 in contrast interacts with a wide range of proteins and localizes to stress granules, similar to the majority of mRNAs. This example also illustrates the difficulty to interpret interactomics data from complexes with various ranges of interactions, that can be direct and indirect (Fig. 3c), and the additional complexity that a given protein can be a bona fide component of several distinct complexes.

Fig. 3 (continued) information based on experimental data are shown as colored dots (green dots = stress granule localization; red dots = not localized in stress granules). Panel **c**: Considerations for interpretation of interactomics data. Most proteins participate in a range of interactions, that can be either direct or indirect. Furthermore, complex composition can vary in a temporally and/or spatially distinct manner, which is difficult to resolve experimentally. Conceptually one can consider a core of tight associations mediating the basic functions of a protein complex (core), and which are readily detectable. However, this is biologically inaccurate as even tight complexes exist in association with other complexes or biological assemblies. These interactions become functionally, as well as physically, more tenuous and will eventually come to include proteins that are off target, but which may still retain a genuine affinity for components of the target complex (lighter colors). In some cases, a given protein can be a bona fide member of more than one complex. The point at which one considers such interactions to represent contaminants is hard to determine and, to some level, is subjective. Full experimental details for the data discussed in panels **a** and **b** are described in ref. 11

4 Notes

1. Control or wild-type samples should always be run on separate gels, ideally in a separate electrophoresis tank. It is very common to have cross-contamination between samples ran on a single gel and this interferes with downstream analysis.
2. SDS must be efficiently removed as it interferes with LC-MSMS analysis.
3. The samples can be stored frozen at −20 °C at this point.
4. The older Orbitrap LTQ technology of the Velos machine offers sufficient sensitivity to detect complexes of low abundance—the use of more sensitive mass spectrometers is possible but will increase the number of nonspecific background binder detections.
5. Download the most recent *T. brucei brucei* TREU927 annotated protein database (currently release 39.0) from TriTrypDB [2]. Define and test parse rules (>([^\s]*) is the Identifier rule for the TriTrypDB file in the tab "*Configuration*" (or, from MaxQuant version 1.6.2. on, this is also embedded in the tab "Global parameters"). Even *when* using the *T. brucei brucei* 427 Lister strain it is usually a better choice to search the *T. brucei brucei* 927 database (due to the overall higher sequence quality). However, the Lister 427 database can be searched separately, to encompass any variant proteins.
6. All other parameters can be used as default presets. Processing with "Match between runs" transfers identifications from one MS run to another, where the same feature was present, thereby increasing the number of available quantifications.
7. The distribution of imputed values can be inspected and compared to the LFQ intensity distribution in plots created using *Visualization/Histogram*. A multi-scatter plot (*Analysis/Visualization/Multi scatter plot)*, visualizing corresponding LFQ intensities between each sample pair, is a useful tool for the quality control of replicates.
8. The cutoff curve is based on the false discovery rate (FDR) and the artificial factor s0. s0 controls the relative importance of the *t*-test *p*-value and difference between means. At $s0 = 0$ only the *p*-value matters, while at nonzero *s*0 the difference of means contributes.

Acknowledgments

Work in our laboratory is supported by the Wellcome Trust (WTI 204697/Z/16/Z to M.C.F.) and the Medical Research Council of the United Kingdom (MR/N010558/1, MR/P009018/ to M.C. F.). We would like to thank Douglas Lamont and the Fingerprints facility (University of Dundee) for excellence in proteome MS, and also Brian Chait (Rockefeller University) who introduced us to the SDS-PAGE method for sample cleanup. M.C.F. is a Wellcome Trust Investigator.

References

1. Ahmad Y, Lamond AI (2014) A perspective on proteomics in cell biology. Trends Cell Biol 24 (4):257–264
2. Aslett M, Aurrecoechea C, Berriman M, Brestelli J, Brunk BP, Carrington M, Depledge DP, Fischer S, Gajria B, Gao X, Gardner MJ, Gingle A, Grant G, Harb OS, Heiges M, Hertz-Fowler C, Houston R, Innamorato F, Iodice J, Kissinger JC, Kraemer E, Li W, Logan FJ, Miller JA, Mitra S, Myler PJ, Nayak V, Pennington C, Phan I, Pinney DF, Ramasamy G, Rogers MB, Roos DS, Ross C, Sivam D, Smith DF, Srinivasamoorthy G, Stoeckert CJ Jr, Subramanian S, Thibodeau R, Tivey A, Treatman C, Velarde G, Wang H (2010) TriTrypDB: a functional genomic resource for the Trypanosomatidae. Nucleic Acids Res 38:D457–D462
3. Urbaniak MD, Guther ML, Ferguson MA (2012) Comparative SILAC proteomic analysis of *Trypanosoma brucei* bloodstream and procyclic lifecycle stages. PLoS One 7(5):e36619
4. Matthews KR (2005) The developmental cell biology of *Trypanosoma brucei*. J Cell Sci 118:283–290
5. Makarov A (2000) Electrostatic axially harmonic orbital trapping: a high-performance technique of mass analysis. Anal Chem 72:1156–1162
6. Keilhauer EC, Hein MY, Mann M (2015) Accurate protein complex retrieval by affinity enrichment mass spectrometry (AE-MS) rather than affinity purification mass spectrometry (AP-MS). Mol Cell Proteomics 14 (1):120–135
7. Cox J, Hein MY, Luber CA, Paron I, Nagaraj N, Mann M (2014) Accurate proteome-wide label-free quantification by delayed normalization and maximal peptide ratio extraction, termed MaxLFQ. Mol Cell Proteomics 13:2513–2526
8. Obado SO, Field MC, Chait BT, Rout MP (2016) High-efficiency isolation of nuclear envelope protein complexes from trypanosomes. Methods Mol Biol 1411:67–80
9. Cox J, Mann M (2008) MaxQuant enables high peptide identification rates, individualized p.p.b.-range mass accuracies and proteome-wide protein quantification. Nat Biotechnol 26:1367–1372
10. Tyanova S, Temu T, Sinitcyn P, Carlson A, Hein MY, Geiger T, Mann M, Cox J (2016) The Perseus computational platform for comprehensive analysis of (prote)omics data. Nat Methods 13(9):731–740
11. Zoltner M, Krienitz N, Field MC, Kramer S (2018) Comparative proteomics of the two *T. brucei* PABPs suggests that PABP2 controls bulk mRNA. PLoS Negl Trop Dis 12(7): e0006679

Chapter 39

Measurement of Energy States of the Trypanosomatid Mitochondrion

Mayke Bezerra Alencar, Richard Bruno Marcel Moreira Girard, and Ariel Mariano Silber

Abstract

The evaluation of mitochondrial functionality is critical to interpret most biological data at the (eukaryotic) cellular level. For example, metabolism, cell cycle, epigenetic regulation, cell death mechanisms, autophagy, differentiation, and response redox imbalance are dependent on the mitochondrial state. In case of parasitic organisms, such as trypanosomatids, it is very often important to have information on mitochondrial functionality in order to assess the mechanisms of actions of drugs being proposed for therapy. In this chapter we present a set of methods that together allow to evaluate with some precision the mitochondrial functionality in *Trypanosoma cruzi* and *Trypanosoma brucei*. We discuss how to determine O_2 consumption, mitochondrial inner membrane potential, ATP production, and the endogenous production of reactive oxygen species.

Key words High-resolution respirometry, Bioenergetics, Trypanosomatids, ATP measurement, OxPhos

1 1 Introduction

The physiological state of mitochondria is determined by a set of key parameters that allow diagnosing the energy state of eukaryotic cells. In this chapter we will discuss those that we judge as being the most relevant. The O_2 consumption, which allows to infer the electron flux in the respiratory chain, and the mitochondrial membrane potential [1] are important to evaluate mitochondrial functions. Trypanosomatids have a single and unusually well-developed mitochondrion per cell that spans the entire cell body [2–4]. This mitochondrion possesses the classical compartments: the outer membrane, the intermembrane space, the inner mitochondrial membrane, and the mitochondrial matrix (reviewed by [5]). In

Mayke Bezerra Alencar and Richard Bruno Marcel Moreira Girard contributed equally to this work.

Paul A. M. Michels et al. (eds.), *Trypanosomatids: Methods and Protocols*, Methods in Molecular Biology, vol. 2116, https://doi.org/10.1007/978-1-0716-0294-2_39, © Springer Science+Business Media, LLC, part of Springer Nature 2020

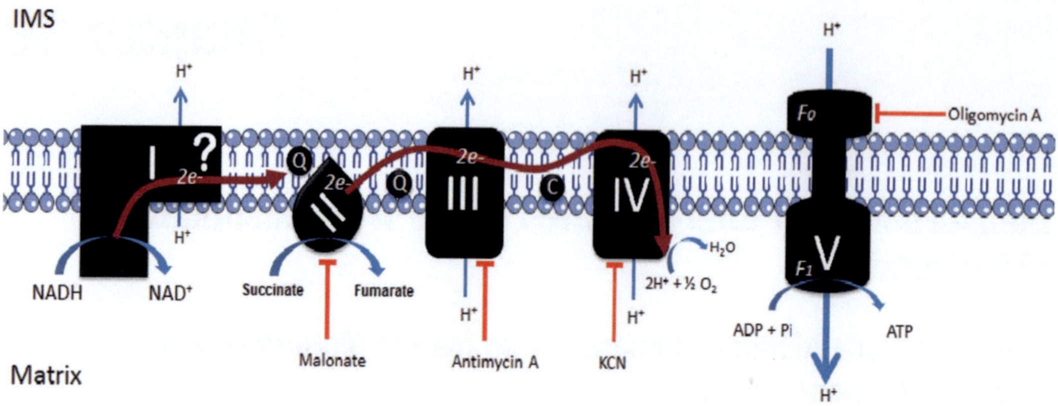

Fig. 1 Schematic representation of the electron transport chain. The major complexes of the electron transport system are present in the inner mitochondrial membrane (although in the trypanosomatids studied so far, the ability of complex I to extrude H^+ could not be demonstrated, as is indicated by its labeling with a question mark), and some enzymes/intermediates are located in the intermembrane space (IMS) or mitochondrial matrix. *Q* ubiquinone, *C* cytochrome c. The F_1F_0 ATP synthase is responsible for OxPhos resulting from the proton-motive force generated through an electrochemical gradient

trypanosomes, different metabolites can be used as intermediates or as fuel for the tricarboxylic acid (TCA) cycle, thus allowing (in principle) their full oxidation to produce reducing power that, ultimately, will feed electrons into the Electron Transfer System (ETS) for ATP production by Oxidative Phosphorylation (OxPhos) (for a schematic overview of ETS and OxPhos, as well as the inhibitors of each protein complex, *see* Fig. 1) [6–11]. Furthermore, the mitochondrial membrane potential ($\Delta\Psi_m$), is the major component of the electrochemical proton gradient (aka. Proton-motive force, comprising $\Delta\Psi_m + \Delta pH$), across the inner mitochondrial membrane, being a crucial indicator of the redox state in the parasites [12]. Here, we describe standardized protocols to measure the ATP production, Reactive Oxygen Species (ROS) formation, O_2 consumption and $\Delta\Psi_m$ in trypanosomatids. This chapter also describes applications of High Resolution Respirometry (HRR). The protocols provide tests for evaluation of the $\Delta\Psi_m$ state (ETS coupled to OxPhos) and respiratory decrease resulting from the inhibition of the F_1F_O ATP synthase (the phosphorylation system). Some general features about OROBOROS Oxygraph-2k use and measurements are also discussed.

2 Materials

2.1 Cells and Culture Conditions

1. *Trypanosoma cruzi* epimastigote forms (CL strain) are cultured in LIT medium (Liver Infusion Tryptose) supplemented with 10% of FBS (Fetal Bovine Serum) and 0.2% of glucose at 28 °C. They are maintained in the exponential growth phase by successive passages every 48 h in fresh LIT medium [13].

2. *Trypanosoma brucei* procyclic forms (PCF) Lister 427 are grown in SDM-79 medium supplemented with 10% fetal calf serum (FCS), penicillin (250 U/mL), streptomycin (250 μg/mL), L-glutamine (300 mg/L), and hemin (7.5 mg/L) at 28 °C [14].

2.2 Equipment

1. Oroboros Oxygraph-2k (Oroboros Instruments, Innsbruck, Austria) equipped with a O2k-Fluo LED2-Module consisting of a Fluorescence-Sensor Green (excitation LED at 525 nm) with a Filter-Cap equipped with a Filter Set Amplex Red (AmR) for ROS measurements or a Fluorescence-Sensor Blue (excitation LED 465 nm) with a Filter-Cap equipped with a Filter sets for Magnesium Green (MgGr) and Rhodamine 123 (Rho123) measurements.
2. Fluorimeter (we use a Hitachi F-7000 spectrofluorimeter (Hitachi High Technologies) equipped with injection system and stirrer). For the fluorimeter a thermoregulation system for temperature control is recommended.
3. Plate spectrofluorimeter reader (we use a SpectraMax i3 (Molecular Devices, Sunnyvale, CA).
4. Quartz cuvettes for fluorescence readings.
5. Hamilton syringes of 10–250 mm^3 (*see* **Note 1**).

2.3 Reagents and Solutions

1. Mitochondrial Cell Respiration Medium (CRM): 125 mM saccharose, 65 mM KCl, 10 mM HEPES, 1 mM $MgCl_2$, 2.5 mM K_2HPO_4, pH 7.2.
2. Mitochondrial Cell Respiration Medium without magnesium (CRM-Mg^-): 125 mM saccharose, 65 mM KCl, 10 mM HEPES, 2.5 mM K_2HPO_4, pH 7.2.
3. Phosphate Buffered Saline (PBS): 137 mM NaCl, 2.6 mM KCl, 8 mM Na_2HPO_4, 1.4 mM KH_2PO_4, pH 7.2.
4. BAG-Mg medium (Buffer A plus Glucose, without Mg): 116 mM NaCl, 5.4 mM KCl, 50 mM HEPES-KOH, 5.5 mM D-glucose, pH 7.2.
5. Cytomix Buffer: 25 mM HEPES-KOH buffer, 120 mM KCl, 0.15 mM $CaCl_2$, 2 mM EDTA, 5 mM $MgCl_2$, 10 mM K^+-phosphate buffer, pH 7.2.
6. Metabolites stocks (ideally stocks should be prepared at high concentration, between 250 and 500 mM) and stored at −20 °C. If it is not possible due to a low solubility or instability, the metabolites must be prepared freshly in CRM buffer. We recommend using each metabolite at concentrations that saturates their uptake system, usually higher than 1 mM (*see* **Note 2**).
7. 0.5 mg/μL Oligomycin A (Omy) stock solution in ethanol.

8. 200 μM Carbonyl cyanide-4-(trifluoromethoxy)phenylhydrazone (FCCP) stock solution in methanol.
9. 5 mM Antimycin A (Antim A) stock solution in ethanol.
10. 5 mM Digitonin stock solution in Milli-Q water.
11. 20% bovine serum albumin (BSA) fatty acid free in water.
12. 1 mM EDTA stock solution in Milli-Q water.
13. 1 mM EGTA stock solution in Milli-Q water.
14. 200 mM ADP stock solution in Milli-Q water.
15. 200 mM ATP stock solution in Milli-Q water.
16. 1 mM MgGr stock solution in Milli-Q water
17. 2.62 mM Rhodamine 123 in ethanol.
18. 0.5 mM Amplex Red in DMSO.
19. 10 U/mL HRR in distilled water.

3 Methods

3.1 Preparation of Cell Samples and the OROBOROS for HRR

1. Collect and wash the parasites (grown until mid-exponential phase) twice in PBS for *T. cruzi* or in BAG for *T. brucei* by centrifugation at 1000 × *g*, 10 min. From this point, to work with *T. brucei*, go to **step 4**.
2. Resuspend the pellets to their original culture volume in PBS and incubate the parasites for 16 h at 28 °C to submit them to metabolic stress (*see* **Note 3**).
3. Wash the parasites twice in PBS by centrifugation at 1000 × *g*, 10 min.
4. Resuspend the pellets in CRM at a cell density of 1×10^9 parasites/mL.
5. Incubate aliquots of 60 μL with an appropriate concentration of the substrates of interest (keep an aliquot to be incubated without substrate as a negative control) during 30 min to 3 h at 28 °C. As positive control, we suggest 5 mM of L-histidine for *T. cruzi* or 5 mM of L-proline for *T. brucei* [6, 7].
6. Add 2 mL of CRM containing (or not for the negative control) the substrates at the concentrations to be tested into the Oroboros O-2K chambers and adjust the stoppers until the bubbles are removed.
7. Set the temperature control of the chamber at the desired temperature for the experiment (*see* **Note 4**).
8. Start recording the O_2 in the chambers until the stabilization of the electrode signal (~20 min).

3.2 Measurements of HRR: Routine Respiration, Leak Respiration, ETS Capacity, and Residual Respiration

It is important to emphasize that the following parameters are acquired in a single experiment: the Routine respiration (R), Leak respiration (L), ETS capacity (E), and Residual respiration (ROX) are obtained sequentially in the same sample of cells.

3.2.1 Routine Respiration

R is the respiratory capacity of intact cells under standard conditions. Respiration is usually regulated by the nonsaturating concentration of ADP and the ratio ADP/ATP inside the cells (this is also known as respiratory control). R is modulated as well by the amount of potentially oxidizable metabolites available in the intact cells, and this is what we propose to measure herein (Fig. 2). In other words, R corresponds to the flux of electrons through the ETS (which corresponds to the consumption of O_2 by respiration) coupled to OxPhos in intact cells.

1. Add 50 μL of cell sample (5×10^7 cells) into the chamber, taking care of not introducing air bubbles. The negative of the derivative of the O_2 consumption with respect to time correspond to R.

3.2.2 Leak Respiration

L corresponds to the O_2 flux occurring under inhibition of the F_1F_O ATP synthase. The proton flow is a property of the inner mitochondrial membrane, and can be inferred from measurement of the respiration rate after inhibition of OxPhos by using inhibitors of the F_1F_O ATP synthase (for example, the classical inhibitor Omy). A proton leak exists in all mitochondria, including those that do not possess uncoupling proteins (UCPs) [15] (which is the case for *T. cruzi* and *T. brucei* mitochondria). The molecular basis of L is still unclear. It has been suggested that the proton leak may occur through the adenine nucleotide translocator (ANT) and membrane–protein junctions [16]. In general, L can be defined as the remaining respiration after F_1F_O ATP synthase inhibition. In the case of *T. brucei*, an organism having in its PCF in addition to the cytochrome-containing respiratory chain also an active trypanosome alternative oxidase, the inhibition of such an oxidase with Ascofuranone (AF) [17] or Salicylhydroxaminic acid (SHAM) [18] should thus be warranted to obtain appropriate values for L. Proton leak can dissipate partially or completely the $\Delta\Psi_m$ due to its contribution to the break-down of the transmembrane H^+ gradient. The proton-motive force at the L state is observed at its maximum capacity when no other uncoupling systems are operative [19].

1. Start the Omy titration with successive additions of 1 μL of Omy from the stock sample (0.5 mg/μL) by waiting at least 4 min between additions. L can be evidenced after reaching a final concentration of approximately ~0.8–1.2 μg/mL (*see* **Note 5**).

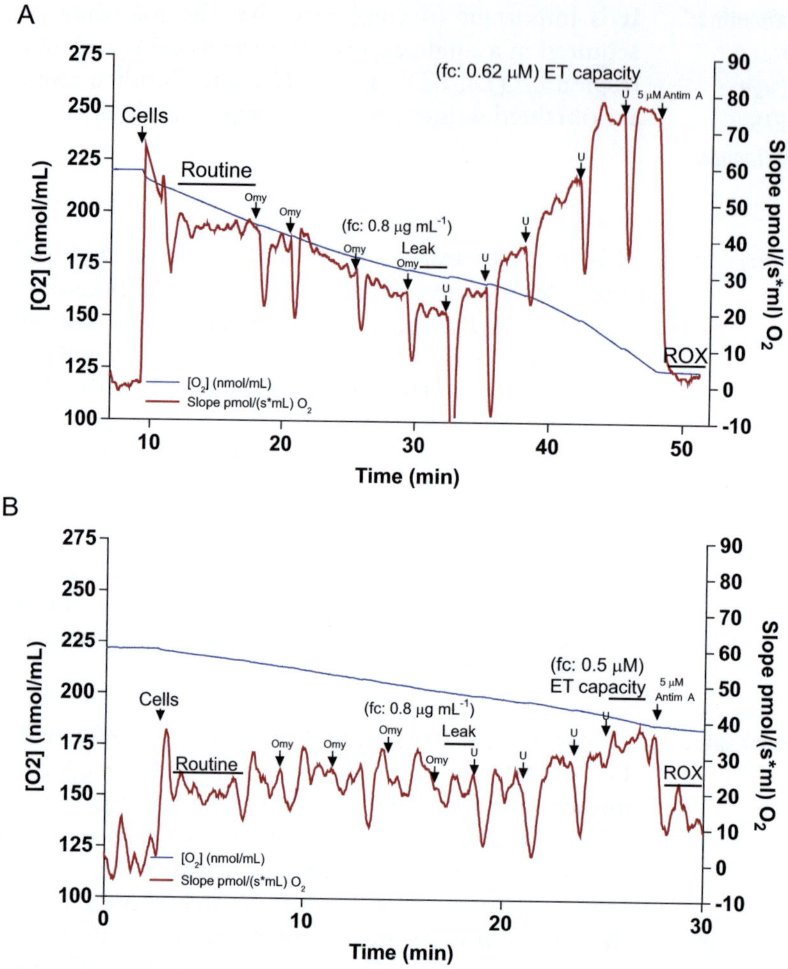

Fig. 2 (**a**) Typical tracing of HRR performed with *T. cruzi* epimastigotes. In this condition, 5×10^7 cells nutritionally stressed for 16 h were stimulated for 30 min with 5 mM L-histidine and added to the O2k chamber. (**b**) Typical tracing of a negative control, where cells were nutritionally stressed for 16 h, and incubated (in the absence of exogenous substrates) in O2k chambers. Soon after the routine (R), the F_1F_o ATP synthase is inhibited by Omy to induce the nonphosphorylative LEAK state. U (uncoupler) indicates successive additions of the FCCP protonophore to obtain the maximum flow through the ETS. Finally, the ETS III complex is inhibited by 5 μM of Antim A in order to quantify the O_2 consumption by side reactions. The blue line represents the oxygen concentration (left axis) in the chamber and the red line represents the negative time derivative of the oxygen concentration (right axis). The cells were prepared as described in the methods (Subheading 3.1)

3.2.3 Electron Transfer Capacity

E is the respiratory capacity of the ETS triggered by the inhibition of OxPhos (Omy treatment from the previous step) followed by the chemical uncoupling of the transmembrane proton gradient. Under this condition, maximal respiration is induced. The uncoupled state is reached by adding optimal concentrations of a protonophore (FCCP or CCCP—compounds which allow the free passage of protons through the inner mitochondrial membrane—

are the most frequently used). At this state respiration occurs at its maximum rate, as it is not coupled anymore to the proton motive force and thus is not dependent on the proton flux through the F_1F_o ATP synthase.

1. Start the FCCP titration with successive additions of 2 μL of Omy from the stock solution (100 μM), while waiting at least 3 min between additions. *E* can be evidenced after reaching a final concentration of approximately ~0.4 μM (*see* **Note 5**).

3.2.4 Residual Respiration Measurement

ROX is the respiration rate remaining after inhibition of the ETS, due to oxidative side reactions. No O_2 consumption has been observed in *T. cruzi* after inhibition of complex III of the respiratory chain with Antim A. However, as previously explained, *T. brucei* PCF has also a functional trypanosome alternative oxidase, which may bypass the cytochrome-containing respiratory chain and contributes to heat generation instead of proton-motive force generation with subsequent ATP production [20, 21]. The use of Antim A allows distinguishing ROX from the respiration rate responsible for the formation of ATP by OxPhos.

1. Add 2 μL Antim A from the stock sample (5 mM, final concentration: 5 μM). Record the O_2 consumption for about 5 min.
2. Clean the equipment by washing the chambers three times with 2 vol of 70% ethanol and three times with 2 vol of distilled H_2O. If intending to continue with a new experiment, reinitiate the protocol at **step 6** of Subheading 3.1. To end the experiment, add 2 mL of 70% ethanol to each chamber and close them with the Stoppers.

3.3 ATP Measurements

MgGr is a fluorescent indicator exhibiting Mg^{2+} dependent fluorescence. The fluorescence increases in an exponential way for concentrations between 0.1 and 10 mM. As Mg^{2+} has differential affinity for ADP and ATP, the use of MgGr has been proposed to measure the rate of change in the free extra-mitochondrial Mg^{2+} concentration [22]. The use of MgGr was validated by measuring for example the ATP–ADP exchange rate mediated by the ANT in isolated mitochondria from mammalian cells [22]. The rate of change in free [Mg^{2+}] can be converted into ATP concentrations by using differential standard binding equations for ADP and ATP (Fig. 3) [22].

3.3.1 Kd Determination of ATP and ADP for Mg^{2+}

In order to determine the *K*d for ATP and ADP, a measurement chamber (OROBOROS O-2K) or a fluorescence cuvette must be prepared as follows

1. Add 2 mL of CRM-Mg^- buffer, 5 μM EGTA and 5 μM EDTA. Add 1 μM of MgGr and record the signal for about 60 s.

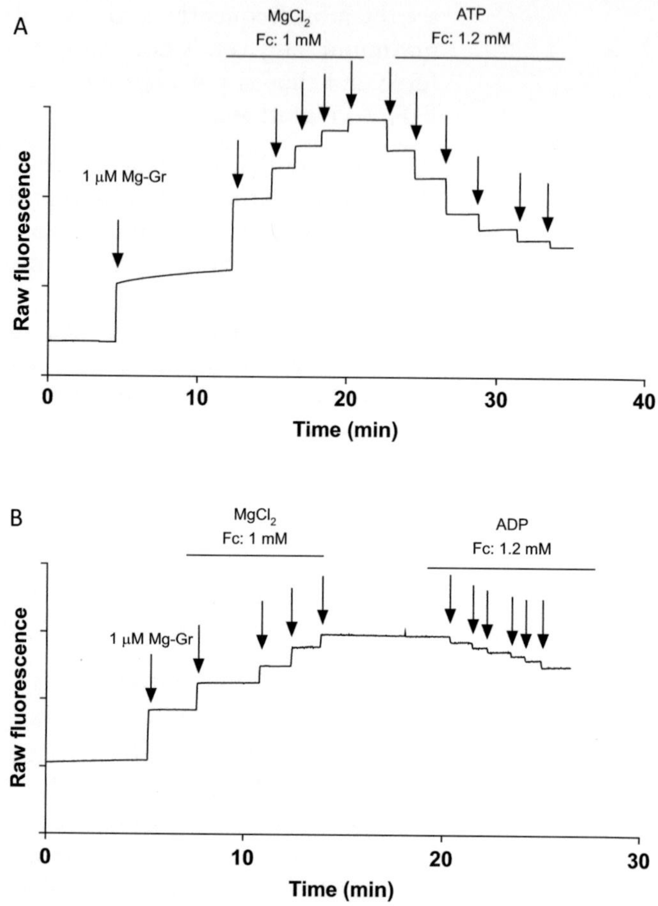

Fig. 3 Sensitivity of Magnesium Green to the ATP and ADP concentrations. The fluorescence emitted by Magnesium Green changes dependent on the ATP (**a**) and ADP (**b**) concentrations which allows to construct a calibration curve

2. Make successive additions of 2 μL of 200 mM $MgCl_2$ until a final concentration of 1 mM. The fluorescence changes should be recorded for at least 30 s after each addition.
3. Add 0.2 mM ATP in subsequent steps for a final concentration of 1.2 mM (Stock 200 mM). Record the signal about 40 s per addition.
4. Repeat the whole procedure using ADP instead of ATP.

The *K*d of ADP for Mg^{2+} and the *K*d of ATP for Mg^{2+} can be calculated from the data obtained (*see* an example in Fig. 3) in order to quantify the ATP production as described in detail in [23].

3.3.2 ATP Net Production Measurement

For the preparation of the parasites follow the protocol as described in Subheading 3.1, **steps 1–4**.

1. Add 2 mL of CRM-Mg^- buffer, 5 μM EGTA and 5 μM EDTA (*see* **Note 6**), 20 μL 20% w/v fatty-acid free BSA. Add 1 μM of MgGr and record the signal for about 60 s.
2. Add 1 mM of $MgCl_2$ for a final concentration of 1 mM (Stock 200 mM). The fluorescence changes should be recorded for at least 30 s after each addition.
3. Add 1.2 mM of ADP (considered as a saturated concentration according to [24]). Record the signal for about 60 s per addition.
4. Add 50 μL of cell sample (5×10^7 cells) into the chamber. Record the signal for about 60 s per addition.
5. Add digitonin sequentially to reach a final concentration of 10 μM (*see* **Note 7**). Record the signal for about 60 s per addition.
6. Add the metabolite of interest. Record the signal for at least 60 s per addition.
7. Add Antim A at final concentration of 5 μM. Record the signal for at least 60 s per addition.

The net ATP synthesis triggered by the metabolite of interest (in this case, 5 mM proline [7]) is evidenced by an acceleration of the fluorescence decrease (a change in the slope, *see* Fig. 4). The addition of Antim A (5 μM) blocks the synthesis of ATP (by blocking the electron flux through the ETS at the level of complex III). In order to calculate the net ATP synthesis, we recommend following protocols and mathematical treatments of data described in [23].

3.3.3 ATP Assessment (Luciferase-Based Assay)

The intracellular levels of ATP in each sample can be measured by using a luciferase assay. The luciferase enzyme converts luciferin into oxyluciferin, a reaction that involves emitting light by luminescence. This reaction requires ATP. If luciferin is at nonlimiting concentrations, the intensity of emitted light is dependent on the ATP concentrations. By comparison with a calibration curve, ATP can be quantified through this reaction (Fig. 5). This protocol is available to be used with several commercial kits.

1. Wash the cells (5×10^6) twice in PBS by centrifugation at $1000 \times g$, 10 min at 4 °C.
2. Resuspend the pellets in 100 μL of PBS.
3. Add 100 μL of Lysis Buffer (according to the manufacturer's instructions) and keep the tubes in ice.

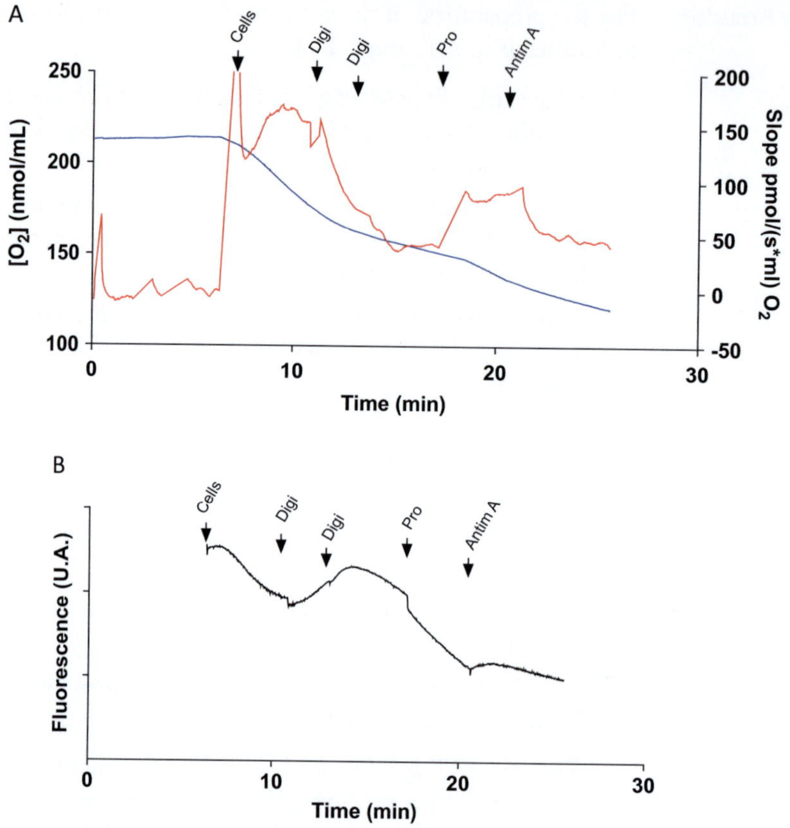

Fig. 4 Simultaneous measurements of respiratory rates (**a**) and net ATP synthesis (**b**) triggered by L-proline (5 mM) following the protocol in Subheading 3.3.1. The red lines indicate the variation in the oxygen concentration as a function of time (right axis) in (**a**). The blue line represents the oxygen concentration (left axis) in the chamber and the red line represents the negative time derivative of the oxygen concentration (right axis)

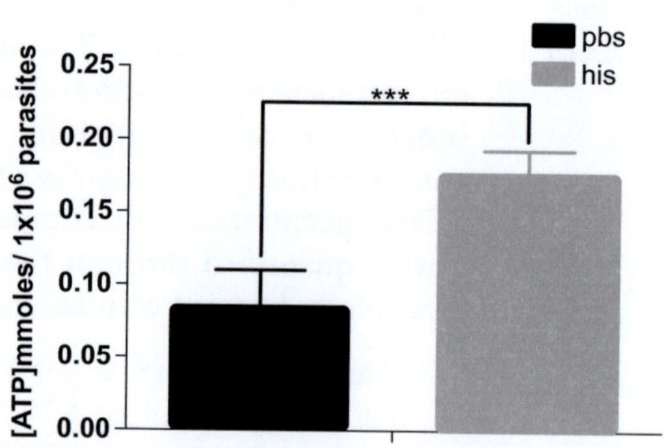

Fig. 5 Measurement of the intracellular ATP content by using the luciferase assay method. Typical values obtained for a negative control, where cells were nutritionally stressed for 16 h (in PBS) and recovered from stress by incubation for 30 min in the presence of 5 mM His (his). Data correspond to average values of three independent experiments made in triplicates each, and bars represent SD. $***p < 0.001$ (*t*-Student test)

4. Dilute the luciferase 1:20 in the Reaction Buffer 1× (luciferase solution).
5. Add 50 μL of from each sample in three wells.
6. Add 50 μL of luciferase solution in triplicate and read in the luminometer.

3.3.4 ATP Calibration Curve

1. Prepare a 1 mM ATP standard.
2. Perform a serial dilution to obtain: 0; 0.01; 0.1; 0.25; 0.5 and 0.1 mM.
3. Prepare and read the calibration curve sample as described in previously.

The ATP concentration for each condition is calculated by using the calibration curve [10].

3.4 ROS Measurement

Measurements of H_2O_2 production can unveil valuable information on the mitochondrial physiological state as well can be useful for evaluating diverse cellular functions and the effect of drugs triggering redox imbalance. In the following protocol, as an example, we will use Omy which triggers endogenous ROS production. Other drugs can be evaluated by following the same procedures. H_2O_2 production can be quantified in real time mode by using a peroxidase reaction which catalyzes the reduction of a probe (in this case, AmR) able to emit light by fluorescence when in its reduced state. This emission is dependent on the produced peroxide and makes it is possible to quantify this production. Noteworthy, with this system it is possible to measure H_2O_2 production over time in a live cell or isolated mitochondria.

3.4.1 H_2O_2 Calibration

1. Add 2 mL of CRM into the chambers.
2. Add of 10 μM AmR and 0.01 U/mL of Horse Radish Peroxidase (HRP).
3. Add H_2O_2 repeatedly (0.1 μM each addition) as shown in Fig. 6.

The successive addition of H_2O_2, which reacts with AmR catalyzed by HRP, is used for calibration by adjusting the data to the linear equation:

$$F = a \times [H_2O_2] + b.$$

where F is the fluorescence measured at 590 nm and $[H_2O_2]$ is the concentration of H_2O_2. The measured fluorescence values obtained for each treatment can be converted into H_2O_2 concentration by using this calibration function.

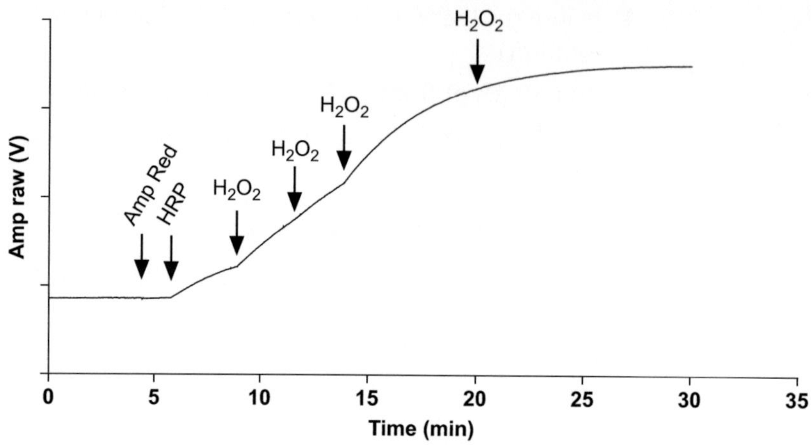

Fig. 6 Sensitivity of Amplex Red to the H_2O_2 concentration. The fluorescence emitted by Amplex Red changes dependent on the H_2O_2 concentration which allows to construct a calibration curve

3.4.2 Measurement of ROS Production Triggered by Omy

For the preparation of the parasites follow the protocol as described in Subheading 3.1, **steps 1–4**.

1. Add to the chamber 10 μM of AmR and 0.01 U/mL of HRP. Data acquisition should be followed until the end of the entire experiment (Fig. 7).

3.5 Mitochondrial Inner Membrane Potential ($\Delta\Psi_m$) Measurement (Rhodamine 123 Based Assay)

It is known that mitochondrial energization produces a rapid quenching of Rho 123. This molecule is electrophoretically distributed in the matrix of the mitochondria as a function of the $\Delta\Psi_m$ [25]. Due to the cationic lipophilic character of this molecule, its accumulation in the mitochondrial matrix is linked to the energy state of the organelle. Oxidizable substrates participating in the energy metabolism are able to trigger the generation of a $\Delta\Psi_m$. In the presence of Rho 123, polarized mitochondria promote the accumulation of Rho 123 in the mitochondrial matrix, producing a phenomenon known as self-quenching resulting in a diminution of the probe's fluorescence [25, 26]. The addition of FCCP collapses the $\Delta\Psi_m$, thereby preventing self-quenching of Rho 123.

For the preparation of the parasites follow the protocol as described in Subheading 3.1, **steps 1–4**.

1. Aliquots of 1 mL of cells (5×10^7 cells) will be treated or not (control without substrate) with the desired concentration of the metabolite of interest at the temperature of interest. Here, 5 mM glucose at 28 °C is used as an example.
2. Add 50 nM of Rho 123 to each aliquot of cells and preincubate for 20 min.
3. Add 2 mL of CRM into the OROBOROS O-2K chambers and adjust the stoppers until the air bubbles disappear.

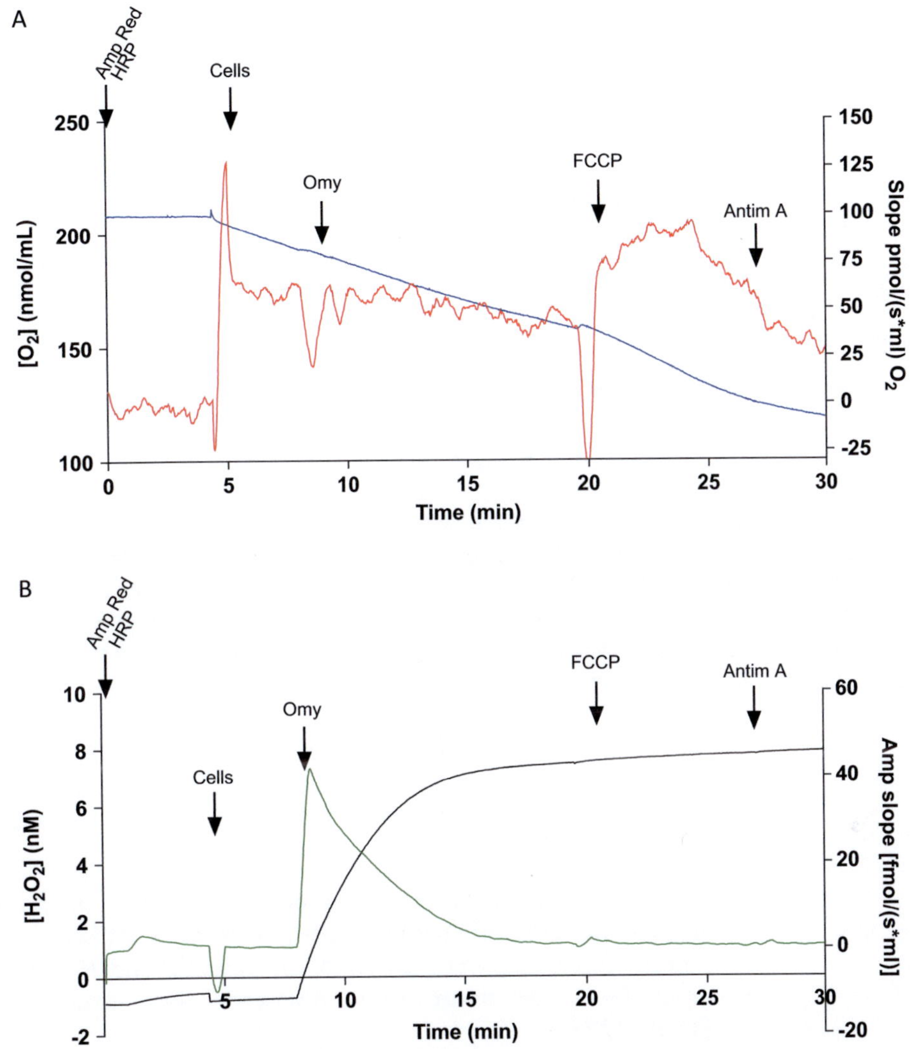

Fig. 7 Simultaneous measurements of respiratory rates (**a**) and ROS production (**b**) as described in Subheading 3.3.2. The red (panel **a**) and green (panel **b**) lines indicate the variation in oxygen and H_2O_2 concentrations, respectively, as a function of time (right axis). The blue (panel **a**) and black (panel **b**) lines represent the O_2 and H_2O_2 concentrations, respectively (scale in the left axis). Note that the addition of Omy triggers the endogenous production of ROS caused by the electron leak at the ETS

4. Add the adequate volume of substrate into the chamber, to reach the desired concentration to be tested (5 mM glucose in this case). As negative control, add the same volume of CRM buffer.
5. Wash the cells twice in CRM buffer (as described in Subheading 3.1) and resuspend the pellets in 50 μL of CRM. Add the cells into the O-2K chambers (at this time, coupled to the O2k-Fluo LED2-Module, with the corresponding filters). Record the signal for at least ~3 min.

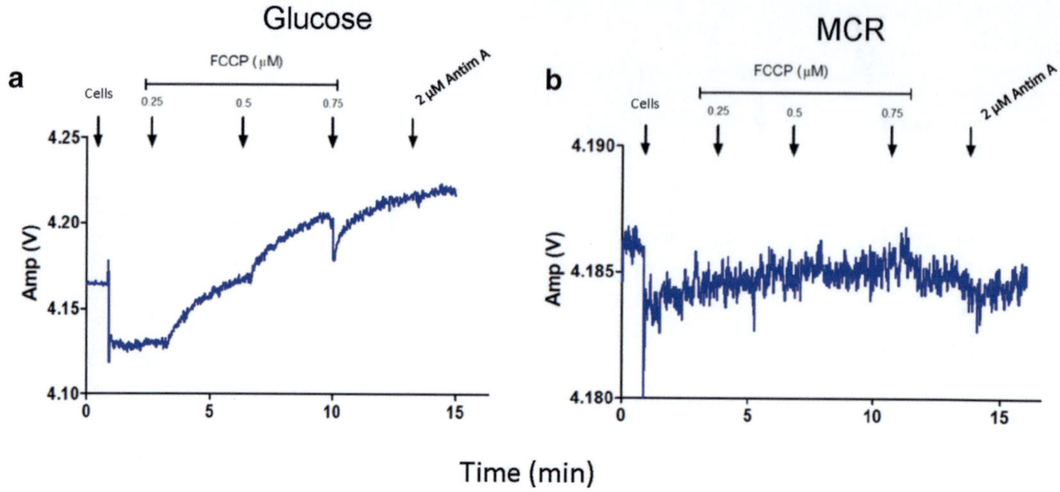

Fig. 8 (**a**) Typical tracing of the mitochondrial inner membrane potential ($\Delta\Psi_m$) assessment with Rhodamine 123, measured in *T. cruzi* epimastigotes. In this example, we used 5×10^7 cells nutritionally stressed for 16 h and further stimulated for 30 min with 5 mM glucose. (**b**) Typical tracing of a negative control, in which cells were nutritionally stressed for 16 h, and incubated in MRC buffer in the absence of any exogenous substrates. Successive additions of the FCCP protonophore led to $\Delta\Psi_m$ collapse, thereby reducing the self-quenching of Rho 123, which is recorded as a fluorescent signal

6. Start the titration by successive additions of 5 μL of 100 μM FCCP until observing the complete collapse of $\Delta\Psi_m$ (*see* **Note 8**). Record the signal for at least 3 min between additions (*see* Fig. 8).

Here, the *F*/Fi fluorescence ratio is used as an estimate of the mitochondrial membrane potential (where Fi is the basal fluorescence before collapsing the membrane potential and *F* is the maximum level of fluorescence obtained after titration with FCCP) [27].

4 Notes

1. It is important to use different Hamilton syringes for each mitochondrial inhibitor, and to keep them adequately labeled. They must be kept correctly cleaned according to the manufacturer's instructions.
2. Check carefully that the metabolite to be used is not toxic at the concentrations to be used for measurements.
3. Metabolic stress reduces the background O_2 consumption (measured by incubating parasites in PBS) due to the oxidation of internal metabolites.

4. Respiration is very sensitive to temperature, so the measurements should be initiated when the chambers reached the desired temperature.
5. Variations can occur between different strains, culture media from which cells are taken, and stages of proliferation (stationary or exponential) [28–30], so it is important to titrate the mitochondrial inhibitors for each kind of cells. Some adjustments to the concentrations suggested in the protocols herein could be necessary.
6. The addition of chelating agents such as EGTA and EDTA is critical, since MgGr can emit fluorescence as a function of small amounts of Ca^{2+} [22, 23].
7. The ideal concentration of digitonin should be determined in advance by titration.
8. The complete collapse of $\Delta\Psi_m$ is observed when fluorescence values become constant after successive additions (fluorescence reaches a plateau).

Acknowledgments

For this work we had the support of the following funding agencies: Fundação de Amparo à Pesquisa do Estado de São Paulo grant 2016/06034-2, Conselho Nacional de Pesquisas Científicas e Tecnológicas (CNPq) grant 308351/2013-4, and the Research Council United Kingdom Global Challenges Research Fund under grant agreement "A Global Network for Neglected Tropical Diseases" (grant MR/P027989/1).

References

1. Sylvester D, Krassner SM (1976) Proline metabolism in *Trypanosoma cruzi* epimastigotes. Comp Biochem Physiol B 55 (3B):443–447
2. Paulin JJ (1975) The chondriome of selected trypanosomatids. A three-dimensional study based on serial thick sections and high voltage electron microscopy. J Cell Biol 66 (2):404–413
3. Paulin JJ (1983) Conformation of a single mitochondrion in the trypomastigote stage of *Trypanosoma cruzi*. J Parasitol 69(1):242–244
4. Brack C (1968) Electron microscopic studies on the life cycle of *Trypanosoma cruzi* with special reference to developmental forms in the vector *Rhodnius prolixus*. Acta Trop 25 (4):289–356
5. Paes LS, Mantilla BS, Barison MJ, Wrenger C, Silber AM (2011) The uniqueness of the *Trypanosoma cruzi* mitochondrion: opportunities to identify new drug target for the treatment of Chagas disease. Curr Pharm Des 17 (20):2074–2099
6. Barison MJ, Damasceno FS, Mantilla BS, Silber AM (2016) The active transport of histidine and its role in ATP production in *Trypanosoma cruzi*. J Bioenerg Biomembr 48(4):437–449. https://doi.org/10.1007/s10863-016-9665-9
7. Mantilla BS, Marchese L, Casas-Sanchez A, Dyer NA, Ejeh N, Biran M, Bringaud F, Lehane MJ, Acosta-Serrano A, Silber AM (2017) Proline metabolism is essential for *Trypanosoma brucei brucei* survival in the tsetse vector. PLoS Pathog 13(1):e1006158.

https://doi.org/10.1371/journal.ppat.1006158

8. Mantilla BS, Paes LS, Pral EM, Martil DE, Thiemann OH, Fernandez-Silva P, Bastos EL, Silber AM (2015) Role of delta1-pyrroline-5-carboxylate-dehydrogenase supports mitochondrial metabolism and host-cell invasion of *Trypanosoma cruzi*. J Biol Chem 290:7767–7790. https://doi.org/10.1074/jbc.M114.574525
9. Paes LS, Mantilla BS, Zimbres FM, Pral EM, Diogo de Melo P, Tahara EB, Kowaltowski AJ, Elias MC, Silber AM (2013) Proline dehydrogenase regulates redox state and respiratory metabolism in *Trypanosoma cruzi*. PLoS One 8(7):e69419. https://doi.org/10.1371/journal.pone.0069419
10. Girard R, Crispim M, Alencar MB, Silber AM (2018) Uptake of L-alanine and its distinct roles in the bioenergetics of *Trypanosoma cruzi*. mSphere 3(4):e00338–e00318. https://doi.org/10.1128/mSphereDirect.00338-18
11. von Brand T, Johnson EM, Rees CW (1946) Observations on the respiration of *Trypanosoma cruzi* in culture. J Gen Physiol 30 (2):163–175
12. Vercesi AE, Bernardes CF, Hoffmann ME, Gadelha FR, Docampo R (1991) Digitonin permeabilization does not affect mitochondrial function and allows the determination of the mitochondrial membrane potential of *Trypanosoma cruzi* in situ. J Biol Chem 266 (22):14431–14434
13. Camargo EP (1964) Growth and differentiation in *Trypanosoma cruzi*. I. Origin of metacyclic trypanosomes in liquid media. Rev Inst Med Trp São Paulo 6:93–100
14. Brun RS (1979) Cultivation and *in vitro* cloning or procyclic culture forms of *Trypanosoma brucei* in a semi-defined medium. Acta Trop 36 (3):289–292
15. Nicholls DG, Ferguson SJ (2013) Bioenergetics 4. Elsevier, London
16. Brand MD, Chien L-F, Ainscowr EK, Rolfe DFS, Porter RK (1994) The causes and functions of mitochondrial proton leak. Biochim Biophys Acta 1187(2):132–139. https://doi.org/10.1016/0005-2728(94)90099-X
17. Minagawa N, Yabu Y, Kita K, Nagai K, Ohta N, Meguro K, Sakajo S, Yoshimoto A (1997) An antibiotic, ascofuranone, specifically inhibits respiration and *in vitro* growth of long slender bloodstream forms of *Trypanosoma brucei brucei*. Mol Biochem Parasitol 84(2):271–280
18. Evans DA, Brown RC (1973) m-Chlorobenzhydroxyamic acid-an inhibitor of cyanide-insensitive respiration in *Trypanosoma brucei*. J Protozool 20(1):157–160
19. Gnaiger E (2009) Capacity of oxidative phosphorylation in human skeletal muscle: new perspectives of mitochondrial physiology. Int J Biochem Cell Biol 41(10):1837–1845. https://doi.org/10.1016/j.biocel.2009.03.013
20. Clarkson AB Jr, Bienen EJ, Pollakis G, Grady RW (1989) Respiration of bloodstream forms of the parasite *Trypanosoma brucei brucei* is dependent on a plant-like alternative oxidase. J Biol Chem 264(30):17770–17776
21. Chaudhuri M, Sharan R, Hill GC (2002) Trypanosome alternative oxidase is regulated post-transcriptionally at the level of RNA stability. J Eukaryot Microbiol 49(4):263–269
22. Chinopoulos C, Vajda S, Csanady L, Mandi M, Mathe K, Adam-Vizi V (2009) A novel kinetic assay of mitochondrial ATP-ADP exchange rate mediated by the ANT. Biophys J 96 (6):2490–2504. https://doi.org/10.1016/j.bpj.2008.12.3915
23. Chinopoulos C, Kiss G, Kawamata H, Starkov AA (2014) Measurement of ADP-ATP exchange in relation to mitochondrial transmembrane potential and oxygen consumption. Methods Enzymol 542:333–348. https://doi.org/10.1016/B978-0-12-416618-9.00017-0
24. Williams N, Frank PH (1990) The mitochondrial ATP synthase of *Trypanosoma brucei*: isolation and characterization of the intact F1 moiety. Mol Bioch Parasitol 43(1):125–132
25. Emaus RK, Grunwald R, Lemasters JJ (1986) Rhodamine-123 as a probe of transmembrane potential in isolated rat-liver mitochondria – spectral and metabolic properties. Biochim Biophys Acta 850(3):436–448. https://doi.org/10.1016/0005-2728(86)90112-X
26. Perry SW, Norman JP, Barbieri J, Brown EB, Gelbard HA (2011) Mitochondrial membrane potential probes and the proton gradient: a practical usage guide. BioTechniques 50 (2):98–115. https://doi.org/10.2144/000113610
27. Baracca A, Sgarbi G, Solaini G, Lenaz G (2003) Rhodamine 123 as a probe of mitochondrial membrane potential: evaluation of proton flux through F(0) during ATP synthesis. Biochim Biophys Acta 1606(1-3):137–146
28. Silva TM, Peloso EF, Vitor SC, Ribeiro LHG, Gadelha FR (2011) O-2 consumption rates along the growth curve: new insights into *Trypanosoma cruzi* mitochondrial respiratory chain. J Bioenerg Biomembr 43(4):409–417. https://doi.org/10.1007/s10863-011-9369-0

29. Stoppani AOM, Docampo R, Deboiso JF, Frasch ACC (1980) Effect of inhibitors of electron-transport and oxidative-phosphorylation on *Trypanosoma cruzi* respiration and growth. Mol Biochem Parasitol 2 (1):3–21. https://doi.org/10.1016/0166-6851(80)90044-4

30. Kalem MC, Gerasimov ES, Vu PK, Zimmer SL (2018) Gene expression to mitochondrial metabolism: variability among cultured *Trypanosoma cruzi* strains. PLoS One 13(5): e0197983. https://doi.org/10.1371/journal.pone.0197983

Chapter 40

Isolation and Characterization of Acidocalcisomes from Trypanosomatids

Guozhong Huang, Silvia N. J. Moreno, and Roberto Docampo

Abstract

Acidocalcisomes are membrane-bounded, electron-dense, acidic organelles, rich in calcium and polyphosphate. These organelles were first described in trypanosomatids and later found from bacteria to human cells. Some of the functions of the acidocalcisome are the storage of cations and phosphorus, participation in pyrophosphate (PP_i) and polyphosphate (polyP) metabolism, calcium signaling, maintenance of intracellular pH homeostasis, autophagy, and osmoregulation. Isolation of acidocalcisomes is an important technique for understanding their composition and function. Here, we provide detailed subcellular fractionation protocols using iodixanol gradient centrifugations to isolate high-quality acidocalcisomes from *Trypanosoma brucei*, which are subsequently validated by electron microscopy, and enzymatic and immunoblot assays with organellar markers.

Key words Trypanosomatids, *Trypanosoma brucei*, Acidocalcisome, Subcellular fractionation, Organellar markers

1 Introduction

Acidocalcisomes are lysosome-related organelles rich in cations and polyphosphate, which were originally identified in trypanosomatids and have been conserved from prokaryotes to eukaryotes [1, 2]. *Trypanosoma brucei*, the causative agent of sleeping sickness or African trypanosomiasis, is an excellent model to study the acidocalcisome because it is the trypanosome that is most amenable to a number of molecular and genetic tools, easy to cultivate, and possesses acidocalcisomes with up to molar levels of PP_i and polyP in the two best-studied life cycle stages: procyclic and bloodstream forms (PCF and BSF) [3]. Studies with this parasite have provided fundamental insights into the acidocalcisome biology and its roles in cation and phosphorus storage, calcium signaling, pH and osmotic regulation, response to stress, autophagy, and growth and infectivity [1–4].

Paul A. M. Michels et al. (eds.), *Trypanosomatids: Methods and Protocols*, Methods in Molecular Biology, vol. 2116,
https://doi.org/10.1007/978-1-0716-0294-2_40,

Subcellular fractionation, a practical approach for obtaining purified organelles, is accomplished by cell membrane lysis and density gradient centrifugation to separate the organelles from other contaminating subcellular structures. Several gradients, such as Nycodenz®, sucrose and Percoll®, have been applied for the isolation of mitochondria, lysosomes, Golgi, glycosomes, or endoplasmic reticulum from parasitic protozoa [5, 6]. Percoll® was initially used to isolate acidocalcisomes from trypanosomes [7], but was effectively replaced by iodixanol (OptiPrep™) in our laboratory [8, 9]. Iodixanol is ideal for density gradient isolation of intact subcellular organelles from tissues or cells [10], since it is a true solute that forms a self-generated gradient capable of maintaining the environment of different organelles close to isoosmoticity, that does not cause co-sedimentation of colloidal silica particles with high-density organelles (such as acidocalcisomes), and that does not interfere with most downstream enzymatic assays and electroblotting analyses without removal. In order to minimize or eliminate other membrane and organelle contaminations, we have recently developed a new iodixanol-based protocol for subcellular fractionation to isolate high-quality acidocalcisomes from PCF trypanosomes through the modification of our previous method [8, 9] using additional gradient centrifugation with higher density iodixanol (Fig. 1). After fractionation, the yield and purity of isolated acidocalcisomes were analyzed by enzymatic and immunoblotting assays using organelle markers for acidocalcisomes (vacuolar proton pyrophosphatase-TbVP1), mitochondria (succinate cytochrome *c* reductase, voltage-dependent anion channel-TbVDAC), glycosomes (hexokinase, pyruvate phosphate dikinase-TbPPDK) and lysosomes (α-mannosidase, Tbp67). The results have validated this method that can efficiently separate acidocalcisomes from other organelles, significantly enhancing their purification (Table 1) by eliminating or decreasing mitochondrial, glycosomal, and lysosomal contaminations (Figs. 2 and 3). Our protocols, described here, have successfully been used for isolation and characterization of acidocalcisomes from *T. brucei*, but can be easily adapted to other trypanosomatids.

2 Materials

Prepare all solutions using ultrapure water (prepared by purifying deionized water, to attain a sensitivity of 18 MΩ cm at room temperature (RT) and analytical grade reagents. Prepare and store all reagents at RT (unless indicated otherwise).

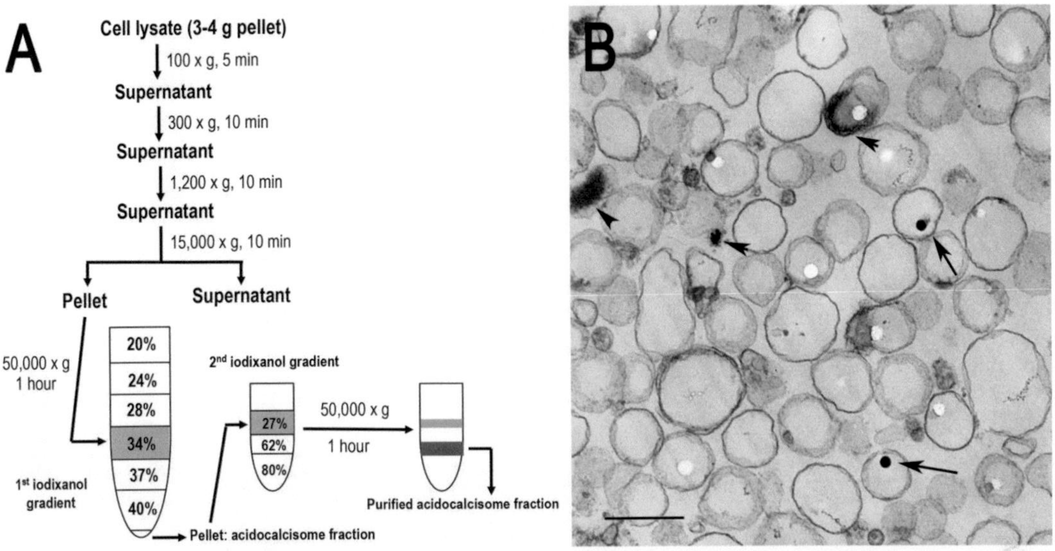

Fig. 1 Subcellular fractionation of acidocalcisomes. (**a**) Trypanosome lysates are obtained by grinding with silicon carbide, decanting by low speed centrifugation to eliminate debris and silicon carbide, and centrifuging at 15,000 × *g* for 10 min to isolate the organellar fraction that is applied to the 34% step of a discontinuous iodixanol gradient. After centrifugation at 50,000 × *g* for 1 h, the pellet is resuspended and applied to the 27% step of a second iodixanol gradient and centrifuged at 50,000 × *g* for 1 h. Aliquots from each fraction are used for enzymatic assays and Western blot analyses. (**b**) Electron microscopy of acidocalcisome fraction prepared by the iodixanol procedure (fraction 5). *Scale bar* = 0.2 μm. Arrows and arrowheads show electron-dense material inside acidocalcisomes (Reproduced from Huang et al. [3] with permission from the Public Library of Science)

Table 1
Purification of acidocalcisomes on iodixanol step gradients

	Yield (%)		Purification-fold	
	First	Second	First	Second
Protein (mg)	0.14 (3)	0.05 (3)		
Pyrophosphatase[a]	9.81 (3)	4.96 (3)	70	99
Succinate cytochrome *c* reductase	0.12 (3)	0.02 (3)	1	0.2
Hexokinase	0.46 (3)	0 (3)	3	0
α-Mannosidase	0.27 (3)	0.08 (3)	2	1.6

Yield values are percentages relative to the 15,000 × *g* pellet fraction and represent averages from number of preparations in parentheses

[a]Pyrophosphatase activities in the 15,000 × *g* pellet, and the first and second gradient acidocalcisome preparations were 0.22 ± 0.09, 15.6 ± 3.2, and 22.6 ± 2.1 μmol/min/mg protein, respectively (mean ± SD) (reproduced from Huang et al. [3]) with permission from the Public Library of Science)

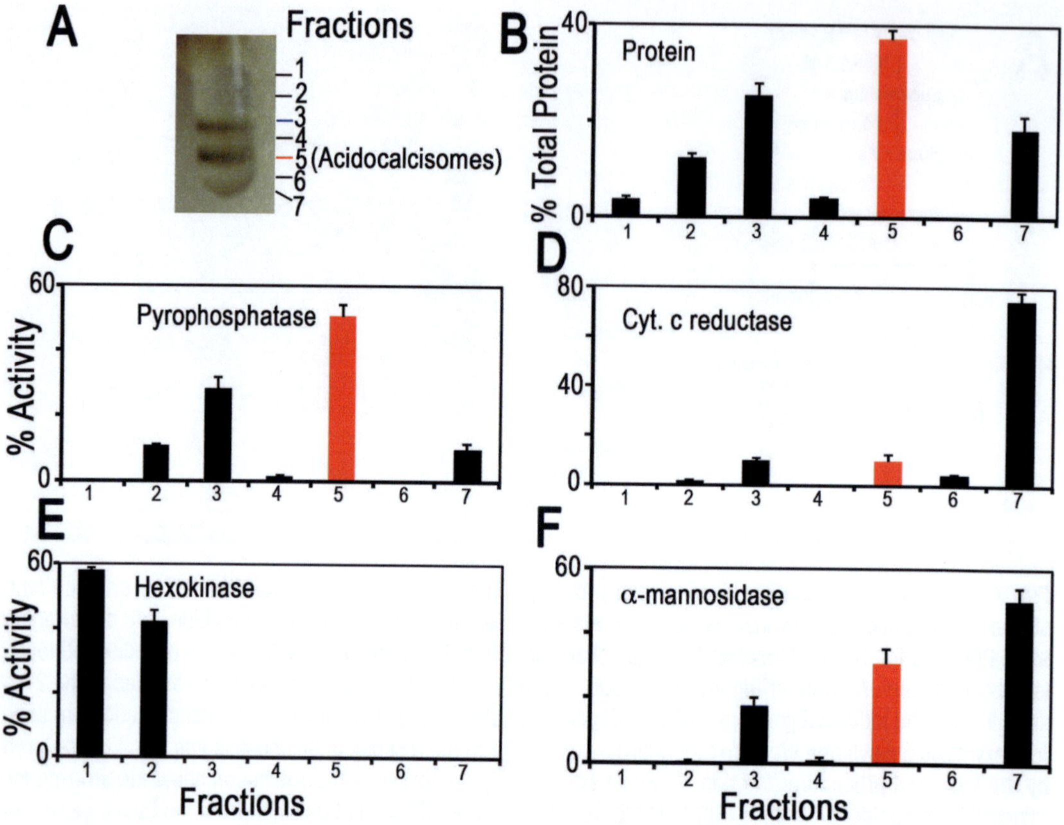

Fig. 2 Distribution on iodixanol gradients of organellar markers from PCF trypanosomes. (**a**) Photograph showing bands obtained after the second iodixanol gradient centrifugation. Fraction 5 corresponds to the purified acidocalcisomes. (**b**) Protein distribution. (**c**) TbVP1 activity (measured as the AMDP-sensitive P_i release) is concentrated in fractions 3 and 5. (**d**) Mitochondrial marker distribution, succinate cytochrome *c* reductase. (**e**) Glycosomal marker distribution, hexokinase. (**f**) Lysosomal marker distribution, α-mannosidase. In (**b–f**) the *y*-axis indicates relative distribution; the *x*-axis indicates fraction number; *bars* show means ± SD (as a percentage of the total recovered activity) from two or three independent experiments (reproduced from Huang et al. [3] with permission from the Public Library of Science)

2.1 Cell Culture and Standard Equipment

1. *T. brucei* procyclic form (PCF) trypanosomes (wild type strain 427) grown in SDM-79 medium [11] supplemented with hemin (7.5 μg/ml) and 10% heat-inactivated fetal bovine serum.
2. Pipettes (20, 200, and 1000 μl, multichannel pipette).
3. Pipet-Aid.
4. Serological pipettes (5, 10, and 25 ml).
5. Pasteur glass pipettes with cotton.
6. Eppendorf tubes (1.5 and 1.8 ml).
7. Glass tubes (disposable culture tubes, 4 and 10 ml).
8. Refrigerated centrifuge for microcentrifuge tubes.

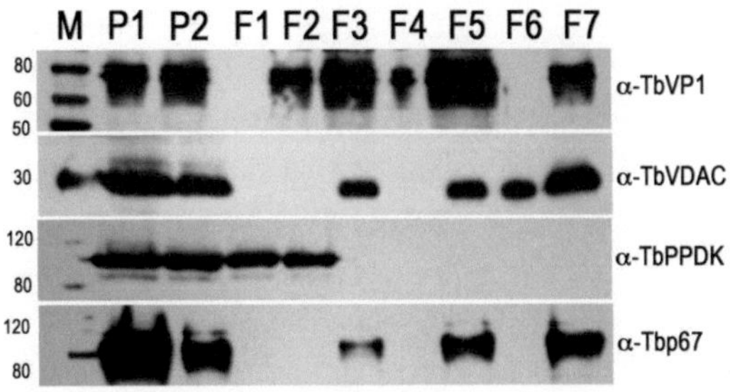

Fig. 3 Western blot analyses of subcellular fractions using antibodies against acidocalcisome marker TbVP1, mitochondrial marker voltage-dependent anion channel (TbVDAC), glycosomal marker pyruvate, phosphate dikinase (TbPPDK), and lysosome marker Tbp67. P1, the 15,000 × *g* pellet (30 μg); P2, the first gradient pellet (2 μg); F1 to F7, the second gradient fractions (2 μg each). M, Magic Marker protein standards (Reproduced from Huang et al. [3] with permission from the Public Library of Science)

9. Centrifuge with fixed angle rotor.
10. Ultracentrifuge with swinging-bucket (SW) rotor.
11. Centrifuge tubes (polycarbonate thick-wall centrifuge tubes, 50 ml).
12. Ultracentrifuge tubes (polycarbonate thick-wall centrifuge tubes, 38 ml; ultra-clear or polyallomer tubes, 5 ml).
13. Stainless steel lab spoon spatula. Precooled at −20 °C.
14. Mortar and pestle. Precooled at −20 °C.
15. Glass tissue homogenizer with tight-fitting pestle (2 and 5 ml). Precooled at 4 °C.
16. Tissue homogenizer mixer with stand.
17. 96-well microplate.
18. No. 5 filter paper.
19. Microplate reader.
20. Microplate incubator shaker.
21. Nitrocellulose membranes.
22. Mini-gel electrophoresis system.
23. Trans-blot apparatus.

2.2 Reagents

2.2.1 Gradient Centrifugations

1. Complete, EDTA-free, protease inhibitor cocktail tablet. Store at 4 °C.
2. Buffer A with glucose (BAG): 116 mM NaCl, 5.4 mM KCl, 0.8 mM $MgSO_4$, 5.5 mM glucose, 50 mM Hepes (free acid), pH 7.2. Store at 4 °C (*see* **Note 1**).
3. Isolation buffer (IB) (*see* **Note 2**): 125 mM sucrose, 50 mM KCl, 4 mM $MgCl_2$, 0.5 mM EDTA, 5 mM dithiothreitol

(DTT), 20 mM Hepes-KOH, pH 7.2, and 1× protease inhibitor cocktails (*see* **Note 3**). Store at 4 °C.

4. OptiPrep™ solution: 125 mM sucrose, 300 mM KCl, 24 mM $MgCl_2$, 3.0 mM EDTA, 30 mM dithiothreitol (DTT) (*see* **Note 3**), 120 mM Hepes-KOH, pH 7.2. Store at 4 °C.
5. OptiPrep™ (60% w/v iodixanol, 1.32 g/ml). Store at 4 °C.
6. Working solution: 50% *w/v* iodixanol: 5 vol of 60% w/v iodixanol plus 1 vol of OptiPrep™ solution (*see* **Note 4**). Freshly prepared. Store at 4 °C.
7. OptiPrep™: 90% w/v iodixanol. Dry 60% *w/v* iodixanol solution completely at 70 °C and then resuspend in IB. Store at 4 °C.
8. Silicon carbide, ~400 mesh. Store at −20 °C.
9. Sucrose solutions: 10% w/v sucrose (5 ml) and 1 M sucrose (5 ml) in IB.
10. RIPA buffer: 150 mM NaCl, 20 mM Tris/HCl, pH 7.5, 1 mM EDTA, 1% SDS, 0.1% Triton X-100, and 1× protein inhibitor cocktails. Freshly prepared.
11. Bovine serum albumin (BSA) standards: 1 mg/ml, dilute to a series of final concentrations of 0, 50, 200, 400, 600, and 800 (μg/ml). Store at 4 °C.

2.2.2 Electron Microscopy

1. 50% Glutaraldehyde solution. Store at 4 °C.
2. 16% Paraformaldehyde, methanol free.
3. 0.2 M Sodium cacodylate buffer, pH 7.4. Store at 4 °C.
4. Fixation solution: 2.5% glutaraldehyde and 4% paraformaldehyde in 0.1 M sodium cacodylate buffer, pH 7.4. Freshly prepared (*see* **Note 5**).

2.2.3 Marker Enzyme Assays

1. 10 mM KH_2PO_4 for phosphate standards. Store at 4 °C.
2. 100 mM Potassium pyrophosphate (PP_i). Store at −20 °C.
3. 10 mM Aminomethylenediphosphonate (AMDP): synthesized by Michael Martin (University of Illinois at Urbana-Champaign). Store at −20 °C
4. PPase reaction buffer: 130 mM KCl, 2 mM $MgCl_2$, 10 mM Hepes-KOH, pH 7.2.
5. 0.045% (w/v) Malachite green (MG): dissolve 45 mg malachite green oxalate salt in 100 ml H_2O and stir for at least 30 min. Store in dark bottle.
6. 4.2% (w/v) Ammonium molybdate (AM) in 4 N HCl: dissolve 4.2 g ammonium molybdate in 100 ml 4 N HCl.

7. 0.2 M Succinate (pH 7.2): dissolve 2.36 g succinic acid in 100 ml H_2O, and then adjust pH to 7.2 with 5 M NaOH.
8. 1 M Hepes-KOH, pH 7.5.
9. 10 mM KCN: dissolve 6.5 mg of KCN in 10 ml H_2O under a fume hood (*see* **Note 6**). Freshly prepared.
10. 5 mM Cytochrome *c* from equine heart. Store at −20 °C.
11. Succinate-cytochrome *c* reductase (SCR) reaction medium: 0.1 mM cytochrome *c*, 0.3 mM KCN, and 40 mM Hepes-KOH pH 7.5. Freshly prepared. Store at 4 °C.
12. 60 mM ATP, disodium salt solution. Freshly prepared. Store at −20 °C
13. 60 mM $NADP^+$. Freshly prepared. Store at −20 °C
14. Glucose-6-phosphate dehydrogenase, type VII, from baker's yeast (250 units). Store at −20 °C.
15. Hexokinase (HK) enzyme solution: 0.5–1 unit/μl of hexokinase in cold H_2O. Prepared immediately before use. Store at −4 °C.
16. Hexokinase (HK) assay medium: 10 mM D-glucose, 0.6 mM ATP, 0.6 mM $NADP^+$, 10 mM $MgCl_2$, 2.5 units/ml glucose-6-phosphate dehydrogenase, and 50 mM Hepes-KOH, pH 7.8. Freshly prepared. Store at 4 °C.
17. 0.4 M Sodium acetate buffer, pH 4.6: dissolve 5.44 g sodium acetate trihydrate in 98 ml H_2O, add 1.2 ml glacial acetic acid, and then adjust pH to 4.6 with NaOH.
18. 12.5 mM *p*-Nitrophenol. Freshly prepared. Store at −20 °C.
19. 60 mM *p*-Nitrophenyl-α-D-mannopyranoside (pNP-Man). Store at −20 °C.
20. 1 M Na_2CO_3.
21. α-Mannosidase (AMA) reaction medium: 200 mM sodium acetate buffer, pH 4.6, and 0.6 mM pNP-Man. Freshly prepared. Store at 4 °C.

2.2.4 Immunoblotting

1. 10% SDS-PAGE gel.
2. SDS-PAGE running buffer: 25 mM Tris–HCl, pH 8.3, 192 mM glycine, 0.1% SDS.
3. MagicMark protein ladder. Store at −20 °C.
4. 2× Laemmli sample buffer.
5. PBS: 137 mM NaCl, 2.7 mM KCl, 10 mM Na_2HPO_4, 1.8 mM KH_2PO_4, pH 7.4.
6. PBS-T: PBS containing 0.1% Tween-20.
7. Blocking buffer: PBS-T containing 10% nonfat milk.

8. Western blot transfer buffer: 25 mM Tris base, 192 mM glycine, 0.01% SDS (*see* **Note 7**), 20% methanol.
9. Horseradish peroxidase conjugated anti-mouse or anti-rabbit IgG (H + L) antibody. Store at −20 °C.
10. Pierce ECL Western blotting substrate. Store at 4 °C.

3 Methods

Isolate and purify acidocalcisomes from trypanosomes using two iodixanol gradient centrifugations (Fig. 1). Carry out all procedures at 4 °C, unless otherwise specified.

3.1 First Gradient Centrifugation

1. Collect late mid-log PCF trypanosomes (1 l, approximately 3–4 g wet weight) by centrifugation at 1000 × *g* for 7 min at room temperature (RT).
2. Wash the trypanosomes twice with BAG at RT.
3. Wash the trypanosomes once in 25 ml cold isolation buffer (IB) supplied with Complete, EDTA-free, protease inhibitor cocktail.
4. Transfer the pellet into a precooled mortar using a precooled spoon spatula.
5. Lyse the washed cells with silicon carbide in IB in a pestle and mortar by grinding for approximately 60 s (*see* **Note 8**).
6. Transfer the lysed cells with silicon carbide into a 38 ml thick-wall centrifuge tube using the spoon spatula.
7. Rinse the mortar, pestle and spoon spatula with 10 ml IB and transfer the lysate-silicon mixture into the 38 ml centrifuge tube (*see* **Note 9**).
8. Resuspend the lysate-silicon mixture (approximately 13 ml) by adding IB to a final volume of 25 ml, incubate it for 20 min to settle some particles out of the mixture, and transfer the supernatant into a new centrifuge tube for centrifugation (*see* **Note 9**).
9. Centrifuge the lysed cells in IB at 100 × *g* for 5 min.
10. Decant the supernatant and centrifuge this at 300 × *g* for 10 min.
11. Decant the supernatant and centrifuge this at 1200 × *g* for 10 min.
12. Centrifuge the supernatant at 15,000 × *g* for 10 min and retain the pellet.
13. Resuspend the pellet in 1 ml IB with a Wheaton homogenizer (*see* **Note 10**) and apply it to the 34% step of a discontinuous gradient.

14. Prepare density gradient solutions (4 ml each) containing 20, 24, 28, 34, 37 and 40% (w/v) iodixanol in 10 ml glass tubes using 50% (w/v) iodixanol working solution and 1 M sucrose with IB (*see* **Note 11**).
15. Load gradient solutions in 38 ml polycarbonate (thick-wall) ultracentrifuge tubes, starting from the bottom with the less dense iodixanol, using a glass pipette with Pipet-Aid (*see* **Note 12**).
16. Centrifuge at 50,000 × *g* for 1 h in a SW Ti rotor in the ultracentrifuge (*see* **Note 13**).
17. Acidocalcisomes form a pellet at the bottom of the gradient (Fig. 1). Aspirate the gradient and resuspend the pellet in IB for the second gradient purification.

3.2 Second Gradient Centrifugation

1. Resuspend the pellet containing crude acidocalcisomes from the first gradient in 700 μl IB with a Wheaton homogenizer (*see* **Note 10**) and apply it to the 27% step of another discontinuous gradient (Fig. 1).
2. Prepare density gradient solutions (1 ml each) containing 27%, 62% and 80% (w/v) iodixanol in 4 ml glass tubes by diluting 90% (w/v) iodixanol (*see* **Note 11**) and 1.4 ml 10% (w/v) sucrose with IB.
3. Load gradient solutions in 5 ml polyallomer centrifuge tube, starting from the bottom with 10% sucrose and the less dense iodixanol, using a glass pipette with Pipet-Aid (*see* **Note 12**).
4. Centrifuge at 50,000 × *g* for 1 h in a SW 55 Ti rotor in the ultracentrifuge (*see* **Note 13**).
5. Collect the separated fractions carefully from the top of the gradient in seven Eppendorf tubes (*see* **Note 14**). Fraction 5 corresponds to the purified acidocalcisomes (Fig. 1).
6. Wash the fractions twice with 3–5 volumes of isolation buffer by centrifugation at 20,000 × *g* for 15 min to remove the iodixanol (*see* **Note 15**).
7. Quantify the protein concentration by Bradford assay (*see* **Note 16**) using a Microplate Reader.
8. Analyze fractions by various organelle marker enzyme assays (*see* **Note 17**) and Western blots (Figs. 2 and 3).

3.3 Electron Microscopy

Observe the morphology and structures of acidocalcisomes (Fig. 1) from fraction 5 of the second gradient by transmission electron microscopy (TEM).

1. Precipitate aliquot (25 μl) of fraction 5 (acidocalcisomes) of the second gradient (Fig. 1) by centrifugation at 20,000 × *g* for 15 min at 4 °C.

2. Fix the pellet in 2.5% glutaraldehyde and 4% paraformaldehyde in 0.1 M sodium cacodylate buffer (pH 7.4) at RT for 1 h.
3. Carefully replace the supernatant with fresh fixative (*see* **Note 5**) without disturbing the pellet and then store it at 4 °C.
4. Process samples for transmission electron microscopy according to the standard procedures [12].

3.4 Marker Enzyme Assays

Detect organelle marker enzymatic activities in the 15,000 × *g* pellet (P1), the first gradient pellet (P2) and the fractions (F1–F7) of the second gradient (Table 1, Fig. 2).

3.4.1 AMDP-Sensitive Vacuolar Proton Pyrophosphatase (V-PPase)

Vacuolar proton (H^+) pyrophosphatase (V-PPase) is an acidocalcisome membrane-associated enzyme, which couples the energy of PP_i hydrolysis to H^+ influx across the organellar membrane. It has been widely used as a specific acidocalcisome marker for subcellular fractionation studies [1–3]. The V-PPase activity assay is based on measuring phosphate (P_i) release using the malachite green assay [13]. Aminomethylenediphosphonate (AMDP) is used to distinguish between vacuolar (sensitive) and soluble (insensitive) PPase activities [14].

1. Prepare phosphate (P_i) standards: 0, 78, 313, 625, and 1250 μM KH_2PO_4.
2. Mix three parts of 0.045% malachite green hydrochloride (MG) and one part of 4.2% ammonium molybdate (AM) (3:1) at RT for at least 20 min and then pass through Whatman No. 5 filter paper.
3. Dilute fraction aliquots to 0.1 μg protein/μl (*see* **Note 18**).
4. Add 5 μl of each P_i standard (duplicated) or each diluted fraction aliquot (in triplicate) into 96-well microplate.
5. Mix reactions by adding 100 μl of PPase reaction buffer only (blank control) or the reaction buffer containing 100 μM PP_i, with or without 40 μM AMDP, using a multichannel pipette.
6. Incubate at 30 °C for 10 min in microplate incubator shaker.
7. Stop the reaction by adding 95 μl of freshly prepared malachite dye solution (MG-AM).
8. Immediately measure the absorbance (A) at 660 nm in microplate reader.
9. Determine the amount of P_i released by comparison with a standard curve, after subtracting blank control values.
10. Calculate the specific activity of V-PPase as μmol P_i released/min/mg of protein (*see* **Note 19**).

3.4.2 Succinate-Cytochrome c Reductase

Succinate-cytochrome *c* reductase (SCR) catalyzes the electron transfer reaction from succinate to cytochrome *c* and involves several oxidation-reduction components in the mitochondrial electron transport chain. The SCR is widely used as a marker of the abundance of mitochondria within a tissue/cell. The enzyme activity of SCR is measured using succinate and cytochrome *c* as the substrates based on the method of Sottocasa et al. [15].

1. Wash fraction aliquots twice and resuspend with IB without DTT (*see* **Note 20**).
2. Add 10 μl of fraction aliquot (in triplicate) into 96-well microplate.
3. Mix the reactions by adding 90 μl of the SCR reaction medium containing 3 mM succinate (pH 7.2), 0.1 mM cytochrome *c*, 0.3 mM KCN, and 40 mM Hepes-KOH pH 7.5. The reaction is started by the addition of the substrate (cytochrome *c*).
4. Incubate at 30 °C for 10 min in microplate incubator shaker.
5. Monitor the increase in the absorbance (A) at 550 nm at every 2 min intervals in the microplate reader. The amount of enzyme resulting in a change in A_{550} of 0.001/min is considered as 1 unit of enzyme.
6. Calculate the activity of SCR as units/mg of protein.

3.4.3 Hexokinase

Hexokinase (HK) is an important glycolytic enzyme in the glycosomes. This enzyme utilizes ATP as phosphoryl donor to catalyze the conversion of D-glucose to glucose 6-phosphate, which is then oxidized to 6-phosphogluconate in the presence of oxidized nicotinamide adenine dinucleotide phosphate ($NADP^+$) by glucose-6-phosphate dehydrogenase (G6PDH). The activity of the glycosomal marker HK is measured spectrophotometrically by following the NADPH formation as an increase of absorbance at 340 nm by coupling the reaction to G6PDH as described previously [16].

1. Prepare HK positive controls for standard curve: 0.1–1.0 units/ml of HK.
2. Add 10 μl of each HK standard or each fraction aliquot (in triplicate) into 96-well microplate.
3. Mix the reactions by adding 90 μl of the HK reaction medium containing 10 mM D-glucose, 0.6 mM ATP, 0.6 mM $NADP^+$, 10 mM $MgCl_2$, 2.5 units/ml glucose-6-phosphate dehydrogenase, and 50 mM Hepes-KOH, pH 7.8. The reaction is started by the addition of ATP.
4. Incubate the reactions at 30 °C for 5 min in microplate incubator shaker.
5. Measure the absorbance (A) at 340 nm in microplate reader.

6. Determine the HK activities by comparison with the standard curve (HK positive controls). One unit of HK is defined as the phosphorylation of 1 μmol of D-glucose/min at pH 7.8 at 30 °C.
7. Calculate the activity of HK as units/mg of protein.

3.4.4 Alpha-Mannosidase

Alpha-mannosidase (AMA) catalyzes the cleavage of the α-form of mannose. This enzyme assists in the breakdown of complex sugars from glycoproteins within the lysosome. The activity of the lysosomal marker AMA is measured spectrophotometrically at 405 nm based on the release of 4-nitrophenol from the synthetic substrate *p*-nitrophenyl-α-D-mannopyranoside (pNP-Man) as described previously [17].

1. Prepare *p*-nitrophenol standards: 0, 25, 75, and 125 μM nitrophenol.
2. Add 10 μl of each fraction aliquot (in triplicate) or IB (blank control) into 96-well microplate.
3. Mix the reactions by adding 90 μl of the AMA reaction medium containing 200 mM sodium acetate buffer (pH 4.6) and 0.6 mM pNP-Man.
4. Incubate the reactions at 30 °C for 30 min in microplate incubator shaker.
5. Stop the reaction by adding 160 μl of 1 M Na_2CO_3.
6. Measure the absorbance (A) at 405 nm in microplate reader.
7. Determine the amount of *p*-nitrophenol released by comparison with a standard curve, after subtracting blank control values. One unit of AMA is defined as the amount of enzyme that releases 1 μmol of *p*-nitrophenol/min at 30 °C and pH 4.6.
8. Calculate the activity of AMA as μmol *p*-nitrophenol released/min × mg protein.

3.5 Western Blot Analyses

Detect the presence of organelle marker proteins in the 15,000 × *g* pellet (P1), the first gradient pellet (P2) and the fractions (F1–F7) of the second gradient by immunoblotting (Fig. 3). Carry out all procedures at RT, unless otherwise specified.

1. Lyse the aliquots of pellets or fractions with RIPA buffer containing protease inhibitor tablet in ice for 1 h.
2. Mix the lysed fractions with 2× Laemmli sample buffer at 1:1 ratio (v/v) and directly load.
3. Transfer the separated proteins onto nitrocellulose membranes using a Trans-Blot apparatus.

4. Block the membranes with 10% nonfat milk in PBS containing 0.5% Tween-20 (PBS-T) at 4 °C overnight.
5. Incubate the blots with antibodies against proteins localized to acidocalcisomes (TbVP1) [18], mitochondria (voltage-dependent anion channel, TbVDAC) [19], glycosomes (pyruvate, phosphate dikinase, TbPPDK) [20], and lysosomes (Tbp67) [21] for 1 h (*see* **Note 21**).
6. After five washings with PBS-T, incubate the blots with horse-radish peroxidase conjugated anti-mouse or anti-rabbit IgG (H + L) antibody at a dilution of 1:20,000 for 1 h.
7. After washing five times with PBS-T, visualize the immuno-blots using Pierce ECL Western blotting substrate according to the manufacturer's instructions.

4 Notes

1. Warm BAG to RT before use, because washing trypanosomes with cold BAG could cause cell lysis or cell aggregation/cell clump formation.
2. Isolation buffer (IB) is also known as lysis buffer (LB) or homogenization buffer (HB), whose osmolality is approximately 300 mOsm.
3. Add DTT and 1× protease inhibitor cocktails just before use.
4. The preparation of the working solution, as described, ensures that the concentrations of KCl, $MgCl_2$, EDTA, DTT, and the buffer (Hepes-KOH, pH 7.2) are constant throughout the gradient.
5. Good fixation requires fresh glutaraldehyde and paraformaldehyde.
6. KCN is highly toxic. Wear a mask to prepare it under fume hood, and avoid skin contact and inhalation.
7. For proteins larger than 80 kDa or membrane proteins, we recommend that SDS be included at a final concentration of 0.01%.
8. Mix the cell pellet (approximately 3–4 g wet weight) with 1.5× wet weight silicon carbide, transfer it to a precooled mortar (−20 °C) using a stainless-steel lab spoon spatula, and then grind with a mortar and pestle on ice until lysis is greater than 99% (generally 45–60 s). Always monitor the efficacy of the grinding or lysis by phase contrast microscopy.
9. Rinse the grinding tools with IB to recover most of the cell-lysates, and also resuspend the lysate-silicon mixtures twice with IB to recover more supernatant, in which acidocalcisome are floating with other organelles.

10. Suspension and homogenization of the pellet should be carried out on ice as gently as possible to avoid damage not only to the target organelles (acidocalcisomes) but also to any other organelles present, particularly those that may release degradative enzymes. In addition, homogenize by approximately six stokes of the pestle (50–70 rpm) using a tissue homogenizer mixer. Aliquots from the homogenizations of the 15,000 × *g* pellet (P1) and the first gradient pellet (P2) are also taken and used for enzymatic assays and Western blot analyses (Table 1, Fig. 3).
11. Glass tubes are better for making up density gradient solutions than plastic tubes. Prepare 4 ml of 20, 24, 28, 34, 37, and 40% (w/v) iodixanol gradient solutions in 10 ml glass tubes, by adding 1.60, 1.92, 2.24, 2.72, 2.96, or 3.20 ml of 50% (w/v) iodixanol working solution to each tube, respectively, supplementing with 166, 200, 233, 283, 308, or 333 μl of 1 M sucrose to maintain each gradient solution isosmotic, and finally add isolation buffer to 4 ml in total, except for the 34% iodixanol gradient (which is mixed with the homogenized pellet in IB). Mix the gradient solutions well and store on ice for the gradient loading.
12. Although overlaying starting from the bottom of an ultracentrifuge tube with the densest layer is the most popular means of creating a discontinuous gradient, underlaying (i.e., starting from the bottom of an ultracentrifuge tube with the least dense layer) using a Pasteur glass pipette with cotton and a pipette aid is easier, more reliable and the recommended method for making discontinuous gradients. The only important requirement is that no air bubbles are introduced which may disturb the lower density layer above, for this reason it requires some practice to maintain a steady liquid flow by pressing the release button slowly.
13. Label the centrifuge tubes and balance exactly.
14. Although a Pasteur pipette or syringe can be used to collect fractions from the top of the ultracentrifuge tube, we prefer using the tip of the pipette to aspirate fractions from the top very slowly, moving it across the diameter of the tube and minimizing the aspiration of any liquid from below the fraction or band.
15. Although iodixanol does not interfere with most downstream analyses (such as SDS-PAGE and enzymatic assays), removal of iodixanol is an absolute requirement for electron microscopy. On the other hand, if it is necessary to concentrate the gradient fractions, TCA precipitation of the proteins is recommended.

16. Bradford and BCA assays are very commonly used protein estimation methods. Bradford is fast because there is 5 min incubation time whereas for BCA its 30 min. In the case of BCA, it is recommended to use a volume of 10–25 μl, which is quite larger than required for Bradford. However, Bradford is less compatible with detergents (such as 1% SDS) than BCA. Since the aliquots of fractions (containing membrane proteins) are lysed with RIPA buffer, we dilute the lysed fractions with IB to reduce the concentration of the RIPA detergents for determination of the protein concentration by Bradford assay.
17. The enzyme activities of succinate-cytochrome *c* reductase (SCR), hexokinase (HK), and α-mannosidase (AMA) are not affected by storage at −80 °C for 2 weeks. However, freezing and storage significantly reduce V-PPase activity, so we recommend that the V-PPase activities of the gradient fractions be assayed just right after the subcellular fractionation.
18. If the protein concentration is below 0.1 μg/μl, concentrate the fraction by TCA first or directly add 5 μl of fraction for assays and finally calculate the enzyme activities based on the original protein concentrations.
19. Calculate the activity of V-PPase as follows: [ΔP_i released (μM) × n]/[incubation time (min) × protein (μg/μl)] = $\Delta P_i \times 0.04$ (μmol/min × mg). The net amount (μM) of P_i released by specific V-PPase (ΔP_i) is obtained by subtracting the value of the (PP_i + AMDP) reaction from that of the PP_i reaction. The incubation time is 10 min. The protein concentration is 0.1 μg/μl, and the dilution factor (n) is 40.
20. Because DTT interferes with SCR activity, we wash the fraction aliquots with IB without DTT before the SCR assay to minimize the interference.
21. Incubate the blots with rabbit antibodies against TbVP1 (1:5000), rabbit antibodies against TbVDAC (1:2000), mouse antibodies against TbPPDK (1:200), and mouse antibodies against Tbp67 (1:3000) at RT for 1 h.

Acknowledgments

We thank Norbert Bakalara for the anti-TbVP1 antibody, Minu Chaudhuri for anti-TbVDAC antibody, Frédéric Bringaud for anti-TbPPDK antibody, James Bangs for anti-Tbp67 antibody, Michael Martin for the AMDP, and Mary Ard and Georgia Electron Microscopy (GEM) facility for assistance with TEM sample preparation and imaging. Work was funded by a grant from the US National Institutes of Health (AI-077358 to R.D.)

References

1. Docampo R, de Souza W, Miranda K, Rohloff P, Moreno SNJ (2005) Acidocalcisomes-conserved from bacteria to man. Nat Rev Microbiol 3:251–261
2. Docampo R, Huang G (2016) Acidocalcisomes of eukaryotes. Curr Opin Cell Biol 41:66–72
3. Huang G, Ulrich PN, Storey M, Johnson D, Tischer J, Tovar JA, Moreno SNJ, Orlando R, Docampo R (2014) Proteomic analysis of the acidocalcisome, an organelle conserved from bacteria to human cells. PLoS Pathog 10: e1004555
4. Huang G, Bartlett PJ, Thomas AP, Moreno SNJ, Docampo R (2013) Acidocalcisomes of *Trypanosoma brucei* have an inositol 1,4,5-trisphosphate receptor that is required for growth and infectivity. Proc Natl Acad Sci U S A 110:1887–1892
5. De Souza W, Morgado-Diaz JA, Cunha-e-Silva NL (2008) Cell fractionation of parasitic protozoa. In: Posch A (ed) 2D PAGE: sample preparation and fractionation. Methods in molecular biology, vol 425. Humana, Totowa, NJ, pp 313–331
6. Jardim A, Hardie DB, Boitz J, Borchers CH (2018) Proteomic profiling of *Leishmania donovani* promastigote subcellular organelles. J Proteome Res 17(3):1194–1215
7. Scott DA, Docampo R, Dvorak JA, Shi S, Leapman RD (1997) In situ composition analysis of acidocalcisomes *Trypanosoma cruzi*. J Biol Chem 272:28020–28029
8. Scott DA, Docampo R (2000) Characterization of isolated acidocalcisomes of *Trypanosoma cruzi*. J Biol Chem 275:24215–24221
9. Ferella M, Nilsson D, Darban H, Rodrigues C, Bontempi EJ, Docampo R, Andersson B (2008) Proteomics in *Trypanosoma cruzi* – localization of novel proteins to various organelles. Proteomics 8:2735–2749
10. Graham J, Ford T, Rickwood D (1994) The preparation of subcellular organelles from mouse liver in self-generated gradients of iodixanol. Anal Biochem 220:367–373
11. Cunningham I (1977) New culture medium for maintenance of tsetse tissues and growth of trypanosomatids. J Protozool 24:325–329
12. Kuo J (ed) (2007) Electron microscopy: methods and protocols (2nd edition). Methods in molecular biology, vol 369. Humana, Totowa, NJ
13. Lanzetta PA, Alvarez LJ, Reinach PS, Candia OA (1979) An improved assay for nanomole amounts of inorganic phosphate. Anal Biochem 100:95–97
14. Zhen R, Baykov AA, Bahuleva NP, Rea PA (1994) Aminomethylenediphosphonate: a potent type-specific inhibitor of both plant and phototrophic bacterial H^+-pyrophosphatases. Plant Physiol 104:153–159
15. Sottocasa GL, Kuylenstierna B, Ernster L, Bergstrand A (1967) An electron-transport system associated with the outer membrane of liver mitochondria. A biochemical and morphological study. J Cell Biol 32:415–438
16. Cannata JJ, Valle E, Docampo R, Cazzulo JJ (1982) Subcellular localization of phosphoenolpyruvate carboxykinase in the trypanosomatids *Trypanosoma cruzi* and *Crithidia fasciculata*. Mol Biochem Parasitol 6:151–160
17. Liao YF, Lal A, Moremen KW (1996) Cloning, expression, purification, and characterization of the human broad specificity lysosomal acid alpha-mannosidase. J Biol Chem 271:28348–28358
18. Lemercier G, Dutoya S, Luo S, Ruiz FA, Rodrigues CO, Baltz T, Docampo R, Bakalara N (2002) A vacuolar-type H^+-pyrophosphatase governs maintenance of functional acidocalcisomes and growth of the insect and mammalian forms of *Trypanosoma brucei*. J Biol Chem 277:37369–37376
19. Singha UK, Sharma S, Chaudhuri M (2009) Downregulation of mitochondrial porin inhibits cell growth and alters respiratory phenotype in *Trypanosoma brucei*. Eukaryot Cell 8:1418–1428
20. Bringaud F, Baltz D, Baltz T (1998) Functional and molecular characterization of a glycosomal PPi-dependent enzyme in trypanosomatids: pyruvate, phosphate dikinase. Proc Natl Acad Sci U S A 95:7963–7968
21. Alexander DL, Schwartz KJ, Balber AE, Bangs JD (2002) Developmentally regulated trafficking of the lysosomal membrane protein p67 in *Trypanosoma brucei*. J Cell Sci 115:3253–3263

Chapter 41

Metabolic Control Analysis for Drug Target Prioritization in Trypanosomatids

Zabdi González-Chávez, Citlali Vázquez, Rafael Moreno-Sánchez, and Emma Saavedra

Abstract

To validate therapeutic targets in metabolic pathways of trypanosomatids, the criterion of enzyme essentiality determined by gene knockout or knockdown is usually being applied. Since, it is often found that most of the enzymes/proteins analyzed are essential, additional criteria have to be implemented for drug target prioritization. Metabolic control analysis (MCA), often in conjunction with kinetic pathway modeling, offers such possibility for prioritization. MCA is a theoretical and experimental approach to analyze how metabolic pathways are controlled. It involves strategies to perform quantitative analyses to determine the degree in which an enzyme controls a pathway flux, a value called flux control coefficient ($C^J_{a_i}$). By determining the $C^J_{a_i}$ of individual steps in a metabolic pathway, the distribution of control of the pathway is established, that is, the identification of the main flux-controlling steps. Therefore, MCA can help in ranking pathway enzymes as drug targets from a metabolic perspective. In this chapter, three approaches to determine $C^J_{a_i}$ are reviewed: (1) In vitro pathway reconstitution, (2) manipulation of enzyme activities within parasites, and (3) in silico kinetic modeling of the metabolic pathway. To perform these methods, accurate experimental data of enzyme activities, metabolite concentrations and pathway fluxes are necessary. The methodology is illustrated with the example of trypanothione metabolism of *Trypanosoma cruzi* and protocols to determine such experimental data for this metabolic process are also described. However, the MCA strategy can be applied to any metabolic pathway in the parasite and general directions to perform it are provided in this chapter.

Key words Metabolic control analysis, Trypanothione, Flux control coefficient, Pathway modeling, γ-Glutamylcysteine synthetase, Trypanothione synthetase, Trypanothione reductase, Tryparedoxin, Tryparedoxin peroxidase

1 Introduction

Identification and validation of enzymes/transporters as drug targets in metabolic pathways of trypanosomatids is not an easy task [1, 2]. Some of the early criteria used for selecting drug targets have been the identification of (1) unique enzymes in the parasite with no counterpart in the host cell, and (2) steps (enzymes/transporters) that have been described as "rate-limiting" in other cellular

Paul A. M. Michels et al. (eds.), *Trypanosomatids: Methods and Protocols*, Methods in Molecular Biology, vol. 2116, https://doi.org/10.1007/978-1-0716-0294-2_41,

systems. Modern strategies rely on the manipulation of the enzyme activities in the parasites through genetic strategies such as knocking out or down the respective genes with screening for consequent negative phenotypes in the parasite physiology. The development of RNAi libraries at genome scale [3] can exponentially increase the number of essential genes identified. Advances in this regard using such genetic approaches have been reported for *Trypanosoma brucei* and *Leishmania* [3, 4]; they have, nevertheless, been difficult to apply to other trypanosomatids such as *Trypanosoma cruzi*, for which the developments of genetic strategies are less advanced.

A limitation of the genetic approach for the identification of drug targets in trypanosomatids is that most of the manipulated enzymes were found to be essential for the parasite function analyzed, particularly when there are no redundant enzymes (*see* for instance [5, 6]). This situation inevitably leads to a number of drug targets similar to that of the pathway enzymes/transporters. Therefore, additional criteria besides genetic essentiality have to be applied to rank the most convenient drug targets in metabolic pathways of parasites. In that regard, a traffic light system of several criteria for proteins to be considered molecular targets for drug intervention has been proposed, which besides essentiality includes druggability, assayability, resistance potential, toxicity potential, and structural information [1]. However, the role that each step has in controlling the flux and intermediary concentrations of its metabolic pathway should also be regarded as a major criterion for drug target prioritization.

Metabolic control analysis (MCA) provides a theoretical and experimental approach to perform quantitative analyses for identifying the most flux-controlling enzymes/transporters in metabolic pathways (*see* for a description of its basic concepts [7], for a review [8], for a specialized book [9]). From this perspective, the steps with the highest control under a variety of physiological conditions can be proposed as the most convenient drug targets for therapeutic intervention against parasites [10, 11]. Through MCA it is possible to quantify the degree of control that each step has to setting the flux through a metabolic pathway; its quantitative expression is called flux control coefficient ($C^J_{a_i}$), in which J is the steady state pathway flux and a is the activity of the pathway enzyme i. The sum of the $C^J_{a_i}$ of all pathway steps must add up to one ("summation theorem"). The experimental results of MCA analyses in several cell types have demonstrated that the control of pathway fluxes is indeed shared in different degrees among all steps, but usually there are two or three steps with the highest control. Furthermore, the $C^J_{a_i}$ values can be somewhat modified depending on the metabolic circumstances. Therefore, the concept of a unique and fixed rate-limiting step in metabolic pathways is misleading and has to be disregarded.

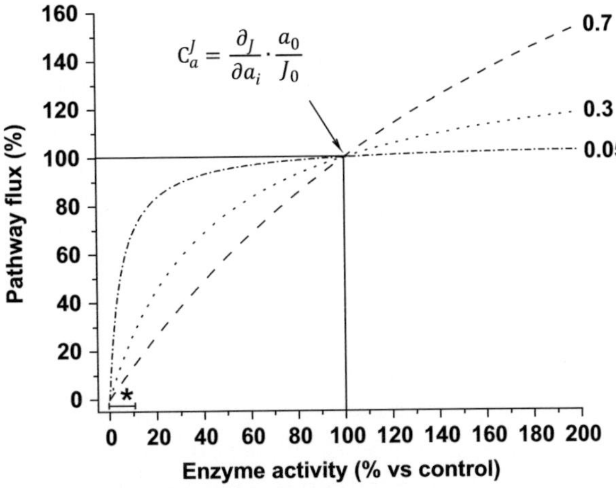

Fig. 1 Determination of flux control coefficients. Plot of normalized pathway flux *versus* enzyme activity for three different enzymes with distinct $C^J_{a_i}$. The $C^J_{a_i}$ is calculated from the slope of the tangent to the curve at 100% enzyme activity. (*Asterisk*) Usual range of residual activity achieved by downregulation of enzyme expression in parasites through genetic methods such as RNA interference

The $C^J_{a_i}$ is determined from the slope of the tangent to a curve (*i.e.*, the derivative $\partial J/\partial a_i$) of a plot of pathway flux *versus* enzyme activity, multiplied by a scalar factor (a_{io}/J_o) of the enzyme activity and pathway flux at the reference metabolic state (Eq. 1) (Fig. 1).

$$C^J_{a_i} = \frac{\partial J}{\partial a_i} \cdot \frac{a_{i_0}}{J_o} \quad (1)$$

To determine the $C^J_{a_i}$, a gradual, individual, and specific (without affecting other pathway steps) titration of the activity of a pathway step (independent variable *x*) has to be carried out, and in parallel the changes in the pathway flux (dependent variable *y*) are measured. By normalizing to the reference metabolic state of enzyme activity and flux (which for drug target validation is the basal level of enzyme activity in the cell), plots such as in Fig. 1 are built and the $C^J_{a_i}$ estimated from the slope of the tangent at the value of 100%. Only by performing simultaneous analyses for all pathway steps, the most controlling enzymes can be identified. In the plot of Fig. 1 it can be seen that relatively low (and probably realistic) percentages of inhibition around 100% enzyme activity (the wild-type level) of a high controlling enzyme may be sufficient to decrease the pathway flux, whereas high (and maybe unrealistic) levels of inhibition are necessary for a low controlling one to achieve the same effect. Furthermore, at high levels of enzyme inhibition (~90%), as those achieved by genetic methods, the pathway flux decreases regardless of the enzymes' $C^J_{a_i}$, which may explain why all pathway steps have proved to be essential. It has to be emphasized that no parameter is as important to influence the

$C^J_{a_i}$, as the actual enzyme activities ($V_{max} = k_{cat} \times [\text{Enzyme}]_{total}$) within the parasites; protein contents or V_{max} of purified enzymes are inadequate descriptors since they do not accurately reflect the physiological content of the active enzyme, which can further vary due to posttranslational and covalent modulation of the enzyme.

The plot of Fig. 1, although simple in concept, requires the design of special experimental strategies for $C^J_{a_i}$ determination. An overview of different approaches can be consulted in [8, 11]. In this chapter, three strategies for determining the $C^J_{a_i}$ are described: (1) in vitro pathway reconstitution with recombinant purified enzymes; (2) manipulation of enzyme activities in the parasites by transgenic techniques; and (3) in silico kinetic pathway modeling. Other strategies such as the use of highly specific inhibitors against each pathway step; or elasticity analysis, which can be performed in live cells without the need of specific inhibitors, genetic manipulation, or knowledge about enzyme kinetic data, require manipulation of the steady-state pathway intermediates (*see* [11]). The examples given in this chapter refer to the determination of the $C^J_{a_i}$ of the enzymes in the trypanothione {$T(SH)_2$} metabolism of *Trypanosoma cruzi* (Figs. 2a and 3a) [5], but the MCA approach can be applied to any metabolic pathway also in other trypanosomatids or any cell or organism of interest and general directions to perform it are provided throughout the sections.

1.1 Determination of $C^J_{a_i}$ by In Vitro Pathway Reconstitution

1.1.1 Example: $T(SH)_2$-Dependent Hydroperoxide Reduction Pathway from *T. cruzi*

This approach (Subheadings 2.1–2.4 and 3.1.1–3.5; Fig. 2) is based on the in vitro reconstitution of segments of the metabolic pathway using purified enzymes. This strategy was previously applied for segments of glycolysis due to the availability of commercial purified enzymes from mammalian sources [12, 13] or recombinant enzymes from the parasite *Entamoeba histolytica* [14]. Nowadays, it is also feasible to obtain purified recombinant enzymes of trypanosomatids from any metabolic pathway. The in vitro pathway reconstitution must simulate as much as possible the in vivo conditions of the pathway within the parasites regarding (1) the ratio of enzyme activities present in the parasite, for which their actual V_{max} values have to be determined at the physiological intracellular pH and growth temperature of the parasite, and (2) the physiological concentrations of substrates and coenzymes.

In case of the hydroperoxide reduction flux in *T. cruzi* (Fig. 2a) the pathway reconstitution is performed with trypanothione reductase (TryR), tryparedoxin (TXN), and tryparedoxin peroxidase (TXNPx) and the experimental conditions of physiological intracellular pH (7.4 for epimastigotes) and environment temperature of the trypomastigotes (37 °C), the infective form in mammalian cells. The hydroperoxide reduction flux is monitored by following the NADPH oxidation. In this setting, it has to be considered that (1) the pathway flux values determined represent the maximal fluxes of peroxide reduction with the amount of the enzymes

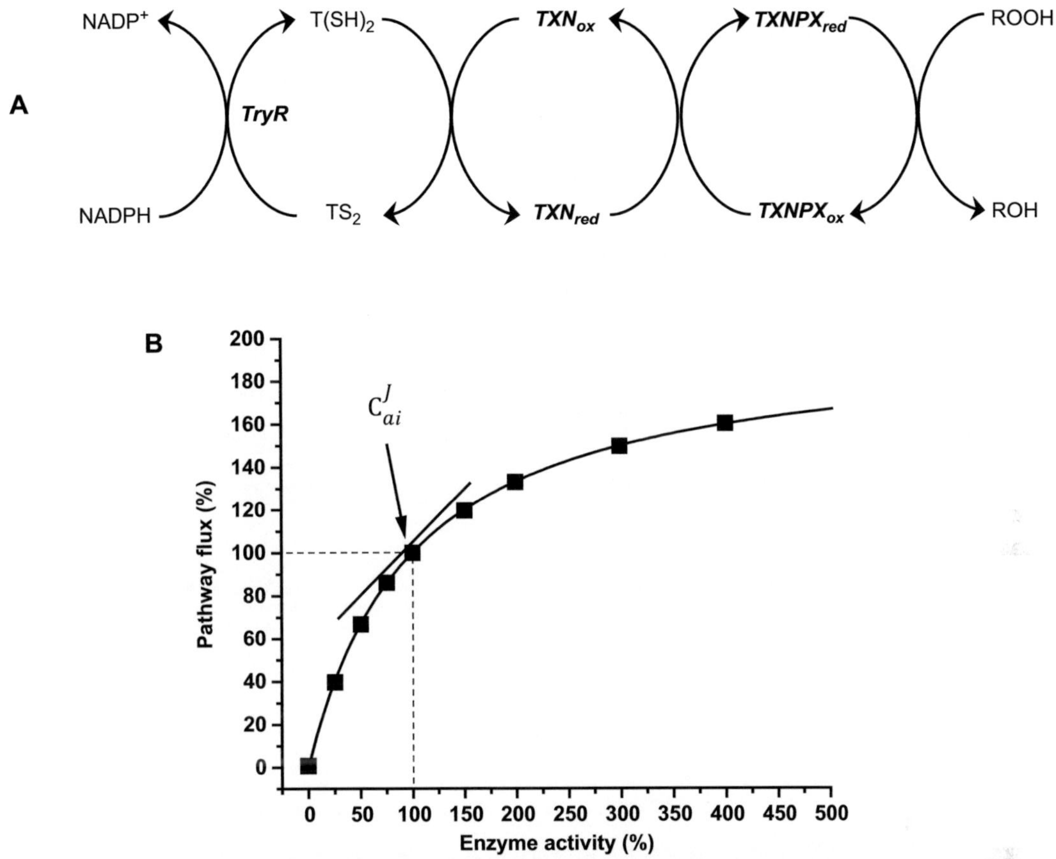

Fig. 2 $C^J_{a_i}$ determination by in vitro reconstitution of the trypanothione-dependent hydroperoxide reduction pathway. (**a**) Hydroperoxide reduction pathway in trypanosomatids. The reductive equivalents are transferred from $T(SH)_2$ to tryparedoxin (TXN) and then to tryparedoxin peroxidase (TXNPx) for peroxide reduction; in parallel, oxidized trypanothione is reduced by trypanothione reductase (TryR). (**b**) Simulated titration curve by pathway reconstitution for $C^J_{a_i}$ determination. Activity of one enzyme is varied from 25% to 400% by adding different concentrations of the purified recombinant enzyme, while the other pathway system components (partner enzymes, substrates, and cofactors) are maintained at the physiological basal (control) level. The changes in pathway flux are determined. A simulation for an enzyme with $C^J_{a_i} = 0.5$ curve is shown, which value is calculated from the slope of the tangent to the curve at 100% enzyme activity

used, because substrates (NADPH, trypanothione, and cumene hydroperoxide (CumOOH)) are at saturating concentrations, and (2) in the in vitro system, some physiological regulatory interactions may be lost. The titration curve of enzyme activity *versus* pathway flux (Fig. 1) has to be constructed by varying the activity of one enzyme at a time while keeping the rest of the system (partner enzymes, substrates, and cofactors) unaltered and in parallel, determining changes in the pathway flux. The TryR, TXN, and TXNPx activities determined for *T. cruzi* epimastigotes are 264, 88, and 177 mU, respectively [15]. Thus, a working reference enzyme ratio of 3:1:2 is used. Enzyme titrations are performed above and below the reference activity found in the parasites.

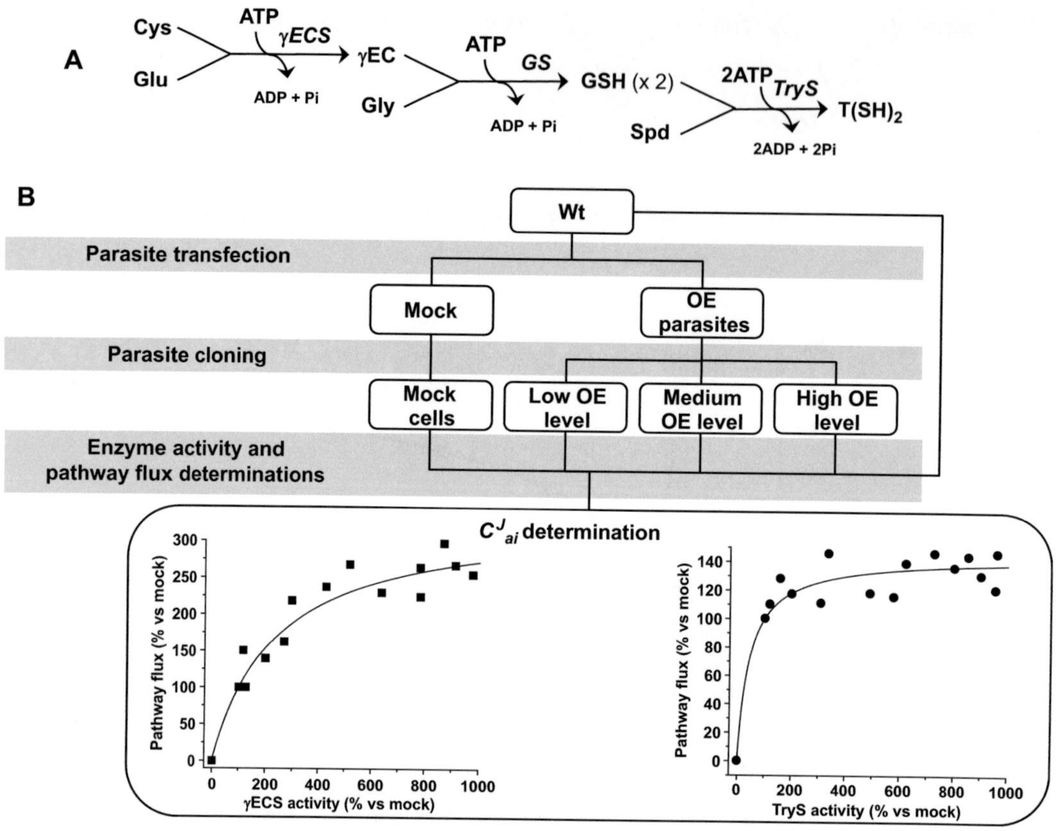

Fig. 3 $C^J_{a_i}$ determination by manipulation of the trypanothione synthesis enzymes in the parasites. (**a**) $T(SH)_2$ synthesis pathway. $T(SH)_2$ is a conjugate of two glutathione (GSH) molecules linked to a spermidine (Spd). Synthesis of $T(SH)_2$ from their precursors is catalyzed by gamma-glutamylcysteine synthetase (γECS), glutathione synthetase (GS) and trypanothione synthetase (TryS), whereas Spd is scavenged from the medium (*T. cruzi*) or de novo synthesized from putrescine (*T. cruzi*) or from ornithine (*T. brucei* and *Leishmania* spp.). $T(SH)_2$ donates its electrons to the peroxide reduction system and is regenerated by TryR (Fig. 2a). (**b**) Experimental design for $C^J_{a_i}$ determination by using overexpressing (OE) clones with different activity levels (low, medium, and high) of the enzymes involved in the $T(SH)_2$ synthesis pathway in parasites. Two titration curves for different enzymes are exemplified

1.2 Determination of $C^J_{a_i}$ by Manipulation of Enzyme Activities in Parasites

1.2.1 Example: Ex vivo $T(SH)_2$ Synthesis Pathway Flux Control Distribution

To determine the $C^J_{a_i}$ that gamma-glutamylcysteine synthetase (γECS) and trypanothione synthetase (TryS) have on the $T(SH)_2$ synthesis flux (Fig. 3a), their wild-type expression is manipulated in the parasites by transfection with plasmids to vary its enzymes activity level, and then determining their effect on the pathway flux (Subheadings 2.5–2.9, Subheadings 3.7–3.12; Fig. 3). Since the basal activities of these enzymes are low in *T. cruzi* and other trypanosomatids [16, 17], variation in their activities in the epimastigotes is performed by overexpressing them, one at a time, and selecting clones with different degrees of enzyme activity (Fig. 3b). Furthermore, $T(SH)_2$ is not a pathway end-product but metabolic intermediate, and its total intracellular pool ($T(SH)_2$ + TS_2) is in a dynamic balance between its synthesis, usage, expulsion, and degradation. Hence, determination of this pathway flux in intact cells requires more sophisticated techniques such as "fluxomics" with radioactive labeling coupled to HPLC-MS, which may be of difficult access to common laboratories. To circumvent this problem, the pathway flux is determined ex vivo using cell extracts or permeabilized cells serving as source of the native enzyme activities expressed in the parasite; then, the flux is determined by feeding the pathway with its precursors at saturating concentrations. For the $T(SH)_2$ synthesis pathway the precursors are cysteine, glutamate, glycine, spermidine (Spd), and ATP. Pyruvate kinase and phosphoenolpyruvate (PEP) are also required in the assay to maintain high and constant the ATP concentration, due to the usual presence of a high spurious ATP-consuming activity in cell extracts. The increases in $T(SH)_2$ in parasite extracts of clones with different levels of enzyme expression are determined by HPLC. In this setting, it has to be considered that (1) the pathway flux values determined represent the maximal fluxes of synthesis with the enzymes expressed in the cell sample and (2) that in the ex vivo system, some physiological regulatory interactions can be lost.

1.3 Determination of $C^J_{a_i}$ by Kinetic Modeling of Metabolic Pathways

1.3.1 Example: Kinetic Model of Trypanothione Metabolism in *T. cruzi*

The $C^J_{a_i}$ can also be determined by kinetic modeling of metabolic pathways (Subheadings 2.10–2.15 and 3.13.1; Fig. 4), a type of mechanistic modeling developed in systems biology [18–20]. Kinetic modeling of metabolic pathways in trypanosomatids has been proposed and applied for drug target prioritization (reviewed in [11, 21]. Kinetic models of metabolic pathways are constructed by using detailed kinetic properties of their enzymes/transporters as well as thermodynamics of their reactions; hence, comprehensive experimental datasets are required to build the metabolic model. Due to the complexity of the approach, only an outline is provided in this chapter and it is recommended to attend specialized courses. A general flowchart to obtain the dataset to build and validate a metabolic pathway model is shown in Fig. 4.

2 Materials

2.1 Enzyme Activity of Recombinant Enzymes

1. Preparations of purified and quantified TryR, TXN, and TXNPx are required (*see* **Note 1**).
2. EDTA solution: 0.5 M EDTA pH 8.0. Weigh 7.3 g EDTA disodium salt dihydrate and add 30 mL distilled water. EDTA is not soluble at low pH. To adjust the EDTA stock solution to pH 8.0, add NaOH pearls under strong stirring, taking care not to exceed pH 8.0. Adjust volume to 50 mL. Store at room temperature.

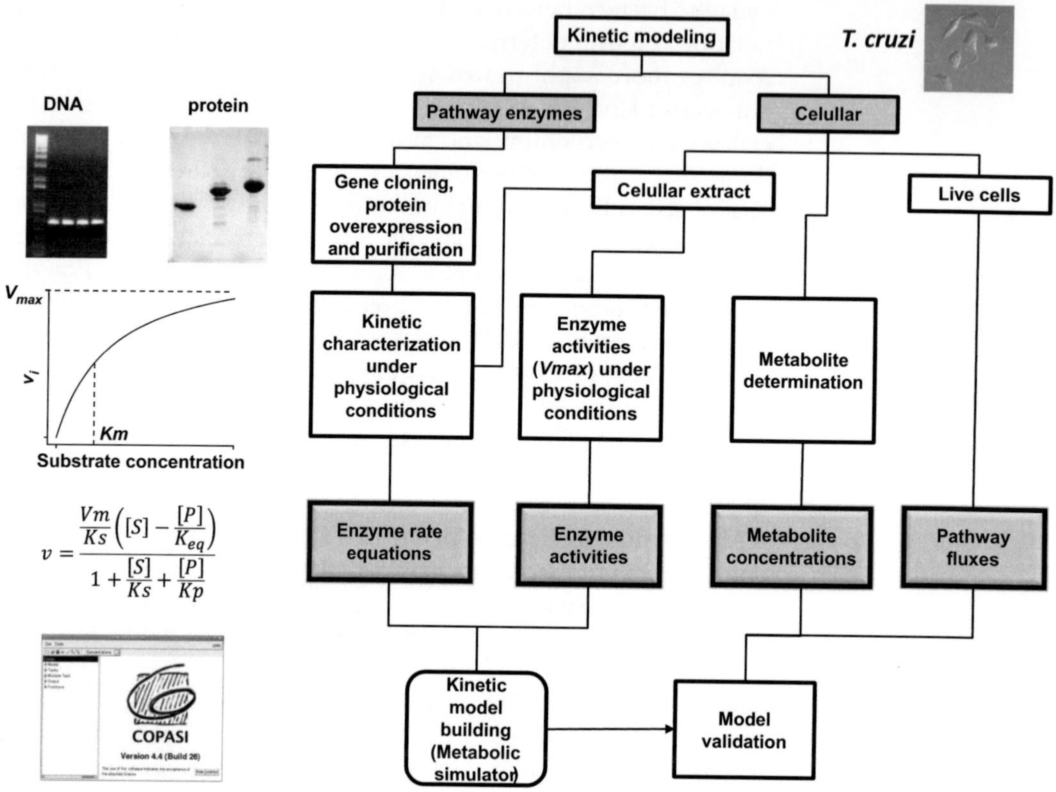

Fig. 4 Workflow chart to construct a kinetic model of a metabolic pathway. For model construction different data are required: (1) dataset of enzyme rate equations, which contains the kinetic parameters of all pathway enzymes/transporters determined using purified (recombinant) enzymes or in cell extracts. (2) Dataset of V_{max} within the parasites, which represents the content of each active enzyme and therefore functional enzyme/transporter. (3) A computer's software for model construction and simulation such as COPASI. (4) Dataset of steady-state pathway intermediates concentrations. (5) Experimental dataset of steady-state pathway fluxes to compare with predictions from model simulations to validate the model. Usually an extensive iterative process of computer simulation and wet experimentation is necessary to obtain a model that can closely simulate the metabolite and fluxes determined in the parasites

3. Assay buffer A: 40 mM Hepes, 1 mM EDTA, pH 7.4. Dissolve 5.2 g Hepes-sodium salt in 450 mL of distilled water, add 1 mL of the EDTA solution prepared in **item 2**, mix and adjust pH to 7.4 with HCl. Adjust volume to 500 mL with distilled water, sterilize by autoclave, and store at 4 °C.
4. Assay buffer for TXNPx: 40 mM Hepes, 1 mM EDTA, pH 7.4, 10% dimethyl sulfoxide (DMSO). Mix 1 mL DMSO with 9 mL of Assay buffer A.
5. Trypanothione solution: trypanothione can be synthesized and purified as in [22] and later lyophilized. With this protocol, a solution of approximately 3 mL yields a mix of reduced trypanothione [T(SH)$_2$] + trypanothione disulfide [TS$_2$] of about 100 mM (*see* **Note 2**).

6. Trypanothione oxidation buffer: 50 mM ammonium acetate, pH 8.0. Dissolve 1.9 g ammonium acetate in 450 mL of distilled water, mix and adjust pH with NaOH. Adjust volume to 500 mL with distilled water and store at 4 °C until use.
7. TS_2 solution (*see* **Note 3**). Once the total concentration of trypanothione $\{T(SH)_2 + TS_2\}$ is determined from the trypanothione solution, synthesized as in **item 5**, transfer enough volume to reach 2 mM of total trypanothione into 50 mL of oxidation buffer and add 435 μL of a 23 mM H_2O_2 solution (*see* **Note 4**). Mix and incubate 2 h at room temperature. Store at −20 °C.
8. NADPH solution: 100 mM NADPH. Weigh 33.3 mg NADPH tetrasodium salt and dissolve in 0.4 mL of milli Q water. Store at −20 °C protected from light.
9. Cumene hydroperoxide: 5.4 mM CumOOH: 10 μL of CumOOH (80% stock solution) are diluted in 1 mL milli Q water. From this first CumOOH solution, withdraw 100 μL and adjust volume to 1 mL with milli Q water. These solutions should be always prepared just before performing the experiment.
10. Spectrophotometer: Diode array Cary 60 from Agilent (Santa Clara, CA, USA). A multicell spectrophotometer (8–18 cells) is preferred, with temperature control set at 37 °C.
11. 0.5 mL spectrophotometer UV-grade cuvettes.

2.2 Parasite Cell Extract Preparation

1. *T. cruzi* epimastigotes culture.
2. PMSF solution: 200 mM phenylmethylsulfonyl fluoride (PMSF). Weigh 0.35 g PMSF and dissolve in 10 mL ethanol (70%). Store at −20 °C.
3. DTT solution: 200 mM dithiothreitol (DTT). Weigh 30 mg DTT and dissolve in 1 mL distilled water. Aliquot and store at −20 °C (*see* **Note 5**).
4. Lysis buffer: 20 mM Hepes, 1 mM EDTA, 0.15 mM KCl, 1 mM PMSF, 1 mM DTT. Dissolve 2.6 g Hepes sodium salt in 450 mL of distilled water, add 1 mL EDTA 0.5 M pH 8.0 (solution from Subheading 2.1), mix and adjust to pH 7.4 with HCl. Adjust volume to 500 mL with distilled water. Store at 4 °C. Just before usage take 1 mL of this solution and add 5 μL PMSF and 5 μL DTT prepared as in **items 2** and **3**.
5. Phosphate buffered saline (PBS): 137 mM NaCl, 2.7 mM KCl, 10 mM Na_2HPO_4, 2 mM KH_2PO_4 pH 7.4. Weigh 4 g NaCl, 0.1 g KCl, 0.68 g Na_2HPO_4, and 0.14 g KH_2PO_4. Dissolve in 450 mL of distilled water, mix and adjust pH 7.4 with HCl. Adjust volume to 500 mL with distilled water, sterilize by autoclave, and store at 4 °C.

6. Liquid nitrogen.
7. Water bath at 37 °C.
8. Reagents and solutions to perform quantification of protein concentration using your preferred methodology.

2.3 Enzyme Activity in Parasite Cell Extracts

1. Same materials as in Subheading 2.1.
2. Same materials for cellular extract preparation as in Subheading 2.2.

2.4 Pathway Reconstitution

1. Same materials as in Subheading 2.1.

2.5 Parasite Transfection

1. LIT broth: 0.5% liver infusion, 0.5% tryptose, 0.2% glucose, 0.4% NaCl, 0.04% KCl, 0.42% Na_2HPO_4. Weigh 4.5 g liver infusion, 4.5 g tryptose, 1.8 g glucose, 3.6 g NaCl, 0.36 g KCl, 3.78 g Na_2HPO_4. Prepare up to 900 mL with milli Q water. Sterilize by autoclaving and store at 4 °C.
2. Hemin solution: 12.5 mg hemin/mL. Weigh 1.25 g hemin and dissolve in 100 mL of 0.1 N NaOH. Mix gently for up to 1 h until completely dissolved. Store at 4 °C protected from light.
3. LIT culture medium: 90% LIT broth, 10% fetal bovine serum (FBS), 25 μg/mL hemin, 10 U/mL penicillin, 10 μg/mL streptomycin. Add 100 mL of heat-inactivated FBS to 900 mL of LIT broth, add 2 mL hemin solution, and 10 mL of penicillin/streptomycin stabilized solution (10,000 U penicillin and 10 mg streptomycin/mL stock solution concentration).
4. Plasmids: 100 μg of purified plasmid construction for mock (empty plasmid) and overexpressing γECS or TryS in *T. cruzi* (*see* **Note 6**) contained in 40 μL milli Q water (*see* **Note 7**).
5. Epimastigotes culture: *T. cruzi* Queretaro strain [23].
6. Electroporator and electroporation cuvettes: Square wave electroporation system BTX ECM 830 Harvard apparatus (Holliston, MA, USA); 2 mm gap BTX electroporation cuvettes.

2.6 Selection and Cloning of Transfected Cells

1. Transfected parasites.
2. LIT culture medium as in Subheading 2.5.
3. G418 (50 mg/mL commercial stock solution).

2.7 Parasite Cell Extract Preparation

1. Material required as in Subheading 2.2.

2.8 Enzyme Activities in Parasites

1. $MgCl_2$ solution: 1 M $MgCl_2$. Weigh 2.03 g $MgCl_2$ hexahydrate and dissolve in 10 mL distilled water. Store at −20 °C.
2. Tris solution: 280 mM Tris (hydroxymethyl)aminomethane: Weigh 1.7 mg Tris and dissolve in 50 mL distilled water. Store at 4 °C.
3. Assay buffer B: 100 mM Hepes pH 7.4, 100 mM KCl, 1 mM EDTA, 5 mM $MgCl_2$: Weigh 13 g Hepes-sodium salt and 3.7 g KCl and dissolve in 450 mL of distilled water. Add 2.5 mL $MgCl_2$ prepared in **item 1**, 1 mL EDTA pH 8.0 (prepared as in Subheading 2.1), mix, and adjust pH to 7.4 with HCl. Adjust to 500 mL with distilled water, sterilize by autoclaving and store at 4 °C.
4. NADH solution: 100 mM NADH. Weigh 28.4 mg β-nicotinamide adenine dinucleotide reduced disodium salt hydrate and dissolve in 400 μL milli Q water. Store at −20 °C and protected from light.
5. L-cysteine solution: 105 mM L-cysteine. Weigh 1.3 mg L-cysteine and dissolve in 100 μL of milli Q water. This solution should be always prepared just before performing the experiment.
6. L-glutamate solution: 65 mM L-glutamate. Weigh 1.2 mg L-glutamate monosodium salt monohydrate, and dissolve in 100 μL milli Q water. Store at −20 °C.
7. γEC solution. 5 mM gamma-glutamylcysteine (γEC). Weigh 12.5 mg γEC and dissolve in 1 mL milli Q water. Store at −20 °C (*see* **Note 5**).
8. Glycine solution: 600 mM glycine. Weigh 4.5 mg glycine and dissolve in 100 μL of milli Q water. Store at −20 °C.
9. L-glutathione solution: 250 mM L-glutathione (GSH). Weigh 7.8 mg GSH and dissolve in 100 μL assay buffer B. Store at −20 °C (*see* **Note 5**).
10. Spermidine solution: 550 mM spermidine (Spd): Dissolve 10 μL Spd (commercial stock solution is 5.5 M) in 100 μL of assay buffer B. This solution should be always prepared just before performing the experiment.
11. ATP solution: 200 mM ATP pH 7.0: Weigh 12.1 mg ATP disodium trihydrate and dissolve in 100 μL Tris solution (prepared in **item 2**; *see* **Note 8**). Store at −20 °C (*see* **Note 5**).
12. Phosphoenolpyruvate solution: 200 mM PEP: Weigh 4.1 mg phosphoenolpyruvate monopotassium salt and dissolve in 100 μL of milli Q water. Store at −20 °C (*see* **Note 5**).
13. Pyruvate kinase/lactate dehydrogenase solution. Stock commercial solution contains 600–1000 U pyruvate kinase/mL, and 900–1400 U lactate dehydrogenase/mL in 50% glycerol with 10 mM Hepes pH 7.0, 100 mM KCl, and 0.1 mM EDTA.

14. DTT solution. 200 mM DTT: Weigh 3.08 mg DTT and dissolve in 100 μL milli Q water. Store at −20 °C for up to 3 months and then discard (*see* **Note 5**).
15. Perchloric acid (PCA) solution: 30% PCA. Dilute 42.8 mL perchloric acid (70% commercial stock) to 100 mL distilled water. Store at 4 °C.
16. Spectrophotometer: Diode Array Cary 60 from Agilent (Santa Clara, CA, USA). A multicell (8–18 cells) spectrophotometer is preferred.

2.9 Ex Vivo Flux

1. Same materials as in Subheading 2.8.
2. Materials for cellular extracts preparation as in Subheading 2.2.
3. HPLC apparatus. Waters (Milford, MA, USA).

2.10 Kinetic Parameters

These are (1) the affinity-related constants for substrates, products, activators, and inhibitors (Km_S, Km_P, Ka, Ki), and (2) V_{max} values (*see* below), of each enzyme/transporter. The former can be obtained using recombinant or purified enzymes, but they can also be determined in cell extracts by ensuring the specificity of the enzymatic assay with appropriate control reactions (*e.g.*, a reaction in the absence of protein added and a reaction lacking a specific substrate whose rates have to be subtracted from the complete one (*see* **Notes 9** and **10**). The kinetic parameters should be determined under near-physiological conditions of environmental temperature, intracellular pH, and ionic strength of the parasite; changes in these three physicochemical parameters may significantly affect the enzyme kinetic parameters. For the $T(SH)_2$ metabolism, the enzymatic assays described in Subheadings 3.1.1 and 3.10 can be used.

2.11 V_{max} Value of Each Enzyme/Transporter in the Parasites

The V_{max} values in the forward and reverse reaction should also be determined under the same physiological conditions. The V_{max} in the cell represents the actual content of active enzyme in the parasite, which is the most influential parameter for a reliable $C^J_{a_i}$ determination. For the $T(SH)_2$ metabolism, the enzymatic assays described in Subheadings 3.2, 3.3, and 3.10 can be used.

2.12 Type of Kinetic Mechanism for Each Enzyme/Transporter

This is to define the rate equation (mechanism) used in the model for each reaction. Enzyme kinetic mechanisms (such as random, ordered, ping-pong; hyperbolic or cooperative) for each enzyme can be found by mining in the literature or in enzyme databases such as BRENDA (https://www.brenda-enzymes.org). Also, the type of inhibition or activation has to be incorporated in the rate equation. General rate equations can be found in [24] and other useful equations for systems biology in [25].

2.13 Software for Model Construction and Simulation

COPASI (http://copasi.org) [26] is a platform of free access and friendly use for model construction, and has the tools to perform MCA.

2.14 Dataset of Metabolite Concentration in the Parasites

This dataset is used as the variables to validate the model simulations. The concentrations of all metabolites defined in the model have to be experimentally determined in parasite extracts. For the $T(SH)_2$ metabolism pathway, they can be determined as described in [16, 27].

2.15 Dataset of Pathway Fluxes

This variable is also used to validate the model simulations. The fluxes can be determined in live parasites, or determined by in vitro reconstitution or ex vivo. For the $T(SH)_2$ metabolism, the fluxes can be determined as described in Subheadings 3.4 and 3.11.

3 Methods

3.1 Determination of $C^J_{a_i}$ by In Vitro Pathway Reconstitution

3.1.1 Determination of Recombinant Enzyme Activities

Previous to the in vitro pathway reconstitution experiment, the actual activities of the recombinant enzymes need to be determined, preferentially just before performing the experiment. To have physiological relevance, the activity assays should be carried out at pH and temperature values that mimic the in vivo conditions of the parasite, rather than the optimal conditions of the purified enzymes. All enzymes must be characterized under the same experimental conditions of buffer assay, just changing the specific substrates. The V_{max} value has to be determined under conditions of initial velocity (in the absence of products) and under saturation concentrations of substrates. In addition, it has to be ensured a linear dependence of velocity *versus* amount of the protein used in the assay. Any spurious reaction should be subtracted from the specific activity (*see* **Note 10**).

3.1.2 Recombinant TryR Activity Assay

1. Mix 3.2 μL of NADPH solution, 230 μL of TS_2 solution and adjust to 2 mL with assay buffer A, and keep it at 37 °C.
2. In four spectrophotometer cuvettes add 0.01, 0.02, 0.04, and 0.08 μg TryR and place them in the spectrophotometer cell holder.
3. Start data acquisition at 340 nm. In each cuvette adjust volume to 0.5 mL with the mix prepared in **step 1**.
4. Follow the NADPH oxidation for about 20 min.
5. The TryR rate is calculated from the slope of the absorbance *versus* time curve at each protein concentration. The specific activity is calculated from the slope of the rate *versus* mg of protein plot (*see* **Note 11**).

6. Convert to enzymatic units using Eq. 2.

$$\frac{\Delta \text{UAbs}}{\text{min}\cdot\text{mg}}\cdot\left(\frac{1\ \mu\text{mol}\cdot\text{cm}}{6.22\ \text{mL}}\right)\cdot\left(\frac{1}{1\ \text{cm}}\right)\cdot\left(\frac{0.5\ \text{mL}}{1}\right)=\frac{\mu\text{mol}}{\text{min}\cdot\text{mg}} \quad (2)$$

3.1.3 Recombinant TXN Activity Assay

1. First, TS_2 in the trypanothione solution has to be reduced. In a separate tube mix the following components in 2.5 mL Assay buffer A: 450 μM trypanothione solution (containing $T(SH)_2$ and TS_2), 75 U of recombinant TryR, and sufficient NADPH to reach an absorbance (A_{340nm}) of 1.0 (*see* **Note 12**), keep it at 37 °C.
2. Prepare five spectrophotometer cuvettes adding 0, 0.1, 0.2, 0.3, and 0.4 μg TXN (*see* **Note 9**), and place them in the spectrophotometer cell holder.
3. Start data acquisition at 340 nm.
4. To the mix of **step 1**, add 75 U TXNPx and 50 μL CumOOH, stir and immediately transfer it to each cuvette to complete their volume to 0.5 mL and mix with a stick.
5. Follow the NADPH oxidation for about 10 min.
6. The TXN rate is calculated from the slope of the absorbance *versus* time curve. The absorbance change is corrected by subtracting the spurious reaction of $T(SH)_2$ with CumOOH (cuvette 1). The activity is obtained from the slope of the rate *versus* mg protein plot (*see* **Note 11**).
7. Convert to enzymatic units using Eq. 2.

3.1.4 Recombinant TXNPx Activity Assay

1. Mix the following components in Assay buffer for TXNPx: 450 μM trypanothione solution (total amount including $T(SH)_2$ and TS_2), 60 U recombinant TryR, and NADPH to reach an $A_{340\ nm}$ of 1.0 (*see* **Note 12**), keep it at 37 °C.
2. Prepare five spectrophotometer cuvettes adding 0, 0.1, 0.2, 0.3, and 0.4 μg TXNPx (*see* **Notes 9** and **13**). Place the two cuvettes with the highest TXNPx concentration in the spectrophotometer cell holder (*see* **Note 14**).
3. Start data acquisition at 340 nm in the spectrophotometer. Of course, no absorbance signal is detected, but this step is required to acquire as many data points as possible under initial rate conditions (*i.e,* linearity) when the reaction is initiated in **step 5**.
4. Add 87.5 U TXN and 50 μL CumOOH to the solution of **step 1** and mix.
5. Immediately transfer 0.5 mL from the solution of **step 4** to the two cuvettes to start the reaction and quickly mix with a stick.

6. Follow the NADPH oxidation for about 1.5–2 min.
7. Remove cuvettes from cell holder (without interrupting data acquisition) and proceed likewise for the other two cuvettes containing TXNPx.
8. Remove these last cuvettes and then proceed to follow the NADPH oxidation in the control cuvette (without TXNPx) for about 5–10 min (*see* **Note 9**).
9. The TXNPx rate is calculated from the slope of the absorbance *versus* time curve, after correcting for the spurious reaction of T $(SH)_2$ with CumOOH (cuvette 1). The activity is obtained from the slope of the rate *versus* mg protein plot.
10. Convert to enzymatic units using Eq. 2.

3.2 Parasite Extracts Production

The enzyme activities in the parasites have to be determined to establish the physiological enzyme ratio that will be used in the pathway reconstitution. Parasite homogenates and the corresponding clarified subcellular fractions need to be prepared ensuring preservation of the activities by assaying (1) different cell disruption procedures; and (2) the adequacy of adding protease inhibitors, reducing agents and glycerol (or other protein stabilizers).

1. Harvest the epimastigotes by centrifuging at 4750 × *g* for 10 min.
2. Discard the supernatant and resuspend the parasites with 10 mL PBS.
3. Centrifuge again at 4750 × *g* for 10 min.
4. Discard the supernatant and resuspend the parasites in 1 mL PBS. Transfer to a 1.5 mL tube.
5. Centrifuge at 6200 × *g* for 10 min.
6. Discard supernatant and resuspend the parasites in ~100 μL (*see* **Note 15**) of lysis buffer.
7. Lyse the parasites by freezing-thawing thrice. Freeze in liquid nitrogen and thaw in a water bath at 37 °C.
8. Centrifuge at 17,000 × *g* for 10 min.
9. Recover the supernatant (cell soluble protein) and discard the pellet. Keep it on ice until use.
10. Immediately proceed to enzyme activity determination. Cellular extracts are always prepared just before activity determination and must not be stored.
11. Perform quantification of cell protein concentration using your preferred methodology.

3.3 Determination of Activities in Parasite Extracts

The same enzymatic assays to determine the activities of the recombinant enzymes under close physiological conditions have to be used to determine the enzyme activities in parasite samples. However, strict additional control reactions have to be performed since very often there are nonspecific activities in cell samples that interfere in the assay, preventing a reliably specific activity determination. Therefore, parallel control reactions have to be performed (*see* **Note 10**).

3.3.1 TryR Activity Assay in Parasite Extracts

1. Mix 3.2 μL of NADPH solution with 230 μL of TS_2 solution and adjust to 2 mL with Assay buffer A; keep it at 37 °C.
2. Add 5, 10, 20, and 40 μg cellular soluble protein to four spectrophotometer cuvettes and place them in the spectrophotometer cell holder.
3. Start data acquisition at 340 nm. Adjust volume to 500 μL to each cuvette, with the mix prepared in **step 1**.
4. Follow the NADPH oxidation for about 60 min (*see* **Note 16**).
5. The TryR rate is calculated from the slope of the absorbance *versus* time curve (*see* **Note 10**). The activity is obtained from the slope of the rate *versus* mg protein plot (*see* **Note 11**).
6. To convert to enzymatic units, use Eq. 2.

3.3.2 TXN Activity Assay in Parasite Extracts

1. Mix the following components in 2.5 mL Assay buffer A: 450 μM trypanothione solution (total amount, including $T(SH)_2$ and TS_2), 75 U recombinant TryR, and NADPH to an $A_{340\ nm}$ of 1.0 (*see* **Note 12**); keep it at 37 °C.
2. Add 0, 50, 100, 200, and 400 μg cell soluble protein to five cuvettes (*see* **Note 9**), and place them in the spectrophotometer cell holder.
3. Start data acquisition at 340 nm.
4. To the mix of **step 1**, add 75 U TXNPx and 50 μL CumOOH and mix.
5. Adjust volume of each cuvette to 500 μL with the mix prepared in **step 4**.
6. Follow the NADPH oxidation for about 10 min.
7. The TXN rate is calculated from the slope of the absorbance *versus* time curve and subtracting the rate of the spurious reaction of $T(SH)_2$ with CumOOH (cuvette 1) (*see* **Note 10**). The activity is obtained from the slope of the rate *versus* protein mg plot (*see* **Note 11**).
8. To convert to enzymatic units, use Eq. 2.

3.3.3 TXNPx Activity Assay in Parasite Extracts

1. Mix the following components with Assay buffer A: 450 μM trypanothione solution (total amount, including $T(SH)_2$ and TS_2), 60 U recombinant TryR, and NADPH at an A_{340nm} of 1.0 (*see* **Note 12**); keep it at 37 °C.
2. Add 0, 30, 60, 120, and 240 μg cellular soluble protein to five spectrophotometer cuvettes (*see* **Notes 9** and **13**). Place the two cuvettes with the highest TXNPx concentration in the spectrophotometer cell holder (*see* **Note 14**).
3. Start data acquisition at 340 nm.
4. To the **step 1** mix, add 87.5 U TXN and 50 μL CumOOH and stir.
5. To start the reaction, immediately transfer the solution prepared in **step 4** to the two cuvettes to complete their volume to 0.5 mL and quickly mix with a stick.
6. Follow the NADPH oxidation for about 2–3 min.
7. Remove cuvettes from cell holder (without interrupting data acquisition) and proceed likewise for the other two cuvettes containing the lower amount of cellular protein.
8. Remove these last cuvettes and then follow the NADPH oxidation in the control cuvette (without protein) for about 5–10 min (*see* **Note 9**).
9. The TXNPx rate is calculated from the slope of the absorbance *versus* time curve, after correcting for the spurious reaction of $T(SH)_2$ with CumOOH (cuvette 1) (*see* **Note 10**). The activity is obtained from the slope of the rate *versus* mg protein plot (*see* **Note 11**).
10. To convert to enzymatic units, use Eq. 2.

3.4 In Vitro Pathway Reconstitution for $C^J_{a_i}$ Determination

For pathway reconstitution of the peroxide reduction pathway of *T. cruzi*, epimastigotes of the Queretaro strain [23] are used because of high biomass yield, which facilitates enzyme activity determination and metabolic studies; the reference activities of TryR, TXN, and TXNPx are 264, 88, and 177 mU, respectively [15]. For other trypanosomatids, parasite cell soluble protein has to be prepared as in Subheading 3.2. Enzyme activities within other trypanosomatids have also to be determined using as guide the methodologies described in Subheadings 3.3.1–3.3.3. Once the activity of the recombinant enzymes is known, the pathway must be reconstituted in the cellular proportion of each enzyme activity present in the parasite. Individual titrations of each enzyme activity above and below the reference activity have to be done and the pathway flux determined.

3.4.1 $C^J_{a_i}$ Determination Assay for TryR

1. Determine TryR, TXN, and TXNPx activities as in Subheading 3.1.1 for the recombinant purified enzymes.
2. Mix the following components in 5 mL Assay buffer A: 450 μM trypanothione solution (total amount, including $T(SH)_2$ and TS_2), 880 mU TXN, and sufficient NADPH to reach an $A_{340\ \mathrm{nm}}$ of 1.0 (*see* **Note 12**); keep it at 37 °C.
3. Prepare eight cuvettes with the following activities of recombinant TryR: 66, 132, 198, 264, 396, 528, 792, or 1056 mU and place them in the spectrophotometer cell holder.
4. Start data acquisition at 340 nm and add the mix prepared in **step 2** to the cuvettes to complete their volume to 500 μL.
5. Incubate until the absorbance signal remains constant, which means TS_2 is completely reduced to $T(SH)_2$ by TryR (*see* **Note 17**).
6. Once a basal line is attained at $A_{340\ \mathrm{nm}} \approx 1.0$, add 10 μL CumOOH to each cuvette and mix with a stick.
7. Monitor the spurious reaction for about 1–2 min (*see* **Note 18**).
8. Add 177 mU TXNPx to each cuvette to start the reaction and quickly mix.
9. Follow the NADPH oxidation for about 30 min.
10. The rate of peroxide reduction is calculated from the difference of the slopes of absorbance *versus* time curves before and after TXNPx addition, at each TryR activity.
11. Convert to units of flux using Eq. 3.

$$\frac{\Delta \mathrm{UAbs}}{\mathrm{min \cdot mg}} \cdot \left(\frac{1\ \mu\mathrm{mol \cdot cm}}{6.22\ \mathrm{mL}}\right) \cdot \left(\frac{1}{1\ \mathrm{cm}}\right) \cdot \left(\frac{0.5\ \mathrm{mL}}{1}\right) \cdot \left(\frac{1000\ \mathrm{nmol}}{1\ \mu\mathrm{mol}}\right) = \frac{\mathrm{nmol}}{\mathrm{min \cdot mg}} \quad (3)$$

3.4.2 $C^J_{a_i}$ Determination Assay for TXN

1. Determine TryR, TXN, and TXNPx activities as in Subheading 3.1.1 for the recombinant purified enzymes.
2. Prepare eight cuvettes with the following activities of recombinant TXN: 22, 44, 66, 88, 132, 176, 264, 352, or 440 mU.
3. Mix the following components in 5 mL Assay buffer A: 450 μM trypanothione solution (total amount, including $T(SH)_2$ and TS_2), 2640 mU recombinant TryR, and sufficient NADPH to reach an $A_{340\mathrm{nm}}$ of 1.0 (*see* **Note 12**); keep it at 37 °C.
4. Place the eight cuvettes containing TXN from **step 2** in the cell holder and start data acquisition at 340 nm.
5. Transfer the mix prepared in **step 3** to each cuvette of **step 4** to complete their volume to 500 μL.
6. Add 10 μL CumOOH to each cuvette and mix.

7. Monitor the spurious reaction for about 1–2 min (*see* **Note 18**).
8. Add 177 mU of TXNPx to each cuvette to start the reaction and quickly stir.
9. Follow the NADPH oxidation for about 30 min.
10. The rate of peroxide reduction is calculated from the difference of the slopes of absorbance *versus* time curves before and after TXNPx addition, at each TXN activity.
11. Convert to units of flux using Eq. 3.

3.4.3 $C^J_{a_i}$ Determination Assay for TXNPx

1. Determine TryR, TXN, and TXNPx activities as in Subheading 3.1.1 for the recombinant purified enzymes.
2. Prepare eight cuvettes with the following activities of recombinant TXNPx: 44, 88, 132, 176, 264, 352, 528, or 704 mU (*see* **Note 13**).
3. Mix the following components in 5 mL Assay buffer A: 450 μM trypanothione solution (total amount, including $T(SH)_2$ and TS_2), 2640 mU recombinant TryR, and sufficient NADPH to reach an A_{340nm} of 1.0 (*see* **Note 12**); keep it at 37 °C.
4. Place the eight cuvettes with TXNPx from **step 2** in the cell holder and start data acquisition at 340 nm.
5. Transfer the mix prepared in **step 3** to each cuvette of **step 4** to complete their volume to 500 μL.
6. Add 10 μL CumOOH to each cuvette and mix.
7. Monitor the spurious reaction for about 1–2 min (*see* **Note 18**).
8. Add 88 mU of TXN to each cuvette to start the reaction and quickly stir.
9. Follow the NADPH oxidation for about 30 min.
10. The rate of peroxide reduction is calculated from the difference of the slopes of absorbance *versus* time curves before and after TXN addition, at each TXNPx activity.
11. Convert to units of flux using Eq. 3.

3.5 Determination of the $C^J_{a_i}$

Plots of pathway flux *versus* enzyme activity are constructed to calculate $C^J_{a_i}$.

3.5.1 Plotting and $C^J_{a_i}$ Calculation for TryR

1. Normalize the TryR activities used in the titration curve of Subheading 3.4.1 considering as 100% the value of 264 mU of activity.
2. Normalize the peroxide reduction fluxes obtained in the titration curve of Subheading 3.4.1, after correcting for the spurious reaction between peroxide and $T(SH)_2$ and considering as

100% the flux attained in the reconstitution experiment with 264 mU TryR (100% TryR activity).

3. Draw a plot of percentage of peroxide reduction flux *versus* percentage of enzyme activity.
4. Fit the data to a two-parameter rectangular hyperbola equation (Michaelis–Menten-like Eq. 4), where C_1 and C_2 are constants with no mechanistic meaning, using appropriate computer software (*see* **Note 19**).

$$\%\text{flux} = \frac{C_1 \cdot \%\text{enzyme activity}}{C_2 + \%\text{enzyme activity}} \tag{4}$$

5. Draw the tangent to the curve at the closest points of 100%. The slope of this tangent corresponds to the $C^J_{a_i}$ (*see* **Note 20**).
6. An example is provided in Fig. 2b.

3.5.2 Plotting and $C^J_{a_i}$ Calculation for TXN

1. Proceed as in Subheading 3.5.1 but normalizing the experimental data obtained in Subheading 3.4.2 considering as 100% the pathway flux obtained with 100% TXN activity (88 mU).
2. An example is provided in Fig. 2b.

3.5.3 Plotting and $C^J_{a_i}$ Calculation for TXNPx

1. Proceed as in Subheading 3.5.1, but normalizing the experimental data obtained in Subheading 3.4.3 considering as 100% the pathway flux obtained with 100% TXNPx (177 mU).
2. An example is provided in Fig. 2b.

3.6 Determination of $C^J_{a_i}$ by Manipulating the Enzyme Activities in Parasites

In order to attain, in the parasites, different levels of activity of the $T(SH)_2$ synthesis pathway enzymes (Fig. 3a), the cells are transfected with plasmids that allow for enzyme overexpression. Afterward, a selection procedure through limited dilution is applied to obtain parasite clones with different degrees of enzyme activity. In each clone, the changes in the enzyme activity and pathway flux are determined. In particular, the enzymes of the $T(SH)_2$ synthesis pathway have low activities within trypanosomatids and thus only enzyme overexpression can yield reliable measurements. However, for other metabolic pathways in which high levels of enzyme activities are present, it is convenient to also gradually decrease the enzyme activity in the parasites by genetic or chemical methods. Hence, experimental data above and below the wild-type enzyme activity level (Figs. 1 and 3b) help to calculate the $C^J_{a_i}$ with less uncertainty.

3.7 Parasite Transfection

Electroporation protocols have to be standardized for each particular *T. cruzi* strain. Procedure optimization can be explored starting from the following protocol:

1. Chill electroporation cuvettes using an ice–water bath.
2. Withdraw 3×10^8 epimastigotes from the culture.
3. Centrifuge the epimastigotes at 4750 × *g* for 10 min.
4. Discard supernatant and resuspend the parasites in 10 mL LIT broth.
5. Centrifuge again at 4750 × *g* for 10 min.
6. Discard supernatant and resuspend the parasites in 350 μL LIT broth. Transfer to a cold 2 mm electroporation cuvette.
7. Add plasmid DNA for mock, γECS, or TryS overexpression (100 μg in 40 μL milli Q water; *see* **Note** 7).
8. Incubate for 10 min in ice–water bath.
9. Place the electroporation cuvette into the electroporator cell holder. Electroporate using one pulse at 300 V for 70 ms (*see* **Note 21**).
10. Incubate for 5 min at room temperature.
11. Transfer the parasites to 5 mL LIT culture medium.
12. Determine parasite viability (motility). High viability may due to low electroporation efficiency. Low viability may result in an unsuccessful selection (*see* **Note 21**).
13. Incubate at 28 °C for 48 h.

3.8 Selection and Cloning of Transfected Cells

1. To the 5 mL of transfected parasites, add 50 μL of G418 solution.
2. Incubate at 28 °C for 12–15 days (*see* **Note 22**).
3. Discard precipitated parasites and centrifuge the supernatant at 4750 × *g* for 10 min.
4. Resuspend the parasites in 5 mL LIT culture medium.
5. Incubate at 28 °C for 5 days (*see* **Note 23**).
6. Determine the number of transfected parasites (*see* **Note 24**).
7. Transfer 500 μL of the culture obtained in **step 5** to a new tube.
8. Complete the volume to 5 mL with LIT culture medium.
9. Add 50 μL G418 solution.
10. Repeat **steps 2–9** until 100% of transfected parasites is reached.
11. Once transfected parasites are completely selected, prepare 50 mL LIT culture medium with 300 μL G418 solution (*see* **Note 25**).
12. Prepare a parasite suspension at a concentration of 290 transfected parasites/mL of LIT culture medium prepared in **step 11**.

13. Prepare a 96 well culture plate by adding 100 μL of LIT culture medium prepared in **step 11** to each well, starting from column 2.
14. Add 200 μL of the parasite suspension prepared in **step 12** in wells of column 1 of the plate.
15. Withdraw 100 μL from the wells of the plate made in **step 14**, and transfer them to the next column. Mix the culture with the LIT culture medium in the wells, making 1:2 serial dilutions.
16. Repeat **step 15** until the wells of the last column contain 200 μL. Stir and discard 100 μL.
17. Incubate at 28 °C (*see* **Note 26**). Occasionally inspect each well searching for cells.
18. After 3 weeks (*see* **Note 27**) check the plate under the microscope. The last well of each row that contains parasites is most probably a culture derived from a single cell and can thus be considered a clone.
19. Transfer the clones of interest to 5 mL LIT culture medium *plus* 30 μL G418.

3.9 Parasite Extracts Production from Overexpressing Clones

1. Method as in Subheading 3.2.

3.10 Determination of Enzyme Activities in Cell Extracts of Overexpressing Parasites

The activities in different clones of an overexpressed enzyme are determined to identify a set of clones with different levels of activity to cover as much as possible an ample range of activities. Once the clones are selected, the activities of the other pathway enzymes have to be determined in order to establish that no significant changes in other enzymes have developed besides for those overexpressed. This is a strict requisite for a proper application of MCA.

3.10.1 γECS Activity Assay

1. Mix the following components in 3.5 mL Assay Buffer B: 5.6 μL NADH, 70 μL L-glutamate, 35 μL ATP, 35 μL PEP, 7 μL pyruvate kinase/lactate dehydrogenase solution; keep at 37 °C.
2. Prepare six cuvettes (numbered 1–6) in the spectrophotometer cell holder grouped in pairs. Each pair of cuvettes is formed by a control reaction (numbers 1, 3, and 5) and complete reaction (numbers 2, 4, and 6) (*see* **Note 28**).
3. Add 10 μL L-Cys to the complete reaction cuvettes (numbers 2, 4, and 6).
4. Add 1 mL of the mix prepared in **step 1** to the control cuvettes (numbers 1, 3, and 5).
5. Add 240, 360, or 480 μg of cellular soluble protein to the control cuvettes and mix.

6. Withdraw 500 μL from each control cuvette and transfer it to its partner complete reaction cuvette and mix.
7. Follow the NADH oxidation for about 20–30 min.
8. The γECS rate is calculated from the slope of the absorbance *versus* time curve, after correcting for the spurious ATP-consuming reaction of its corresponding control cuvette (*see* **Note 10**). The specific activity is obtained from the slope of the rate *versus* mg protein plot (*see* **Note 11**).
9. Convert to enzymatic units using Eq. 2.

3.10.2 GS Activity Assay

1. Mix the following components in 3.5 mL Assay Buffer B: 5.6 μL NADH, 70 μL glycine, 35 μL ATP, 35 μL PEP, 7 μL pyruvate kinase/lactate dehydrogenase solution; keep at 37 °C.
2. Prepare six cuvettes (numbered 1–6) in the spectrophotometer cell holder grouped in pairs. Each pair of cuvettes is formed by a control reaction cuvette (numbers 1, 3, and 5) and complete reaction cuvette (numbers 2, 4, and 6) (*see* **Note 28**).
3. Add 4 μL γEC to the complete reaction cuvette (numbers 2, 4, and 6).
4. Add 1 mL of the mix prepared in **step 1** to the control cuvettes (numbers 1, 3, and 5).
5. Add 200, 300, or 400 μg of cellular soluble protein to the control cuvettes and mix.
6. Withdraw 500 μL from each control cuvette and transfer it to its partner complete reaction cuvette and mix.
7. Follow the NADH oxidation for about 10–20 min.
8. The GS rate is calculated from the slope of the absorbance *versus* time curve, after correcting for the spurious ATP-consuming reaction of its corresponding control cuvette (*see* **Note 10**). The activity is obtained from the slope of the rate *versus* mg protein plot (*see* **Note 11**).
9. Convert to enzymatic units using Eq. 2.

3.10.3 TryS Activity Assay

1. Mix the following components in 3.5 mL Assay Buffer B: 5.6 μL NADH, 70 μL Spd, 35 μL ATP, 35 μL PEP, 7 μL pyruvate kinase/lactate dehydrogenase solution; keep at 37 °C.
2. Prepare six cuvettes (numbered from 1 to 6) in the spectrophotometer cell holder grouped in pairs. Each pair of cuvettes is formed by a control reaction cuvette (numbers 1, 3, and 5) and a complete reaction cuvette (numbers 2, 4, and 6) (*see* **Note 28**).
3. Add 6 μL GSH to the complete reaction cuvette (numbers 2, 4, and 6).
4. Add 1 mL of the mix prepared in **step 1** to the control cuvettes (numbers 1, 3, and 5).

5. Add 80, 160, or 320 μg of cellular soluble protein to the control cuvettes and mix.
6. Withdraw 500 μL from each control cuvette and transfer it to its partner complete reaction cuvette and mix.
7. Follow the NADH oxidation for about 10–20 min.
8. The TryS rate is calculated from the slope of the absorbance *versus* time curve, after correcting for the spurious ATP-consuming reaction of its corresponding control cuvette (*see* **Note 10**). The activity is obtained from the slope of the rate *versus* mg protein plot (*see* **Note 11**).
9. Convert to enzymatic units using Eq. 2. Divide by two to convert to nmol $T(SH)_2$ produced/min·mg of cellular soluble protein.

3.11 Ex Vivo $T(SH)_2$ Synthesis Flux Determination

After clones with different levels of overexpressed γECS or TryS activities have been selected, the ex vivo $T(SH)_2$ synthesis flux is individually determined in a cell extract of each overexpressing clone as well as in extracts of mock-transfected parasites. An ex vivo $T(SH)_2$ synthesis flux determination protocol is used here because of the very low rates of the $T(SH)_2$ synthesis enzymes. However, for other metabolic pathways of interest, any convenient and reliable way to determine the pathway flux even in intact cells (*e.g*, an excreted end-product metabolite such as pyruvate, alanine, ethanol, or lactate for glycolysis) can be applied [8–11].

1. Prepare five 1.5 mL Eppendorf tubes with 10 μL PCA solution to be used in **step 4**.
2. In a 1.5 mL Eppendorf tube mix 400 μL of Assay buffer B with 10 μL Cys, 10 μL Glu, 10 μL Gly, 10 μL Spd, 15 μL ATP, 5 μL PEP, 25 μL DTT, and 10 μL pyruvate kinase/lactate dehydrogenase solution (*see* **Note 29**). Maintain at 37 °C.
3. Add 0.8–1.2 mg of cellular soluble protein and mix to start the reaction (*see* **Note 30**).
4. Immediately transfer 90 μL of the reaction to a tube prepared in **step 1** to stop the reaction. Maintain on ice.
5. Repeat **step 4** at 0.5, 1, 3, and 5 min after starting the reaction.
6. Determine the newly formed $T(SH)_2$ by HPLC as in [27].

3.12 Determination of the $C^J_{a_i}$

Once data of enzyme activity and pathway flux are obtained, a plot of the relationship between these variables is constructed to determine the $C^J_{a_i}$.

3.12.1 Plotting and $C^J_{a_i}$ Calculation for γECS

1. Normalize the γECS activity determined in individual clones overexpressing γECS after correcting for the spurious ATP hydrolysis (Subheading 3.10.1), considering as 100% the

value of γECS activity in mock-transfected parasites (*see* **Note 31**).

2. Normalize the $T(SH)_2$ synthesis fluxes determined by HPLC in the corresponding individual clones of overexpressing γECS (Subheading 3.11) and considering as 100% the flux attained in mock-transfected parasites (*see* **Note 31**).
3. Draw a plot of percentage of $T(SH)_2$ synthesis flux *versus* percentage of enzyme activity obtained from each clone.
4. Fit the data to a two-parameter rectangular hyperbola equation (Michaelis–Menten-like Eq. 4), where C_1 and C_2 are different constants with no mechanistic meaning, using appropriate computer software (*see* **Note 19**).
5. Draw the tangent to the curve at the points nearest to 100%. The slope of this tangent corresponds to the $C^J_{a_i}$ (*see* **Note 20**).
6. An example is provided in Fig. 3b. Due to the use of different clones with different degrees of transfection efficiency, these experimental data exhibit higher biological variability than those of the in vitro pathway reconstitution (Fig. 2b).

3.12.2 Plotting and $C^J_{a_i}$ Calculation for TryS

1. Proceed like in Subheading 3.12.1, but normalizing the activities and pathway fluxes in the clones overexpressing TryS.
2. An example is provided in Fig. 3b.

3.12.3 $C^J_{a_i}$ Calculation for GS

1. By applying the summation theorem of MCA, the $C^J_{a_i}$ of GS is determined from the equation $C^J_{GS} = 1 - (C^J_{\gamma ECS} + C^J_{TryS})$.

3.13 Determination of $C^J_{a_i}$ by Kinetic Modeling of Metabolic Pathways

3.13.1 Model Construction

Instruction manuals for how to construct a kinetic model can be found at the COPASI website (http://copasi.org/Support/). A general outline of the procedure is the following.

1. The reactions that constitute the pathway are coded in the COPASI software.
2. A rate equation is coded for each reaction.
3. The kinetic parameters values determined for each enzyme/transporter are assigned in the rate equation.
4. The concentrations of pathway intermediates determined in the parasites are used as initial metabolite concentrations.
5. The model is run to calculate all the variables for different tasks (*e.g.*, steady-state analysis, time-course simulation, MCA).
6. Usually several rounds of model refinement and experimentation are necessary to obtain a model that can closely simulate the metabolic intermediates concentrations and pathway fluxes

determined in the parasites, which are the variables used for validation.

7. The MCA COPASI task provides the $C^J_{a_i}$ for each reaction included in the model.
8. An interactive database of published kinetic models can be found in the website http://jjj.biochem.sun.ac.za/.

4 Notes

1. Enzymes can be obtained in their recombinant forms using your preferred methodology for gene cloning, and systems for protein overexpression and purification. Purity above 95% is recommended. The protein concentration has to be quantitated using your protocol of preference.
2. $T(SH)_2$ content is determined spectrophotometrically by making it react with the Ellman's reagent (dithionitrobenzoic acid) in a solution of 100 mM KH_2PO_4 at pH 8 and determining the absorbance at 412 nm. The TS_2 content is enzymatically determined by using recombinant TryR and measuring the amount of oxidized NADPH at 340 nm. Alternatively, commercial TS_2 can be used.
3. This procedure is only for trypanothione synthesized according to [22] as in Subheading 2.1 **step 5**, whose product contains a mixture of both TS_2 and $T(SH)_2$ forms.
4. The H_2O_2 solution is prepared in milli Q water and calibrated spectrophotometrically. $A_{240\text{nm}} = 1.0$ is equivalent to 22.9 mM.
5. Prepare as indicated and store until use. Once thawed it is not recommended to freeze again. Prepare aliquots of convenient volumes for one-time use.
6. For a review of different available plasmids for trypanosomatid transfection (*see* [28]).
7. Purify your plasmids using your preferred methodology (cesium chloride or commercial kit). Plasmids are usually stored in Tris–EDTA buffer. Prior to transfection, the plasmids must be precipitated and dissolved in milli Q water.
8. The ATP solution is prepared using a Tris solution. Verify to reach a final pH of 7.0 or slightly lower for longer stability.
9. Cuvette 1 (no protein added) serves as control for the rate of the spurious nonenzymatic reaction of a peroxide (CumOOH) with $T(SH)_2$, which has to be subtracted from the rate values attained in the other cuvettes at the end of experiment.

10. To ensure that the activity measured is specific for the desired enzyme (other than spurious reactions), control assays must be performed. This is done by adding in separate assays the specific substrates in different order; the enzyme-specific activity has to be detected only when all specific substrates are present in the reaction. In addition, the calculated specific activity value of each separate assay (after subtracting any spurious reaction) must be the same. Another control is a full reaction mixture lacking added protein to monitor nonspecific reactions among the reagents.
11. A plot of rate *versus* mg of protein must be prepared (after subtraction of any spurious reaction). Fit a curve to the data according to a linear equation, adjusting the intercept to 0, 0. The slope is obtained from the equation of the linear fitting.
12. A significant fraction of the initial NADPH added is used by TryR for reducing the TS_2 present in the synthesized trypanothione solution. Ensure that the amount of NADPH added to the mix is enough to totally reduce the TS_2, and when necessary, add extra NADPH. Maintain the $A_{340nm} \approx 1.0$ after reducing all TS_2.
13. TXNPx is inhibited by dilution at concentrations <1 μg/mL for the recombinant enzyme and <100 μg protein/mL for cellular extract [15, 29]. If TXNPx dilutions are required, then they must be done in Assay buffer for TXNPx which contains DMSO.
14. Because of the high TXNPx inhibition by dilution, the initial velocity of the reaction at the protein concentrations used in the assay lasts for ≈60 s. Therefore, it is recommended that data acquisition for a single cuvette be <3 s to get as many data points as possible. To achieve this, only two cuvettes must be monitored at the same time.
15. Adjust the volume depending on the number of parasites at a protein concentration of 20–40 mg/mL. Consider that 1×10^9 epimastigotes have ≈300 μg of soluble protein and ≈600 μg of total protein.
16. TryR activity in cellular extracts shows hysteresis (delayed activity). Therefore, it is frequently difficult to observe changes in the absorbance for at least 20 min. Avoid adding more cell protein, since this will result in activity underestimation.
17. The time needed to obtain a basal line depends on the activity of TryR added, being greater when less TryR is present. When TryR is varied (reconstitution assays), the required time to reach $A_{340nm} = 1.0$ will be different for each cuvette.

18. The spurious reaction between $T(SH)_2$ and CumOOH must be determined before starting the experimental reaction, and must be subtracted from the flux determined. The time of monitoring may vary, particularly when TryR is being varied. Usually, the time to decrease 0.2 U of absorbance below the initial absorbance is enough to have a reliable slope to determine this rate.
19. A computational software such as Origin 8 Pro can be used.
20. Alternatively, create the derivative curve of the fitted curve of **step 4**. The derivative (*Y* value) at the 100% value on the *X* axis is the $C^J_{a_i}$.
21. Electroporation conditions are different for distinct trypanosomatids or even different *T. cruzi* strains. Consider to adjust the electroporation protocol by first varying the time pulse and later the voltage.
22. The incubation time depends on the epimastigotes growth. It is recommended to daily monitor parasite growth after 10 days culture to avoid sample loss due to cell death.
23. Parasite growth must be monitored for up to 7 days to verify cell viability.
24. In order to have a control of the electroporation procedure, prepare an overexpression plasmid construct with a gene coding for a fluorescent protein, and electroporate the same batch of parasites in parallel to the experimental ones. The efficiency of parasite transfection is determined by fluorescence microscopy as the number of fluorescent parasites *versus* total viable (motile) parasites.
25. Transfected parasites are selected with 500 μg G418/mL. For parasite growth maintenance use 300 μg G418/mL.
26. Take care of evaporation. Cover the border of the plate with Parafilm. Use a humid camera to control evaporation.
27. The time needed for cloning is variable, and cell growth must be monitored throughout the cloning procedure.
28. Parasite extracts have a spurious ATPase reaction, which accounts for 150–300 mU ADP produced/mg cell protein [17]. The control and complete reactions have to be derived from the same assay mixture (without the thiol specific substrate) to avoid that differences in NADH oxidation are due to variations in protein sampling. The control reactions lack the thiol specific substrate and are used for determining this ATPase activity, which must always be subtracted from the complete reaction.
29. For this protocol lactate dehydrogenase is not necessary, since $T(SH)_2$ is directly determined by thiol derivatization and HPLC. Alternatively, purified commercial pyruvate kinase can be used.

30. The soluble cell protein should be adjusted to ensure that the ex vivo pathway flux is linear with respect to the amount of protein used in the assay.
31. Alternatively, the enzyme activities and pathway fluxes can be determined in nontransfected parasites and these values are then used as control and can be normalized.

Acknowledgments

The research in the author's laboratory is supported by CONACyT grants 272941 and 282663 to E.S. Z.G.-C. was supported by CONACyT Ph.D. fellowship No. 355168 and acknowledges to Programa de Posgrado en Ciencias Bioquímicas of the Universidad Nacional Autónoma de México for academic preparation.

References

1. Gilbert IH (2014) Target-based drug discovery for human African trypanosomiasis: selection of molecular target and chemical matter. Parasitology 141(1):28–36
2. Field MC, Horn D, Fairlamb AH, Ferguson MAJ, Gray DW, Read KD, De Rycker M, Torrie LS, Wyatt PG, Wyllie S, Gilbert IH (2017) Anti-trypanosomatid drug discovery: an ongoing challenge and a continuing need. Nat Rev Microbiol 15(7):217–231
3. Glover L, Alsford S, Baker N, Turner DJ, Sanchez-Flores A, Hutchinson S, Hertz-Fowler C, Berriman M, Horn D (2015) Genome-scale RNAi screens for high-throughput phenotyping in bloodstream-form African trypanosomes. Nat Protoc 10 (1):106–133
4. Jones NG, Catta-Preta CMC, Lima APCA, Mottram JC (2018) Genetically validated drug targets in *Leishmania*: current knowledge and future prospects. ACS Infect Dis 4 (4):467–477
5. Olin-Sandoval V, Moreno-Sánchez R, Saavedra E (2010) Targeting trypanothione metabolism in trypanosomatid human parasites. Curr Drug Targets 11(12):1614–1630
6. Flohé L (2012) The trypanothione system and the opportunities it offers to create drugs for the neglected kinetoplast diseases. Biotechnol Adv 30(1):294–301
7. Nelson DL, Cox MM (2008) Lehninger principles of biochemistry, 6th edn. W. H. Freeman, New York, NY, p Chapter 15.2
8. Moreno-Sanchez R, Saavedra E, Rodriguez-Enriquez S, Olin-Sandoval V (2008) Metabolic control analysis: a tool for designing strategies to manipulate metabolic pathways. J Biomed Biotechnol 2008:597913
9. Fell D (1997) Understanding the control of metabolism. Portland Press, London, p 301
10. Bakker BM, Westerhoff HV, Opperdoes FR, Michels PA (2000) Metabolic control analysis of glycolysis in trypanosomes as an approach to improve selectivity and effectiveness of drugs. Mol Biochem Parasitol 106(1):1–10
11. Saavedra E, Gonzalez-Chavez Z, Moreno-Sanchez R, Michels PAM (2019) Drug target selection for *Trypanosoma cruzi* metabolism by metabolic control analysis and kinetic modeling. Curr Med Chem 26(36):6652–6671. https://doi.org/10.2174/0929867325666180917104242
12. Torres NV, Souto R, Meléndez-Hevia E (1989) Study ofthe flux and transition time control coefficient profiles in a metabolic system in vitro and the effect of an external stimulator. Biochem J 260(3):763–769
13. Giersch C (1995) Determining elasticities from multiple measurements of flux rates and metabolite concentrations. Application of the multiple modulation method to a reconstituted pathway. Eur J Biochem 227(1–2):194–201
14. Moreno-Sánchez R, Encalada R, Marín-Hernández A, Saavedra E (2008) Experimental validation of metabolic pathway modeling. An illustration with glycolytic segments from *Entamoeba histolytica*. FEBS J 275 (13):3454–3469
15. González-Chávez Z, Olin-Sandoval V, Rodíguez-Zavala JS, Moreno-Sánchez R, Saavedra

E (2015) Metabolic control analysis of the *Trypanosoma cruzi* peroxide detoxification pathway identifies tryparedoxin as a suitable drug target. Biochem Biophys Acta 1850:263–273

16. Olin-Sandoval V, González-Chávez Z, Berzunza-Cruz M, Martínez I, Jasso-Chávez R, Becker I, Espinoza B, Moreno-Sánchez R, Saavedra E (2012) Drug target validation of the trypanothione pathway enzymes through metabolic modelling. FEBS J 279(10):1811–1833
17. González-Chavez Z, Vázquez C, Mejia-Tlachi-M, Martínez-Cuevas T, Márquez-Dueñas C, Encalada R, Manning-Cela R, Rodríguez-Enríquez S, PAM M, Moreno-Sánchez R, Saavedra E (2019) Gamma-glutamylcysteine synthetase and tryparedoxin 1 exert high control on the antioxidant system in *Trypanosoma cruzi* contributing to drug resistance and infectivity. Redox Biol 26:101231
18. Bruggeman FJ, Westerhoff HV (2007) The nature of systems biology. Trends Microbiol 15(1):45–50
19. Westerhoff HV (2011) Systems biology left and right. Methods Enzymol 500:3–11
20. Saa PA, Nielsen LK (2017) Formulation, construction and analysis of kinetic models of metabolism: a review of modelling frameworks. Biotechnol Adv 35(8):981–1003
21. Haanstra JR, Bakker BM (2015) Drug target identification through systems biology. Drug Discov Today Technol 15:17–22
22. Comini MA, Dirdjaja N, Kaschel M, Krauth-Siegel RL (2009) Preparative enzymatic synthesis of trypanothione and trypanothione analogues. Int J Parasitol 39:1059–1062
23. López-Olmos V, Pérez-Nasser N, Piñero D, Ortega E, Hernández R, Espinoza B (1998) Biological characterization and genetic diversity of mexican isolates of *Trypanosoma cruzi*. Acta Trop 69(3):239–254
24. Segel IH (1975) Enzyme Kinetics. Wiley, New York, NY
25. Tummler K, Lubitz T, Schelker M, Klipp E (2014) New types of experimental data shape the use of enzyme kinetics for dynamic network modeling. FEBS J 281(2):549–571
26. Hoops S, Sahle S, Gauges R, Lee C, Pahle J, Simus N, Singhal M, Xu L, Mendes P, Kummer U (2006) COPASI—a COmplex PAthway SImulator. Bioinformatics 22(24):3067–3074
27. Vázquez C, Mejia-Tlachi M, González-Chávez Z, Silva A, Rodríguez-Zavala JS, Moreno-Sánchez R, Saavedra E (2017) Buthionine sulfoximine is a multitarget inhibitor of trypanothione synthesis in *Trypanosoma cruzi*. FEBS Lett 591(23):3881–3894
28. Taylor MC, Huang H, Kelly JM (2011) Genetic techniques in *Trypanosoma cruzi*. Adv Microbiol 75:231–250
29. Flohé L, Steinert P, Hecht JH, Hofmann B (2002) Tryparedoxin and tryparedoxin peroxidase. Methods Enzymol 347:244–258

Part VI

Biomarkers and Diagnosis

Chapter 42

Establishment of a Standardized Vaccine Protocol for the Analysis of Protective Immune Responses During Experimental Trypanosome Infections in Mice

Magdalena Radwanska, Hang Thi Thu Nguyen, Sangphil Moon, Emmanuel Obishakin, and Stefan Magez

Abstract

To date, trypanosomosis control in humans and animals is achieved by a combination of parasitological screening and treatment. While this approach has successfully brought down the number of reported *T. b. gambiense* Human African Trypanosomosis (HAT) cases, the method does not offer a sustainable solution for animal trypanosomosis (AT). The main reasons for this are (i) the worldwide distribution of AT, (ii) the wide range of insect vectors involved in transmission of AT, and (iii) the existence of a wildlife parasite reservoir that can serve as a source for livestock reinfection. Hence, in order to control livestock trypanosomosis the only viable long-term solution is an effective antitrypanosome vaccination strategy. Over the last decades, multiple vaccine approaches have been proposed. Despite repeated reports of promising experimental approaches, none of those made it to a field applicable vaccine format. This failure can in part be attributed to flaws in the experimental design that favor a positive laboratory result. This chapter provides a vaccine protocol that should allow for a proper outcome prediction in experimental anti-AT vaccine approaches.

Key words Vaccination, Memory, B cell

1 Introduction

One of the main defense systems that trypanosomes have developed to escape destruction by the mammalian immune system is the suppression of an effective antibody immune response in combination with antigenic variation [1]. The latter involves the interplay between the expression of a major variant specific glycoprotein on the surface of the parasite, that is, Variant Surface Glycoprotein (VSG), and the induction of anti-VSG antibodies by the host. The regular alterations of VSG epitopes ensure that the parasite population as a whole is never in danger of total elimination [2]. Besides VSG molecules, trypanosomes express a range of immunologically conserved molecules [3]. Under natural conditions, infection-

Paul A. M. Michels et al. (eds.), *Trypanosomatids: Methods and Protocols*, Methods in Molecular Biology, vol. 2116, https://doi.org/10.1007/978-1-0716-0294-2_42,

associated antibodies against these constant epitopes are being generated, but are unable to eliminate the parasite. Different reasons can explain the latter, with lack of surface accessibility and surface clearance being major contributors [4, 5].

Host–pathogen coevolution results from the complex interplay between the two, in which immune diversion is a major pathogen weapon. Hence, antigens that evoke strong antibody responses de facto are those that function as immunological decoy targets, while vital conserved molecular epitopes will typically evolve towards low immunogenicity. This principle is possibly best described in the field of anti-influenza immunity [6]. In general, there are four ways that vaccination technology can unbalance the host–pathogen interplay, in favor of the host. Firstly, targeting major surface antigens ensures the host goes through a cycle of B cell maturation (including somatic hypermutation, class switching and memory B cell generation) so that upon a first pathogen encounter, the response is better both in terms of quality and quantity as compared to a first exposure in a natural infection. This is how most vaccines work. Secondly, providing a single unique antigen during vaccination will eliminate the negative effect of competition with other immuno-dominant molecules that would be present during a natural infection. Thirdly, vaccinating with pathogen signal molecules that are involved in the establishment of the initial phase of infection, will allow the induction of a unique full scale antibody response early on in infection. Hence, this vaccination approach might reverse the order of antigen-antibody appearance and disrupt the natural host–pathogen interplay, interfering with the onset of infection. Finally, antipathology vaccination can be considered as a fourth immune intervention strategy. This approach targets pathogen compounds that drive various infection-associated pathologies, rather than targeting the infection itself. Combined, these approaches might one day be part of the solution for the global control of trypanosomosis.

To date, an antitrypanosome vaccination literature review will result in data on several promising candidates [7, 8]. However, not a single vaccine has so far been shown to be successful in a field setting. One explanation could be that the general use of experimental mouse trypanosomosis models in vaccine trials does not reflect the correct immune-parasite interplay of the natural host (be it cattle or man). Equally likely is that in many experimental vaccine studies, conditions are used that bias a favorable experimental outcome from the start, and do not respect some of the basic immunological principles that underlie vaccinology success in general. One of the main issues here is that the aim of a vaccine is not per se to induce antibodies upon antigen exposure, but to induce a memory response that results in a complex recall activation upon pathogen challenge [9, 10]. A second issue concerns the definition of 'protection' while interpreting the results. In case of trypanosomosis, only sterile protection can be considered as a success. Delayed onset of parasitemia or reduced first peak parasitemia still will result in 100% death of the animals and consequently should not be considered as protection. Borderline protection, observed only when challenges are done with low dose parasite inoculation, should also not be considered as true protection [11]. Finally, protection that is only obtained within days after the final boost should also not be considered as a promising result [7, 11–15]. This chapter delivers a protocol that ensures the sterile protection as well as memory recall responses can be assessed in experimental mouse vaccination models for trypanosomosis.

2 Materials

2.1 Vaccine Materials

1. Purified trypanosome proteins, or purified recombinant proteins. The challenge dose for mouse is typically 10 μg/mouse, at a concentration of 0.1 mg/mL PBS.
2. PBS: Start with 800 mL of distilled water, add 8 g NaCl, 0.2 g KCl, 1.44 g Na_2HPO_4, 0.24 g KH_2PO_4, adjust the pH to 7.4 with HCl and finally add distilled water to a total volume of 1 L.
3. Complete Freund's Adjuvant (CFA) (Sigma F5881) and Incomplete Freund's Adjuvant (IFA) (Sigma F5506), or alternatives (*see* **Notes 1–3**).
4. Mock vaccine material: purified or recombinant protein used at same concentration as an actual vaccine compound (*see* **Notes 4–7**).
5. Locking Eppendorf 1.5 mL microtubes.
6. Vortex Mixer.
7. Glass Syringe 1 mL with Luer-lock tip.

2.2 Mice and Parasites

1. Eight-week-old C57BL/6 mice are the most commonly used strain in trypanosome vaccine trials (*see* **Notes 8–10**).
2. Mice are infected by intraperitoneal (IP) injection using 5×10^3–5×10^4 parasites (*see* **Notes 11–17**). Parasites stocks (heparinized infected mouse or rat blood) can be preserved at −80 °C as 50 μL aliquots of 1:1 diluted infected blood in Alsever's solution supplemented with 10% glycerol (cell culture grade). Frozen aliquots should be dissolved/diluted in PBS prior to infection, adjusting the volume to obtain a correct parasite inoculum dose in 100 μL. If desired, a single mouse can be infected with the stabilates. Within 4–5 days infected blood can subsequently be used to initiate the actual experiment, using blood dilution in PBS, PSG (PBS + 1% glucose), or

medium (i.e., DMEM or RPMI) to obtain the required parasite concentration. This ensures that mainly viable parasites are being used in the challenge setup.

3. DEAE Sepharose Fast Flow resins (GE Healthcare 17-0709-01).
4. NaOH (50% H_2O stock).
5. Heparin (Sigma H3393) 1000 U/mL dissolved in PBS (stored at −20 °C in 1 mL aliquots).
6. 15 mL conical centrifuge tubes.

2.3 Antibody Readout Reagents

1. Nunc-Immuno MicroWell 96-well solid plates are suitable for antigen coating and subsequent testing of vaccine induced antibody titers.
2. PBS pH 7.4 or carbonate buffer can be used to coat target antigen at a saturation concentration of 10 μg/mL. Titration might be needed to find the optimal coating concentration using serial dilutions between 10 μg/mL and 0.5 μg/mL (*see* **Note 18**).
3. Carbonate buffer: Start with 800 mL of distilled water, add 8.4 g $NaHCO_3$, 3.56 g Na_2CO_3, adjust to pH 9.5 with NaOH (50% H_2O) and finally add distilled water to a total volume of 1 L.
4. PBS/Tween: 0.5 mL of Tween 20 in 1 L PBS.
5. Blocking Solution: 1% BSA (1:30 dilution of BSA solution Sigma A9576) in PBS.
6. TMB reagent (Sigma RABTMB3).
7. TMB stop solution 2 N H_2SO_4.
8. Polyclonal HRP Goat-anti-mouse IgG (minimal x-reactive) antibody (Biolegend 405306—or equivalent) should be titrated 1:2000–1:5000, to determine optimal conditions.

2.4 FACS Readout Reagents

1. Dulbecco's Modified Eagle Medium (DMEM): 10% fetal bovine serum (FBS), 1% penicillin/streptomycin. Store at 4 °C and use at room temperature.
2. GentleMACS dissociator with C tubes (Milenyi Biotec).
3. Red Blood Cell (RBC) lysis solution: pH 7.2. Add 1 volume of 10× stock RBC lysis solution (Biolegend 420301) to 9 volumes distilled water. Store at 4 °C and use at room temperature.
4. Trypan Blue dead cell exclusion dye (Sigma 302643).
5. Neubauer improved hemocytometer cell counting chamber.
6. Inverted microscope (Olympus CKX31) with 20× objective (Olympus LCAch N 20×/0.40 Plan), or equivalent.

7. FACSAria II or Accuri C6 (BD Bioscience) or equivalent, allowing to detect FITC, PE, PE-CY7, and APC fluorochromes.
8. FACS buffer: pH 7.2, 0.5% FBS using BD FACS Sheath fluid (BD 342003). Store at 4 °C and use at room temperature.
9. 5 mL polystyrene Round-Bottom tubes.
10. Anti-Fc blocking, using CD16/32 antibody (BD 553141).
11. Fluorochrome-conjugated antibodies (Biolegend): B220-FITC (clone RA3-6B2), CD1d-PE (clone 1B1), CD138-PE/Cy7 (clone 281-2), and CD93-APC (clone AA4.1), CD4-FITC (clone RM4-4), CD8-PE (clone 53-6.7), NK1.1-APC (clone PK136), Ly6G-FITC (clone 1A8), Ly6C-PE (clone HK1.4), CD11b-APC (clone M1/70).

3 Method

3.1 Vaccination and Challenge Protocol

Mice should be housed according to guidelines of the Institutional Committee for Ethical Use of Experimental Animals, an Institutional Animal Care and User Committee or an equivalent committee that reviews and approves all protocols prior to execution of the experiment. During the experiment mice should be kept under optimal conditions with free access to food and water, and ambient temperature of 18–23 °C and an air humidity of 40–60%. Mice should be provided with cage enrichment to decrease overall stress levels and health should be checked daily. Humane endpoints for the experiment must be set prior to the start of the experiment.

In order to get a complete insight into the vaccination result, several experimental groups should be prepared, including proper controls. As outlined in Fig. 1 and Table 1, there are 26 basic control conditions that should be tested in order to fully understand the outcome of a vaccine result, when vaccine efficacy is tested week 8–12 post parasite challenge. Results for some of these control groups might be found in literature, but a good standard protocol should at least include an assessment of all groups in similar conditions as the actual vaccine target groups. Finally, when challenging vaccinated mice with live parasites, control groups should be challenged with dead parasites, rather than PBS. This ensures that also the control groups are exposed to a proper antigen challenge prior to analysis.

1. Prepare antigen (Ag)–adjuvant mix at a concentration that allows subcutaneous injection of 10 μg/mouse in 200 μL total volume (i.e., 100 μL – 0.1 mg/mL Ag/PBS + 100 μL adjuvant). Use 1.5 mL cone-shaped microtubes, adding 500 μL antigen solution and 500 μL CFA.

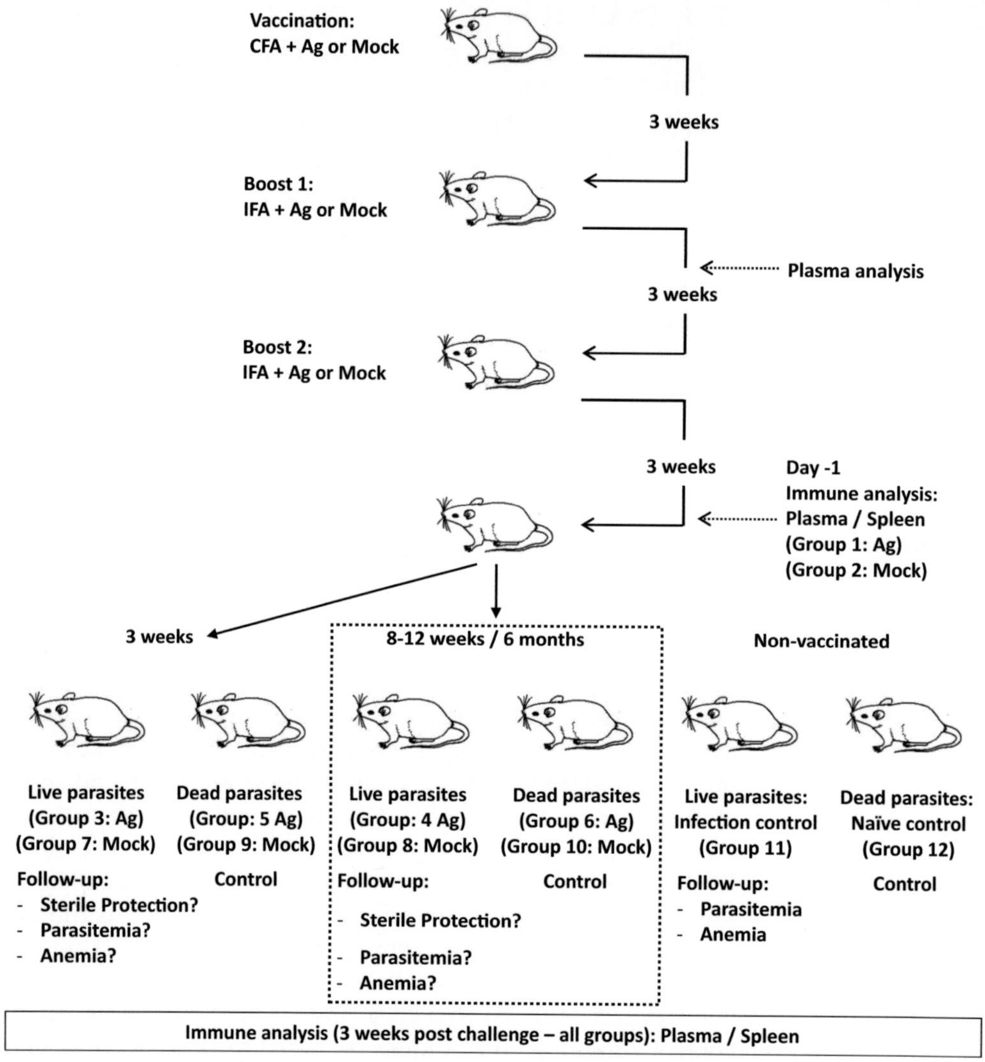

Fig. 1 A prototype vaccine experiment includes three subsequent exposures to antigen–adjuvant formulations followed by a resting period that allows vaccine induced antibody titers to decline to background levels. After 8–12 weeks (or eventually 6 months), mice can be challenged with parasites in order to assess true vaccine-induced protective memory responses. In order to obtain preliminary data, a parasite challenge can be performed 3 weeks after the second vaccine boost. This will allow to assess whether vaccine-induced immune effector mechanisms offer any significant level of short-term protection. Nonvaccinated mice should be used as controls in both settings. Additional control groups should be challenged with dead parasites to assure antigen exposure at the same time that the actual target groups are receiving an exposure to live parasites. Including these controls will allow for a proper immune profiling of the vaccine response 3 weeks post parasite challenge

2. Vortex the emulsion till a homogenous white appearance is obtained (2–3 min) at maximum speed. Alternatively, the emulsion can be obtained by mixing the antigen solution and adjuvant between two glass syringes using silicone tubing or two sterile Luer-lock syringes joined by a stopcock (*see* **Note 19**).

Table 1
Vaccine trial control groups

Group	Adjuvant	Antigen	Mock	Live parasite challenge 3 weeks	Dead parasite challenge 3 weeks	Live parasite challenge 8–12 weeks (or 6 months)	Dead parasite challenge 8–12 weeks (or 6 months)
13	+	–	–	–	–	–	–
14	–	+	–	–	–	–	–
15	–	–	+	–	–	–	–
16	+	–	–	+	–	–	–
17	+	–	–	–	+	–	–
18	+	–	–	–	–	+	–
19	+	–	–	–	–	–	+
20	–	+	–	+	–	–	–
21	–	+	–	–	+	–	–
22	–	+	–	–		+	–
23	–	+	–	–	–	–	+
24	–	–	+	+	–	–	–
25	–	–	+	–	+	–	–
26	–	–	+	–	–	+	–
27	–	–	+	–	–	–	+

Multiple control groups are required for the proper immune profiling of a vaccine trial result, including (1) mice that receive adjuvant, target antigen, and mock antigen exposure separately without being exposed to a subsequent parasite challenge (groups 13–15), (2) mice that receive adjuvant devoid of target or mock antigens and are subsequently challenged with parasites (groups 16–19) and (3) mice that are exposed to target antigen or mock antigen in the absence of adjuvant, and are subsequently challenged with parasites (groups 20–27)

3. Using a 21 G needle and suitable glass syringe, inject 200 μL Ag/CFA emulsion subcutaneously. The fold of skin from the scruff of the neck down the back is the ideal injection location (*see* **Note 20**).
4. Allow a 3-week rest period after the first vaccine challenge, prior to challenging the mice with a vaccine boost containing the antigen and Incomplete Freund's Adjuvant (*see* **Note 21**).
5. Repeat **step 1**, this time using antigen and Incomplete Freund's Adjuvant in a 1:1 ratio mixed into a white emulsion. Use a 21 G needle and suitable glass syringe to inject 200 μL Ag/IFA emulsion subcutaneously.
6. Ten days after the boost, take a blood sample from the tail vain, collecting 25 μL in a 1.5 mL cone-shaped microtube containing 2.5 μL heparin. Plasma can now be analyzed by ELISA for the presence of vaccine induced antibodies. Alternatively, plasma can be stored at –20 °C for future analysis.

7. Allow a 3-week rest period after the first vaccine boost, prior to administering a second vaccine boost. Repeat **steps 5** and **6**.
8. After 20 days (1 day prior to parasite challenge) take a blood sample from the tail vain, collecting 25 μL in a 1.5 mL cone-shaped microtube containing 2.5 μL heparin. Plasma can now be analyzed by ELISA or stored at −20 °C for future analysis.
9. Allow a 3-week rest after the second boost, and subsequently challenge the mice with 5×10^3 or 5×10^4 parasites/100 μL PBS by IP injection. Control groups can be injected with an equal dose of dead parasites (for preparation, *see* below, and *see* **Note 22**).
10. In a second experimental setup, allow an 8- to 12-week rest period after the second vaccine boost, prior to challenging the mice with 5×10^3 parasites/100 μL PBS by IP injection. For the third setup, wait the same 8- to 12-week period of time and challenge the mice with 5×10^4 parasites/100 μL PBS by IP injection. Alternatively, if results of the second setup were successful, the 8–12 week waiting period might be pushed to a 6 month waiting period (*see* **Note 23**).
11. Make a comparative follow-up study between antigen vaccinated and mock vaccinated mice (*see* **Note 24**), including parasitemia development, the occurrence of anemia, and immunological parameters at spleen level (*see* below).
12. Vaccine-induced protection should be measured as the fraction of mice that exhibit sterile protection against the parasite challenge (*see* **Note 25**).

3.2 Preparation of Purified Dead Parasites for Vaccination Control Groups

The procedure below has been optimized for *T. brucei* AnTat 1.1. The principle is based on the use of ion exchange column chromatography. At pH 8.0 this allows to separate trypanosomes from infected blood. For other trypanosomes, the functional pH might be slightly adjusted for optimal results.

1. Prepare 500 mL of PS and 500 mL PSG (Phosphate Saline—Glucose) pH 8.0: Start with 400 mL of distilled water, add 0.53 g NaCl, 2.11 g Na_2HPO_4, and 0.12 g NaH_2PO_4. For PSG, add 4.23 g glucose. Add distilled water to a total volume of 500 mL. If properly prepared the pH should be 8.0 exactly.
2. Agitate stock DEAE Sepharose to resuspend the resin particles. Check the pH of resin using a pH strip. Initially, the pH is around 6–6.5.
3. Allow 150 mL of the resin to settle for a few hours in a glass flask, and remove the layer of top buffer using a 10 mL pipette. Add 200 mL of fresh PS buffer pH 8.0 to the settled resin. Shake vigorously to mix and then adjust the pH to pH 8.0 using NaOH (50% H_2O stock).

4. Repeat **steps 4** and **5** twice a day for 2–3 days till the resin reaches a constant pH 8.0. Keep the resin at 4 °C during this procedure. Do not stir the resin during the pH adjustment procedure, as it will "grind" the resin particles and will prevent a proper column flow rate in the next step.
5. Place a 20 mL syringe (no needle) fit on a stand in vertical position with the nozzle facing downwards. Use cotton to block the nozzle of the syringe.
6. Add up to 10 mL of equilibrated DEAE resin slowly using a spoid. Allow the resin to settle and excess buffer to flow out from the syringe.
7. Add 10 mL of PSG buffer over the resin to equilibrate the DEAE ion exchange column. Allow the column to adjust to room temperature.
8. Collect infected blood from CO_2 euthanized *T. brucei* infected mice (peak parasitemia) through cardiac puncture and supplement the blood with 1% heparin in PBS in a 1.5 mL microtube.
9. Load the heparinized blood sample on the column drop-by-drop using a spoid and allow the blood to penetrate the resin.
10. Wash the column with PSG buffer pH 8.0 and collect 12 mL from the nozzle of the syringe in a 15 mL centrifuge tube. Only trypanosomes will flow through the column.
11. Centrifuge the flow-through fraction at approx. 1500 × *g* for 10 min at 4 °C.
12. Aspirate the supernatant and resuspend the pellet in a minimal volume of PBS, and count the parasites. Dilute parasites to the required concentration.
13. Lyse the parasites by three freeze–thaw cycles and store the lysed parasites at −80 °C for later use.

3.3 Vaccine Induced Antibody Titer Determination (ELISA)

1. Coat the plate: dilute the target antigen to the proper concentration (*see* above) and transfer 100 μL to each well of a high affinity, protein-binding ELISA plate. Seal the plate to prevent evaporation. Incubate at 4 °C overnight.
2. Block the plate: Bring the plate to room temperature, flick off the capture antibody solution, wash three times with PBS/Tween, and block nonspecific binding sites by adding 250 μL of Blocking Solution to each well.
3. Seal the plate and incubate at room temperature for 1 h.
4. While incubating the plate, prepare serial dilutions of all plasma samples that need to be analyzed. Use blocking solution as sample diluent. Start with a dilution of 1:50 and prepare subsequent 1:2 dilutions.

5. Wash the plate three times with PBS/Tween. Firmly blot the plate against clean paper towels.
6. Add 100 μL plasma sample dilution per well to the ELISA plate.
7. Seal the plate and incubate at room temperature for 2–4 h or at 4 °C overnight.
8. Flick off the plasma sample dilutions and wash the plate three times with PBS/Tween.
9. Dilute the goat anti-mouse-HRP conjugate to its predetermined optimal concentration in Blocking Buffer. Add 100 μL per well.
10. Seal the plate and incubate at room temperature for 30 min.
11. Wash the plate five times with PBS/Tween.
12. Add 100 μL TMB reagent into each well. Incubate at room temperature (room temperature for 30 min) for color development. To stop the color reaction, add 100 μL of TMB Stop Solution.
13. Read the optical density (OD) for each well with a microplate reader set to 450 nm.
14. Compare the results from plasma obtained D10 post second boost, D1 prior to parasite challenge and samples obtained after parasite challenge. This will indicate whether or not a memory recall immune activation took place.

3.4 Overall Spleen Immunopathology Assessment (FACS)

Trypanosome infections have a detrimental effect on spleen organization and cellular composition. Assessing the latter 3 weeks after parasite exposure will provide a very clear view on whether or not mice have been infected. Even with parasitemia levels below microscopic detection, alterations in composition of spleen cell populations can be recorded in this manner [16–19].

Perform all steps on ice water (4 °C), unless otherwise stated. All centrifugation steps are conducted at 314 × *g* for 7 min at 4 °C.

1. Euthanize mice according the protocol according to guidelines of the Institutional Committee for Ethical Use of Experimental Animals, the Institutional Animal Care and User Committee or an equivalent committee.
2. Isolate the spleens and place them separately in 6 mL DMEM.
3. Generate a single cell suspension by homogenizing the spleen in a C-tube, using a GentleMACS dissociator.
4. Prerinse a 70 μm cell strainer with 1 mL DMEM and pass the obtained cell suspension through the cell strainer to remove any residual cell clumps and tissue debris. Rinse the C-tube twice with 3 mL DMEM and apply it onto the cell-strainer.

5. Spin down the cells and gently remove the supernatant.
6. Perform RBC lysis by resuspending the "reddish" pellets in 5 mL 1× RBC lysis solution and incubate for 5 min on ice, occasionally shaking in 1 min intervals.
7. Stop RBC lysis by diluting the solution with 30 mL FACS buffer and spin down the cells.
8. Remove the supernatant, wash the cells with 5 mL FACS buffer, and spin them down once again.
9. Discard the supernatant and suspend the cells in 1 mL FACS buffer. Take a 10 μL aliquot and dilute the cells 1:5 with Trypan Blue. Count the cell concentration using a hemocytometer.
10. Distribute cells at 5×10^5 cells/100 μL in 5 mL polystyrene Round-Bottom tubes. Add 1 μL of anti CD16/32 Fc blocking antibody and incubate 20 min at 4 °C.
11. Prepare antibody cocktails for staining of (a) B cells, (b) T cells and NK cells and (c) monocytes and granulocytes. Prepare 1/200 dilutions (in FACS buffer) of (a) anti-B220-FITC+ anti-CD1d-PE + anti-CD138-PE/Cy7 + CD93-APC, (b) CD4-FITC + CD8-PE + NK1.1-APC, and (c) Ly6G-FITC + Ly6C-PE + CD11b-APC.
12. Mix 50 μL of antibody cocktail with the 100 μL cell suspension of **step 11**, resulting in a 1:600 final dilution of all antibodies. Incubate cells 20 min at 4 °C.
13. Analyze individual tubes and compare solenocyte profiles between targets-vaccinated and mock-vaccinated groups, challenged with either living or dead parasites (*see* **Note 26**). Include all other relevant controls indicated at the top of this protocol.

4 Notes

1. The combination of Complete Freund's Adjuvant (CFA) and Incomplete Freund's Adjuvant (IFA) cannot be used in the final host species (livestock or human) but the use of these compounds in experimental mouse vaccination trials allows to refer to a wealth of previous data. Complete Freund's Adjuvant is a water in oil emulsion which is composed of inactivated and dried mycobacteria, usually *Mycobacterium tuberculosis* (the pathogenic agent of tuberculosis). Incomplete Freund's Adjuvant is Freund's adjuvant without the mycobacteria component. If used improperly, the use of CFA can result in the induction of chronic inflammation and granuloma formation at the site of injection. Oil droplets might produce systemic

granulomas and chronic wasting disease. To avoid these side effects, the concentration of mycobacteria in CFA is advised to be kept below 0.1 mg/mL. Injection intervals should be kept at 2–3 weeks for the same reason, and not shortened. The adjuvant should be injected subcutaneously in small doses (0.1 mL for mice).

2. Gerbu is an adjuvant that has been formulated both for use in experimental mouse conditions and in larger animal breeds. It should be considered as a real alternative for the CFA/IFA vaccination method as it is equally effective, causing potentially less morbidity. At this moment, there, however, are no published trypanosome vaccine data using this adjuvant [20].
3. For specific purposes, adjuvants such as synthetic oligodeoxynucleotides (ODNs) containing unmethylated CpG motifs have been used [21, 22]. Some preliminary antitrypanosome vaccination data have indicated this might a promising adjuvant approach. However, besides the problem of being significantly more expensive than CFA/IFA or Gerbu, such approach poses the problem of translation from the experimental model to a real-world livestock infection. In addition, using more exotic vaccine additives makes it harder to understand the fundamental working mechanisms of the vaccine, needed for future translation to an applicable vaccine format.
4. Vaccination protocols need a multitude of control groups. One major control group is the mock vaccination. Often PBS is being used. This should be avoided and ideally a mock target most similar in molecular mass and production methods should be used in comparison to the actual vaccine target.
5. In case of the use of recombinant antigens (target and mock), the expression system can affect the result. Using bacterial expression systems does not allow assessing the influence of carbohydrate moieties. These have been shown to be important in trypanosome pathology [15]. Hence, when taking an antidisease vaccination approach this might affect the obtained results.
6. Using yeast or mammalian expression systems might provide an alternative to *Escherichia coli*, when glycosylation effects are to be expected. However, one must consider that glycosylation patterns can still be different when comparing recombinant antigen and natural antigen. Hence, when glycosylation is a key factor, backup data are needed to generate a relevant vaccine target.
7. Using bacterial expression systems could result in the presence of lipopolysaccharides (LPS) in the target preparation. This is, however, acceptable in preclinical research. Indeed, the only requirement in this context for commercial vaccines is that they

have been proven to be safe. Commercial vaccines have been reported to contain LPS at doses ranging from 'undetected' to 10^6 EU/mL (Endotoxin Units/mL) [23]. In addition, it could be argued that in experimental mouse vaccinations using Freund's Adjuvant, the presence of a limited amount of LPS in the recombinant target preparation will not affect the vaccination outcome. Still, knowledge of the LPS content could be important to understand the overall result.

8. The C57BL/6 mouse strain is characterized by a strong Th1 driven immune response, that results in relatively good parasitemia control accompanied by inflammatory pathology such anemia and cachexia. These are all hallmarks of livestock trypanosomosis. A very large collection of C57BL/6 gene knockout mice is available, opening the possibility for further research in case a vaccine result needs to be assessed at a functional gene level.
9. BALB/c mice have been used for particular experimental trypanosome applications. These mice are extremely susceptible for *T. congolense* infections. C3H/HeJ mice offer the advantage of being hypo-responsive to LPS, show high parasitemia susceptibility and shortened survival time in case of *T. brucei* infections. C3H/HeN mice show a similar phenotype but have a regular susceptibility to LPS. CBA/Ca mice exhibit low parasite burdens accompanied with low inflammatory pathology and have been used for specific studies of *T. brucei* infections.
10. Gene knockout mice can be used in vaccination set-ups. The most extreme example is the use of B cell knockout mice as a tool to prove the involvement of B cell memory in the functionality of the approach. This can be a very valuable approach to discover artifacts induced by immunomodulation activities of the vaccine target [24].
11. Experimental trypanosome vaccine research is mainly focused on *T. brucei* and *T. congolense*. During natural tsetse transmission, the inoculum size has been estimated to range from 5×10^3 to 5×10^4. Hence, it is important to stay within this range when exposing vaccinated mice to a parasite challenge. Previous research has shown that borderline protection can occur when the parasite challenge is dropped below 10^3/mouse [11]. Partial protective vaccine outcome under these conditions should be considered irrelevant for field conditions.
12. For more natural parasite exposure, infection by tsetse offer a relevant alternative over IP injection, but only very few laboratories have access to this technology.

13. Intradermal infections could possibly be considered as more 'natural' as compared to IP, but so far this position is not being supported by published data. In any case, natural tsetse fly saliva compounds that play a crucial role during the onset of infection will always be a missing factor in any nontsetse challenge. This is an important limitation of any experimental trypanosome challenge that omits the use of a natural vector [25–27].
14. The human and cattle infective *T. b. rhodesiense* is a serum-resistance associated (SRA) variant of *T. b. brucei*. As the SRA factor itself has no role in the mouse-trypanosome interaction, the biosafety risk associated to the use of *T. b. rhodesiense* in a primary vaccine trial is a significant burden. The human infective *T. b. gambiense* variants have in general the issue of very slow parasitemia growth in mice, but can have their unique value in vaccine studies [28]. Some laboratory clones of *T. brucei* have been adapted to monomorphic strains, but this has completely disrupted the relevant host–parasite interaction dynamics. Hence, these parasites should be considered irrelevant targets for vaccine research. They do not exist in natural infection conditions.
15. *T. evansi* infections have become a world-wide problem that threaten the livestock industry in regions including South America, North Africa, the Middle East, Southern Europe and Asia, including the Russian territories, China and several countries in South-East Asia. From a genetic point of view, however, they can be considered very similar to *T. brucei*. In fact, it is now widely accepted that *T. evansi* is not one group of parasites, but rather a result of *T. brucei* adaptations that have occurred several times independently during trypanosome evolution [29]. Nevertheless, taken the unique host–parasite interaction that governs *T. evansi* infections, and the fact that many *T. evansi* parasites are able to infect mice, they should be considered valuable candidates for future vaccine research. *T. equiperdum* is a sexually transmitted parasite causing pathology in equines. There is no relevant mouse model for this infection, and the parasite is considered closely related to *T. evansi*. Hence, at this stage they are not to be considered as main targets for experimental vaccine research.
16. *T. suis* is a trypanosome mainly affecting pigs. At this stage there are only limited data available on host–pathogen interaction biology and no relevant mouse models seem to be available that would allow to initiate vaccine research at this stage.
17. *T. musculi* is a natural rodent trypanosome. While this parasite would be the most relevant to study vaccine interventions in the most natural host–parasite vaccination context, *T. musculi*

only causes very limited pathology and is considered self-healing in mice. Hence the model does not offer a relevant advantage in research that focusses on the pathogenic trypanosomes that cause either HAT or AAT [30].

18. Optimal antigen coating depends on factors including the coating surface. Manufacturers might indicate a suggested coating concentration as 600 ng/cm^2. A typical 96-well surface is 0.33 cm^2, resulting in a 200 ng coating capacity + additional capacity on the side of the wells. Protein size and charge might affect coating efficiency.
19. Avoid the use of disposable plastic syringes with a rubber plunger, as the adjuvant will interfere with plunger movement and mixing will become impossible after a few seconds.
20. Using the lower neck skin as injection side ensures the mouse has only limited access to the injection site preventing grooming or interfering with the vaccination. In addition, the location provides ample physical space for a 200 μL injection. Avoid using CFA/IFA as adjuvant for IP vaccination. The adjuvant will cause limited granuloma formation when used in a subcutaneous setup, providing a slow release of the antigen. IP injection will result in local inflammation, systemic granuloma formation, and antigen dilution and will not allow proper longer-term retention.
21. Antibody induction after a first challenge takes 4–10 days (IgM-IgG) and the half-life of IgM and IgG antibodies is estimated to be between 5 and 21 days, respectively. Memory B cell formation requires antigen stimulation, B cell expansion, immunoglobulin class switching and B cell differentiation of mature naive B cells to germinal center B cells, plasma cells and memory cells. This process will take up to 2 weeks. Considering the half-life of the Ig production and the time needed for memory B cell formation, a 3-week interval period ensures that Abs start to decline but are still circulating at the time of secondary antigen exposure. This ensures a competition between the Abs of the first generation and newly formed B cells as well as reactivated memory cells. Only cells with a B cell receptor (BCR) exhibiting a higher affinity than the circulating antibodies will be favored and activated in the second challenge, hence improving the immune response in terms of BCR quality/affinity.
22. Infection should be executed in mice challenged with the actual vaccine target antigen as well as the mock vaccine target. Additional control groups are listed at the start of this protocol and Table 1. In a first experiment, vaccinated mice can be infected with 5×10^3 parasites, a dose which can be considered a moderate challenge. In a repeat experiment, mice should be

challenged with a high dose of 5×10^4 parasites, as this is considered the upper limit of parasite transmission by the tsetse. This step will allow to see if vaccine induced antibodies (if present—see below) offer a significant level of protection.

23. The 8–12 week interval between the second boost and the parasite challenge will allow to assess the vaccination potential of the target. After this period of time, antibody titers induced by the second boost will have resided and protection now will rely on the capacity of the immune system to deliver a memory recall response. If results are promising, the 12-week waiting period can be extended to a 6-month waiting period. In the past, several papers were published where the waiting time between the last challenge and parasite exposure was limited to less than 1 week (reviewed in ref. [7]). In this case the onset of infection will be significantly affected by the immune modulation caused by the adjuvant. Such protocol does not allow assessing the true meaning of a vaccine, as it excludes the assessment of any memory recall response activation.
24. A proper mock vaccination includes at least a group of mice that have undergone the same vaccine procedure, using a proper mock target to replace the actual vaccine target. When a proper immune profiling, however, is planned as part of the investigation, a multitude of additional groups have to be considered, including (a) mice that received adjuvant or antigen the absence of a final parasite challenge, (b) mice that were exposed to adjuvant challenges devoid of target of mock antigen, and subsequently exposed to parasites, and (c) mice that were exposed to repeated target or mock antigen exposer in the absence of adjuvant, prior to the parasite challenge.
25. Vaccine induced protection should be measured as number of mice in which the parasite cannot establish an infection. A reduced parasite burden is not protection, as eventually all infected animals will succumb. Using a reduced first peak parasitemia as promising positive result has so far never given rise to a method with field applicability. Borderline protection is obtained when protection is seen at low-dose challenge only, but not the higher 5×10^4 parasites challenge.
26. Trypanosome infections have a detrimental effect on spleen organization and cellular composition. Assessing the latter will provide a very clear view on whether or not mice have been infected. Even with parasitemia levels below microscopic detection, alterations in composition of spleen cell populations can be recorded. Challenging a group of mice with dead parasites rather than PBS as control, will ensure all mice have seen a final exposure to parasite antigen. This is a more useful control than using a PBS sham injection in the control group.

Acknowledgments

Trypanosome vaccine research at the Magez laboratory is being supported by two grants of the FWO (Fonds voor Wetenschappelijk Onderzoek—Vlaanderen) # G015016 N and #G013518 N.

References

1. Cnops J, Magez S, De Trez C (2015) Escape mechanisms of African trypanosomes: why trypanosomosis is keeping us awake. Parasitology 142(3):417–427. https://doi.org/10.1017/S0031182014001838
2. Pinger J, Chowdhury S, Papavasiliou FN (2017) Variant surface glycoprotein density defines an immune evasion threshold for African trypanosomes undergoing antigenic variation. Nat Commun 8(1):828. https://doi.org/10.1038/s41467-017-00959-w
3. Koumandou VL, Boehm C, Horder KA, Field MC (2013) Evidence for recycling of invariant surface transmembrane domain proteins in African trypanosomes. Eukaryot Cell 12 (2):330–342. https://doi.org/10.1128/EC.00273-12
4. Ziegelbauer K, Multhaup G, Overath P (1992) Molecular characterization of two invariant surface glycoproteins specific for the bloodstream stage of *Trypanosoma brucei*. J Biol Chem 267(15):10797–10803
5. Engstler M, Pfohl T, Herminghaus S, Boshart M, Wiegertjes G, Heddergott N, Overath P (2007) Hydrodynamic flow-mediated protein sorting on the cell surface of trypanosomes. Cell 131(3):505–515. https://doi.org/10.1016/j.cell.2007.08.046
6. Altman MO, Angeletti D, Yewdell JW (2018) Antibody immunodominance: the key to understanding influenza virus antigenic drift. Viral Immunol 31(2):142–149. https://doi.org/10.1089/vim.2017.0129
7. La Greca F, Magez S (2011) Vaccination against trypanosomiasis: can it be done or is the trypanosome truly the ultimate immune destroyer and escape artist? Hum Vaccin 7 (11):1225–1233. https://doi.org/10.4161/hv.7.11.18203
8. Black SJ, Mansfield JM (2016) Prospects for vaccination against pathogenic African trypanosomes. Parasite Immunol 38(12):735–743. https://doi.org/10.1111/pim.12387
9. Wong R, Bhattacharya D (2018) Basics of memory B-cell responses: lessons from and for the real world. Immunology. https://doi.org/10.1111/imm.13019
10. Lambert PH, Liu M, Siegrist CA (2005) Can successful vaccines teach us how to induce efficient protective immune responses? Nat Med 11(4 Suppl):S54–S62. https://doi.org/10.1038/nm1216
11. Radwanska M, Magez S, Dumont N, Pays A, Nolan D, Pays E (2000) Antibodies raised against the flagellar pocket fraction of *Trypanosoma brucei* preferentially recognize HSP60 in cDNA expression library. Parasite Immunol 22 (12):639–650
12. Li SQ, Yang WB, Ma LJ, Xi SM, Chen QL, Song XW, Kang J, Yang LZ (2009) Immunization with recombinant actin from Trypanosoma evansi induces protective immunity against *T. evansi*, *T. equiperdum* and *T. b. brucei* infection. Parasitol Res 104(2):429–435. https://doi.org/10.1007/s00436-008-1216-9. Erratum in: Parasitol Res. 104(2):493. Lun, Zhao-Rong [removed]
13. Li SQ, Fung MC, Reid SA, Inoue N, Lun ZR (2007) Immunization with recombinant beta-tubulin from *Trypanosoma evansi* induced protection against *T. evansi*, *T. equiperdum* and *T. b. brucei* infection in mice. Parasite Immunol 29(4):191–199. https://doi.org/10.1111/j.1365-3024.2006.00933.x
14. Lubega GW, Byarugaba DK, Prichard RK (2002) Immunization with a tubulin-rich preparation from *Trypanosoma brucei* confers broad protection against African trypanosomosis. Exp Parasitol 102(1):9–22
15. Stijlemans B, Baral TN, Guilliams M, Brys L, Korf J, Drennan M, Van Den Abbeele J, De Baetselier P, Magez S (2007) A glycosylphosphatidylinositol-based treatment alleviates trypanosomiasis-associated immunopathology. J Immunol 179(6):4003–4014
16. Radwanska M, Guirnalda P, De Trez C, Ryffel B, Black S, Magez S (2008) Trypanosomiasis-induced B cell apoptosis results in loss of protective anti-parasite antibody responses and abolishment of vaccine-induced memory responses. PLoS Pathog 4 (5):e1000078. https://doi.org/10.1371/journal.ppat.1000078
17. Bockstal V, Guirnalda P, Caljon G, Goenka R, Telfer JC, Frenkel D, Radwanska M, Magez S,

Black SJ (2011) *T. brucei* infection reduces B lymphopoiesis in bone marrow and truncates compensatory splenic lymphopoiesis through transitional B-cell apoptosis. PLoS Pathog 7 (6):e1002089. https://doi.org/10.1371/journal.ppat.1002089

18. Cnops J, Bockstal V, De Trez C, Miquel MC, Radwanska M, Magez S (2015) Curative drug treatment of trypanosomosis leads to the restoration of B-cell lymphopoiesis and splenic B-cell compartments. Parasite Immunol 37 (9):485–491. https://doi.org/10.1111/pim.12209
19. Cnops J, Kauffmann F, De Trez C, Baltz T, Keirsse J, Radwanska M, Muraille E, Magez S (2016) Maintenance of B cells during chronic murine *Trypanosoma brucei gambiense* infection. Parasite Immunol 38(10):642–647. https://doi.org/10.1111/pim.12344
20. Stills H Jr (2005) Adjuvants and antibody production: dispelling the myths associated with Freund's complete and other adjuvants. ILAR J 46(3):280–293
21. Bode C, Zhao G, Steinhagen F, Kinjo T, Klinman DM (2011) CpG DNA as a vaccine adjuvant. Expert Rev Vaccines 10(4):499–511. https://doi.org/10.1586/erv.10.174
22. Harris TH, Mansfield JM, Paulnock DM (2007) CpG oligodeoxynucleotide treatment enhances innate resistance and acquired immunity to African trypanosomes. Infect Immun 75 (5):2366–2373. https://doi.org/10.1128/IAI.01649-06
23. Brito LA, Singh M (2011) Acceptable levels of endotoxin in vaccine formulations during preclinical research. J Pharm Sci 100(1):34–37. https://doi.org/10.1002/jps.22267
24. Stijlemans B, Radwanska M, De Trez C, Magez S (2017) African trypanosomes undermine humoral responses and vaccine development: link with inflammatory responses? Front Immunol 24(8):582. https://doi.org/10.3389/fimmu.2017.00582
25. Caljon G, Van Den Abbeele J, Stijlemans B, Coosemans M, De Baetselier P, Magez S (2006) Tsetse fly saliva accelerates the onset of *Trypanosoma brucei* infection in a mouse model associated with a reduced host inflammatory response. Infect Immun 74(11):6324–6330. https://doi.org/10.1128/IAI.01046-06
26. Caljon G, De Ridder K, De Baetselier P, Coosemans M, Van Den Abbeele J (2010) Identification of a tsetse fly salivary protein with dual inhibitory action on human platelet aggregation. PLoS One 5(3):e9671. https://doi.org/10.1371/journal.pone.0009671
27. Magez S, Caljon G (2011) Mouse models for pathogenic African trypanosomes: unravelling the immunology of host-parasite-vector interactions. Parasite Immunol 33(8):423–429. https://doi.org/10.1111/j.1365-3024.2011.01293.x
28. Coustou V, Plazolles N, Guegan F, Baltz T (2012) Sialidases play a key role in infection and anaemia in *Trypanosoma congolense* animal trypanosomiasis. Cell Microbiol 14 (3):431–445. https://doi.org/10.1111/j.1462-5822.2011.01730.x
29. Carnes J, Anupama A, Balmer O, Jackson A, Lewis M, Brown R, Cestari I, Desquesnes M, Gendrin C, Hertz-Fowler C, Imamura H, Ivens A, Kořený L, Lai DH, MacLeod A, McDermott SM, Merritt C, Monnerat S, Moon W, Myler P, Phan I, Ramasamy G, Sivam D, Lun ZR, Lukeš J, Stuart K, Schnaufer A (2015) Genome and phylogenetic analyses of *Trypanosoma evansi* reveal extensive similarity to *T. brucei* and multiple independent origins for dyskinetoplasty. PLoS Negl Trop Dis 9(1):e3404. https://doi.org/10.1371/journal.pntd.0003404
30. Albright JW, Jiang D, Albright JF (1997) Innate control of the early course of infection in mice inoculated with *Trypanosoma musculi*. Cell Immunol 176(2):146–152

Chapter 43

Isolation of *Trypanosoma brucei brucei* Infection-Derived Splenic Marginal Zone B Cells Based on CD1d^{High}/B220^{High} Surface Expression in a Two-Step MACS-FACS Approach

Nick Vereecke, Magdalena Radwanska, and Stefan Magez

Abstract

Magnetic- and fluorescent-activated cell sorting (MACS and FACS) are used for isolation of distinct cell populations for subsequent studies including transcriptomics. The latter allows for the analysis of infection-induced alterations in gene expression profiles. MACS and FACS both use antibodies against cell surface molecules to isolate populations of interest. Standardized methods for both approaches exist for use in mouse models. These protocols, however, do not account for the fact that infection-associated immunopathology can significantly modulate the cell surface expression of targeted molecules. This is the case for *Trypanosoma brucei brucei* infection, where downregulation of CD23 surface expression on B cells has been reported. This hallmark of progressing infection interferes with the commercially available MACS technique for B cell purification, as CD23 expression is the target for the separation between Marginal Zone (MZ) and Follicular (Fo) B cells. Here, we provide a robust alternative method for isolation of infection-derived MZ B cells using CD1d and B220 surface molecules in a two-step MACS-FACS approach. The method yields 99% pure viable infection-derived MZ B cells, allowing extraction of a high quality total RNA suitable for subsequent RNA sequencing.

Key words Marginal zone B cells, Magnetic-activated cell sorting (MACS), Fluorescent-activated cell sorting (FACS), RNA isolation, cell isolation, RNA sequencing

1 Introduction

Magnetic-activated cell sorting (MACS) and fluorescent-activated cell sorting (FACS) facilitate isolation of specific cell populations. Both techniques use antibodies recognizing specific cell surface markers to differentiate between various cell populations. While the MACS method relies on antibodies conjugated to magnetic particles, antibodies coupled to fluorochromes are used in FACS. In case of a MACS approach, the cell population of interest is sorted using a magnetic field. This technique is fast but cannot be controlled with high accuracy. In contrast, FACS separation is using a laser to excite fluorochromes in order to separate labeled cells. This

Paul A. M. Michels et al. (eds.), *Trypanosomatids: Methods and Protocols*, Methods in Molecular Biology, vol. 2116, https://doi.org/10.1007/978-1-0716-0294-2_43,

allows for a very high control of accuracy, but in contrast to MACS it is a slow technique when it comes to isolating minor cell populations. Both isolation techniques are characterized by a limited cell recovery yield [1, 2]. Choosing a good cell isolation protocol is of major importance when considering downstream RNA sequencing applications, which allows studying infection-associated cellular mechanisms underlying immunopathology. Moreover, those methods require the isolation of sufficient cell quantity and high population purity, which is challenging when working with cell populations that only account for a small fraction of an immunological organ. This is the case for the isolation of splenic Marginal Zone (MZ) B cells, a cell population that accounts for less than 5% of the total splenocytes. These cells play a key role in immune defense against blood-borne extracellular pathogens, mainly but not exclusively by mounting T cell-independent antibody responses [3, 4]. Previously it was demonstrated that *Trypanosoma brucei brucei* infection triggers B cell pathology, resulting in complete MZ B cell depletion at early onset infection [5]. Multiple mechanisms were proposed to be involved in the trypanosomosis-induced B cell depletion, including (1) interferon-gamma induced inflammation, (2) natural killer mediated toxicity, or (3) parasite-cell contact induced apoptosis [5–10]. However, due to the lack of comprehensive transcriptomics, proteomics, and metabolomics data, the exact mechanisms involved remain to be elucidated. Currently, only Miltenyi Biotec GmbH (Bergisch Gladbach, Germany) provides a negative MACS-based selection protocol for the isolation of splenic MZ B cells using the conventional differential surface expression of CD23 on Follicular (Fo) and MZ B cells [11, 12]. Besides this surface marker, mature naive MZ B cells express a variety of molecules ($B220^{+}IgM^{High}IgD^{Int}CD21\text{-}35^{High}\text{-}CD23^{Low}CD1d^{High}$) which are different from those found on mature naive Fo B cells ($B220^{+}IgM^{Low}IgD^{High}CD21\text{-}35^{low}\text{-}CD23^{High}CD1d^{low}$) [3, 5]. However, the use of a commercially available CD23-based MACS MZ B cell isolation protocol on *T. b. brucei* derived samples results in significantly reduced performance due to altered CD23 surface expression, and infection-associated fluctuations of cell numbers. The latter include erythrocytes, transitional B cells, MZ and Fo B cells, plasma B cells, and T lymphocytes [5, 9, 13]. Similar events occur when observing progressing immunopathology in other parasitic infections such as *Plasmodium* sp. and *Leishmania* sp., but also in *Staphylococcus* sp. and Simian Immunodeficiency Virus (SIV) infections [14–19].

Here we demonstrate that infection-derived splenic MZ B cells can be efficiently isolated using a combined MACS-FACS approach. The advantage of speed offered by MACS is used to eliminate the major non B cell populations, followed by the precision of FACS to purify MZ B cells from the total B cell pool. The included MACS pre-enrichment step shortens significantly the overall time needed for purification, allowing for the optimal recovery of viable cells and subsequently the isolation of high-quality total RNA. Rather than using CD23, we developed the combined purification protocol relying on $CD1d^{High}/B220^{High}$ surface marker expression of MZ B cells [3, 5]. Hence, the established MACS-FACS method includes the first step of a MACS-based pre-enrichment for MZ and Fo B cells, while the second FACS step allows isolation of MZ B cells from this pre-enriched fraction. The resulting MZ B cell population is 99% pure, which can be subsequently used for extraction of a high-quality total RNA for downstream RNA-based applications.

2 Materials

Prepare all reagents following general laboratory sterility rules in a laminar flow. All reagents are kept at 4 °C, unless stated otherwise.

Mice should be housed according to guidelines of the Institutional Committee for Ethical use of Experimental Animals, an Institutional Animal Care and User Committee or an equivalent committee that reviews and approves all protocols *prior* to the execution of experiments. During the experiment, mice should be kept under optimal conditions with free access to food and water, ambient temperature of 18 °C to 23 °C, and an air humidity of 40–60%. Mice should be provided with cage enrichment to decrease overall stress levels and health should be checked daily. Humane endpoints for the experiment must be set prior to the start of the experiment.

2.1 Mice, Infection, and Single Cell Suspensions

1. C57Bl/6N mice, 8-week-old female. Perform intraperitoneal injection using 5000 live pleomorphic AnTat 1.1E *T. b. brucei*, resuspended in PBS pH 7.2 [20] (*see* **Note 1**).
2. Dulbecco's Modified Eagle Medium (DMEM): 10% fetal bovine serum (FBS), 1% Penicillin/Streptomycin. Store at 4 °C and use at room temperature.
3. GentleMACS dissociator with C tubes (Milenyi Biotec, Germany).
4. Red Blood Cell (RBC) lysis solution: pH 7.2, containing ammonium chloride, potassium carbonate, and EDTA. Add 1 volume of 10× stock RBC lysis solution (Biolegend, USA) to 9 volumes deionized water. Store at 4 °C and use at room temperature.
5. FACS buffer: pH 7.2, 0.5% FBS using BD FACS Sheath fluid. Store at 4 °C and use at room temperature (*see* **Note 2**).
6. Trypan Blue dead cell exclusion dye.
7. Neubauer improved hemocytometer cell counting chamber.
8. Inverted microscope with 20× objective.

2.2 MACS-Based MZ B Cell Pre-enrichment

1. Separation buffer: pH 7.2, 2 mM EDTA, 0.5% FBS using autoMACS rinsing solution (Miltenyi Biotec, Germany).
2. Non B cell biotinylated antibody cocktail and anti-biotin microbeads available in MZ and Fo B cell isolation kit (Miltenyi Biotec, Germany) (*see* **Note 3**).
3. MidiMACS separator with LS column purchased from Miltenyi Biotec, Germany.
4. FACS buffer: pH 7.2, 0.5% FBS using BD FACS Sheath fluid. Store at 4 °C and use at room temperature.
5. Trypan Blue dead cell exclusion dye.
6. Neubauer improved hemocytometer cell counting chamber.
7. Inverted microscope with 20× objective.

2.3 CD1d^{High}/B220^{High}-Based MZ B Cell Isolation Using FACS

1. FACSAria II (BD Biosciences, USA), allowing to detect FITC, PE, PE-CY7, and APC fluorochromes.
2. FACS buffer: pH 7.2 using BD FACS Sheath fluid. Store at 4 °C and use at room temperature.
3. Pre-Sort Buffer (BD Biosciences, USA). Store at −20 °C, protected from light, and use at 4 °C.
4. 5 mL polystyrene Round-Bottom tubes purchased from Corning, USA.
5. 5 mL polystyrene Round-Bottom tubes with cell-strainer cap purchased from Corning, USA.
6. Anti-Fcγ blocking, using CD16-32 antibody (clone 93) purchased from Biolegend, USA.
7. Fluorochrome-conjugated antibodies: B220-FITC (clone RA3-6B2), CD1d-PE (clone 1B1), CD138-PE/Cy7 (clone 281-2), and CD93-APC (clone AA4.1), all purchased from Biolegend, USA.
8. *post*-FACS buffer: pH 7.2, 0.5% FBS, using BD FACS Sheath fluid, supplemented with 20 U/mL RNase Inhibitor (Roche, Switzerland).

2.4 RNA Isolation and 1.2% Agarose Formaldehyde Denaturing Electrophoresis

1. TRIzol reagent.
2. Direct-Zol RNA MiniPrep Plus RNA isolation kit (Zymo Research, USA), containing Zymo-Spin IIICG Column, Direct-zol RNA PreWash Buffer, RNA Wash Buffer, DNase I (6 U/μL), and DNA Digestion Buffer (*see* **Note 4**).
3. 95–100% ethanol, RNase/DNase free.
4. *in-column* DNase I reagent: Add 5 μL of DNase I to 75 μL DNA Digestion Buffer.
5. Microcentrifuge at 15,000 × *g*.
6. NanoDrop spectrophotometer.

7. 10× FA buffer: Add MOPS to a final concentration of 200 mM in 100 mL DEPC-treated water. Add 5 mL of 0.5 M sodium acetate and adjust the pH to 7.0 with NaOH. Finally, add EDTA (pH 8.0) to a final concentration of 10 mM and make up to 250 mL with DEPC-treated water. Autoclave prior to use (*see* **Note 5**).
8. 1× FA running buffer: Add 100 mL 10× FA buffer and 20 mL formaldehyde (37%) to 880 mL DEPC-treated water in a fume hood.
9. 1.2% agarose FA denaturing gel (for a 10 × 7 cm gel tray): Weigh 0.72 g agarose E and dissolve into 6 mL 10× FA buffer and 54 mL DEPC-treated water. Cool down to 65 °C and add 1 mL formaldehyde (37%) in a fume hood (*see* **Note 6**).
10. Riboruler RNA ladder (Invitrogen, USA), 1:3 diluted in RNase/DNase-free water and 2× Loading Dye (*see* **Note 7**).
11. Heat block at 70 °C.
12. Gel electrophoresis apparatus and power supply (75 and 100 V required).

3 Methods

3.1 Mice, Infection, And Single Cell Suspensions

Perform all steps at room temperature, unless otherwise stated. All centrifugation steps are conducted at 314 × *g* for 7 min at room temperature.

1. Perform intraperitoneal injection containing 5000 *T. b. brucei* AnTat1.1E parasites. Four infected and four naive control mice should be used for isolation of MZ B cells (*see* **Note 8**).
2. Isolate the spleens and place them separately in 6 mL DMEM.
3. Generate a single cell suspension by homogenizing the spleen in a C-tube, using a GentleMACS dissociator (*see* **Note 9**).
4. Prerinse a 70 μm cell strainer with 1 mL DMEM and pass the obtained cell suspension through the cell strainer to remove any residual cell clumps and tissue debris. Rinse the C-tube twice with 3 mL DMEM and apply it onto the cell-strainer.
5. Spin down the cells and gently remove the supernatant.
6. Perform RBC lysis by resuspending the "reddish" pellets in 5 mL 1× RBC lysis solution and incubate for 5 min on ice, occasionally shaking in 1 min intervals.
7. Stop RBC lysis by diluting the solution with 30 mL FACS buffer and spin down the cells.
8. Remove the supernatant, wash the cells with 5 mL FACS buffer, and spin them down once again (*see* **Note 10**).

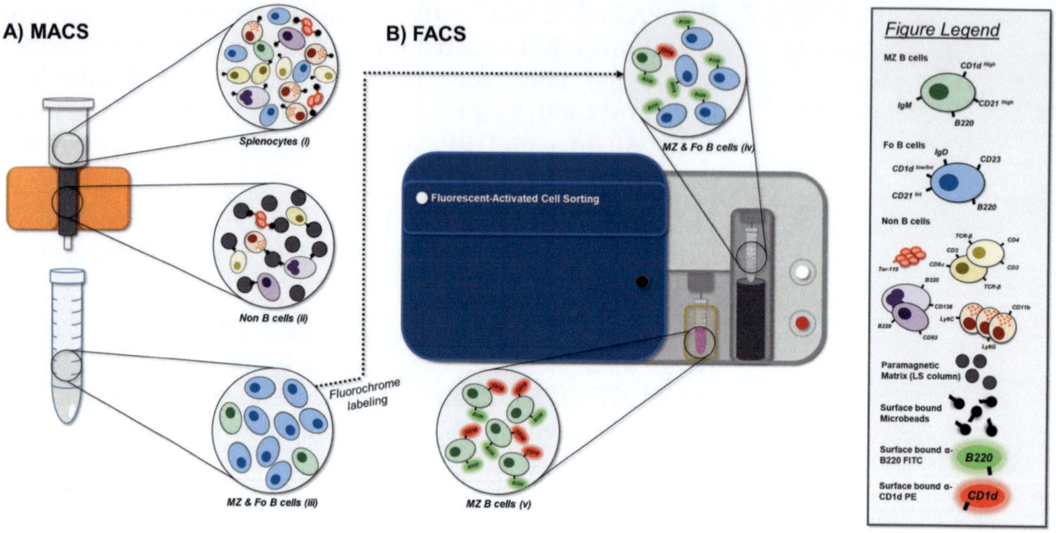

Fig. 1 Schematic overview of MACS-FACS protocol for the isolation of MZ B cells. Single cell suspensions were prepared after red blood cell lysis of a spleen cell suspension. Four hundred million splenocytes were labeled with a biotin-antibody cocktail targeting all spleen non B cells and anti-biotin MicroBeads. This suspension was loaded onto a first Miltenyi Biotec LS column (i), retaining the non B cell population (ii). The flow-through MZ and Fo B cell fraction (iii) was labeled with a fluorochrome-conjugated antibody cocktail containing B220-FITC, CD1d-PE, CD138-PE/CY7, and CD93-APC (iv) and used for CD1d^{High}/B220^{High} FACS-based MZ B cell (v) isolation

9. Discard the supernatant, pool the obtained four single cell suspensions containing RBC-depleted splenocytes into a single tube, and take a small aliquot (typically 10 μL). Dilute the aliquot of the cells 1:5 with Trypan Blue and count the cell concentration using a hemocytometer (*see* **Note 11**).

3.2 MACS-Based MZ B Cell Pre-enrichment

Perform all steps at 4 °C, unless stated otherwise. All centrifugation steps are conducted at 314 × *g* for 7 min at 4 °C. A schematic overview is given in Fig. 1a.

1. Take 4×10^8 RBC-depleted splenocytes, spin them down, and remove the supernatant.
2. Resuspend the pellet in 400 μL separation buffer and mix with 100 μL of the non B cell biotinylated antibody cocktail. Incubate for 5 min (*see* **Note 12**).
3. Add 300 μL separation buffer and 200 μL anti-biotin microbeads to the tube and mix gently. Incubate for 10 min.
4. Wash the cells with 10 mL separation buffer and spin them down to remove any unbound antibodies and microbeads.
5. Place a LS column in the MidiMACS magnet and prerinse with 3 mL separation buffer (*see* **Note 13**).

6. Resuspend the pellet in 500 μL separation buffer, place a new 15 mL Falcon tube under the LS column and apply the cells (*see* **Note 14**).
7. Wash the tube with 3 mL separation buffer and apply onto the LS column. The pre-enriched MZ and Fo B cells are present in the flow-through (*see* **Note 15**).
8. Determine the concentration of the pre-enriched MZ and Fo B cell fraction by diluting a small aliquot (typically 10 μL) 1:5 with Trypan Blue. Spin the cells down and bring them to a final concentration of 5×10^7 cells/mL using Pre-Sort Buffer (*see* **Note 16**).

3.3 FACS-Based MZ B Cell Isolation

Keep all cell preparations on ice water (4 °C), unless stated otherwise. A schematic overview is given in Fig. 1b.

1. Add 20 U/mL RNase inhibitor to the pre-enriched MZ and Fo B cells to prevent any RNase activity in the subsequent sorting procedure (*see* **Note 17**).
2. Add anti-CD16-32 to a final 1:400 dilution and incubate for 20 min, followed by the addition of the four fluorochrome-conjugated antibodies using a final dilution of 1:300 in FACS buffer. Incubate cells with antibodies for 30 min in the dark.
3. Establish compensation settings and gating strategies using the nonstained cells, single-, double-, and quadruple-stained cells. First, determine the live gate, followed by the exclusion of $CD93^+$ and $CD138^+$ immature and plasma cells, respectively. Subsequently, sort MZ B cells using their $CD1d^{High}/B220^{High}$ profile. Figure 2 shows and explains the gating strategy in more detail (*see* **Notes 18** and **19**).
4. Prepare six 5 mL polystyrene Round-Bottom tubes with 100 μL *post*-FACS buffer to collect the MZ B cell fractions.
5. Prior to FACS, dilute each fraction (750 μL) of the stained pre-enriched MZ and Fo B cell in 1250 mL FACS buffer and filter them through a cell-strainer cap of a 5 mL polystyrene Round-Bottom tube.
6. Apply the tube onto the FACS and sort MZ B cells in 20 to 40 min intervals, resulting in sorting of 200,000–400,000 MZ B cell events, varying when working with naive and infection-derived samples.
7. Immediately transfer the sorted MZ B cell fractions into a 2 mL microcentrifuge tubes, rinse the 5 mL polystyrene Round-Bottom tube with 500 μL TRI reagent, and mix it with the fraction present in the 2 mL microcentrifuge tube. Keep tubes at room temperature.

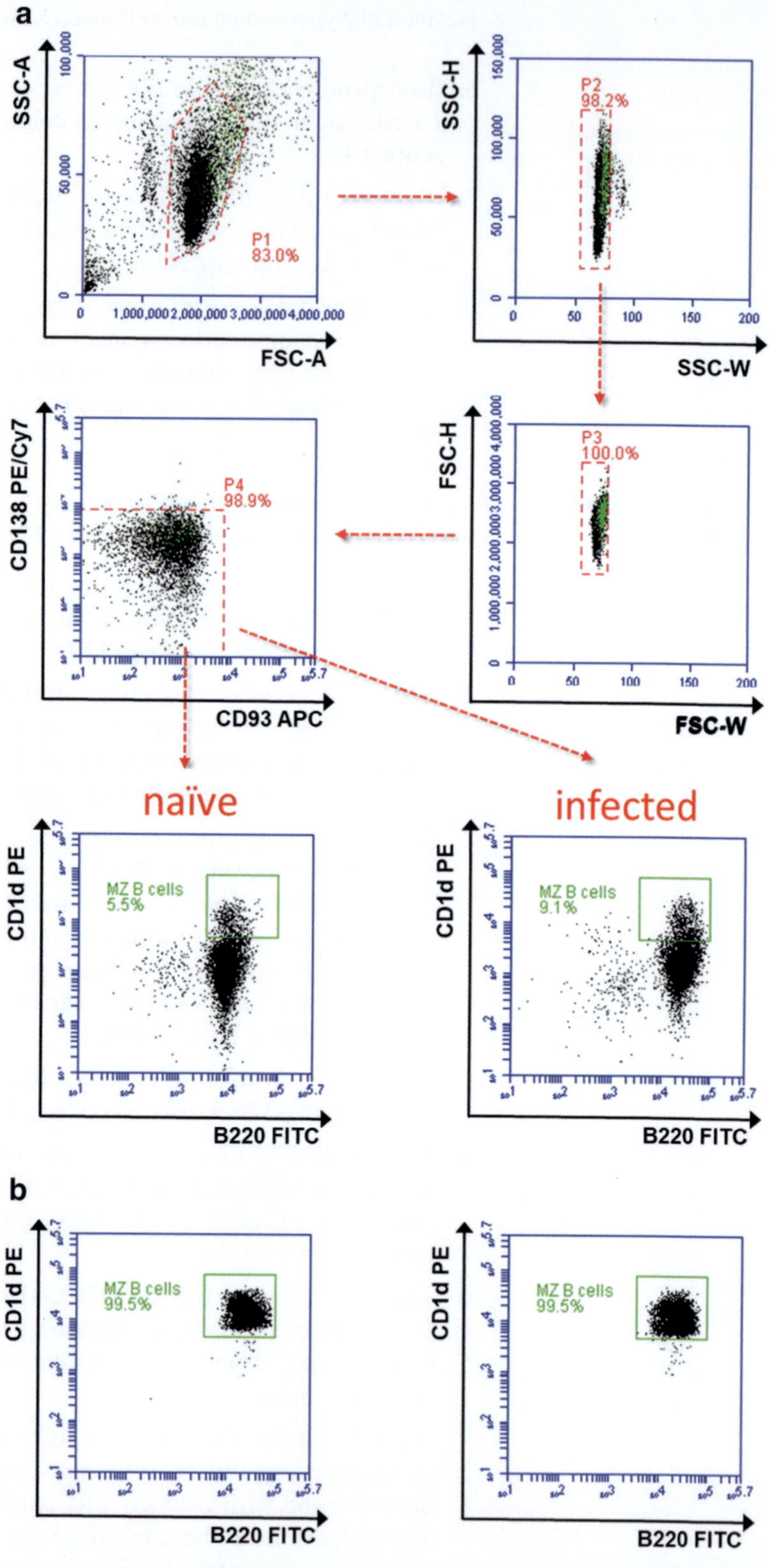

Fig. 2 CD1d^{High}/B220^{High}-based FACS MZ B cell isolation gating strategy for naive and infection-derived samples (**a**), for the isolation of a highly pure MZ B cell population (**b**). In both naive and infection-derived settings, cells were gated

3.4 RNA Isolation and 1.2% Agarose Formaldehyde Denaturing Electrophoresis

Perform all steps at room temperature, unless stated otherwise. All centrifugation steps are conducted at 15,000 × *g* programmed "at set speed." This allows the centrifuge to first reach the required 15,000 × *g*, followed by a spin for the requested time. The RNA isolation and denaturing agarose electrophoresis procedures are executed as indicated by the Direct-Zol RNA MiniPrep Plus RNA isolation protocol (Zymo Research, USA) and Qiagen's RNeasy Mini Handbook (Qiagen, Germany), respectively.

1. Disrupt and homogenize the TRIzol-submerged MZ B cells by vortexing them for 1 min.
2. Add an equal volume (typically 700 μL) of 95–100% ethanol to each fraction and mix thoroughly.
3. Transfer 800 μL of the lysed cell mixture onto a Zymo-Spin IIICG column, placed into a collection tube, and centrifuge for 30 s.
4. Repeat **step 3** until all fractions have been applied on the same Zymo-Spin IIICG column (*see* **Note 20**).
5. Add 400 μL RNA Wash buffer to the column and centrifuge for 30 s.
6. Gently add 80 μL of the *in-column* DNase I reagent onto the column matrix and incubate for 15 min at room temperature.
7. Add 400 μL Direct-zol RNA PreWash and centrifuge for 30 s.
8. Discard the flow-through and repeat **step** 7.
9. Add 700 μL RNA Wash Buffer and centrifuge 2 min to ensure complete removal of the wash buffer.
10. Transfer the column carefully into an RNase-free microcentrifuge tube and add 50 μL RNase/DNase-free water in the center of the column matrix and centrifuge for 30 s. Immediately place the tube on ice (*see* **Note 21**).
11. Repeat **step 10** to collect a second eluate.
12. Determine the concentration using NanoDrop and verify A_{260}/A_{280} and A_{260}/A_{230} ratios (*see* **Note 22**).
13. Subsequently prepare MZ B cell isolated RNA, 1:3 diluted Riboruler RNA ladder, a positive control (100 ng A20 B cell lymphoma RNA), and a negative control (RNase/DNase-free

Fig. 2 (continued) on their forward scatter area (FSC-A) and side scatter area (SSC-A), excluding dead cells and debris from the live gate. Next, doublets were excluded based on width, forward, and side scatter height (FSC-H and SSC-H, respectively). This is followed by gating out any residual $CD93^+$ Immature and $CD138^+$ Plasma cells before sorting the final $CD1d^{High}/B220^{High}$ MZ B cell population, resulting in MZ B cell populations reaching above 99% purity in both naïve and infection-derived setting (**b**)

Table 1
Quantitative and qualitative RNA yield analyses of total RNA isolated from MACS-FACS purified MZ B cells using the Zymo Research Direct-Zol RNA isolation kit

Sample	Naive		Infected	
MZ B cells (events)	2,153,422	2,152,507	1,863,594	1,517,228
Total RNA yield (μg)	1.760	1.745	1.685	1.305
RIN	7.9	7.4	7.8	7.6
rRNA ratio	1.8	1.9	2.2	2.0
gDNA contamination[a]	No	No	No	No

Number of MZ B cell events as indicated by FACSAria II (BD Bioscience), RNA yield, RNA quality based on RIN and rRNA ratios obtained from 2100 Expert Bioanalyzer (Agilent) at DNA-link (Seoul, South-Korea), and gDNA contamination

[a]gDNA contamination determined based on 1.2% agarose formaldehyde denaturing gel electrophoresis

water), for 1.2% formaldehyde denaturing gel electrophoresis by mixing with 2× Loading Dye in a 1:1 ratio in separate microcentrifuge tubes (*see* **Note 23**).

14. Incubate the tubes at 70 °C for 10 min.
15. Immediately place the tubes on ice for 3 min.
16. Load 4 μL of the Riboruler RNA ladder and 8 μL of the sample, positive, and negative control in the corresponding lanes.
17. Run the 1.2% agarose formaldehyde denaturing gel for 15 min at 75 V, followed by 45 min at 100 V.
18. Rinse the gel with distilled water and visualize the RNA bands (28S and 18S) using a UVsolo Imager system (*see* **Note 6** and Table 1).
19. Store RNA samples at −80 °C for further downstream applications.

4 Notes

1. We use AnTat 1.1E *T. b. brucei* (EATRO 1125 stock) parasites in our experimental setup. The stabilate (trypanosomes in 25–50 μL whole blood) is thawed from −80 °C or liquid nitrogen, resuspended in PBS, PSG, or medium (i.e., DMEM or RPMI), and subsequently applied onto a hemocytometer to determine viability and concentration. We recommend to first establish a parasitemia experiment to determine first peak day, as this might vary upon the stabilate used, mouse strain, and parasite viability. Subsequently perform splenectomies either *pre-* or *post*-first-parasitemia peak. Four naive 8 weeks old, female C57Bl/6N mice are used as a control group.

2. Preparation of single cell suspensions at room temperature using FACS buffer supplemented with FBS results in increased cell viability. It is recommended to continue working at 4 °C when proceeding with the MACS-based MZ and Fo B cell pre-enrichment and subsequent FACS procedure.
3. This two-step MACS-based MZ and Fo B cell isolation kit includes the first antibody cocktail that eliminates non B cells using biotin labeled anti-Ter-119 (erythrocyte removal), anti-CD4 ($CD4^+$ T lymphocyte removal), anti-CD43 (monocyte, granulocyte, $CD8\alpha^+$ T cell, pre-pro-, pre-, and pro-B cell removal), and anti-CD93 (immature and Transitional B cell removal) antibodies. This pre-enrichment step performs equally well using naive and *T. b. brucei* derived samples. However, the second anti-CD23-based MZ and Fo B cell separation step shows impaired isolation performance when using cells from the *T. b. brucei* infection. The use of a pre-enriched MZ and Fo B cell fraction, increases the throughput of subsequent FACS-based MZ B cell isolation.
4. We recommend using the Zymo Research RNA isolation kit instead of the Qiagen RNA isolation kit, as in our hands this routinely yields up to five times more total RNA of high quality.
5. When autoclaving, 10× FA buffer turns slightly yellowish and can be stored up to 2 months at 4 °C. Importantly, only use RNase/DNase-free graded reagents or perform 0.1% DEPC treatment on solutions and glassware by incubating them for 12 h at 37 °C, followed by DEPC-inactivation through autoclaving (20 min at 120 °C). Any used glassware should be baked at 240 °C for at least 4 h, followed by autoclaving. Additionally, we suggest using only filter tips and RNaseZAP (Sigma-Aldrich, USA) to clean pipettes, gloves, benches, etc.
6. Use formaldehyde strictly in a fume hood. Pour the gel in the fume hood to avoid inhalation of and potential irritations due to volatile fumes of the formaldehyde. Once the 1.2% agarose formaldehyde denaturing gel is poured, allow it to solidify for 20 min in the fume hood and then transfer it into the 1× running buffer used for electrophoresis. Allow both gel and 1× running buffer to cool down to a room temperature for at least 30 min before running the gel.
7. Wear gloves when working with the 2× Loading Dye as this contains 95% formamide, 0.025% SDS, 0.025% bromophenol blue, 0.025% xylene cyanol FF, 0.025% ethidium bromide, and 0.5 mM EDTA. Ethidium bromide is a carcinogen and care should be exercised when working with the 2× Loading Dye and any reagent that was brought into contact with the 2× Loading Dye. Follow biohazard disposal rules. Alternatively, 6 μL of 10,000× GelRed Nucleic Acid Gel Stain

(Biotium, USA) can be added to the molten agarose, followed by the use of an ethidium bromide-free 2× RNA Loading Dye (New England Biolabs, USA) to load the RNA samples.

8. It is essential to use flow cytometry first to determine the total numbers of MZ B cells present in the spleen on different days of infection before selecting the exact day for their isolation. The sufficient number of MZ B cells can be obtained up to *post*-first-peak day. It has to be taken into account that *T. b. brucei* infection results in full depletion of MZ B cells by day 10 of infection [5]. Moreover, in order to obtain a sufficient amount of total RNA for downstream applications approximately two million of MZ B cells have to be collected by FACS resulting in on average 1.8 μg. In order to reach 1.8 μg of purified total RNA, 4×10^8 of total splenocytes have to be pooled from both naive and infection-derived samples.
9. We recommend using a GentleMACS dissociator as it results in higher cell yields and more reproducible outcomes. Use the "m_spleen_04.01" program to obtain complete single cell suspensions. When no GentleMACS dissociator is available, splenocyte suspensions can be prepared by placing them in a cell culture dish and crushing vigorously with the back of a 20 mL syringe.
10. RBC lysis allows proper RBC removal up to 10 days *post* infection. It is not recommended to perform an additional RBC lysis as this step usually results in decreased cell viability.
11. Based on our experiments and the number of recuperated cells, splenocyte pellets obtained from the naive mice should be resuspended in 2 mL separation buffer, and for splenocytes extracted from infected mice it is recommended to use 3–4 mL for cellular pellets prepared prior to the first peak of parasitemia, and 6 mL for any other day of infection onward.
12. Even though manufacturer's protocol suggests using 100 μL non-B cell biotinylated antibody cocktail and 200 μL anti-biotin microbeads per 1×10^8 total splenocytes to remove contaminants, the same volumes can be used for up to 4×10^8 total splenocytes for both naive and up to *post*-first-parasitemia peak samples.
13. It is highly recommended to prerinse the LS column during the washing step in **step 4**. Prevent the column from running dry, paying attention to the fact that it takes approximately 1 min for a volume of 1 mL to run through the LS column.
14. We recommend reusing the pipette tip. We observe high cell loss when changing the pipette tip, which is related to the highly concentrated cell suspension ($1–2 \times 10^8$ cells in 500 μL). To increase the cell yields, reuse the same tip for the subsequent 3 mL washing step in **step 7**.

15. When performing this procedure, it is recommended to check the enrichment efficiency by verifying various cell populations (e.g., B lymphocytes, T lymphocytes, granulocytes, and other cell populations) within the non B cells (*see* Fig. 1a). To recuperate the latter fraction, remove the LS column from the magnetic field, transfer it into a new 15 mL Falcon tube and flush the LS column with 5 mL of a separation buffer.
16. Optimal cell sorting is performed when using a Ca^{2+}/Mg^{2+} free buffer, which prevents cells from aggregating. Additionally, the used sort buffer should have minimal background signal and/or interference with antibody staining in FACS. We suggest the use of Pre-Sort Buffer (BD) or 1× PBS, supplemented with 1 mM EDTA, 25 mM HEPES, pH 7.0, and 1% FBS.
17. To prevent RNA degradation after FACS, an RNase inhibitor is added to the MZ B cell collection tube. This inhibitor prevents the total RNA from being degraded by RNases which are released during cellular lysis.
18. Before conducting a FACS staining, it is recommended to take a sample (5×10^6 cells) to determine compensation settings and gating strategies. This requires nonstained cells, single-stained cells (B220-FITC, CD1d-PE, CD138-PE/CY7, and CD93-APC), double-stained cells (B220-FITC and CD1d-PE, B220-FITC and CD138 PE/Cy7, and CD1d-PE and CD138 PE/Cy7), and quadruple-stained cells (B220-FITC and CD1d-PE and CD138-PE/Cy7 and CD93-APC) using a separate 5 mL polystyrene Round-Bottom tube. Perform a Fcγ blocking step for 20 min at a final dilution of 1:1000, followed by a staining with fluorochrome-conjugated antibodies at 1:600 final dilution for 30 min in the dark. Stop staining by adding 200 μL FACS buffer.
19. We use the alternative $CD1d^{High}/B220^{High}$ MZ B cell staining since we observed downregulation of CD23 surface expression throughout *T. b. brucei* infection. In our FACS gating strategy we gate out any Immature $CD93^+$ B cell and Plasma $CD138^+$ B cells in order to select only the MZ B cell population.
20. Applying multiple fractions onto a single column is suggested by the manufacturer's protocol (Zymo Research, USA). We obtain high yield of total RNA in combination with high quality when pooling up to six different fractions (max. 1 mL TRIzol-submerged MZ B cells) onto a single Zymo-Spin IIICG Column.
21. It is important to apply the RNase/DNase-free water in the center of the column matrix to obtain a maximum RNA yield in the first eluate. Perform additional elution steps to assure all RNA has been collected. Typically, second elution has lower

RNA quality A_{260}/A_{280} (protein/phenol contamination) and A_{260}/A_{230} (EDTA/phenol/carbohydrate contamination) ratios. If impaired total RNA quantity or quality is observed, we suggest using the Zymo Research RNA concentrator and cleanup kit (Zymo Research, USA).

22. When working with low concentrations (<20 ng/μL), OD ratios obtained from NanoDrop become difficult to interpret. As such, we would recommend relying on the results of a bioanalyzer (e.g., 2100 Expert Bioanalyzer (Agilent, USA)) to determine RNA quality. Alternatively, more accurate concentrations can be determined using Qubit™ RNA HS Assay Kit (Invitrogen).
23. Here a 10 × 7 cm gel tray (Edvotek, USA) is used with a 10-lane comb (Edvotek, USA), allowing up to 10 μL per lane. It is recommended to dilute the Riboruler ladder 1:3 times using DNase/RNase-free water and load only 4 μL, instead of 8 μL as for the samples, negative, and positive control. As such avoiding the UV overexposure of the gel picture due to a high concentration of the ladder.

Acknowledgments

Trypanosome research is being supported by a grant of the FWO (Fonds voor Wetenschappelijk OnderzoekVlaanderen) #G013518 N. N.V. is a Ph.D. fellow supported by an individual grant of the FWO-Vlaanderen # 1107619N.

References

1. Almeida M, García-Montero AC, Orfao A (2004) Cell purification: a new challenge for biobanks. Pathobiology 81:261–275. https://doi.org/10.1159/000358306
2. Davies D (2012) Cell separations by flow cytometry. Cancer Res 878:185–199. https://doi.org/10.1007/978-1-61779-854-2_12
3. Cerutti A, Cols M, Puga I (2013) Marginal zone B cells: virtues of innate-like antibody-producing lymphocytes. Nat Rev Immunol 13:118–132. https://doi.org/10.1038/nri3383
4. Zouali M, Richard Y (2011) Marginal zone B-cells, a gatekeeper of innate immunity. Front Immunol 2:63. https://doi.org/10.3389/fimmu.2011.00063
5. Radwanska M, Guirnalda P, De Trez C, Ryffel B, Black S, Magez S (2008) Trypanosomiasis-induced B cell apoptosis results in loss of protective anti-parasite antibody responses and abolishment of vaccine-induced memory responses. PLoS Pathog 4. https://doi.org/10.1371/journal.ppat.1000078
6. Schnaufer A, Domingo GJ, Stuart K (2001) Natural and induced dyskinetoplastic trypanosomatids: how to live without mitochondrial DNA. Int J Parasitol 32:1071–1084. https://doi.org/10.1016/S0020-7519(02)00020-6
7. Radwanska M, Vereecke N, Deleeuw V, Pinto J, Magez S (2018) Salivarian trypanosomosis: a review of parasites involved, their global distribution and their interaction with the innate and adaptive mammalian host immune system. Front Immunol 9:1–20. https://doi.org/10.3389/fimmu.2018.02253
8. Stijlemans B, Radwanska M, De Trez C, Magez S (2017) African trypanosomes undermine humoral responses and vaccine development:

link with inflammatory responses? Front Immunol 8:582. https://doi.org/10.3389/fimmu.2017.00582

9. Bockstal V, Guirnalda P, Caljon G, Goenka R, Telfer JC, Frenkel D, Radwanska M, Magez S, Black SJ (2011) *T. brucei* infection reduces B lymphopoiesis in bone marrow and truncates compensatory splenic lymphopoiesis through transitional B-cell apoptosis. PLoS Pathog 7: e1002089. https://doi.org/10.1371/journal.ppat.1002089
10. Frenkel D, Zhang F, Guirnalda P, Haynes C, Bockstal V, Radwanska M, Magez S, Black SJ (2016) *Trypanosoma brucei* co-opts NK cells to kill splenic B2 B cells. PLOS Pathog 12: e1005733. https://doi.org/10.1371/journal.ppat.1005733
11. White HN, Meng QH (2012) Recruitment of a distinct but related set of VH sequences into the murine CD21hi/CD23-marginal zone B cell repertoire to that seen in the class-switched antibody response. J Immunol 188:287–293. https://doi.org/10.4049/jimmunol.1101264
12. Turchinovich G, Vu TT, Frommer KJ, Schmid S, Alles M, Loubert JB, Goulet JP, Zimber-Strobl U, Schneider P, Bachl J, Pearson R, Crossley M, Agenes F, Kirberg J (2011) Programming of marginal zone B-cell fate by basic Kruppel-like factor (BKLF/KLF3). Blood 117:3780–3792. https://doi.org/10.1182/blood-2010-09-308742
13. Dempsey WL, Mansfield JM (1983) Lymphocyte function in experimental African trypanosomiasis. VI. Parasite-specific immunosuppression. J Immunol 130:2896–2898
14. Teirlinck AC, Roestenberg M, Bijker EM, Hoffman SL, Sauerwein RW, Scholzen A (2015) *Plasmodium falciparum* infection of human volunteers activates monocytes and CD16+ dendritic cells and induces upregulation of CD16 and CD1c expression. Infect Immun 83:3732–3739. https://doi.org/10.1128/IAI.00473-15
15. Cadman ET, Abdallah AY, Voisine C, Sponaas AM, Corran P, Lamb T, Brown D, Ndungu F, Langhorne J (2008) Alterations of splenic architecture in malaria are induced independently of Toll-like receptors 2, 4, and 9 or MyD88 and may affect antibody affinity. Infect Immun 76:3924–3931. https://doi.org/10.1128/IAI.00372-08
16. Santana CC, Vassallo LAR d FJ, Oliveira GGS, Pontes-de-Carvalho LC, Dos-Santos WLC (2008) Inflammation and structural changes of splenic lymphoid tissue in visceral leishmaniasis: a study on naturally infected dogs. Parasite Immunol 30:515–524. https://doi.org/10.1111/j.1365-3024.2008.01051.x
17. Goodyear CS, Silverman GJ (2003) Death by a B cell superantigen: In vivo VH-targeted apoptotic supraclonal B cell deletion by a Staphylococcal Toxin. J Exp Med 197:1125–1139. https://doi.org/10.1084/jem.20020552
18. Peruchon P, Chaoul N, Burelout C, Delache B, Brochard P, Laurent P, Cognasse F, Prévot S, Garraud O, Le Grand R, Richard Y (2009) Tissue-specific B-cell dysfunction and generalized memory B-cell loss during acute SIV infection. PLoS One 4:e5966. https://doi.org/10.1371/journal.pone.0005966
19. Viau M, Longo NS, Lipsky PE, Zouali M (2005) Staphylococcal protein a deletes B-1a and marginal zone B lymphocytes expressing human immunoglobulins: an immune evasion mechanism. J Immunol 175:7719–7727. https://doi.org/10.1007/978-1-61779-854-2_12
20. Van Meirvenne N, Magnus NE, Buscher P (1995) Evaluation of variant specific trypanolysis tests for serodiagnosis of human infections with Trypanosoma brucei gambiense. Acta Trop 60:189–199. https://doi.org/10.1016/0001-706X(95)00127-Z

Chapter 44

Cellular Markers for the Identification of Chemoresistant Isolates in *Leishmania*

Maritza Padrón-Nieves and Alicia Ponte-Sucre

Abstract

Markers to diagnose chemoresistance in infecting *Leishmania* parasites are urgently required. This is fundamental for patients who do not heal during or after treatment, as they are unresponsive, or patients who relapse at the end of the therapy, suffering from therapeutic failure. Glucose utilization is an indicator of cell viability that closely associates with metabolic activity. In *Leishmania*, glucose is a source of carbon atoms and is imported into the cell through specific transporters. In experimentally developed chemoresistant *Leishmania* parasites a significant decrease of the expression of glucose transporters as well as in the cellular accumulation glucose has been described. Alternatively, the electrical membrane potential is an essential parameter for the formation of the electromotive force needed for the acquisition of important nutrients and solutes (e.g., glucose) by cells, and changes in glucose concentration are suggested to constitute a physiological adaptation associated with a chemoresistant phenotype of *Leishmania* parasites. Here we describe easy methods to measure glucose uptake and the membrane potential in isolates from patient suffering leishmaniasis. Correlation between both parameters might be helpful to identify chemoresistant parasites. Results suggest that the measured kinetics of glucose utilization rate can be correlated with the plasma membrane potential and together used to differentiate between the performance of wild-type and reference parasites on the one hand and parasites isolated from patients with therapeutic failure on the other.

Key words Bis-oxonol, Drug resistance, Drug resistance markers, Glucose uptake, *Leishmania*, Plasma membrane potential, Therapeutic failure

1 Introduction

Chemotherapy research exploits qualitative and quantitative differences between host and pathogenic agents to design drugs that affect pathogen survival, while not affecting host integrity. The molecules eventually transform into human medicines that promote elimination of pathogenic agents [1]. However, therapeutic efficacy may not be adequate and consequently, the ghost of therapeutic failure (TF)—cases that do not heal during or after treatment, or do not respond from the beginning (unresponsiveness) and those which fail in their response after receiving the

Paul A. M. Michels et al. (eds.), *Trypanosomatids: Methods and Protocols*, Methods in Molecular Biology, vol. 2116, https://doi.org/10.1007/978-1-0716-0294-2_44,

corresponding therapy (relapses)—might emerge [2–4]. Among the multiple reasons that can support the existence of TF, that is, factors associated with the drug (presentation, route of administration, toxicity, pharmacokinetics, and cost) [5, 6], host (immunosuppression, comorbidity, noncompliance with the therapeutic regimen), or epidemiological conditions (risk of reinfection), only those associated with a pathogenic agent less susceptible to the drug—natural or acquired (under drug pressure)—favor the persistence of chemoresistant parasites [3].

Resistance implies that although a large percentage of pathogens living under drug pressure may die, selected parasites genetically different from "wild" cells survive. The selected cells express mutations that favor their persistence in the presence of the compounds and these mutations are transmitted to the offspring. The problems associated with this situation represent a public health challenge involving many diseases, including leishmaniasis. In fact, increases in the incidence of cases of leishmaniasis with TF and the need to identify which cases are related to parasite chemoresistance highlight the urgency of identifying easy-to-implement resistance markers, to be used in the laboratory routine for identifying infective parasites that express resistant phenotypes.

In the present chapter we describe how the correlation of results obtained by two methods could be implemented as easy-to-use resistance markers, that is, glucose uptake and plasma membrane potential.

Trophic activity is fundamental in the processes of transmission, development, adaptation, and survival of *Leishmania* [7]. Thus, the adaptive success of the parasite depends, to a large extent, on its ability to use substrates such as glucose [8]. In environments with high oxygen tension the parasites proliferate rapidly producing ATP through aerobic glycolysis, whereas when the oxygen level is low, they do so by anaerobic glycolysis [9]. The use of glucose has been shown to be restricted in media with low oxygen availability [10], as in the intracellular environment and in the intestine of the invertebrate vector, where the environment is hypoxic [7, 8, 11, 12].

Glucose uptake by the cell, independently of its subsequent metabolism [13, 14], offers a simple parameter to study the way how the cell's physiological state is affected. The determination of glucose is carried out in the supernatant of the culture at a determined time, for which the enzymatic method of Trinder [15] can be used. This reaction involves the oxidation of glucose in the presence of glucose oxidase to gluconic acid and hydrogen peroxide, and the formation of a red quinonimine, by reaction of the peroxide with 4-aminoantipyrine and phenol, in the presence of peroxidase. The amount of red quinonimine formed is proportional to the concentration of glucose in the sample and is determined spectrophotometrically (*see* Fig. 1). Specifically, we adapted the methodology originally described by Seyfang and Duszenko

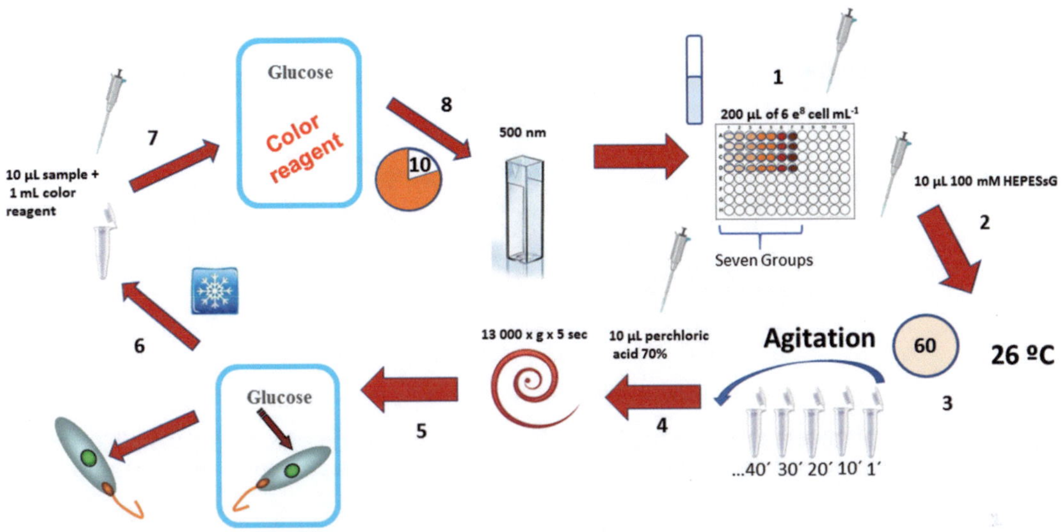

Fig. 1 Determination of glucose utilization rate

[16], to study glucose uptake in *Leishmania* parasites isolated from diffuse cutaneous leishmaniasis (DCL) patients with TF [17]. It may be a good cellular marker to differentiate chemosensitive and chemoresistant strains of *Leishmania*.

Differences in the electrical potential across membranes is a common characteristic both in prokaryotic and eukaryotic cells. These differences in plasma membrane potential ($\Delta\Psi p$) occur as a consequence of ionic concentration gradients (Na^+, K^+, H^+, Cl^-, ...) across membranes involving the action of different pumps [18–20]. In the case of *Leishmania* (*L.*) *donovani*, $\Delta\Psi p$ seems to be set by hydrogen and potassium ion diffusion gradients, while sodium does not seem to have a primary role [21]. Even more, as has been primarily demonstrated by Zilberstein and colleagues, *Leishmania* creates a protonmotive force across their plasma membrane that drives nutrient transport [22, 23].

At rest, mammalian cells have a $\Delta\Psi p$ in the range of 40–90 mV (~70 mV), the interior being negative with respect to the exterior [20]. By convention, the negative interior $\Delta\Psi p$ is expressed with a minus sign (−40 to −90 mV). In protists such as *Leishmania*, the $\Delta\Psi p$ depends on the energy metabolism and the life cycle of the parasite, varying between −75 mV in amastigotes [22–24] and −113 mV in promastigotes [25]. Hyperpolarization occurs as an increase in the magnitude of the $\Delta\Psi p$ at rest and it is expressed with a lower value than the previous one, while depolarization represents the opposite situation.

The $\Delta\Psi p$ is fundamental for the formation of the protonmotive force necessary for nutrient and other important solute acquisition by the parasites, as well as for permitting the interaction with the

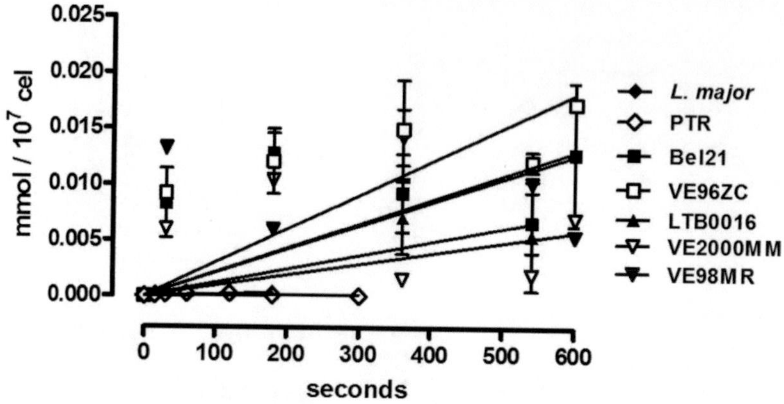

Fig. 2 Comparison of the rate of glucose uptake by reference strains and parasites isolated from DCL patients (Reprinted by permission from Nature/Springer/Palgrave, Parasitology Research 2014; 113(6):2121–2128)

host [18, 19, 22, 24–26]. Thus, the $\Delta\Psi p$ may reflect the state of energy metabolism, cellular homeostasis, and the physical integrity of the plasma membrane.

Some fluorescent markers, such as the lipophilic anion bis-oxonol [bis-(1,3-diethylthiobarbituric acid) trimethinaoxonol], can be used to indirectly measure $\Delta\Psi p$ in *Leishmania* (*see* Fig. 2) [27, 28]. In the presence of cellular depolarization, bis-oxonol undergoes a conformational change, increasing its emission of light by fluorescence. When the cells repolarize, the anion dissociates from the membrane and decreases the emission [27, 28]. To measure the $\Delta\Psi p$ of *Leishmania*, we use the bis-oxonol fluorescent compound according to the methodology initially described by Vieira et al. [25], with modifications. This technique has been used to study the leishmanicidal effect of peptide antibiotics on promastigotes of *Leishmania* (*L.*) *donovani* [29] and $\Delta\Psi p$ in New World *Leishmania* parasites isolated from DCL patients with TF [17] and may be a good cellular marker to differentiate chemosensitive and chemoresistant strains of *Leishmania*. To measure the $\Delta\Psi p$, it is mandatory to perform some calibration procedures to determine the optimal cell density to be used, as well as the extracellular and intracellular bis-oxonol concentration.

For the herein described methods, the parasites isolated from lesions (isolates) were obtained from three patients that regularly attended the Dermatology Department of the Institute of Biomedicine, MPPS-UCV-Caracas-Venezuela. The patients suffered DCL with TF to treatment with meglumine antimonate. The isolates were identified by molecular biology [30] as belonging to the *Leishmania* (*L.*) *mexicana* and *Leishmania* (*L.*) *amazonensis* groups and were kept frozen in liquid nitrogen until their use to minimize changes in their phenotype. Further details are given in the Methods section.

2 Materials

All solutions should be prepared either with double distilled water or deionized water (impedance of 18 MΩ cm at 25 °C) and analytical grade reagents. Each method describes the storage characteristics of the solutions to be used. Follow strictly the instructions and be aware to dispose of in an appropriate way the waste, following suitable regulations.

2.1 Solutions

1. Biphasic medium of blood agar (modified NNN medium) prepared according to standard procedures. Solid phase: base agar with 15% defibrinated rabbit blood and sodium penicillin (100 U/mL). Liquid phase: glucose solution 1.5% w/v, NaCl 0.85% w/v, male urine 5% v/v, and bovine fetal serum (inactivated at 56 °C for 30 min) 10% v/v (*see* **Note 1**).
2. Saline phosphate buffer solution (PBS): 136 mM NaCl, 2.6 mM KCl, 10 mM $Na_2HPO_4 \cdot 2H_2O$, 1.7 mM KH_2PO_4 (*see* **Note 1**).
3. HEPES salts (HEPESs): 10 mM HEPES, 132 mM NaCl, 3.5 mM KCl, 1 mM $CaCl_2$, 0.5 mM $MgCl_2$, pH 7.3 (*see* **Note 2**).
4. HEPES salts glucose (HEPESsG): 10 mM HEPES, 132 mM NaCl, 3.5 mM KCl, 1 mM $CaCl_2$, 0.5 mM $MgCl_2$, 5 mM glucose, pH 7.3 (*see* **Note 2**).
5. Perchloric acid 70% (70-PA) (*see* **Note 3**).
6. *N*-methylglucamine (NMGCl): 10 mM HEPES, 140 mM NMGCl, 0.5 mM $MgCl_2$, 11 mM glucose, pH 7.3 (*see* **Note 2**).
7. Bis-oxonol [bis-(1,3-diethylthiobarbituric acid)trimethinaoxonol] (Molecular Probes) [28] 10 μM (stock solution dissolved in DMSO) (*see* **Note 4**).
8. Valinomycin 100 μM (stock solution in DMSO) (*see* **Notes 4** and **10**).
9. KCl 4 mM (stock solution in water).

2.2 Parasites

2.2.1 Reference Species Certified by the World Health Organization (WHO)

1. *L. amazonensis* (MHOM/BR/77/LTB0016).
2. *Leishmania* (*L.*) *major* (MHOM/IL/81).
3. *L. major* (MHOM/SU/73/5ASKH).
4. *L. mexicana* (MHOM/BR/82/Bel21).
5. *L. major PTR* (MHOM/IL/80/Friedlin/PTR, a cosmid transfected strain containing PRP1, an ABC transporter conferring pentamidine resistance in *L. major* [31].

2.2.2 Parasites Isolated from Patient Lesions

6. *L. mexicana*—MHOM/VE/ 1996/ZC-(VE96ZC).
7. *L. amazonensis*-MHOM/VE/1998/MR-(VE98MR).
8. *L. amazonensis*-MHOM/VE/2000/MM-(VE2000MM).

Parasites of species 1 and 2 were donated by Dr. Lionel Schnur, The Hebrew University-Hadassah Medical School, Jerusalem; species 3, 4, 6, 7, and 8 by Dr. Noris Rodríguez, Instituto de Biomedicina, Universidad Central de Venezuela, Caracas, Venezuela; and species 5 by Dr. Paulo Cotrim Dpto. Moléstias Infecciosas e Parasitárias, Instituto de Medicina Tropical de São Paulo, São Paulo, Brazil.

3 Methods

3.1 Parasite Culture and Estimation of Cell Density

1. Parasites are thawed according to conventional protocols and subcultured weekly in NNN semisolid blood agar, at 26 °C, with glucose solution. The parasites are seeded at 5×10^5 cells/mL and cultivated until growth reaches the initial stationary phase, just before the plateau.
2. Dilute an aliquot, 10 μL of a culture suspension with 0.04% trypan blue in PBS and place it under a microscope (40× magnification) using a Neubauer chamber. Count live (colorless) parasites. Calculate cell density using the following formula according to the manufacturer's recommendation: *N*° of cells/mL = *N*° of cells $\times 10^4 \times$ dilution factor.

3.2 Glucose Utilization Rate

Glucose uptake is determined in the exponential phase of parasite growth by measuring the import of the substrate into the cell independently of its subsequent metabolism [13, 14]. Specifically, glucose disappearance from the medium with time is measured by an adaptation of a methodology previously described [15]. The identity of the transporters involved has been demonstrated previously [32]. Figure 1 illustrates the glucose uptake method herein used step by step as follows:

1. After centrifugation (500 × *g* for 10 min) and washing promastigotes three times with PBS, resuspend the cells (gently, using Pasteur pipettes) in 200 μL of HEPESs, at a density of 2×10^8 cells/mL.
2. Place 200 μL of 2×10^8 cells/mL resuspended in HEPESs in a 96 well plate. Make seven groups of quadruplicates.
3. Add 10 μL of HEPESsG to obtain a final concentration of 5 mM glucose (*see* **Note 5**).
4. Incubate at 26 °C with agitation. Withdraw the first group of tubes from the bath at min 1 and then the remaining groups every 10 min until completion at 1 h.

5. To the withdrawn tubes add 10 μL of 70-PA to stop the reaction (*see* **Note 3**).
6. Centrifuge for 5 s at 13,000 × *g* at room temperature (RT).
7. Store the supernatant at 4 °C until glucose determination.
8. To 10 μL of each sample, including the reference glucose standard, add 1 mL of the Cromatest® Kit color reagent.
9. Incubate for 10 min at RT, measure the absorbance at 500 nm to determine the glucose concentration (*see* **Note 6**).

Perform each experiment determining glucose utilization at least three times in quadruplicate. Include blank and controls: i.e. one tube with 5 mM glucose concentration as standard; one tube including only the color reagent and one tube including only HEPESsG.

The rate of glucose utilization is estimated from the decrease of glucose levels in the medium. For curve analysis, we use the Microsoft Excel® 2007 and Prism Graph-Pad 5® programs.

Figure 2 depicts an example of the time course of glucose uptake by strains and isolates. The slope of each curve represents the rate of glucose uptake for each case. In all cases and for all strains and isolates a linear incorporation of glucose into the cells during the first 600 s was demonstrated. The slopes obtained for each reference strain or isolate, expressed as mmol of glucose × $10^{-5}/10^7$ cells sec, and 95% confidence intervals, are summarized in Table 1. The data represented in this table compare the rates of glucose import for each isolate and its corresponding reference strain. The results indicate that cells accumulate glucose following the order *L. mexicana* (VE96ZC > Bel21) = *L. amazonensis* (VE98MR) > *L. amazonensis* (LTB0016=VE2000MM) ≫ *L. major* (*L. major* > PTR).

3.3 Plasma Membrane Potential (ΔΨp)

In eukaryotic cells, membrane potentials occur in several organelles, including mitochondria. The membrane potential probe bis-oxonol only fluoresces in the microenvironment of a membrane, and enters and exits the cell in response to the charge on the plasma membrane. It can enter depolarized cells and bind to

Table 1
Rate of glucose utilization by reference strains and patient isolates

mmol of glucose × $10^{-5}/10^7$ cells second (95% confidence intervals)						
L. major		*L. mexicana*		*L. amazonensis*		
*L. major**	PTR*	Bel21**	VE96ZC**	LTB0016***	VE2000MM	VE98MR***
0.19 + 0.002 (0.11–0.27)	0.06 + 0.004 (0.00–0.015)	2.12 + 0.05 (0.98–3.25)	3.02 + 0.04 (2.00–3.90)	1.23 + 0.03 (0.3–2.13)	0.97 + 0.5 (0.00–0.22)	2.17 + 0.06 (0.53–3.81)

*, **$p < 0.001$, ***$p < 0.005$

intracellular proteins or membranes, exhibiting an enhanced (brighter) fluorescence. As the inner leaflet becomes more negative (hyperpolarized), bis-oxonol leaves the cell and its signal decreases [33]. Although bis-oxonol should be largely excluded from mitochondria because of their overall negative charge, the signal produced by this dye provides a ratio that includes these (and other) organelles.

Before performing the experimental protocol, calibrations should be accomplished: that is, the conditions for linearity of fluorescence *vs.* cell density and the optimal extracellular and intracellular concentration of bis-oxonol. This allows the linear relationship with the fluorescence to be determined.

3.3.1 Calibration of Cell Density vs. Fluorescence (ΔF)

1. Place cells at variable densities (from 10^5 to 10^7 in 200 μL of HEPESsG) in a 96-well plate.
2. Add bis-oxonol (2 μL of 10 μM stock solution) to reach a concentration of 0.1 μM.
3. Incubate at RT for 10 min in darkness. Record the fluorescence changes (540 nm (exc); 580 nm (emi)) for 60 s.
4. Establish linearity between cell density and fluorescence changes (*see* **Note** 7).

3.3.2 Calibration of Extracellular and Intracellular Concentration of Bis-Oxonol vs. Δf

1. Place cells at the optimal density in 200 μL of HEPESsG in a 96-well plate.
2. Add bis-oxonol, [varying volumes (1–10 μL) stock solution] to reach concentrations (0.05–0.5 μM).

   Skip **steps 3** and **4** from Fig. 3.

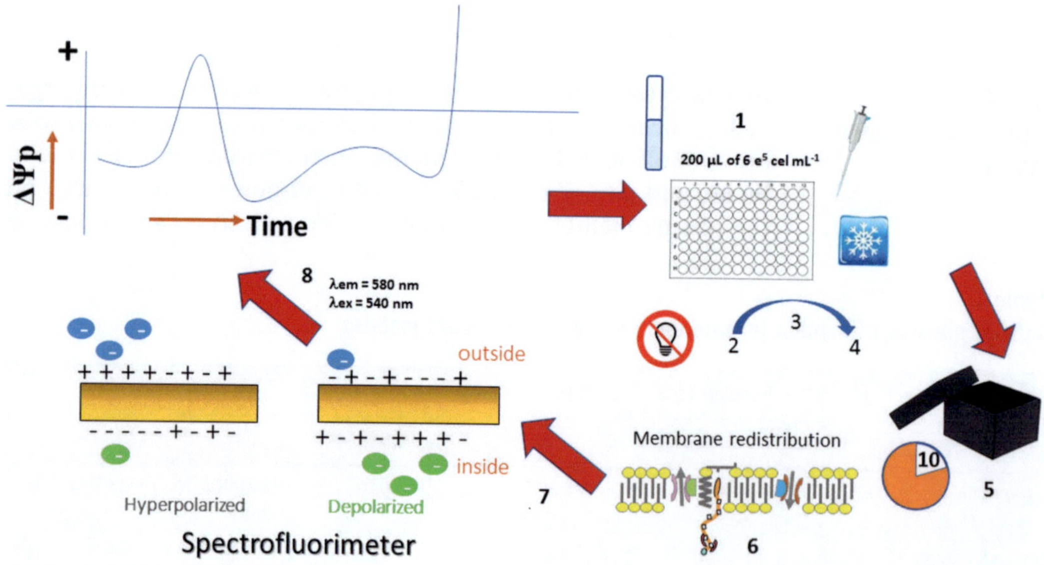

Fig. 3 Determination of $\Delta\Psi p$

5. Incubate at RT for 10 min.
6. Record the fluorescence changes (540 nm (exc)/580 nm (emi)) for 60 s (*see* **Note 7**).
7. Establish the linearity between bis-oxonol concentration and fluorescence changes (*see* **Notes 8** and **9**).

3.3.3 Experimental Protocol for the Evaluation of $\Delta\Psi p$

Figure 3 illustrates the method herein used to determine $\Delta\Psi p$ step by step as follows:

1. Place cells at the optimal density as determined from the calibration curve (described in Subheading 3.3.2) in 200 μL NMGCl solution in a 96-well plate (*see* **Notes 8** and **9**).
2. Add valinomycin (2 μL of 100 μM stock solution) to reach a concentration of 1 μM (*see* **Notes 3** and **10–12**) [34].
3. Add bis-oxonol (2 μL of 10 μM stock solution) to reach a concentration of 0.1 μM.
4. Add KCl. From the original stock perform dilutions in water to prepare KCl solutions of 25–3000 μM. Add 2 μL of each dilution to successive wells to obtain varying KCl concentrations from 0.25 to 20 mM (*see* **Note 13**).
5. Incubate at RT in the darkness for 10 min.
6. Record the fluorescence changes (540 nm (exc); 580 nm (emi)) for 60 s.
7. Establish the linearity between fluorescence and estimated plasma membrane potential $\Delta\Psi p$ according to the extracellular KCl concentration.
8. Determine the basal $\Delta\Psi p$ and its depolarizing behavior in increasing concentrations of KCl for each isolate, to later compare with the reference species (*see* **Note 14**).

Perform each experiment to determine the $\Delta\Psi p$ (please follow instructions as depicted in Fig. 3) at least four times in quadruplicate, in each case with positive and negative controls included.

Figure 4 and Table 2 present experimental results obtained using these protocols for our reference strains and parasites isolated from DCL patients. First, a linear correlation was established between bis-oxonol fluorescence and KCl concentration. For the Student *t* test analysis of the effect of inhibitors on $\Delta\Psi p$, the Microsoft Excel® 2007 and Prism Graph-Pad 5® programs were used. The calibration curves of plasma membrane potential for each strain are depicted in Fig. 4, displaying the linear correlation between fluorescence (540 nm/580 nm) and plasma membrane potential. Additionally, Table 2 summarizes the $\Delta\Psi p$ determined from the corresponding slopes for each strain tested. The determined data demonstrate that $\Delta\Psi p$ spans from −170 to −200 mV

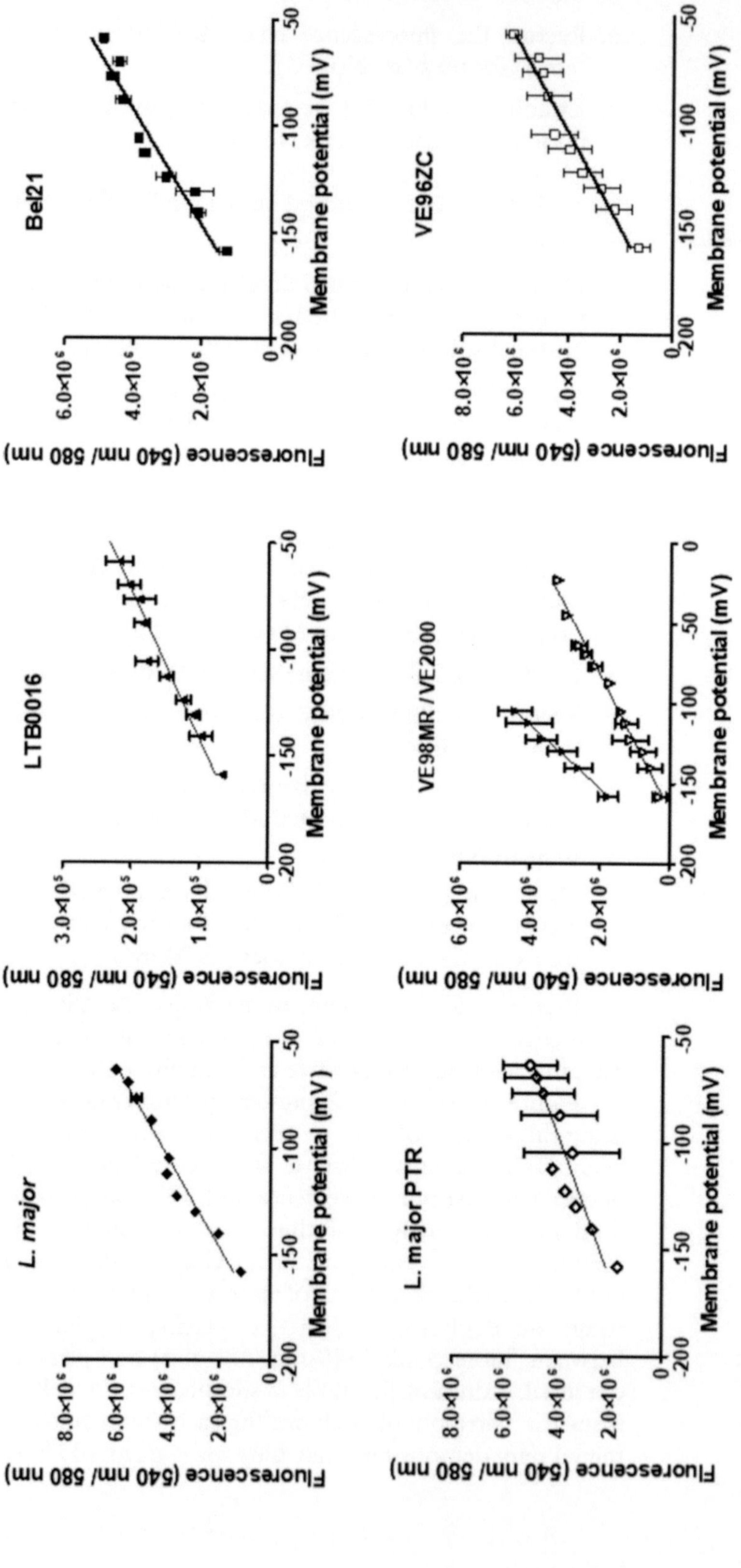

Fig. 4 The linear relationship between plasma membrane potential and measured fluorescence in reference strains and parasites isolated from DCL patients

Table 2
Membrane potential (Vm) in reference strains and in parasites isolated from DCL patients

Species	Vm [mv] (95% confidence interval)	Goodness of fit (R^2)
L. major	−180 (−196/−169)	0.99
L .major (PTR)	−200 (−219/−186)	0.96
L. mexicana (Bel 21)	−200 (−220/−190)	0.84
VE96ZC	−195 (−240/−168)	0.54
L. amazonensis (LTB0016)	−212 (−230/−198)	0.89
VE2000MM	−170 (−190/−150)	0.73
VE98MR	−190 (−240/−170)	0.54

R^2 correlation coefficient

for strains and isolates used herein. $\Delta\Psi p$ of reference strains and isolates VE96ZC and VE98MR remain at values close to −200 mV. However, $\Delta\Psi p$ significantly deviates toward depolarizing values in isolate VE2000MM.

3.4 Conclusion

Glucose utilization by parasites is an indicator of cell viability, as it is closely associated with metabolic activity. On the other hand, the plasma membrane potential is an essential parameter in the formation of the protonmotive force needed for the acquisition of important nutrients and solutes (e.g., glucose) in many organisms and cells, including *Leishmania*. Results obtained by the herein described methods suggest that: (1) *L. major*, responsible for cutaneous leishmaniasis (CL) in the Old World, accumulate glucose at a lower rate than *L. amazonensis* and *L. mexicana*, both responsible for DCL in America; (2) in the pentamidine-resistant strain PTR, glucose accumulation is lower than in its *L. major* reference strain; and (3) in *L. amazonensis* and *L. mexicana* parasites isolated from DCL patients, glucose accumulation either increases or remains at similar values as in their corresponding reference strains. Additionally, as the plasma membrane potential is the force needed for import of nutrients and other solutes into cells, results suggest that parasites accumulate glucose without a significant modification of the $\Delta\Psi p$, a result which could constitute a physiological change that may reflect an adaptation of the parasite against chemotherapeutic agents [35], initially defined as "fitness" [36]. As these results thus suggest that chemoresistance may involve a physiological response to the drug pressure—a metabolic adaptation—that modulates the use of energy substrates, the herein described and standardized methods for evaluating both parameters and their correlation, could be helpful in the identification of chemoresistant infecting parasites. It is interesting to note that previously we have used these two methods together to identify which ions are responsible for the plasma membrane potential in *Leishmania* parasites, and if these ions differ in chemosensitive and chemoresistant parasites [17], as well as to analyze the mechanism of action of natural products and semisynthetic molecules derived from them and designed as potential antileishmania products (Alcazar, personal communication), and the mechanisms by which neuropeptides may exert their action as chemotactic agents (Giammarressi, personal communication). Thus, the ease of their implementation makes them treasured for laboratory routine as well as for the molecular laboratory.

4 Notes

1. Store at 4 °C.
2. The osmolarity of this solution should be checked to have the adequate physiological value of 298 mOsm/L.
3. Perchloric acid is strongly oxidizing. Thus, when you work with it, please use fume hoods with a wash-down capability to prevent accumulation of oxidizers in the ductwork.
4. DMSO is a liquid that should be handled with precaution. If working in cold climates remember that pure DMSO has a melting point of 18.5 °C (64 °F) and if frozen DMSO must be thawed before it can be used. To preserve the purity of the solution it is wise to transfer an aliquot to a small tube and use it rather than the big flask, since it very easily captures water. Please use fume hoods with a wash-down capability to prevent accumulation of DMSO gases.
5. Calibration curves should be performed in the range of 0–5 mM glucose.
6. Glucose concentrations (mM) should be calculated according to instructions supplied by the company. Glucose concentration = 5.5 × sample OD/standard OD = mmol/L.
7. It is recommended to make a minimum of four replicates of each condition.
8. To establish the linearity between intracellular bis-oxonol concentration and fluorescence, the cells must be heated for 15 min at 60 °C to collapse the plasma membrane potential; under these conditions bis-oxonol freely distributes in the cell so that both fluorophore concentrations [internal and external] are similar.
9. These cells must be resuspended in the NMGCl solution where all cations are replaced by NMGC1 and therefore cells are dissolved in monovalent cation-free solution.

10. Since this compound increases the fluorescence background, you should be very careful when using it; background values must be subtracted from the values of fluorescence.
11. Valinomycin is a selective dodecadepsipeptide antibiotic ionophore specific for potassium [34].
12. These cells must be resuspended in the HEPESs.
13. KCl working solutions.

Sol.	[KCl] (μM)	Solute (μL)	Solvent distilled H_2O (μL)	Total (μL)	(2 μL in 200 μL) (1:100) (mM)
0	*4000*	*KCl 0.5964 g (MW 74.56 g/mol)*	*2000*	*2000*	–
12	3000	375 Sol. 0	125	500	30
11	2000	250 Sol. 0	250	500	20
10	1000	125 Sol. 0	375	500	10
9	800	100 Sol. 0	400	500	8
8	600	75 Sol. 0	425	500	6
7	400	50 Sol. 0	450	500	4
6	*200*	*100 Sol. 0*	*1900*	*2000*	2
5	150	375 Sol. 6	125	500	1.5
4	100	250 Sol. 6	250	500	1
3	75	187.5 Sol. 6	312.5	500	0.75
2	50	125 Sol. 6	375	500	0.5
1	25	62.5 Sol. 6	437.5	500	0.25

14. The plasma membrane potential ($\Delta\Psi p$) is calculated according to the KCl concentration added to the wells using the Nernst equation: $\Delta\Psi p = -59.16 \log([K^+]i/[K^+]o)$, where $[K^+]i$ is the intracellular potassium concentration (considered as 120 mM) [22] and $[K^+]o$ is the KCl concentration added. A linear correlation is established between bis-oxonol fluorescence and KCl concentration.

Acknowledgments

The authors are grateful to Dr. Emilia Diaz, Med. Vet. Wilmer Alcazar, and Med. Doc. Michelle Giammarressi for details related to the methods herein described and to Mrs. Pilar Rodríguez for her technical assistance. Likewise, they are grateful for the support conferred by the Alexander von Humboldt Foundation and the

Siebold-Collegium Institute for Advanced Studies, University of Würzburg, Germany, to Alicia Ponte-Sucre. The authors are grateful to the Universidad Central de Venezuela Council for Research, grants CDCH-UCV PI-09-8717-2013/1 and PG-09-8646-2013/1. This project was approved by the Ethical Committee of the Institute of Biomedicine, Universidad Central de Venezuela.

References

1. Barret M Bolelart M, Castillo-Riquelme M et al. (2010) Research priorities for Chagas disease, human African *Trypanosomiasis* and *Leishmaniasis*. Technical report of the TDR Disease Reference Group on Chagas disease, Human African Trypanosomiasis and Leishmaniasis
2. Salaam-Blyther T. (2013) Neglected tropical diseases: background, responses, and issues. R41607 CRS report for Congress Congressional Research Service. www.crs.gov
3. G-Science Academies Statements (2013) Drug resistance in infectious agents – a global threat to humanity innovation. www.who.int/pmnch/media/membernews/2011/20110407_who_whd/en/
4. Ponte-Sucre A, Gamarro F, Dujardin JC et al (2017) Drug resistance and treatment failure in leishmaniasis: a 21st century challenge. PLoS Negl Trop Dis 11(12):e0006052. https://doi.org/10.1371/journal.pntd.0006052
5. Reveiz L, Maia-Elkhoury ANS, Nicholls RS et al (2013) Interventions for american cutaneous and mucocutaneous leishmaniasis: a systematic review update. PLoS One 8:1–14
6. Croft SL, Sundar S, Fairlamb AH (2006) Drug resistance in leishmaniasis. Clin Microbiol Rev 19:111–126
7. Durán C, Quiroga MF, Díaz-bello Z et al (2009) *Leishmania chagasi* y *Trypanosoma cruzi*: conducta trófica en cultivos axénicos puros y mixtos. Bol Malariol y Salud Ambient 49:97–106
8. Subramanian A, Jhawar J, Sarkar RR (2015) Dissecting *Leishmania infantum* energy metabolism – a systems perspective. PLoS One 10:e0137976. (1–34)
9. Michels PAM, Bringaud F, Herman M et al (2006) Metabolic functions of glycosomes in trypanosomatids. Biochim Biophys Acta 1763:1463–1477
10. Furuya T, Kessler P, Jardim A et al (2002) Glucose is toxic to glycosome-deficient trypanosomes. Proc Natl Acad Sci U S A 99:14177–14182
11. Saunders EC, Ng WW, Kloehn J et al (2014) Induction of a stringent metabolic response in intracellular stages of *Leishmania mexicana* leads to increased dependence on mitochondrial metabolism. PLoS Pathog 10:e1003888. (1–15)
12. Burchmore RJS, Hart DT (1995) Glucose transport in amastigotes and promastigotes of *Leishmania mexicana mexicana*. Mol Biochem Parasitol 74:77–86
13. Seyfang A, Landfear SM (1999) Substrate depletion upregulates uptake of myo-inositol, glucose and adenosine in *Leishmania*. Mol Biochem Parasitol 104:121–130
14. Machuca C, Rodríguez A, Herrera M et al (2006) *Leishmania amazonensis*: metabolic adaptations induced by resistance to an ABC transporter blocker. Exp Parasitol 114(1):1–9
15. Trinder P (1969) Determination of glucose in blood using glucose oxidase with an alternative oxygen aceptor. Ann Clin Biochem 6:24–27
16. Seyfang A, Duszenko M (1991) Specificity of glucose transport in *Trypanosoma brucei*. Effective inhibition by phloretin and cytochalasin B. Eur J Biochem 202:191–196
17. Padrón-Nieves M, Diaz E, Machuca C et al (2014) Correlation between glucose uptake and membrane potential in *Leishmania* parasites isolated from DCL-patients with therapeutic failure: a proof of concept. Parasitol Res 113(6):2121–2128
18. Konings W, Albers S-V, Koning S et al (2002) The cell membrane plays a crucial role in survival of bacteria and archaea in extreme environments. Antonie Van Leeuwenhoek 81:61–72
19. Nolan DP, Voorheis HP (2000) Factors that determine the plasma-membrane potential in bloodstream forms of *Trypanosoma brucei*. Eur J Biochem 267:4615–4623
20. Purves D, Augustine GJ, Fitzpatrick D et al (2001) Electrical signals of nerve cells. In: Purves D, Augustine GJ, Fitzpatrick D et al (eds) Neuroscience. Sinauer Associates, Sunderland, MA, pp 31–46

21. Glaser TA, Utz GL, Mukkada AJ (1992) The plasma membrane electrical gradient (membrane potential) in *Leishmania donovani* promastigotes and amastigotes. Mol Biochem Parasitol 51:9–15
22. Zilberstein D, Dwyer DM (1985) Protonmotive force-driven active transport of D-glucose and L-proline in the protozoan parasite *Leishmania donovani*. Proc Natl Acad Sci U S A 82:1716–1720
23. Zilberstein D, Dwyer DM (1988) Identification of a surface membrane proton-translocating ATPase in promastigotes of the parasitic protozoan *Leishmania donovani*. Biochem J 256:13–21
24. Marchesini N, Docampo R (2002) A plasma membrane P-type H^+-ATPase regulates intracellular pH in *Leishmania mexicana amazonensis*. Mol Biochem Parasitol 119:225–236
25. Vieira L, Slotki I, Cabantchik ZI (1995) Chloride conductive pathways which support electrogenic H+ pumping by *Leishmania major* promastigotes. J Biol Chem 270:5299–5304
26. Souto-Padron T (2002) The surface charge of trypanosomatids. An Acad Bras Cienc 74:649–675
27. Bene L (2013) Oxonol has the potential to probe membrane fields. Cytometry A 83:608–611
28. DiSBAC2(3) (bis-(1,3-diethylthiobarbituric acid)trimethine oxonol). https://www.thermofisher.com/order/catalog/product/B413?SID=srch-srp-
29. Vanaerschot M, Maes I, Ouakad M et al (2010) Linking in vitro and in vivo survival of clinical *Leishmania donovani* strains. PLoS One 8(8): e12211. https://doi.org/10.1371/journal.pone.00122
30. Rodríguez N, De Lima H, Aguilar CM et al (2002) Molecular epidemiology of cutaneous leishmaniasis in Venezuela. Trans R Soc Trop Med Hyg 96(S1):105–109
31. Coelho AC, Beverley SM, Cotrim PC (2003) Functional genetic identification of PRP1, an ABC transporter superfamily member conferring pentamidine resistance in *Leishmania major*. Mol Biochem Parasitol 130:83–90
32. Uzcategui NL, Figarella K, Camacho N et al (2005) Substrate preferences and glucose uptake in glibenclamide-resistant *Leishmania* parasites. Comp Biochem Physiol C Toxicol Pharmacol 140(3–4):395–402
33. Adams DS, Levin M (2012) Measuring resting membrane potential using the fluorescent voltage reporters DiBAC4(3) and CC2-DMPE. Cold Spring Harb Protoc 4:459–464. https://doi.org/10.1101/pdb.prot067702.
34. Díaz-Achirica P, Ubach J, Guinea A et al (1998) The plasma membrane of *Leishmania donovani* promastigotes is the main target for CA(1-8)M(1-18), a synthetic cecropin A-melittin hybrid peptide. Biochem J 330:453–460
35. Padrón-Nieves M, Machuca C, Díaz E et al (2014) Correlation between glucose uptake and membrane potential in *Leishmania* parasites isolated from DCL patients with therapeutic failure: a proof of concept. Parasitol Res 113:2121–2128
36. Natera S, Machuca C, Padrón-Nieves M et al (2007) *Leishmania* spp.: proficiency of drug resistant parasites. Int J Antimicrob Agents 29:637–642

Part VII

Drug Discovery for Trypanosomatid-Borne Diseases

Chapter 45

In Vitro Image-Based Assay for *Trypanosoma cruzi* Intracellular Forms

Amanda G. Eufrásio and Artur T. Cordeiro

Abstract

The advances in development and popularization of automated fluorescence microscopes and pipetting robots allowed scientists to establish high-throughput compound screening using image-based assays for *Trypanosoma cruzi* intracellular forms, which are associated to chronic Chagas disease. An intracellular *T. cruzi* image-based assay is a valuable tool to early stage drug discovery for Chagas disease, because it allows scientists to assess a compound's efficacy and safety in the same experiment. During the last 10 years, several improvements have been incorporated into intracellular *T. cruzi* assay protocols to make them more predictable in what happens with parasites within an infected organism. In the present chapter, a protocol will be presented for an intracellular *T. cruzi* assay, but at a low-throughput scale, more compatible with facilities in many academic laboratories.

Key words Drug discovery, Chagas disease, Image-based assay, *Trypanosoma cruzi*, Amastigote

1 Introduction

Chagas disease is caused by infection with the protist *Trypanosoma cruzi*. The World Health Organization (WHO) estimates that eight million people worldwide are infected with *T. cruzi*. Benznidazole and nifurtimox are the only drugs currently available for treatment of Chagas disease. However, both drugs require long treatement periods, cause severe adverse effects and show reduced eficacy against the chronic stage of disease. This scenario reinforces the need for better drugs.

Projects on drug discovery usually start with an in vitro assay for identification of hit compounds. Still at in vitro scale, hits will be optimized to gain drug-like proprieties without losing efficacy and safety. After hit optimization, compounds will be submitted to in vivo experiments for proof of concept. In the case of Chagas disease, the establishment of bioluminescent *T. cruzi* linages allowed the development of in vivo imaging of animal models for both acute and chronic stages of the disease [1]. The development

Paul A. M. Michels et al. (eds.), *Trypanosomatids: Methods and Protocols*, Methods in Molecular Biology, vol. 2116,
https://doi.org/10.1007/978-1-0716-0294-2_45,

of image-based assays at the in vitro scale for quantification of intracellular forms *T. cruzi* represented a remarkable breakthrough in the traditional process of drug discovery for Chagas disease [2–4], which previously was dependent on viability assays with the epimastigote form for selection of compounds with anti-*T.cruzi* activity.

The present chapter brings a detailed protocol to run in vitro image-based assays for intracellular *T. cruzi* forms. This protocol is based on the method reported by Alonso-Padilla and colleagues [4], with modifications to make it more susceptible to trypanocidal rather than trypanostatic compounds. The protocol is described for a 96-well microplate format, more common in academic laboratories. This method can be used to screen compounds at unique concentratrions and to determine EC_{50} values from a variable concentration response experiment.

2 Materials

1. H9c2 rat cardiomyocytes (*see* **Note 1**).
2. LLC-MK2 green monkey kidney epithelial cells.
3. *T. cruzi* (Y strain) (*see* **Note 2**).
4. Growth Medium: Dulbecco's Modified Eagle's Medium (DMEM) supplemented with 10% heat-inactivated fetal bovine serum (FBS), penicillin (100 U/mL), and streptomycin (100 μg/mL).
5. Maintenance Medium: same as Growth Medium, but with 2% FBS.
6. Liver Infusion Tryptose (LIT) Medium: dissolve 9 g Liver Infusion Broth, 5 g Tryptose, 1 g NaCl, 8 g Na_2HPO_4, 0.4 g KCl, 10 mg hemin, and 1 g glucose in 950 mL of milliQ water, adjust pH to 7.2, complete volume to 1 L and filter-sterilize through a 0.2 μm membrane. Prior to use, supplement LIT medium with 10% heat-inactivated FBS and penicillin (100 U/mL) and streptomycin (100 μg/mL).
7. Phosphate-buffered saline (PBS).
8. Trypsin solution: Trypsin-EDTA (0.25%) with Phenol Red solution.
9. Dimethyl sulfoxide anhydrous ≥99.9% (DMSO).
10. PFA: 4% paraformaldehyde in PBS (filter-sterilized).
11. Staining solution: 4 μg/mL Hoechst 33342 in PBS.
12. Multichannel pipette plastic reservoir.
13. 75 cm^2 (T-75) and 25 cm^2 (T-25) cell culture flasks
14. 50 mL and 0.5 mL sterile tubes.

15. Serological pipettes of 25, 10, and 1 mL.
16. Neubauer chamber.
17. Assay plate: sterile 96-well microplate with lid, flat and clear bottom.
18. Intermediary plate: 96-well microplate with V-bottom.
19. Laminar flow cabinet.
20. Cell incubator with temperature, humidity, and CO_2 control.
21. Centrifuge with adaptors for 50 and 0.5 mL tubes.
22. Automated Cell Counter, cell counting chamber slides and Trypan blue stain (0.4%).
23. Inverted light microscope.
24. Operetta (PerkinElmer) automated fluorescence microscope with 20× objective.
25. Harmony (PerkinElmer) software for high content image analysis.
26. Prism (GraphPad), software for numerical data analysis and graphical representation.

3 Methods

3.1 *T. cruzi* Differentiation

1. Thaw a vial with *T. cruzi* epimastigotes in an ice bath and start the culture with a cell density of 1×10^6 parasites/mL in LIT medium at 28 °C (*see* **Note 2**).
2. Count daily the number of parasites in a Neubauer chamber. When the culture density reaches 1×10^7 parasites/mL, transfer 1 mL of the culture to a new T-25 flask with 9 mL of fresh LIT medium.
3. A healthy doubling time for an epimastigote culture is about 16 h. Repeat **step 2** until the parasites reach a typical doubling rate. Then incubate the culture for 2 weeks at 28 °C to allow *T. cruzi* epimastigotes to differentiate into metacyclic trypomastigotes.

3.2 LLC-MK2 Infection

1. Transfer the metacyclic trypomastigotes culture to a 15 or 50 mL tube and centrifuge at 1250 × *g* for 10 min.
2. Discard the supernatant, resuspend cells in 5 mL of Growth Medium and transfer to a T-75 flask with adhered LLC-MK2 cells and 10 mL of Growth Medium.
3. After 24 h, replace the Growth Medium by 15 mL of Maintenance Medium (*see* **Note 3**).
4. After 4 days, replace the Maintenance Medium.

5. On the seventh day post infection (dpi), transfer the culture with trypomastigotes to a 50 mL tube, centrifuge at 1250 × *g* for 10 min, discard the supernatant, add 5 mL of Growth Medium, repeat the previous centrifuge step and incubate the tube for 4 h at 37 °C, 5% CO_2 to allow trypomastigotes to swim out of the pellet.
6. Transfer the supernatant with active trypomastigotes to a new LLC-MK2 culture and repeat **steps 3–6** to maintain the LLC-MK2 infection.

3.3 Intracellular Image-Based Assay

Day 1

1. At day 01, add 2×10^6 H9c2 cells to a T-75 flask with 15 mL of Growth Medium and incubate for at least 4 h at 37 °C, 5% CO_2 to allow cells adhesion to the flask surface (Fig. 1).
2. Collect trypomastigotes from the supernatant of the LLC-MK2 infected culture, transfer them to a 50 mL tube, centrifuge (1250 × *g* for 10 min) and allow the parasites to swim out of the pellet for 4 h (like **step 5** in Subheading 3.2). Then, transfer the supernatant to another tube.
3. Count trypomastigotes in the Neubauer chamber and transfer 2×10^6 parasites to the H9c2 culture flask. Incubate the culture overnight at 37 °C, 5% CO_2 (infection period).

Day 2

4. After 18 h (overnight), wash cells with 10 mL PBS, add 2 mL of trypsin solution and incubate for 2 min to allow cellular detachment.
5. Add 4 mL of Growth Medium and transfer the H9c2 cells to a 50 mL tube. Count the cells (in an automated cell counter or Neubauer chamber) and use fresh Growth Medium to prepare a Host Cell Solution with 1.1×10^5 cells/mL.
6. Use a sterile plastic reservoir and a multichannel pipette to transfer 90 μL of the Host Cell Solution to a 96-well microplate (Assay Plate).
7. Incubate the Assay Plate for 48 h at 37 °C, 5% CO_2 (parasite growth period) (*see* **Note 4**).

Day 4

8. Prepare a "compound intermediary plate" by transferring 1 μL of samples from stock solution (in 100% DMSO) to wells containing 99 μL of Maintenance Medium. Plate layout should be defined according to assay purpose, primary screening or dose–response curve for EC_{50} calculation (Fig. 2) (*see* **Note 5**).

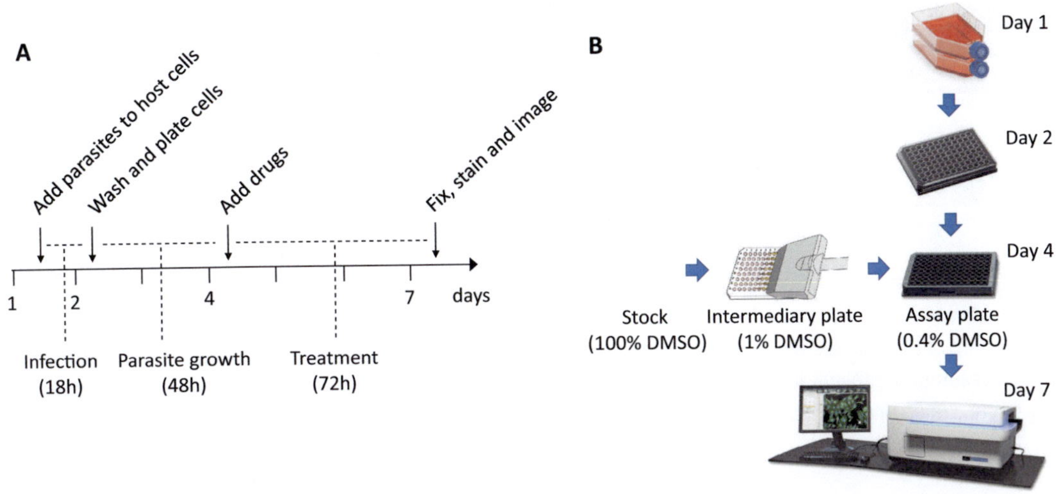

Fig. 1 *T. cruzi* intracellular image-based assay. (**a**) Assay timeline indicating most relevant actions and (**b**) assay schematic representation

A

	1	2	3	4	5	6	7	8	9	10	11	12
A	P	S1	S2	S3	S4	S5	S6	S7	S8	S9	S10	N
B	P	S11	S12	S13	S14	S15	S16	S17	S18	S19	S20	N
C	P	S21	S22	S23	S24	S25	S26	S27	S28	S29	S30	N
D	P	S31	S32	S33	S34	S35	S36	S37	S38	S39	S40	N
E	P	S41	S42	S43	S44	S45	S46	S47	S48	S49	S50	N
F	P	S51	S52	S53	S54	S55	S56	S57	S58	S59	S60	N
G	P	S61	S62	S63	S64	S65	S66	S67	S68	S69	S70	N
H	P	S71	S72	S73	S74	S75	S76	S77	S78	S79	S80	N

B

	1	2	3	4	5	6	7	8	9	10	11	12
A	N	N	N	N	N	N	S7	S7	S7	S7	S7	S7
B	P	P	P	P	P	P	S8	S8	S8	S8	S8	S8
C	S1	S1	S1	S1	S1	S1	S9	S9	S9	S9	S9	S9
D	S2	S2	S2	S2	S2	S2	S10	S10	S10	S10	S10	S10
E	S3	S3	S3	S3	S3	S3	S11	S11	S11	S11	S11	S11
F	S4	S4	S4	S4	S4	S4	S12	S12	S12	S12	S12	S12
G	S5	S5	S5	S5	S5	S5	S13	S13	S13	S13	S13	S13
H	S6	S6	S6	S6	S6	S6	S14	S14	S14	S14	S14	S14

Fig. 2 Intermediary plate layout options according to assay purpose: (**a**) primary screening layout with 80 compounds per plate at the same concentration and (**b**) dose-response curve layout with 14 compounds at six different concentrations (*see* **Note 5**). *N* negative control (no drug, but 0.4% DMSO), *P* positive control (reference drug, Benznidazole), *S* samples

9. Use a multichannel pipette to transfer 60 μL from the intermediary plate to the Assay Plate (preloaded with 90 μL). Final volume and DMSO concentration will be 150 μL and 0.4%, respectively (*see* **Note 6**).
10. Incubate the Assay Plate at 37 °C, 5% CO_2 for an additional 72 h (treatment period).

Day 7

11. Use a multichannel pipette (or another aspiring device) to remove medium from the Assay Plate, wash the adhered cells with PBS and fix them with 4% PFA solution. Incubate the

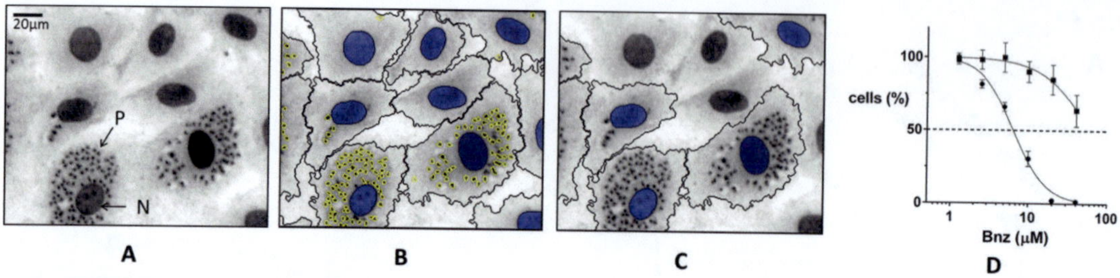

Fig. 3 Image analysis and benznidazole dose–response curves. (**a**) Raw image with arrows pointing to the nuclei of a host cell (N) and intracellular parasites (P). (**b**) Host nuclei (blue mask), host plasma membrane (black line), and parasites (contoured yellow) identified by raw image analysis. (**c**) Host nuclei (blue mask) and plasma membrane (black line) of infected cells. (**d**) Benznidazole (Bnz) dose–response curves. Drug concentration at *x*-axis and normalized values of total (squares) and infected cells (circles) at *y*-axis

Assay Plate at room temperature for 45–60 min. Wash the Assay Plate with PBS to remove PFA solution.

12. Add 100 μL of Staining solution and incubate the Assay Plate at room temperature for 30 min. Keep the plate protected from light exposure by covering it with aluminum foil.
13. Image the cells by automated fluorescence microscopy, with a 20× objective (Fig. 3a). Capture multiple fields for each well to assure a minimum count of 1.0×10^3 cells/well.
14. Load negative controls images in the Harmony software and create an Analysis Script (Primary Analysis) using the Building Blocks commands: Find Nuclei, Find Cytoplasm and Find Spots (in cytoplasm area) (Fig. 3b). Define Results as: Total Cells = number of nuclei, Infected Cells = cells with at least three spots in the cytoplasm area (Fig. 3c) and Infection rate = Infected Cells/Total Cells. Save the Analysis Script (*see* **Note** 7).
15. Apply the Analysis Script to the entire plate. Save the Results in a table format.
16. For secondary analysis, open results table in Prism software, normalize data using values of negative control and zero to define 100% and 0%, respectively; fit normalized values of Total Cells and Infection Rate to a sigmoidal curve to obtain EC_{50} values (Fig. 3d) (*see* **Note 8**).

4 Notes

1. Attention is required to the passage number of the H9c2 culture. Changes in cell morphology might be observed after the tenth passage [5]. If that happens, restart a new culture from frozen stocks.

2. *T. cruzi* samples from curated collections (like ATCC and COLPROT) are usually maintained as epimastigote forms and are distributed in frozen vials. In order to get infective forms, it is necessary to first differentiate epimastigotes into metacyclic trypomastigotes (metacyclogenesis) which can be used to infect a host cell lineage.
3. Reduction of FBS to 2% in Maintenance Medium will slow down cell growth and retard culture confluency.
4. The "parasite growth period" is important to allow for differentiation of trypomastigotes into amastigotes and replication of parasites within the cytoplasm of infected host cells.
5. For primary screening, compounds are usually assayed at 10 μM (final assay concentration, FAC). In this case, stock solutions have to be prepared at 2.5 mM (in 100% DMSO). For a dose-response curve, the compound highest assay concentration is usually 40 μM (FAC) and in this case stock solution will be 10 mM (in 100% DMSO).
6. Check the highest concentration of every compound under an inverted microscope. If you see small crystals or amorphous precipitates, these are signals of poor sample solubility. This is not good. In the case of precipitation try to increase the amount of DMSO in the intermediary plate, but do not exceed 2%, otherwise DMSO-mediated cell toxicity in the assay can arise.
7. Check if the Analysis Script applies well to the positive control (treated with a reference drug).
8. EC_{50} and TC_{50} are parameters that indicate compound efficacy and toxicity, respectively, and correspond to the compound concentrations that give 50% inhibition of infection rate and total cell number, respectively.

Acknowledgments

ATC received financial support from São Paulo Research Foundation (FAPESP) research grant number 2016/14271-4.

References

1. Lewis MD, Francisco AF, Taylor MC, Kelly JM (2015) A new experimental model for assessing drug efficacy against *Trypanosoma cruzi* infection based on highly sensitive in vivo imaging. J Biomol Screen 20(1):36–43
2. Engel JC, Ang KK, Chen S et al (2010) Image-based high-throughput drug screening targeting the intracellular stage of *Trypanosoma cruzi*, the agent of Chagas' disease. Antimicrob Agents Chemother 54(8):3326–3334

3. Sykes ML, Avery VM (2013) Approaches to protozoan drug discovery: phenotypic screening. J Med Chem 56(20):7727–7740
4. Alonso-Padilla J, Cotillo I, Presa JL et al (2015) Automated high-content assay for compounds selectively toxic to *Trypanosoma cruzi* in a myoblastic cell line. PLoS Negl Trop Dis 9(1): e0003493. https://doi.org/10.1371/journal.pntd.0003493
5. Witek P, Korga A, Burdan F et al (2016) The effect of a number of H9C2 rat cardiomyocytes passage on repeatability of cytotoxicity study results. Cytotechnology 68(6):2407–2415

Chapter 46

In Vitro Drug Efficacy Testing Against *Trypanosoma brucei*

Marcel Kaiser and Pascal Mäser

Abstract

The recent endorsement of fexinidazole by the European Medicines Agency for the treatment of human African trypanosomiasis has demonstrated the high predictive value of cell-based assays for parasite chemotherapy. Here we describe three in vitro drug susceptibility tests with *Trypanosoma brucei* that have served as the basis for the identification of fexinidazole as a promising lead: (1) a standard assay with end-point measurement to determine drug efficacy; (2) a wash-out assay to test for reversibility and speed of drug action; (3) isothermal microcalorimetry for real-time measurement of onset of drug action and time to kill. Together, these assays allow to estimate pharmacodynamic parameters in vitro and to devise appropriate treatment regimens for subsequent in vivo experiments.

Key words *Trypanosoma brucei*, African trypanosomes, Parasite chemotherapy, Drug discovery, Cell-based assay, Drug sensitivity testing, Pharmacodynamics, Isothermal microcalorimetry

1 Introduction

Cell-based assays remain a mainstay in the research and development pipelines for chemotherapeutic agents. This is particularly true for parasiticides, where the majority of new drug candidates has been developed from cell-based screening campaigns as the starting point [1]. This also applies to fexinidazole, the first drug for human African trypanosomiasis (HAT, sleeping sickness) that is orally applicable and active against both stages of the disease [2]. In the following, we describe three in vitro assays that were key to the identification of fexinidazole, among a large set of nitroimidazoles, as a lead for HAT [3]. These are (*see* Subheading 3.1) a standard assay with resazurin as an end-point indicator of cell number and viability to determine the dose–response curve and calculate 50% inhibitory concentration (IC_{50}) and Hill slope [4] (*see* Subheading 3.2); a wash-out assay to determine the speed of drug action and test for reversibility [5] (*see* Subheading 3.3); noninvasive, real-time monitoring of cell proliferation by isothermal microcalorimetry to determine pharmacodynamic parameters such as onset of drug

Paul A. M. Michels et al. (eds.), *Trypanosomatids: Methods and Protocols*, Methods in Molecular Biology, vol. 2116, https://doi.org/10.1007/978-1-0716-0294-2_46, © Springer Science+Business Media, LLC, part of Springer Nature 2020

action and time to kill [6]. These assays are based on the in vitro systems developed for axenic cultivation of *Trypanosoma brucei* spp. bloodstream forms [7–9], which are the relevant life cycle stages for chemotherapy.

2 Materials

2.1 Cultivation Medium for T. brucei

The medium for cultivation of bloodstream-form *T. b. brucei* and *T. b. rhodesiense* consists of HMI-9 [10] supplemented with 15% serum (*see* **Note 1**), 1% of a 200 mM ß-mercaptoethanol stock solution (*see* **Note 2**), and 1% of a 100 mM hypoxanthine/100 mM sodium pyruvate /150 mM L-cysteine/5 mM bathocuproine sulfonate/16 mM thymidine stock solution (*see* **Note 3**). The medium is sterilized by filtration and stored at 4 °C for up to 1 week. The medium for *T. b. gambiense* is the same, except that it requires the addition of human serum [11]. We use 5% human serum plus 10% fetal bovine serum.

2.2 Test Compounds

Test compounds are dissolved in dimethyl sulfoxide (DMSO) at 10 mg/ml and stored at −20 °C. The maximal final concentration of DMSO in the test should not exceed 0.5%. As a positive reference compound we use melarsoprol (Arsobal, kindly provided by the WHO), which has an IC_{50} of 0.004 μg/ml in the 72 h standard assay (described in Subheading 3.1).

2.3 Cell Lines

Our reference cell lines are *T. b. rhodesiense* STIB900, *T. b. gambiense* STIB930, and *T. b. gambiense* K03048. STIB900 is a derivative of *T. b. rhodesiense* STIB704, isolated from a patient in Ifakara, Tanzania, in 1982 [12]. STIB930 is a derivative of the *T. b. gambiense* TH1/78E (031) strain isolated from a patient in Côte d'Ivoire in 1978 [13]. K03048 was isolated from a patient in South Sudan in 2003 [14]. All have been adapted to axenic culture.

2.4 Equipment

Cultivation of *T. brucei* bloodstream forms requires a humidified incubator. Cell cultures and assay plates are inspected with an inverted phase contrast microscope. A fluorescence plate reader is required for the resazurin test (Subheading 3.1) and the wash-out assay (Subheading 3.2). Real-time monitoring of cultures (Subheading 3.3) requires an isothermal microcalorimeter; we use a TAM III (Thermal Activity Monitor, model 249) from TA Instruments. All work with live *T. brucei* has to be carried out in a biosafety level 2 laboratory.

3 Methods

3.1 Low Inoculation, Long Incubation Test (LILIT)

This 72-h test is the standard in vitro assay we use to quantify drug efficacy against African trypanosomes.

1. Dilute the drug stock solution (Subheading 2.2) with cultivation medium (Subheading 2.1) to twice the maximal concentration that is to be tested. Add 75 μl thereof to the first column of a 96-well microtiter plate (flat bottom).
2. To all other columns, add 50 μl per well of medium that has been prewarmed to 37 °C.
3. Using a multichannel pipette, perform a dilution series of 1:3 as follows: transfer 25 μl from column one to column two, mix well, transfer 25 μl to the next column, and so on. The last 25 μl are discarded. Leave at least one column (i.e., column 12) drug-free, as a control to determine 100% growth (cells but no drug).
4. Add 50 μl medium to those rows that will not be inoculated with trypanosomes, as a control to determine the background fluorescence (drug but no cells).
5. To all other rows, add 50 μl per well of a cell suspension that has been made by diluting a log-phase trypanosome culture to 4×10^4 cells/ml (*see* **Note 4**) in prewarmed medium.
6. Incubate the plate for 69 h at 37 °C, 5% CO_2 in a humidified atmosphere.
7. Before quantitative evaluation, inspect the plate under an inverted microscope to ensure that the trypanosomes have multiplied, the drug-free control wells are not overgrown, and there are no drug precipitates or contaminations (*see* **Note 5**).
8. Add 10 μl of resazurin (*see* **Note 6**) solution (12.5 mg in 100 ml H_2O) to each well. Incubate for 3 h at 37 °C, 5% CO_2 in a humidified atmosphere.
9. Read the plate in a fluorescence scanner at an excitation wavelength of 536 nm and an emission wavelength of 588 nm. As a quality check, the values of the positive control wells (cells but no drug) should be 5–10 times higher than those of the background controls (drug but no cells).
10. Subtract background values, convert to percent growth, and plot with a logarithmic concentration scale to obtain the dose–response curve. The Hill slope and the 50% and 90% inhibitory concentrations (IC_{50} and IC_{90}) can be calculated by nonlinear regression (*see* **Note 7**).

3.2 Wash-Out Assay

This assay determines the reversibility and speed of drug action. For each time point, prepare a 96-well microtiter plate (V-bottom) as follows.

1. Add 75 μl prewarmed medium (*see* Subheading 2.1) to all wells of column 1, and 50 μl prewarmed medium to all wells of columns 2–12.
2. Add 1.5 μl of the appropriate compound stock solution (*see* Subheading 2.2) to the wells of column one. Eight compounds can be tested on one plate, one in each row.
3. Using a multichannel pipette, perform a dilution series of 1:3 as follows: transfer 25 μl from column one to column two, mix well, transfer 25 μl to the next column, and so on. The last 25 μl is discarded. Leave the last column drug-free, as control to determine 100% growth (cells but no compound) and background (no cells, no compound).
4. Add 50 μl prewarmed medium without parasites to wells A12, B12, G12, and H12, which will serve as controls to provide the background signal in the fluorescence plate reader.
5. To all other wells, add 50 μl per well of a cell suspension that has been made by diluting a log-phase trypanosome culture to 2×10^5 cells/ml in prewarmed medium.
6. Incubate the plates for the respective time windows (e.g., 3 h/6 h/24 h/48 h; *see* Fig. 1) at 37 °C, 5% CO_2 in a humidified atmosphere.
7. At the designated time, centrifuge the plate at 2000 × *g* for 3 min to sediment the cells.

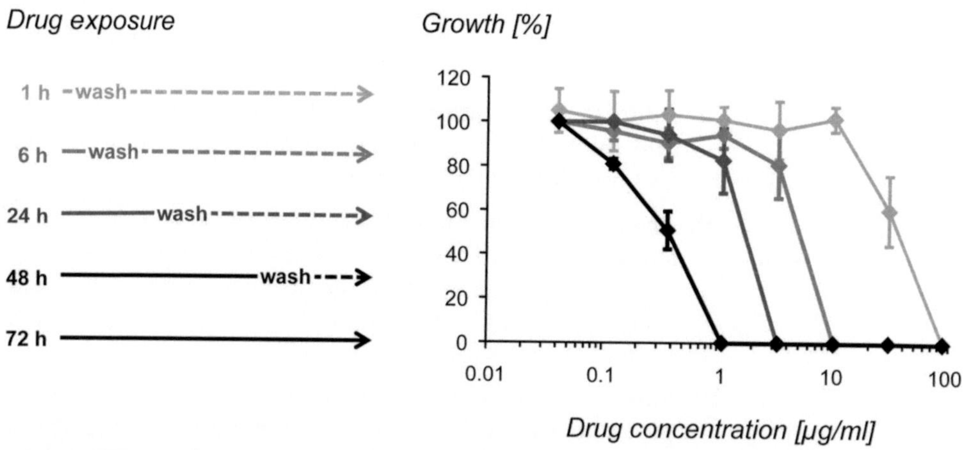

Fig. 1 Wash-out assay with fexinidazole sulfone, the major metabolite of fexinidazole; data are from [5]. The different time windows of drug exposure (solid lines, left) were followed by incubation without drug (dashed lines) to a total of 72 h. The dose–response curves (right) after 48 and 72 h of drug exposure (in black) coincided, indicating that fexinidazole sulfone reaches maximal activity after 48 h. The assay also demonstrates that 1 μg/ml fexinidazole sulfone is irreversibly cidal after 48 h, but not after shorter exposure periods

8. Using a multichannel pipette, aspirate 50 μl of the supernatant of each well, discard, and add 150 μl prewarmed medium (without serum and additives).
9. Centrifuge the plate again. Aspirate 150 μl from the supernatant and replace it with 150 μl fresh, prewarmed medium.
10. Repeat the wash step [9] once more. Add 150 μl prewarmed complete medium.
11. Centrifuge the plate and remove 150 μl of the supernatant. Add 50 μl prewarmed medium to obtain a total volume of 100 μl per well.
12. From each plate containing washed cell suspension, prepare triplicate assay plates (96 well, flat bottom) by transferring the following volumes of cell suspension: 25 μl per well for the 3 h and 6 h compound exposure periods; 10 μl for 24 h compound exposure; 5 μl for 48 h compound exposure. Complete the volume to 100 μl per well with prewarmed medium.
13. Further incubate the assay plates to a total of 69 h (dashed lines, Fig. 1) at 37 °C, 5% CO_2 in a humidified atmosphere (*see* **Note 8**).
14. Before quantitative evaluation, inspect the plate under an inverted microscope to ensure that the trypanosomes have multiplied, the drug-free control wells are not overgrown (*see* **Note 4**), and there are no drug precipitates or contaminations.
15. Add 10 μl of resazurin (*see* **Note 6**) solution (12.5 mg in 100 ml H_2O) to each well. Incubate for 3 h at 37 °C, 5% CO_2 in a humidified atmosphere.
16. Read the plate in a fluorescence scanner at an excitation wavelength of 536 nm and an emission wavelength of 588 nm. As a quality check, the values of the positive control wells (cells but no drug) should be ten times higher than those of the background controls (drug but no cells).
17. Take averages of triplicate values, subtract background values, convert to percent growth, and plot with a logarithmic concentration scale to obtain the dose–response curve (Fig. 1) and calculate the 50% and 90% inhibitory concentrations (IC_{50} and IC_{90}) (*see* **Note 5**).

3.3 Isothermal Microcalorimetry

Microcalorimetry uses heat flow data as a proxy for the number of viable parasites [15]. This allows to monitor drug action in real time. The following protocol is designed for a microcalorimeter that uses ampoules with a total volume of 4 ml.

1. Prepare compound solutions in prewarmed medium (37 °C) at concentrations of 1×, 3×, 10×, and 30× the IC_{50} as determined under Subheading 3.1. The final DMSO concentration must not exceed 0.2% (vol/vol). For each concentration, prepare 4 ml compound solution in a 10 ml tube.

2. Prepare 20 ml of a cell suspension that has been made by diluting a log-phase trypanosome culture to 2×10^5 cells/ml in prewarmed medium.
3. To each of the tubes with compound solution, add 4 ml cell suspension to obtain 8 ml test sample per concentration with a density of 10^5 trypanosomes/ml.
4. For the positive control (cells without compound), place 4 ml prewarmed medium in a 10 ml tube and add 4 ml cell suspension. For the negative control (background), use 8 ml prewarmed medium.
5. For each sample, test or control, prepare triplicate ampoules by transferring 2 ml of sample into a 4 ml glass ampoule that has been prewarmed to 37 °C (*see* **Note 9**).
6. Seal the ampoules airtight and insert them into the isothermal microcalorimetry instrument. Heat flow (in μW) is continuously measured (1 reading/s) at 37 °C for up to 7 days.
7. Data analysis: The recorded data are reduced to one data point per 90 s interval and exported, for example, into a Microsoft Excel spreadsheet or an R object. The time required for the preparation of the ampoules is added to all timepoints. The three replicates are averaged and the curves are smoothed using a bicubic spline [16] to avoid perturbations due to metabolic oscillation. The final curve allows to estimate parameters of cell growth and drug action (*see* Fig. 2 and **Note 10**).

4 Notes

1. Commercial fetal bovine serum (FBS) works fine. However, the use of fetal serum is not necessary for bloodstream-form trypanosomes, which naturally proliferate in the mammalian blood. We have obtained best results for cultivation of *T. brucei* bloodstream forms with heat-inactivated horse serum, which we prepare ourselves from horse blood obtained from the butchery.
2. As first demonstrated by Baltz et al., ß-mercaptoethanol is necessary as a reducing agent since the trypanosomes are cysteine auxotrophs [17] and cannot import cystine [7]. Prepare the stock solution by dissolving 14 μl ß-mercaptoethanol in 10 ml H_2O. Prepare fresh but leave at room temperature for at least 2 h before use (or use it directly but leave the medium at 4 °C for 24 h, or 37 °C for 2 h, before use).
3. Like most obligate parasites, *T. brucei* are purine auxotrophs and require addition of a purine source. Why pyruvate needs to be added is not clear (at least not to us); the trypanosomes actually secrete pyruvate [18]. For the stock solution, dissolve

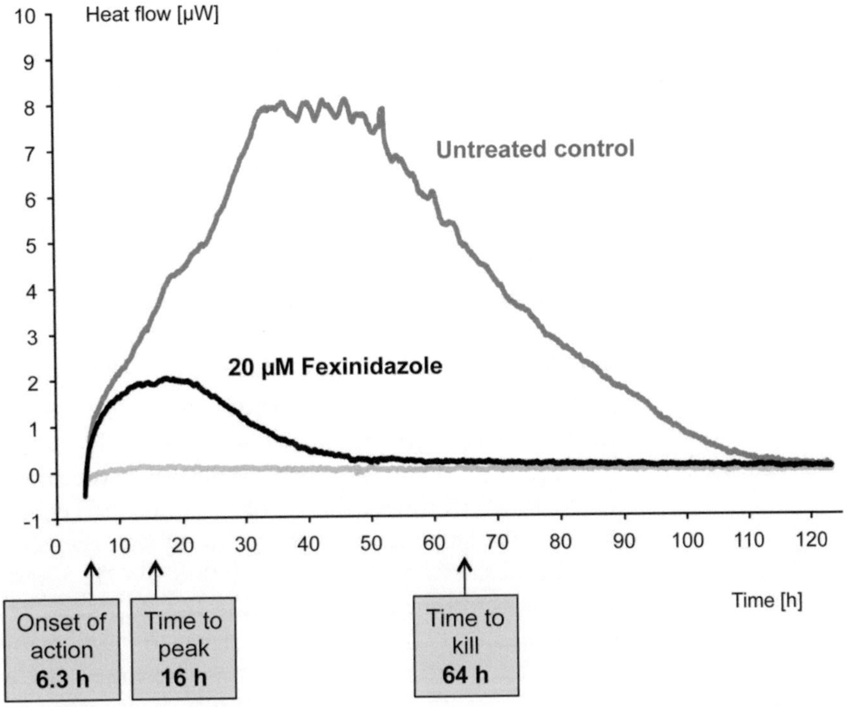

Fig. 2 In vitro determination of pharmacokinetic parameters by isothermal microcalorimetry. Bloodstream-form *T. b. rhodesiense* STIB900 were exposed to 20 μM fexinidazole, corresponding to 10× the IC_{50}. The heat flow emitted by the cultures was recorded in real time (black, drug-exposed cells; dark gray, drug-free control cells; light gray, background control, no cells). Pharmacodynamic parameters that can be estimated from this approach are onset of drug action, time to peak, and time to kill. *See* **Note 10** for details

3.4 g hypoxanthine in a small amount of 1 M NaOH. Add 2.75 g sodium pyruvate, 5.9 g L-cysteine, 0.71 g bathocuproine sulfonate, 0.98 g thymidine, and 250 ml H_2O. Adjust pH to 9.7, sterilize by filtration (pore size 0.2 μm), aliquot and store at −20 °C. Do not use adenine as a purine source as this is toxic to trypanosomes [19].

4. The trypanosome density is determined with a Cell Analysis System (CASY, Schärfe System) or by counting with a hemocytometer. The optimal inoculum depends on the growth characteristics of the cultures. If the drug-free control wells are overgrown after 72 h incubation, the inoculum will need to be decreased.

5. The minimal inhibitory concentration (MIC) can be determined by eye, defined as the lowest concentration at which either no parasites have normal shape and motility or all parasites are dead.

6. Resazurin is also sold, at a much higher price, under the brand name alamarBlue™. We use resazurin sodium salt from Sigma.

7. By monitoring the effect of increasing serum concentrations in the medium on the IC_{50}, this assay can also be used to qualitatively assess serum protein binding of the test compounds; for an example *see* [20].
8. To test for cidality of drug action, modify the protocol as follows: use 5 μl of cell suspension for all plates, add 95 μl medium, and incubate for an additional 69 h. Proceed with **step 14**.
9. For microcalorimetric experiments it is important that all material, solutions, and medium are prewarmed to 37 °C, and all samples kept at 37 °C until insertion into the instrument.
10. To estimate the maximum growth rate μ, the heat flow over time curve is fitted with a logistic model [21] using the grofit package [22]. Time to peak is calculated as the timepoint that corresponds to the maximum of the smoothed curve. Time to kill is calculated as the timepoint where the slope of the smoothed curve flattens below 0.005 μW/h. Onset of drug action is determined by comparing the slopes of the curves of the drug-free control with the drug-containing sample. We define the onset of drug action as the timepoint where the slopes diverge by more than 0.04 μW/h. R scripts to calculate onset of action and time to kill are provided in the supplement of ref. 23.

References

1. Mäser P, Wittlin S, Rottmann M et al (2012) Antiparasitic agents: new drugs on the horizon. Curr Opin Pharmacol 12:562–566
2. Mesu V, Kalonji WM, Bardonneau C et al (2018) Oral fexinidazole for late-stage African *Trypanosoma brucei gambiense* trypanosomiasis: a pivotal multicentre, randomised, non-inferiority trial. Lancet 391:144–154
3. Torreele E, Bourdin Trunz B, Tweats D et al (2011) Fexinidazole—a new oral nitroimidazole drug candidate entering clinical development for the treatment of sleeping sickness. PLoS Negl Trop Dis 4:e923
4. Räz B, Iten M, Grether-Bühler Y et al (1997) The Alamar Blue assay to determine drug sensitivity of African trypanosomes in vitro. Acta Trop 68:139–147
5. Kaiser M, Bray MA, Cal M et al (2011) Antitrypanosomal activity of fexinidazole, a new oral nitroimidazole drug candidate for treatment of sleeping sickness. Antimicrob Agents Chemother 55:5602–5608
6. Wenzler T, Steinhuber A, Wittlin S et al (2012) Isothermal microcalorimetry, a new tool to monitor drug action against *Trypanosoma brucei* and *Plasmodium falciparum*. PLoS Negl Trop Dis 6:e1668
7. Baltz T, Baltz D, Giroud C et al (1985) Cultivation in a semi-defined medium of animal infective forms of *Trypanosoma brucei*, *T. equiperdum*, *T. evansi*, *T. rhodesiense* and *T. gambiense*. EMBO J 4:1273–1277
8. Brun R, Kunz C (1989) In vitro drug sensitivity test for *Trypanosoma brucei* subgroup bloodstream trypomastigotes. Acta Trop Basel 46:361–368
9. Hirumi H, Hirumi K (1994) Axenic culture of african trypanosome bloodstream forms. Parasitol Today 10:80–84
10. Hirumi H, Hirumi K (1989) Continuous cultivation of *Trypanosoma brucei* blood stream forms in a medium containing a low concentration of serum protein without feeder cell layers. J Parasitol 75:985–989
11. Brun R, Baeriswyl S, Kunz C (1989) In vitro drug sensitivity of *Trypanosoma gambiense* isolates. Acta Trop Basel 46:369–376
12. Brun R, Schumacher R, Schmid C et al (2001) The phenomenon of treatment failures in

Human African Trypanosomiasis. Tropical Med Int Health 6:906–914

13. Felgner P, Brinkmann U, Zillmann U et al (1981) Epidemiological studies on the animal reservoir of gambiense sleeping sickness. Part II. Parasitological and immunodiagnostic examination of the human population. Tropenmed Parasitol 32:134–140
14. Maina N, Maina KJ, Mäser P et al (2007) Genotypic and phenotypic characterization of *Trypanosoma brucei gambiense* isolates from Ibba, South Sudan, an area of high melarsoprol treatment failure rate. Acta Trop 104:84–90
15. Braissant O, Wirz D, Gopfert B et al (2010) Use of isothermal microcalorimetry to monitor microbial activities. FEMS Microbiol Lett 303:1–8
16. Legendre P, Legendre LFJ (2012) Numerical ecology. Elsevier, Amsterdam
17. Duszenko M, Muhlstadt K, Broder A (1992) Cysteine is an essential growth factor of *Trypanosoma brucei* bloodstream forms. Mol Biochem Parasitol 50:269–273
18. Mazet M, Morand P, Biran M et al (2013) Revisiting the central metabolism of the bloodstream forms of *Trypanosoma brucei*: production of acetate in the mitochondrion is essential for parasite viability. PLoS Negl Trop Dis 7:e2587
19. Geiser F, Luscher A, de Koning HP et al (2005) Molecular pharmacology of adenosine transport in *Trypanosoma brucei:* P1/P2 revisited. Mol Pharmacol 68:589–595
20. Kaiser M, Maes L, Tadoori LP et al (2015) Repurposing of the open access malaria box for kinetoplastid diseases identifies novel active scaffolds against trypanosomatids. J Biomol Screen 20:634–645
21. Braissant O, Bonkat G, Wirz D et al (2013) Microbial growth and isothermal microcalorimetry: growth models and their application to microcalorimetric data. Thermochim Acta 555:64–71
22. Kahm M, Hasenbrink G, Lichtenberg-Frate H et al (2010) Grofit: fitting biological growth curves with R. J Stat Software 33:1–21
23. Gysin M, Braissant O, Gillingwater K et al (2018) Isothermal microcalorimetry – a quantitative method to monitor *Trypanosoma congolense* growth and growth inhibition by trypanocidal drugs in real time. Int J Parasitol Drugs Drug Resist 8:159–164

Chapter 47

In Vitro Growth Inhibition Assays of *Leishmania* spp.

Sarah Hendrickx, Guy Caljon, and Louis Maes

Abstract

In vitro growth (inhibition) assays have a dual application, either supporting the discovery of novel drugs or as a monitoring tool of drug resistance in patient isolates. From an experimental design point of view, both are quite different with regard to the infecting *Leishmania* species and strain, the wide variety of permissive host cells (primary cells versus cell lines), drug exposure times, detection methods and endpoint criteria. Recognizing the need for enhanced assay standardization to decrease interlaboratory variation and improve proper interpretation of results, a detailed description is given of the basic fundamental procedures and requirements for routine in vitro growth of *Leishmania* spp. with specific focus on the intracellular amastigote susceptibility assay. Although the described experimental procedures focus on visceral *Leishmania* species, the same assay principles may apply for the cutaneous species as well.

Key words *Leishmania*, Amastigote, Drug discovery, Drug susceptibility, Laboratory/field strains, Macrophages, Assay harmonization

1 Introduction

Leishmaniasis is caused by various species of the protozoan genus *Leishmania* and represents one of the more important neglected tropical diseases [1, 2]. Two particular challenges hamper the long-term efficient control of the disease: (1) the reliance on relatively few, mostly old drugs that are not devoid of side effects [3, 4] and (2) the increasing incidence of treatment failures and posttreatment relapses particularly in visceral leishmaniasis (VL) [5–7]. To take both into consideration, in vitro growth inhibition assays are indispensable for supporting novel drug discovery and for monitoring drug susceptibility of clinical field isolates to the current antileishmanial drugs [8–10]. Recognizing that VL represents the prime medical need and is also confronted with increasing treatment failures and drug resistance [10], the described experimental procedures will uniquely focus on *L. donovani* or *L. infantum*, although the same assay principles may also apply to *Leishmania* species that cause cutaneous leishmaniasis (CL) [11].

Paul A. M. Michels et al. (eds.), *Trypanosomatids: Methods and Protocols*, Methods in Molecular Biology, vol. 2116, https://doi.org/10.1007/978-1-0716-0294-2_47,

Over the last decades, many in vitro growth inhibition models and procedures have indeed been described, but they all show subtle differences with regard to selection of the species/strain, type of macrophage (mφ) host cell and culture, infecting stage, level of infection, assay duration, and end point parameters. Yet unsatisfactory progress is being made in assay standardization to decrease interlaboratory variation and improve interpretation of results [12]. This triggered us to publish a detailed overview of the standard laboratory procedures to evaluate drug resistance in VL [10]. A recent follow-up study compared primary cells (mouse peritoneal exudate cells (PEC), mouse bone-marrow derived macrophages (BMM), human peripheral blood monocyte derived macrophages) and commercially available cell lines (THP-1, J774, RAW) for their susceptibility to infection, their role in supporting intracellular amastigote multiplication and overall feasibility/accessibility of experimental protocol [13]. The materials and methods of the recommended assay procedures of the latter study are elaborated in greater detail here (Fig. 1). As shown, two distinct paths for the intracellular amastigote susceptibility assay need to be considered: (1) using *laboratory strains* that have already been adapted to in vitro culture conditions and are available as metacyclic promastigote or as ex vivo (spleen-derived) amastigote (*see* **Note 1**), and (2) using *clinical field isolates* that are generally available only as promastigote upon primary isolation and are not adapted to laboratory culture methods. Their mere differences in intrinsic growth, infectivity and intracellular multiplication potential will have profound consequences on the design and interpretation of the growth inhibition assay, highlighting that one universal standard operating procedure will likely remain unachievable.

2 Materials

2.1 Materials for Standard In Vitro Culture of Macrophage (mφ) Host Cells

Sodium bicarbonate solution ($NaHCO_3$) 7.5%, L-glutamine 200 mM (100×), NH_4Cl, $KHCO_3$, Na_2EDTA, sodium pyruvate, phosphate buffered saline (PBS), MEM nonessential amino acids (NEAA, 100×), penicillin–streptomycin (P/S) 10,000 U/mL for cell culture, phorbol 12-myristate 13-acetate (PMA), MEM 10×, RPMI-1640, fetal bovine serum heat inactivated at 56 °C for 30 min (FBSi), THP-1 cell line, demineralized water (demi-H_2O), membrane filter (0.22 μm) for filter sterilization, 15 mL centrifuge tube, T25 or T75 cell culture flasks, cell counting chamber, 37 °C water bath, CO_2-incubator (37 °C, 5% CO_2), 70% ethanol as disinfectant, light microscope (50× immersion-oil objective and 10 or 12.5× ocular), inverted microscope (20×, 40× objectives—10 or 12.5× ocular).

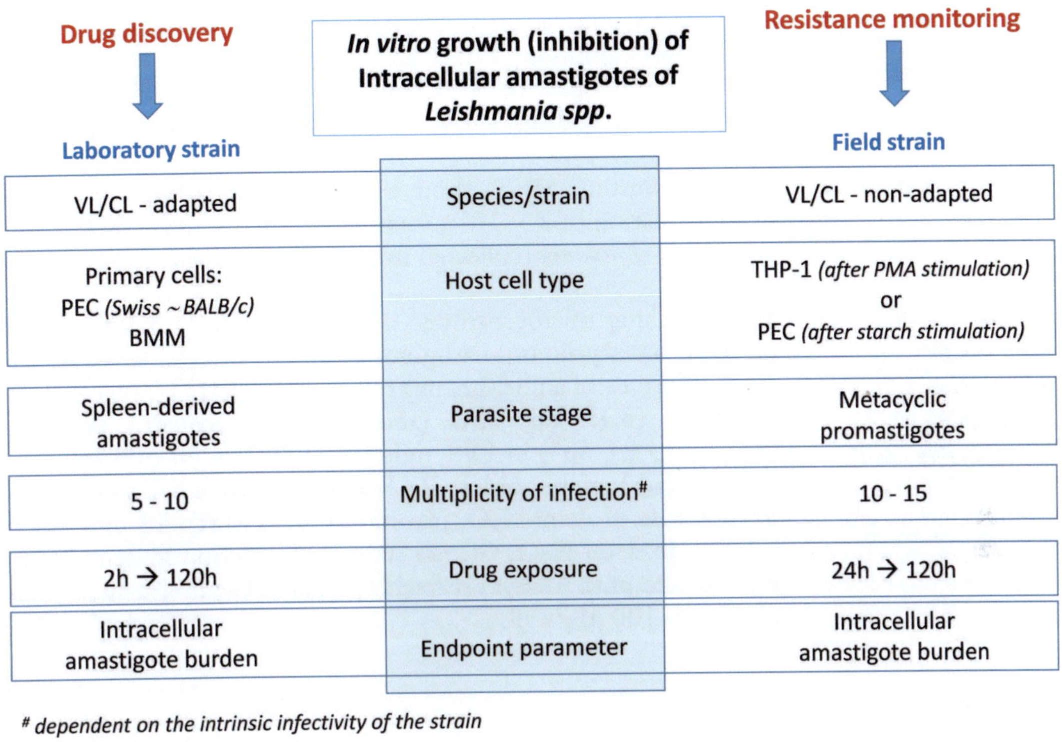

Fig. 1 Recommended conditions for the intracellular amastigote susceptibility assay for clinical isolates and/or laboratory-adapted strains [14] (*see also* **Note 3**)

2.2 Materials for Harvesting Primary Cells from Mice

Dissection material (scalpel, scissors, forceps), 15 mL conical centrifuge tubes, filter tips, disposable syringes and needles (25 G, 21 G), cell counting chamber, multiwell cell culture plates, 2% potato starch suspension (0.2 g starch in 10 mL PBS) for PEC isolation.

Ammonium chloride potassium (ACK) buffer: 8.29 g NH_4Cl, 1 g $KHCO_3$, 37.2 mg Na_2EDTA in 1 L demi-H_2O, pH adjusted 7.2 and filter-sterilized; dissociation buffer: 1% EDTA, 20 mM HEPES in PBS).

2.3 Additional Materials for Obtaining Infective Stages of Leishmania for Infection

2.3.1 For Metacyclic Promastigotes

1. *Adenine solution*: 200 mg adenine, 2.5 mL 1 N NaOH, 17.5 mL demi-H_2O.
2. *Folic acid solution*: 15 mg folic acid, 200 μL 1 N NaOH, 19.8 mL demi-H_2O.
3. *D-Biotin solution*: 10 mg D-biotin, 500 μL 1 N NaOH, 19.5 mL demi-H_2O.
4. *Hemin solution*: 37.5 mg hemin, 15 mL 50% triethanolamine, 15 mL demi-H_2O.
5. *Complete HOMEM promastigote medium*: add 50 mL MEM 10× to 450 mL demi-H_2O and supplement with 9 mL 7.5% $NaHCO_2$, 10 mL 200 mM L-glutamine, 1.5 g D-glucose, 5 g

HEPES, 2 mL adenine solution, 2 mL folic acid solution, 2 mL D-biotin solution, 2 mL hemin solution, and 50 mL FBSi. Adjust to pH 6.5–7.0 with 1 N NaOH, filter-sterilize (0.22 μm) and store at 4 °C. Parasites are cultured at 25 °C.

2.3.2 For Spleen-Derived Amastigotes

Golden hamsters (M/F), about 6–8 weeks infected upon intracardial inoculation of 2 × 10^7 spleen-derived amastigotes of *L. donovani* or *L. infantum* (collected from a donor hamster).

2.4 Additional Materials for Intracellular Amastigote Susceptibility Assay

Sterile locking microcentrifuge tubes (Eppendorf), multichannel pipettes, metacyclic promastigotes or spleen-derived amastigotes, stock solutions of antileishmania reference drugs [11]: pentavalent antimony (3.19 mg SSG (sodium stibogluconate) per mL (eq. 1 mg/mL Sb^V) in PBS, miltefosine (MIL): 20 mM solution in demi-H_2O, amphotericin-B (AmB): 5.4 mM stock solution in 5% dextrose in demi-H_2O, paromomycin (PMM): 20 mM stock solution in demi-H_2O, Giemsa stain (1/5 dilution in demi-H_2O, filtered 0.22 μm). Always use freshly prepared Giemsa, stain 96-well plate with 100 μL/well.

3 Methods

3.1 In Vitro Culture of Macrophage (mφ) Host Cells (See also Note 2)

3.1.1 MEM Culture Medium

Add 450 mL sterile demi-H_2O to 50 mL MEM (10×), supplement with 10.6 mL 7.5% $NaHCO_3$ 7.5%, 25 mL FBSi, and 5 mL 200 mM L-glutamine. If necessary, filter-sterilize (0.22 μm) and store at 4 °C.

3.1.2 Complete RPMI-1640 Culture Medium

For cell lines, add 50 mL FBSi to 500 mL RPMI-1640. For primary cells, supplement the basic medium with 2% penicillin/streptomycin (P/S) and 1% L-glutamine solution. Store at 4 °C.

3.1.3 THP-1 Cell Culture

THP-1 human monocyte cell line is cultured at 37 °C and 5% CO_2 in RPMI-1640 medium supplemented with 10% FBSi and subcultured every 2 days with particular attention not to exceed a cell density of 10^6 mL^{-1}. Before use for infection, 30,000 cells/well are plated in 96-well plates and simultaneously stimulated with PMA (100 ng/mL). The PMA stimulus is removed after 72 h by renewing the medium.

3.1.4 Harvesting and Culture of Primary Peritoneal Exudate Cells (PEC)

1. Before intraperitoneal injection (1 mL 2% starch suspension) of the mice, make sure the starch is completely suspended and is at 37 °C.
2. For collection of the PECs 2 days after stimulation, euthanize the mouse with a CO_2 overdose or cervical dislocation and

disinfect the skin with 70% ethanol. All further actions are carried out under a laminar air flow.

3. Inject 10 mL prewarmed (37 °C) complete RPMI-1640 intraperitoneally and gently massage the abdomen to distribute the fluid and suspend the cells.
4. Remove the ventral skin with sterile scissors and tweezers and disinfect the exposed peritoneum with 70% ethanol.
5. Aspirate all the abdominal fluid and use 10 μL subsample for cell counting.
6. Macrophages easily attach to plastic and even glass surfaces, which can be reduced by prechilling the recipients on ice.
7. Seed the PECs in a 96-well plate at 3×10^5 cells/well.

3.1.5 Harvesting and Culture of Primary Bone-Marrow Derived Macrophages (BMM)

1. Euthanize the mouse with a CO_2 overdose or cervical dislocation and disinfect the skin with 70% ethanol. All further actions are carried out under a laminar air flow.
2. Remove the hind legs and most of the skin and muscles until the femur and tibia are completely clean.
3. Cut both ends of the bone until a small red dot (bone-marrow) is seen and flush with 1 mL basic RPMI-1640 until the cavity is white. Collect in a sterile 15 mL Falcon tube on ice.
4. To further separate the cells, aspirate through a 21 G needle and eject through a 25 G needle. Do not repeat this more than two times to avoid damage of the cells.
5. Centrifuge for 10 min at $200 \times g$ and remove the supernatant.
6. Use ACK buffer for lysis of red blood cells during isolation of BMM and stop cell lysis after 3 min by adding an excess of complete RPMI-1640 medium.
7. Centrifuge again and dissolve the pellet in 5 mL of complete RPMI-1640 medium.
8. Distribute 1 mL of the cell suspension into petri dishes, each with 9 mL complete RPMI-1640 culture medium (additionally supplemented with 15% L929 supernatant containing M-CSF) and incubate for 7 days at 37 °C in 5% CO_2.
9. Remove the medium and detach the cells for 5 min with dissociation buffer.
10. Centrifuge at $200 \times g$ for 5 min and count the collected cells in a counting chamber.
11. Adjust to the right concentration and seed in a 96-well plate at 3×10^5 cells/well.

3.2 Obtaining Leishmania Stages for Infection

3.2.1 Metacyclic Promastigotes

1. Promastigotes are cultured at 25 °C in complete HOMEM promastigote medium [11] and are subcultured twice weekly. The passage number should be kept as low as possible to avoid a decrease in virulence due to prolonged cultivation in vitro [10] (*see* **Note 1**).
2. Most promastigote strains grow better in a slightly acidic environment (pH 6.5–7).

   The time required to reach stationary culture containing infective metacyclics is dependent on the *Leishmania* species/strain. If the option for preconditioning is considered [14], 5-day-old cultures can be used (*see* **Note 3**).

3.2.2 Ex Vivo Spleen-Derived Amastigotes (Only for Adapted Strains)

1. Sacrifice the hamster with a CO_2 overdose and disinfect the abdomen with 70% ethanol.
2. Aseptically remove the spleen and place it in a sterile petri dish.
3. Cut a small piece of spleen and remove excess blood with absorbing paper.
4. Make a number of smear impressions on a microscopic slide and dry to air.
5. Upon fixation (2 min) in methanol and Giemsa staining (15 min), allow the slide to dry to the air.
6. Determine the net weight of the spleen (accuracy 0.01 g) and put in 10 mL complete RPMI-1640 medium in a Tenbroeck tissue grinder.
7. Transfer the splenic cell suspension in a sterile 15 mL centrifugation tube and centrifuge for 10 min at 200 × *g* and 4 °C.
8. Transfer the supernatant to a sterile 15 mL centrifugation tube and centrifuge for 30 min at 3000 × *g* (if the supernatant is not clear after 30 min, centrifuge another 5–10 min to make sure all amastigotes are in the pellet).
9. Discard the supernatant and suspend the pellet in complete RPMI-1640 (= infection inoculum).
10. To calculate the correct volume of RPMI-1640, microscopically count 500 nuclei and the corresponding number of amastigotes on the Giemsa-stained slide (prepared earlier) and use the Stauber method [15] to quantify the number of amastigotes.
11. For infection of hamsters, 2×10^7 amastigotes in 100 μL are used (intracardial injection under isoflurane inhalation anaesthesia).

3.3 Intracellular Amastigote Susceptibility Assay

As indicated in Fig. 1, two paths can be followed, depending whether adapted (Fig. 2a) or nonadapted (Fig. 2b) strains are used.

1. Add 100 μL infection inoculum (suspension in complete RPMI-1640 of metacyclic promastigotes for nonadapted strains or spleen-derived amastigotes for adapted strains) in each well already containing 100 μL macrophage culture.
2. The multiplicity of infection may differ according to the *Leishmania* species/strain and generally varies between 5 and 10 for lab strains and 10 and 15 for field strains.
3. Incubate at 37 °C and 5% CO_2 for 2 or 24 h to remove the noninternalized stages by discarding the medium.
4. Replenish by adding 200 μL complete RPMI-1640 medium to each well.
5. With a multichannel pipette, transfer 10 μL test compound or reference drug dilution onto the infected macrophages, avoiding to touch the monolayer.
6. Incubate in a CO_2 incubator for 5 days at 37 °C.
7. For Giemsa staining, discard the medium from the test plates and allow the plates to dry to the air in the laminar flow.
8. Dispense 100 μL absolute methanol to each well and fix for 10 min, discard the methanol and allow the plates to dry to the air.
9. Finally, dispense 100 μL Giemsa work solution in each well and stain for 15 min, discard the Giemsa solution, rinse the plates under running tap water and allow to dry.
10. Reading of the test is performed by microscopic reading (*see* **Note 4**).
11. The parasite burden is determined by counting an adequate number of microscopic fields with the total parasite burden = % infected mφ × mean number of amastigotes/mφ.
12. The degree of reduction of infection in the drug-treated wells is compared to the control wells to calculate the IC_{50} or IC_{90}.

4 Notes

1. During long term laboratory maintenance of strains, the phenotype may alter depending on the way of serial passage. If passaged in vitro as promastigote, they may lose the capacity to infect in vivo. Alternatively, ex vivo (hamster) spleen-derived amastigotes may lose the capacity to backtransform to multiplying promastigotes. For this reason, it is advised to cryopreserve the strains [10] at the lowest possible passage number.

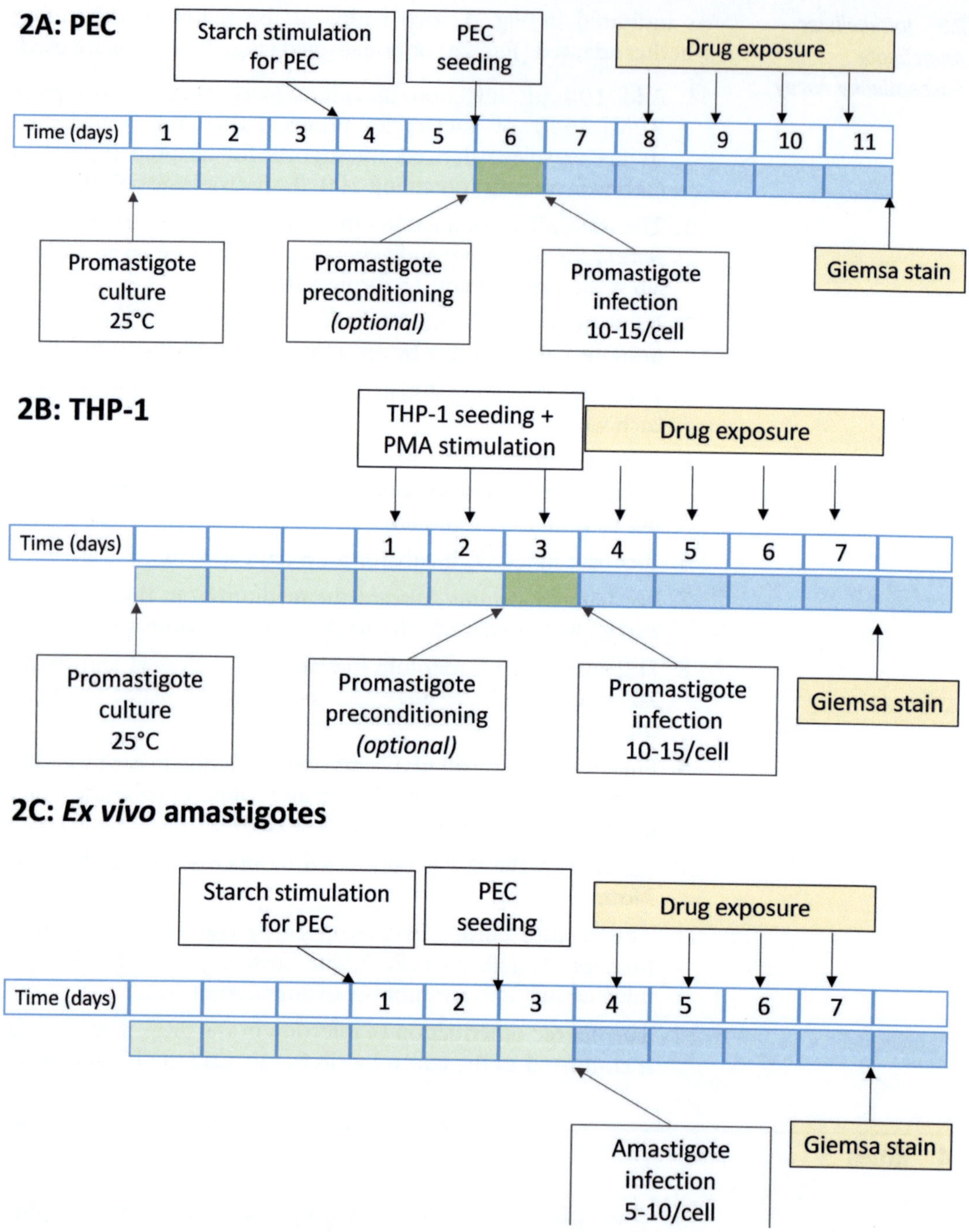

Fig. 2 Standard intracellular susceptibility protocol: experimental design related to the application of different host cells and different parasite stages for infection. (**a**) For nonadapted strains using metacyclic promastigotes for infection of PECs. (**b**) For nonadapted strains using metacyclic promastigotes for infection of THP-1. (**c**) For adapted strains using ex vivo (spleen-derived) amastigotes for infection of PEC [14] (*see also* **Note 2**)

2. Primary cells are recommended for drug susceptibility evaluation and PECs can be proposed as a pragmatic second option (less complicated and technically demanding). There are no relevant differences between cells derived from Swiss mice (cheap) and BALB/c mice (expensive). If mice are not available, THP-1 cells are the only valid option. The rapidly multiplying macrophage cell lines J774 and RAW tend to outgrow the *Leishmania* infected cells, obscuring proper readout of the assay [14].
3. Although mostly not required, promastigotes can be preconditioned for metacyclogenesis to enhance their infectivity for mφ [14]: Centrifuge the promastigote culture for 10 min at 200 × *g* and discard the supernatant, resuspend the pellet in 5 mL sterile promastigote medium at pH 5.4 and incubate at 25 °C for 24 h before using for infection.
4. Although alternative "imaging" methods have been proposed for assay endpoint reading (using reporter strains, DNA staining), we still recommend the (unfortunately quite labor-intensive) microscopic reading of Giemsa-stained cultures as more in-depth information is obtained, incl. Cytotoxicity on the macrophage host cell.

Acknowledgement

Funding: The authors and their research in this particular area are funded by the Research Fund Flanders (FWO: project G051812N and 12I0317N) and research funds of the University of Antwerp (TT-ZAPBOF 33049 and TOP-BOF 35017). LMPH is a partner of the Antwerp Drug Discovery Network (ADDN, www.addn.be) and the Excellence Centre "Infla-Med" (www.uantwerpen.be/infla-med).

References

1. Bern C, Maguire JH, Alvar J (2008) Complexities of assessing the disease burden attributable to leishmaniasis. PLoS Negl Trop Dis 2(10): e313
2. Davies CR, Kaye P, Croft SL, Sundar S (2003) Leishmaniasis: new approaches to disease control. BMJ 326(7385):377–382
3. Alves F, Bilbe G, Blesson S, Goyal V, Monnerat S, Mowbray C, Muthoni Ouattara G, Pecoul B, Rijal S, Rode J, Solomos A, Strub-Wourgaft N, Wasunna M, Wells S, Zijlstra EE, Arana B, Alvar J (2018) Recent development of visceral Leishmaniasis treatments: successes, pitfalls, and perspectives. Clin Microbiol Rev 31(4):pii: e00048-18
4. Croft SL, Olliaro P (2011) Leishmaniasis chemotherapy—challenges and opportunities. Clin Microbiol Infect 17(10):1478–1483
5. Croft SL (2001) Monitoring drug resistance in leishmaniasis. Trop Med Int Health 6 (11):899–905
6. Sundar S (2001) Drug resistance in Indian visceral leishmaniasis. Trop Med Int Health 6 (11):849–854
7. Rijal S, Ostyn B, Uranw S, Rai K, Bhattarai NR, Dorlo TP, Beijnen JH, Vanaerschot M, Decuypere S, Dhakal SS, Das ML, Karki P,

Singh R, Boelaert M, Dujardin JC (2013) Increasing failure of miltefosine in the treatment of kala-azar in Nepal and the potential role of parasite drug resistance, reinfection, or noncompliance. Clin Infect Dis 56 (11):1530–1538

8. Fumarola L, Spinelli R, Brandonisio O (2004) In vitro assays for evaluation of drug activity against Leishmania spp. Res Microbiol 155 (4):224–230. https://doi.org/10.1016/j.resmic.2004.01.001
9. Gupta S (2011) Visceral leishmaniasis: experimental models for drug discovery. Indian J Med Res 133:27–39
10. Hendrickx S, Guerin PJ, Caljon G, Croft SL, Maes L (2016) Evaluating drug resistance in visceral leishmaniasis: the challenges. Parasitology 145:453–463. https://doi.org/10.1017/s0031182016002031
11. Maes L, Cos P, Croft S (2013) The relevance of susceptibility tests, breakpoints and markers. In: Ponte-Sucre A, Diaz E, Padrón-Nieves M (eds) Drug resistance in Leishmania parasites. Springer, Vienna, pp 407–429
12. Hendrickx SML, Croft SL, Caljon G (2018) The challenges of effective leishmaniasis treatment. In: Sucre AP (ed) Drug resistance in Leishmania parasites. Springer, Vienna
13. Van den Kerkhof M, Van Bockstal L, Gielis JF, Delputte P, Cos P, Maes L, Caljon G, Hendrickx S (2018) Impact of primary mouse macrophage cell types on Leishmania infection and in vitro drug susceptibility. Parasitol Res 117 (11):3601–3612
14. Inocencio da Luz RA, Vermeersch M, Dujardin JC, Cos P, Maes L (2009) In vitro sensitivity testing of Leishmania clinical field isolates: preconditioning of promastigotes enhances infectivity for macrophage host cells. Antimicrob Agents Chemother 53(12):5197–5203
15. LS (1955) Leishmaniasis in the hamster. In: Cole WH (ed) Some physiological aspects and consequences of parasitism. Rutgers University Press, New Brunswisck, NJ, pp 76–90

Chapter 48

In Vivo Bioluminescence Imaging to Assess Compound Efficacy Against *Trypanosoma brucei*

Ryan Ritchie, Michael P. Barrett, Jeremy C. Mottram, and Elmarie Myburgh

Abstract

Traditional animal models for human African trypanosomiasis rely on detecting *Trypanosoma brucei brucei* parasitemia in the blood. Testing the efficacy of new compounds in these models is cumbersome because it may take several months after treatment before surviving parasites become detectable in the blood. To expedite compound screening, we have used a *Trypanosoma brucei brucei* GVR35 strain expressing red-shifted firefly luciferase to monitor parasite distribution in infected mice through noninvasive whole-body bioluminescence imaging. This protocol describes the infection and in vivo bioluminescence imaging of mice to assess compound efficacy against *T. brucei* during the two characteristic stages of disease, the hemolymphatic phase (stage 1) and the encephalitic or central nervous system phase (stage 2).

Key words Firefly luciferase, *Trypanosoma brucei brucei*, In vivo imaging, Bioluminescence

1 Introduction

Human African trypanosomiasis (HAT), also called sleeping sickness, occurs in two clinical stages: a hemolymphatic phase (stage 1), where parasites are detected in blood and lymph, and an encephalitic phase (stage 2) involving the central nervous system (CNS). Established mouse models for HAT rely on detection of blood parasites, usually of monomorphic *T. brucei* strain Lister 427 during the first few days of infection (to mimic stage 1 disease), and of pleomorphic *T. brucei* strain GVR35 after 21 days of infections (to mimic stage 2 disease) [1, 2]. This involves sampling of blood for parasite detection by light microscopy and does not allow real-time detection of parasites that are extravascular and within tissues such as the spleen, lymph nodes, adipose tissue, and brain.

In vivo imaging is highly sensitive, noninvasive, and quantifiable, and has become an indispensable and valuable tool for the monitoring of disease progression in live animals. This technology has been applied to investigate infection dynamics and to screen

Paul A. M. Michels et al. (eds.), *Trypanosomatids: Methods and Protocols*, Methods in Molecular Biology, vol. 2116, https://doi.org/10.1007/978-1-0716-0294-2_48,

drugs against *Plasmodium* spp. [3–5], *Mycobacterium tuberculosis* [6], *Leishmania* spp. [7, 8], *Trypanosoma cruzi* [9], and *Trypanosoma brucei* [10, 11]. To make use of this technology for the screening of novel trypanocidal compounds, bioluminescent *Trypanosoma brucei brucei* cell lines were generated [12, 13] and an imaging method that is highly sensitive, reproducible and expedites the screening process was developed [14]. The optimized bioluminescence imaging model using *T. b. brucei* GVR35 expressing red-shifted firefly luciferase has been valuable for the identification of novel compounds against stage 2 HAT [15]. This bioluminescence GVR35 model can also be utilized to screen for in vivo activity during stage 1 disease. Infection of mice with pleomorphic *T. brucei* strains is characterized by waves of parasitemia that can be difficult to detect in the blood. However, sensitive bioluminescence imaging tracks live parasites over the whole body making it possible to assess compound activity even with fluctuating and low blood parasitemia. Using one parasite strain and method to screen for both stage 1 and 2 efficacy saves limited time and resources routinely spent to assess compounds in multiple parasite strains and infection models.

In this protocol, we describe the generation and testing of bioluminescent *T. b. brucei* GVR35 stabilates to be used for reproducible infections of mice. We describe the imaging model (Fig. 1) for screening of compounds against pleomorphic *T. b. brucei* GVR35 during stage 1 (day 7 postinfection) or stage 2 (day 21 postinfection) trypanosomiasis. We provide details on infection of donor and experimental mice, bioluminescence imaging of mice (using the IVIS imaging system from PerkinElmer), determination of blood parasitemia, treatment of mice with compounds, blood sampling for pharmacokinetic analysis and end-point imaging and harvesting of organs to allow parasite quantification by PCR (*see* **Note 1**).

2 Materials

2.1 Generation and Testing of Bioluminescent *T. brucei* Stabilates

2.1.1 Culturing of *T. b. brucei* GVR35 Bloodstream form Trypanosomes

1. *Trypanosoma brucei brucei* GVR35-VSL2 [12] (*see* **Note 2**).
2. IMDM (Iscove's Modified Dulbecco's Medium, Gibco) supplemented with 20% heat-inactivated fetal calf serum, 20% Serum Plus, 0.75 mM hypoxanthine in 0.1 N NaOH, 4.1 mM glucose, 0.12 mM thymidine, 1.5 mM sodium pyruvate, 0.037 mM bathocuproine disulfonic acid, 0.2 mM β-mercaptoethanol, 1.1 mM L-cysteine, 0.38 mM adenosine, 0.38 mM guanosine, 0.83 g/L methylcellulose, 0.04 mM kanamycin, 75 units/mL penicillin, and 0.075 mg/mL streptomycin (all Sigma-Aldrich), pH 7.4.
3. 25 cm^3 vented flasks.

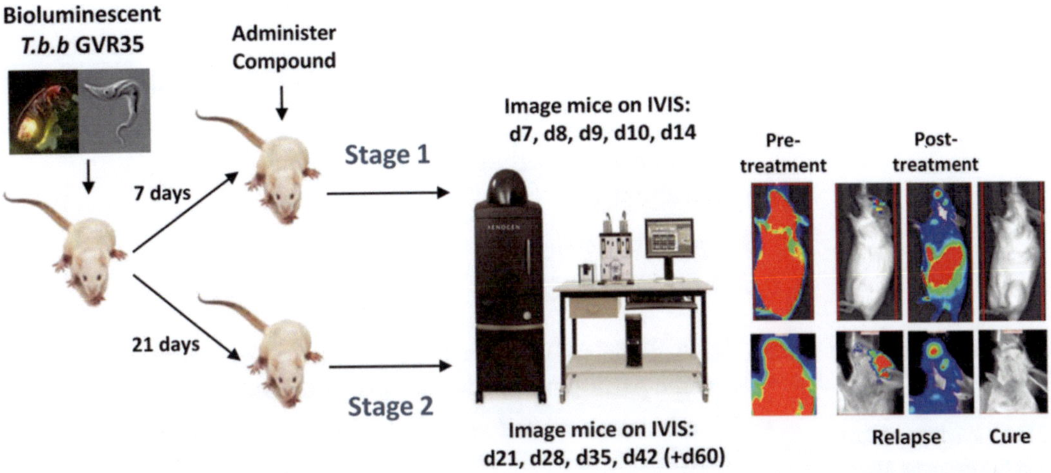

Fig. 1 Schematic of the *T. brucei brucei* GVR35-VSL2 imaging model. CD1 mice are infected with 3×10^4 bloodstream form *T. b. brucei* GVR35-VSL2 and treated with compounds from day 7 (d7) or day 21 (d21) postinfection to screen for activity during stage 1 or stage 2 trypanosomiasis, respectively. Whole body bioluminescence imaging is performed using an IVIS imaging system before treatment and daily (stage 1) or weekly (stage 2) after treatment to monitor parasite burden

2.1.2 Generation of Bioluminescent T. brucei *Stabilates*

1. Trypanosome dilution buffer (TDB): 20 mM Na_2HPO_4, 2 mM $NaH_2PO_4.2H_2O$, 80 mM NaCl, 5 mM KCl, 1 mM $MgSO_4.7H_2O$, 20 mM D-glucose, pH 7.4.
2. Adult, female CD1 (ICR) mice (~25 g body weight) maintained under specific pathogen free conditions (*see* **Note 3**).
3. 1 mL syringes and 25 G needles.
4. 0.9% NH_4Cl.
5. Blood lancets.
6. CBSS heparin solution: 25 mM HEPES, 120 mM NaCl, 5.4 mM $CaCl_2{\cdot}H_2O$, 0.5 mM $MgSO_4{\cdot}7H_2O$, 5.6 mM Na_2HPO_4, 11.1 mM D-glucose, pH 7.4, 10 units heparin/mL.
7. Light microscope and hemocytometer within the animal facility.
8. CO_2 euthanasia apparatus.
9. Fine bore polythene tubing (0.58 mm internal diameter, 0.96 mm external diameter).
10. Monoject aluminum hub blunt needles (0.6 mm × 25.4 mm).
11. Cryovial tubes.
12. Glycerol.
13. “Mr frosty” freezing container.

2.1.3 Testing of Bioluminescent *T. brucei* Stabilates

1. *Trypanosoma brucei brucei* GVR35-VSL2 [12] blood straws (*see* Subheading 3.1.2).
2. Trypanosome dilution buffer (TDB) (*see* Subheading 2.1.2).
3. Adult, female CD1 mice (~25 g body weight) maintained under specific pathogen free conditions (*see* **Note 3**).
4. 0.9% NH_4Cl.
5. Blood lancets.
6. 1 mL syringes and 25 G needles.

2.2 In Vivo Imaging Model

2.2.1 Infection of Donor and Experimental Mice

- Adult, female CD1 mice (~25 g body weight) maintained under specific pathogen free conditions (*see* **Note 3**).
- Blood straws of *T. b. brucei* strain GVR35-VSL2 (red-shifted) luciferase expressing cell line (*see* Subheading 3.1.2).
- Trypanosome dilution buffer (TDB) (*see* Subheading 2.1.2).
- CBSS heparin solution (*see* **item 7** in Subheading 2.1.1).
- 0.9% NH_4Cl.
- Blood lancets.
- 1 mL syringes and 25 G needles.
- Light microscope and hemocytometer in the animal facility.
- CO_2 euthanasia apparatus.
- Ear punch tool.

2.2.2 Bioluminescence Imaging

1. IVIS spectrum In Vivo Imaging System from PerkinElmer (*see* **Note 4**).
2. $MgCl_2$ and $CaCl_2$ free Dulbecco's PBS purchased from Gibco.
3. Beetle luciferin potassium salt (1 g) from Promega—Prepare 15 mg/mL working stock by resuspending 1 g beetle luciferin (D-luciferin) potassium salt in 66.66 mL of $MgCl_2$ and $CaCl_2$ free Dulbecco's PBS, freeze 1 mL aliquots at −20 °C.
4. Isoflurane gaseous anesthesia equipment including gas vaporizer, scavenger, and oxygen generator (e.g., XGI-8 Gas Anesthesia System connected to an oxygen tank or generator).
5. Lacri-Lube ocular lubricant from Allergan pharmaceuticals.
6. PBS-G: $MgCl_2$ and $CaCl_2$ free Dulbecco's PBS with 10 mM glucose, pH 7.4.

2.2.3 Determine Blood Parasitemia

1. Blood lancets.
2. 0.9% NH_4Cl.
3. Light microscope and hemocytometer in the animal facility.

2.2.4 In Vivo Compound Treatments

1. Diminazene aceturate (control treatment).
2. Distilled H_2O to solubilize diminazene aceturate.
3. 0.22 μm syringe filters.
4. 1 mL syringes.
5. Mouse feeding tubes—plastic or metal.
6. Lacri-Lube ocular lubricant from Allergan pharmaceuticals.
7. PBS-G: $MgCl_2$ and $CaCl_2$ free Dulbecco's PBS with 10 mM glucose, pH 7.4.
8. Test compounds and suitable vehicle.
9. Weighing scales.

2.2.5 Blood Sampling for Pharmacokinetic Analysis

1. Blood lancets.
2. Thermostatically controlled heated chamber.
3. Mouse restraining apparatus.
4. Heparinized tubes.
5. Screwcap sample tubes.
6. Antimicrobial solution (e.g., chlorhexidine).

2.2.6 End Point Imaging

1. In Vivo Imaging System (IVIS).
2. Beetle luciferin (D-luciferin), 15 mg/mL working stock (*see* **item 3** in Subheading 2.2.2).
3. PBS-G: $MgCl_2$ and $CaCl_2$ free Dulbecco's PBS with 10 mM glucose added, pH 7.4.
4. Heparinized tubes.
5. Dissection kit.
6. Petri dishes.
7. Liquid nitrogen and benchtop liquid nitrogen container.

3 Methods

3.1 Generation and Testing of Bioluminescent T. brucei Stabilates

The bioluminescence imaging model requires infection of donor mice from *T. brucei* blood stabilates. These blood stabilates can be generated from cultured parasites (Subheadings 3.1.1 and 3.1.2) or from F1 blood stabilate stocks that should be tested (Subheading 3.1.3) and then used for infection and generation of new blood stabilates (Subheading 3.1.2 from **step 5** onward) (*see* **Note 5**).

3.1.1 Culturing of T. b. brucei GVR35-VSL2 Bloodstream form Trypanosomes

1. Defrost a culture stabilate of *T. b. brucei* GVR35-VSL2 bloodstream form trypanosomes [12] and transfer the cell suspension to a 25 cm^3 vented flask containing 10 mL pre-warmed supplemented IMDM medium.

2. Leave to recover for around 72 h by culturing cells in vitro at 37 °C, 5% CO_2 in an upright flask.
3. Count cells and subpassage in supplemented IMDM to 5×10^4 cells/mL (*see* **Note 6**).
4. Following the first passage, count cells every 3–4 days and subpassage to ensure that the culture is maintained between 5×10^4 and 1×10^6 cells/mL (*see* **Note 7**).
5. Keep in vitro culture to a minimum to avoid effects on virulence.

3.1.2 Generation of Bioluminescent T. brucei *Blood Stabilates*

1. *For infection from cultured parasites*: Count cells of a log-stage *T. b. brucei* GVR35-VSL2 culture (between 5×10^5 and 1×10^6 cells/mL) to determine cell density.
2. Transfer 5×10^5 cells to a sterile tube, add 5 mL trypanosome dilution buffer (TDB) and centrifuge at 1500 × *g* for 10 min at room temperature.
3. Carefully remove supernatant, repeat centrifugation as above in 5 mL fresh TDB.
4. Carefully remove supernatant, leaving ~500 μL in tube. Resuspend pellet in remaining TDB, count cells and adjust final concentration to 1.2×10^5 parasites/mL. Proceed to **step 6**.
5. *For infection from blood stabilates*: Defrost required amount of F2 blood straws for infection of two donor mice (determined in Subheading 3.1.3) into 500 μL TDB and mix well.
6. Inject two CD1 mice intraperitoneally with 250 μL (3×10^4 parasites) per mouse using a 1 mL syringe and 25 G needle (*see* **Note 8**).
7. Monitor parasitemia of infected mice daily as follows: Dilute 4 μL of blood (taken via a tail vein venipuncture using a lancet or needle, *see* **Note 9**) in 16 μL of 0.9% ammonium chloride to lyse the blood cells. Determine parasite density in blood by counting on a hemocytometer.
8. When parasitemia reaches the first peak (~1×10^7 parasites/mL) cull the mouse by exposure to CO_2 in a rising concentration, and remove all blood by cardiac puncture using a syringe pre-loaded with 200 μL of CBSS heparin buffer (this prevents coagulation of the blood) (*see* **Note 10**).
9. Add 71.4 μL of glycerol to every 500 μL of blood and mix with a vortex.
10. Using a 1 mL syringe and blunt needle inject blood/glycerol mix into fine bore polythene tubing and cut into ~2.5 cm sections, placing "blood straws" into cryovials.

11. Place cryovials in a "Mr Frosty" or cotton wool lined box and freeze at −80 °C overnight before transferring to liquid nitrogen for long-term storage (this is designated as the F1 storage stock).

3.1.3 Testing of Bioluminescent *T. brucei* Stabilates

1. Remove three frozen straws from liquid nitrogen and dilute in 500 μL TDB.
2. Count parasites with a hemocytometer to calculate the parasite number in one straw and the number of straws required to achieve a count of 1.2×10^5 parasites/mL.
3. Inject 250 μL (3×10^4 parasites) into a CD1 mouse by intraperitoneal injection.
4. Monitor parasitemia daily to calculate the length of time before the first parasitemia peak.
5. A second stock of blood straws (F2 working stocks) should be made from the F1 stock as in Subheading 3.1.2 (**steps 5–11**)—this F2 stock should also be tested as above and used for infections of donor mice for reproducible infections.

3.2 In Vivo Imaging Model

3.2.1 Infection of Donor and Experimental Mice

1. Select appropriate infection day of donor mice based on when mice are expected to develop the first peak of parasitemia (determined in Subheading 3.1.3) (*see* **Note 11**).
2. Defrost required amount of F2 blood straws for infection of two donor mice (determined in Subheading 3.1.3) into 500 μL TDB and mix well.
3. Inject each mouse intraperitoneally with 250 μL of TDB/blood straw mixture.
4. Monitor parasitemia daily as described in Subheading 3.1.2 (**step 7**) until the first peak of parasitemia is achieved (5×10^6–1.0×10^7 parasites/mL).
5. Harvest blood by cardiac puncture under terminal anesthesia using a syringe prefilled with 200 μL of CBSS heparin to prevent coagulation of the blood.
6. Determine the blood parasitemia and dilute blood with CBSS heparin to achieve a concentration of 1.2×10^5 parasites/mL before injecting each experimental mouse with 250 μL (3×10^4 parasites/mouse).
7. Ear mark mice for identification and weigh all mice.
8. Assign mice to treatment groups (*see* **Note 12**).

3.2.2 Bioluminescence Imaging (See **Note 4**)

1. At day 7 (stage 1 model) or day 21 (stage 2 model) postinfection (*see* **Note 13**) image mice before treatment using the IVIS spectrum as described below. Posttreatment imaging should be done daily or weekly after start of treatment (*see* **Note 14**). Determine blood parasitemia (*see* Subheading 3.2.3) on the same day as imaging.

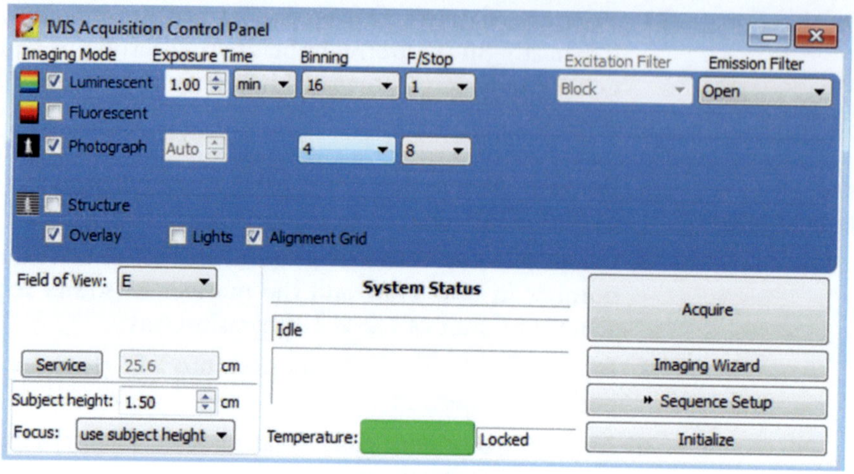

Fig. 2 IVIS Acquisition Control panel in the Living Image Software. An example of the image settings for acquisition of bioluminescence is shown. In this case, exposure time of 1 min, binning of 16, F/stop of 1 and field of view E is selected for imaging of the whole body after compound treatment (*see* Table 1)

2. Defrost the appropriate number of beetle luciferin (15 mg/mL working stock) vials (10 μL/g of mouse is required).
3. Start the Living Image software. Enter initials or select from the list when prompted to do so by the software.
4. Create an appropriate folder on the computer hard drive to save the data generated.
5. Once the program opens initialize the system using the "Initialize" tab in the bottom right corner of the control panel (Fig. 2).
6. Once the system is initialized the "System Status" in the control panel will show "Idle" and the "Temperature" box will be green (Fig. 2, bottom middle).
7. Place a black XFM-1 low fluorescence mat inside the imaging chamber with the matt side facing upward (the black mat is required for bioluminescence and fluorescence imaging but may have been removed by others when doing trans-illumination imaging).
8. Start the anesthesia/isoflurane system—this should be connected to the IVIS and to an induction chamber. Make sure that the system receives O_2 (for example from an open O_2 tank or oxygen generator) and that the isoflurane level is full. If not then these will need to be filled/replaced before proceeding.
9. Turn on the O_2 supply and the waste gas scavenger.
10. Transfer 3–5 mice to the induction chamber and close it tightly (*see* **Note 15**).

11. Initiate anesthesia using 1.5 L per minute O_2 with 4% isoflurane. Ensure that the flow of isoflurane is toward the induction chamber.
12. Inject 150 mg/kg beetle luciferin subcutaneously (using 10 μL of the 15 mg/mL stock per gram of mouse) and record the time of luciferin injection (*see* **Notes 16** and **17**).
13. Mice are usually imaged from 10 to 12 min after luciferin injection (*see* **Note 18**)—while waiting for this time to pass choose the appropriate predetermined settings on the Living Image software control panel (Fig. 2, top and left panels). For imaging in this model and using subcutaneous injection of luciferin we use the settings shown in Table **1**. The time of image acquisition and sequence of images are shown below:

    Time of image acquisition: start 12 min after luciferin injection (the bioluminescent signal plateau is from 15 to 20 min).

    Sequence of imaging: (1) one ventral whole body image, (2) one side whole body image (with spleen facing upward), mice are then imaged individually for (3) one dorsal head image, (4) one side head image (*see* **Note 19**).

    Ensure that the "Overlay" and "Alignment Grid" boxes (middle of control panel) are ticked.
14. Using a cotton swab, gently apply Lacri-lube ocular lubricant directly to the eyes of each mouse to prevent eyes from drying out.
15. Transfer mice to the IVIS imaging chamber and place each mouse with its nose in a nose cone; ensure that unused nose pieces are closed with black plugs (*see* **Note 21**).

Table 1
Image acquisition settings used for the *T. b. brucei* GVR35-VSL2 imaging model

Field of view (FOV)	Imaging mode	Exposure time	Binning	f/stop	Excitation
Untreated mice/whole body					
E	Luminescence	1 s	Small (4)	1	Block
Untreated mice/head					
A	Luminescence	1 s	Small (4)	1	Block
Treated mice/whole body (*see* **Note 20**)					
E	Luminescence	1 min	Large (16)	1	Block
Treated mice/head					
A	Luminescence	1 min	Large (16)	1	Block

16. Place light absorbing dividers between mice to avoid signal contamination (*see* **Note 22**).
17. Reduce isoflurane to 1.5% and direct the flow of anesthetic to the IVIS system (using the ON/OFF switch or turning the knob toward the IVIS system—this mechanism depends on the system being used).
18. Acquire images by clicking "Acquire" on bottom left side of the control panel.
19. Upon acquisition of the first image after initialization the software will offer the option of auto-saving and allow selection of the location for the saved files. Select auto-save.
20. Various input boxes are available to record data, such as time point, mouse strain and general comments. Useful information to record are the treatment group, mouse numbers, time-point, type of image (e.g., ventral body or dorsal head), and the luciferin injection time (this allows easier selection later of images that were acquired at exactly the same time after luciferin injection).

3.2.3 Determination of Blood Parasitemia

1. Dilute 4 μL of blood (taken via a tail vein venipuncture using a lancet or needle) in 16 μL of 0.9% ammonium chloride to lyse the blood cells. Determine parasite density in blood by counting on a hemocytometer.

3.2.4 In Vivo Compound Treatments

1. The optimal vehicle and dosing route for drug treatment should be determined in advance (*see* **Note 23**). Diminazene aceturate is administered intraperitoneally in water as a single dose at 40 mg/kg in distilled water.
2. Prepare the vehicle and compounds one day before treatment (if compound stability allows for this). Diminazene aceturate should be prepared fresh on the day of treatment and filtered using a 0.22 μm syringe filter.
3. Store treatment compounds as aliquots at 4 °C during treatment regime. Bring to room temperature and mix well before each treatment.
4. Treatment starts at day 7 (stage 1 model) or day 21 (stage 2 model) after infection (*see* **Note 13**); mice should be weighed and dosed according to weight (*see* **Note 24**).
5. If required take blood samples for pharmacokinetic analysis as described in Subheading 3.2.5.
6. Weigh mice and monitor daily for adverse effects of infection or treatment.

3.2.5 Blood Sampling for Pharmacokinetic Analysis

1. Blood sampling (site, volume and frequency) should be done in accordance with animal welfare legislation and as approved by the relevant Ethics Committee. If needed this may require additional animals or alternating bleeding of mice to minimize stress and stay within ethical guidelines.
2. Prepare labeled collection tubes in advance.
3. Heat mice in a thermostatically controlled warm air box to dilate blood vessels (in this case, the tail vein).
4. Disinfect the blood sampling site by washing with an antimicrobial solution (e.g., 2% water-based chlorhexidine).
5. Restrain the mouse and puncture the skin and underlying blood vessel using a needle or lancet.
6. Withdraw the appropriate amount of blood into a heparinized collection tube.
7. Stop blood flow by applying finger pressure on the site for ~30 s and return the animal to its cage.
8. Mix the blood in the collection tube, transfer the appropriate volume(s) to fresh nonheparinized tubes and freeze at −20 °C for pharmacokinetic analysis.

3.2.6 End Point Imaging

1. For the stage 1 model the end point may range between day 14 and 21. For the stage 2 model the untreated controls should be culled at day 28–30 postinfection (*see* **Note 25**), while diminazene aceturate controls and treatment group mice will be culled upon relapse of parasitemia in blood. If no relapse occurs in the treated group, mice may be monitored for longer periods until a defined end point (e.g., day 100 or day 180).
2. At the chosen end point image mice as described in Subheading 3.2.2.
3. Cull mice by cervical dislocation or exposure to a rising concentration of CO_2 (the latter is advised if perfusion of mice is required).
4. Optional: Perfuse mice with PBS-G to remove all blood from the brain for quantification of the brain-resident parasites.
5. Remove the brain and place into a petri dish; add 100 μL of beetle luciferin (15 mg/mL stock) onto the brain surface and image ex vivo, using 1-min exposure time, large binning and f stop 1. The signal peaks ~8 min after luciferin application; however, images are taken continuously up to 10 min after application.
6. Optional: Rinse brains with PBS, snap-freeze in liquid nitrogen and store at −80 °C for qPCR analysis [13, 16].

3.3 Image Analysis

1. Analyze images using Living Image software from PerkinElmer as described in the software manual.

4 Notes

1. All animal procedures described in this chapter are in accordance with the guidelines of the UK Home Office under authorized Home Office licenses and approved by the relevant Animal Welfare and Ethics Committees. Its implementation in other laboratories will require approval from relevant government and institutional committees before commencing work.
2. *T.b.b.* GVR35-VSL2 lines can be obtained from the corresponding author as culture stabilates or as blood stabilates for infection of donor mice.
3. Outbred CD1 (ICR) mice tolerate infection with *T. brucei* GVR35 well. Pilot studies with inbred BALB/c mice indicated that this strain is more susceptible to secondary infections when infected with *T. brucei.*
4. The GVR35 imaging model described here makes use of bioluminescence imaging (Subheading 3.2.2) with the IVIS spectrum imaging system (PerkinElmer) and Living Image analysis software (Subheading 3.3); the model can also be adapted for use with other in vivo small animal imaging systems and analysis software.
5. In vitro culturing will affect the virulence of *T. brucei* GVR35; use of F1 blood stabilates for the generation of new blood stabilate working stocks is recommended.
6. Cells may grow very slowly after the first passage. Some cells will die while others continue to divide resulting in no net increase in cells in the first couple of days. The culture will recover and grow normally (~three fold overnight) between 1 and 2 weeks after thawing of the stabilate. Cells will start growing faster (growth of fivefold overnight) over time but may also become more virulent so this should be avoided to ensure reproducibility of the model.
7. The cells will start dying from 1.5–2 $\times$ 10^6 cells/mL so are best kept at a density below 1 $\times$ 10^6 cells/mL.
8. Mice will develop parasitemia at different times and parasites harvested from blood may vary in their infectivity. It is therefore advised to infect two mice for harvesting of parasites and to make two sets of stabilates for later selection of the set which results in the most reliable infections (Subheadings 3.1.2 and 3.1.3).

9. Single-use needles and lancets should be used to avoid contamination and additional injury to mice.
10. It is important to harvest parasites from mice while parasitemia is increasing. Once parasitemia has reached its peak and decreases again the parasites will be less infective. Harvest parasites when parasitemia is in the range of 5×10^6–1.5×10^7 parasites/mL of blood.
11. Parasites will be harvested from donor mice during their first peak of parasitemia and then used to infect experimental mice (designated as day 0). Imaging and treatment of mice is usually done from day 7 (stage 1 model) or day 21 (stage 2 model) after infection and should ideally fall on a convenient day that will also allow for preparation of compounds one day in advance. For example, our blood straws produce an infection in donor mice with the first peak of parasitemia developing 4–5 days postinfection. By infecting donor mice on a Thursday blood and parasites can usually be harvested on the following Tuesday for infection of experimental mice. This allows for preparation of compounds on Monday and imaging as well as start of compound treatment on Tuesday.
12. We routinely set mice up in groups of six per treatment with three diminazene aceturate-treated controls and three untreated controls. These animal numbers have been determined using a power analysis with variables estimated from previous experiments. The variables and calculated group sizes may change depending on the mice used, the bioluminescence of the parasites and sensitivity of the imaging systems. Pilot studies should be performed when setting up a new model to estimate the variables for power analysis.
13. The GVR35 mouse model mimics stage 1 disease at day 7 postinfection. By day 21 the parasites become established in the CNS and infections can only be cured by compounds active in the brain [16, 17]. For screening in stage 2, mice should always be treated after 21 days of infection. Treatment can also be delayed by 1 or 2 days if required for logistical reasons (e.g., day 8 or 9 for stage 1 and day 22 or 23 for stage 2) with subsequent delay in the posttreatment imaging time points.
14. The imaging schedule should be determined in advance and will depend on what is feasible and what analysis is to be done. To analyze in vivo kill kinetics daily imaging after treatment may be needed. For stage 1, imaging usually starts on day 7 and can be done daily afterward up to day 14 (e.g., day 7, 8, 9, 10, 14). For stage 2, imaging usually starts at day 21 and is done weekly, or later (usually after day 63), 2-weekly intervals following start of treatment (e.g., day 21, 28, 35, 42, 49, etc.).

15. The number of animals to be imaged will depend on the IVIS imaging system being used. We prefer to image three mice at a time to allow space between mice.
16. It is preferable to inject luciferin subcutaneously or intraperitoneally. While subcutaneous injection results in a slightly lower signal compared with intraperitoneal injection it has a longer and flatter signal kinetics making it more suitable for taking multiple images of the whole body or head. Furthermore, there is a higher risk of failure for intraperitoneal injection (where injection is placed into a site other than the peritoneal cavity, such as the lumen of the stomach or bowel, or injection is subcutaneous, retroperitoneal or intravascular), particularly in trypanosome-infected mice where spleens are enlarged. A failed injection may reduce the luciferin concentration in tissues resulting in lower bioluminescence or result in death.
17. Luciferin can be injected once the animal is anesthetized; however, this will alter the kinetics of the signal compared with an animal that is awake. This should be taken into account when establishing acquisition timings and setting.
18. Imaging acquisition settings and the timing of imaging after luciferin injection need to be determined in advance. This will depend on the site of luciferin injection, strength of the signal, and location of the signal. To establish the imaging start time calculate a kinetic curve during a pilot study—this is done by taking multiple images over time and determining when the signal peaks and falls.
19. The mouse to be imaged is moved to the middle nose cone while the other two remain on outer nose cones. For head images the "Field of view (FOV)" on the IVIS acquisition panel should be set on A—this increases resolution by moving the stage upward but will only allow imaging of the middle mouse (e.g., for the IVIS spectrum FOV A is 3.9 × 3.9 cm). Once head images of the middle mouse are completed it is transferred to a holding box and another mouse is moved to the middle for imaging of head (any open nose cones should be blocked with black plugs as mice are transferred from the imaging chamber).
20. Mice may have low bioluminescence signal after treatment with a trypanocidal compound; to detect these low signals increase the exposure time and the binning. In untreated mice, or mice with relapsed parasitemia, signal may be saturated at high exposure and binning; in these instances the exposure time and binning should be decreased or the F/stop increased.
21. Transparent nose cones ensure gas delivery to individual mice from the anesthesia manifold. Black rubber plugs seal unused ports of the anesthesia manifold. Nose cones and plugs should be provided with the IVIS gas anesthesia system.

22. XMD-2 manifold dividers are available in different heights and can be purchased from PerkinElmer or may have been provided with the IVIS system. We cut dividers from black Lexan plastic sheets. In cases where high signal from a mouse still spills over to other mice with low signal it may be necessary to re-image mice separately (e.g., this may occur when parasites have recrudesced in one mouse while others remain clear of parasite signal).
23. The vehicle and dosing regimen for compounds should be determined in advance and tested for toxicity in uninfected mice before used for treatment in the *T. b. brucei* infection model.
24. Compound administration should be done in volumes as specified in the appropriate animal project license or as recommended by animal research advisory boards. For example for oral dosing it is considered good practice to administer compounds in 10 mL vehicle/kg of mouse [18].
25. CD1 mice infected with *T. b. brucei* GVR35 may develop symptoms related to infection of the CNS such as hind-leg paralysis and paresis. This usually occurs from day 28–35 postinfection. To avoid these adverse effects from developing untreated mice should be culled at day 28–30 postinfection (e.g., after the imaging session, 7 days after start of treatment) or when symptoms become visible.

Acknowledgments

This work was supported by the Wellcome Trust [104976, 104111] and the Bill and Melinda Gates Foundation ([OPPGH5337] (http://www.gatesfoundation.org/).

References

1. Jennings FW, Gray GD (1983) Relapsed parasitaemia following chemotherapy of chronic *T. brucei* infections in mice and its relation to cerebral trypanosomes. Contrib Microbiol Immunol 7:147–154
2. Jennings FW, Rodgers J, Bradley B, Gettinby G, Kennedy PG, Murray M (2002) Human African trypanosomiasis: potential therapeutic benefits of an alternative suramin and melarsoprol regimen. Parasitol Int 51 (4):381–388. doi:S1383576902000442
3. Franke-Fayard B, Waters AP, Janse CJ (2006) Real-time in vivo imaging of transgenic bioluminescent blood stages of rodent malaria parasites in mice. Nat Protoc 1(1):476–485. https://doi.org/10.1038/nprot.2006.69
4. Miller JL, Murray S, Vaughan AM, Harupa A, Sack B, Baldwin M, Crispe IN, Kappe SH (2013) Quantitative bioluminescent imaging of pre-erythrocytic malaria parasite infection using luciferase-expressing *Plasmodium yoelii*. PLoS One 8(4):e60820. https://doi.org/10.1371/journal.pone.0060820
5. Ploemen IH, Prudencio M, Douradinha BG, Ramesar J, Fonager J, van Gemert GJ, Luty AJ, Hermsen CC, Sauerwein RW, Baptista FG, Mota MM, Waters AP, Que I, Lowik CW, Khan SM, Janse CJ, Franke-Fayard BM (2009) Visualisation and quantitative analysis of the rodent malaria liver stage by real time imaging. PLoS One 4(11):e7881. https://doi.org/10.1371/journal.pone.0007881

6. Zelmer A, Carroll P, Andreu N, Hagens K, Mahlo J, Redinger N, Robertson BD, Wiles S, Ward TH, Parish T, Ripoll J, Bancroft GJ, Schaible UE (2012) A new in vivo model to test anti-tuberculosis drugs using fluorescence imaging. J Antimicrob Chemother 67 (8):1948–1960. https://doi.org/10.1093/jac/dks161
7. Lang T, Goyard S, Lebastard M, Milon G (2005) Bioluminescent *Leishmania* expressing luciferase for rapid and high throughput screening of drugs acting on amastigote-harbouring macrophages and for quantitative real-time monitoring of parasitism features in living mice. Cell Microbiol 7(3):383–392. https://doi.org/10.1111/j.1462-5822.2004.00468.x
8. Michel G, Ferrua B, Lang T, Maddugoda MP, Munro P, Pomares C, Lemichez E, Marty P (2011) Luciferase-expressing *Leishmania infantum* allows the monitoring of amastigote population size, *in vivo*, *ex vivo* and *in vitro*. PLoS Negl Trop Dis 5(9):e1323. https://doi.org/10.1371/journal.pntd.0001323
9. Lewis MD, Fortes Francisco A, Taylor MC, Burrell-Saward H, McLatchie AP, Miles MA, Kelly JM (2014) Bioluminescence imaging of chronic *Trypanosoma cruzi* infections reveals tissue-specific parasite dynamics and heart disease in the absence of locally persistent infection. Cell Microbiol 16(9):1285–1300. https://doi.org/10.1111/cmi.12297
10. Claes F, Vodnala SK, van Reet N, Boucher N, Lunden-Miguel H, Baltz T, Goddeeris BM, Buscher P, Rottenberg ME (2009) Bioluminescent imaging of *Trypanosoma brucei* shows preferential testis dissemination which may hamper drug efficacy in sleeping sickness. PLoS Negl Trop Dis 3(7):e486
11. Giroud C, Ottones F, Coustou V, Dacheux D, Biteau N, Miezan B, Van Reet N, Carrington M, Doua F, Baltz T (2009) Murine models for *Trypanosoma brucei gambiense* disease progression: from silent to chronic infections and early brain tropism. PLoS Negl Trop Dis 3(9):e509. https://doi.org/10.1371/journal.pntd.0000509
12. McLatchie AP, Burrell-Saward H, Myburgh E, Lewis MD, Ward TH, Mottram JC, Croft SL, Kelly JM, Taylor MC (2013) Highly sensitive in vivo imaging of *Trypanosoma brucei* expressing "red-shifted" luciferase. PLoS Negl Trop Dis 7(11):e2571. https://doi.org/10.1371/journal.pntd.0002571
13. Myburgh E, Coles JA, Ritchie R, Kennedy PG, McLatchie AP, Rodgers J, Taylor MC, Barrett MP, Brewer JM, Mottram JC (2013) In vivo imaging of trypanosome-brain interactions and development of a rapid screening test for drugs against CNS stage trypanosomiasis. PLoS Negl Trop Dis 7(8):e2384. https://doi.org/10.1371/journal.pntd.0002384
14. Burrell-Saward H, Rodgers J, Bradley B, Croft SL, Ward TH (2015) A sensitive and reproducible in vivo imaging mouse model for evaluation of drugs against late-stage human African trypanosomiasis. J Antimicrob Chemother 70 (2):510–517. https://doi.org/10.1093/jac/dku393
15. Khare S, Nagle AS, Biggart A, Lai YH, Liang F, Davis LC, Barnes SW, Mathison CJ, Myburgh E, Gao MY, Gillespie JR, Liu X, Tan JL, Stinson M, Rivera IC, Ballard J, Yeh V, Groessl T, Federe G, Koh HX, Venable JD, Bursulaya B, Shapiro M, Mishra PK, Spraggon G, Brock A, Mottram JC, Buckner FS, Rao SP, Wen BG, Walker JR, Tuntland T, Molteni V, Glynne RJ, Supek F (2016) Proteasome inhibition for treatment of leishmaniasis, Chagas disease and sleeping sickness. Nature 537(7619):229–233. https://doi.org/10.1038/nature19339
16. Rodgers J, Jones A, Gibaud S, Bradley B, McCabe C, Barrett MP, Gettinby G, Kennedy PG (2011) Melarsoprol cyclodextrin inclusion complexes as promising oral candidates for the treatment of human African trypanosomiasis. PLoS Negl Trop Dis 5(9):e1308. https://doi.org/10.1371/journal.pntd.0001308
17. Jennings FW, Whitelaw DD, Holmes PH, Chizyuka HG, Urquhart GM (1979) The brain as a source of relapsing *Trypanosoma brucei* infection in mice after chemotherapy. Int J Parasitol 9(4):381–384. doi:0020-7519(79)90089-4
18. Diehl KH, Hull R, Morton D, Pfister R, Rabemampianina Y, Smith D, Vidal JM, van de Vorstenbosch C, European Federation of Pharmaceutical Industries A, European Centre for the Validation of Alternative M (2001) A good practice guide to the administration of substances and removal of blood, including routes and volumes. J Appl Toxicol 21 (1):15–23

INDEX

Paul A.M. Michels et al. (eds.), *Trypanosomatids: Methods and Protocols*, Methods in Molecular Biology, vol. 2116, https://doi.org/10.1007/978-1-0716-0294-2, © Springer Science+Business Media, LLC, part of Springer Nature 2020

M

N

O

P

Q

R

S

MIX
Papier aus verantwortungsvollen Quellen
Paper from responsible sources
FSC® C105338

If you have any concerns about our products,
you can contact us on
ProductSafety@springernature.com

In case Publisher is established outside the EU,
the EU authorized representative is:
Springer Nature Customer Service Center GmbH
Europaplatz 3, 69115 Heidelberg, Germany

Printed by Libri Plureos GmbH
in Hamburg, Germany